Pathology
for the
Surgeon

Pathology for the Surgeon

Peter M. Banks, M.D.
Townsend Professor and Director of Anatomic Pathology
Department of Pathology
The University of Texas
Health Science Center at San Antonio
San Antonio, Texas

William G. Kraybill, M.D.
Associate Professor of Surgery
State University of New York at Buffalo
Chief, Soft Tissue-Melanoma-Bone Service
Department of Surgery
Roswell Park Cancer Institute
Buffalo, New York

W.B. SAUNDERS COMPANY
A Division of Harcourt Brace & Company
Philadelphia London Toronto Montreal Sydney Tokyo

W.B. SAUNDERS COMPANY
A Division of Harcourt Brace & Company

The Curtis Center
Independence Square West
Philadelphia, Pennsylvania 19106

Library of Congress Cataloging-in-Publication Data

Pathology for the surgeon / [edited by] Peter M. Banks, William G. Kraybill. — 1st ed.

p. cm.

ISBN 0–7216–5288–3

1. Pathology, Surgical. I. Banks, Peter M. II. Kraybill, William G.
[DNLM: 1. Pathology, Surgical. WO 142 P2995 1996]

RD57.P34 1996 616.07—dc20

DNLM/DLC 95-11487

Pathology for the Surgeon ISBN 0–7216–5288–3

Printed in the United States of America.

Last digit is the print number: 9 8 7 6 5 4 3 2 1

To the many surgeons and pathologists
from whom we have learned

Contributors

Jorge Albores-Saavedra, M.D.
Professor of Pathology, Department of Pathology, University of Texas Southwestern Medical School; Director, Division of Anatomic Pathology, Parkland Memorial Hospital and Zale Lipshy University Hospital, Dallas, Texas
The Liver, Biliary Tract, and Pancreas

Peter M. Banks, M.D.
Townsend Professor and Director of Anatomic Pathology, Department of Pathology, The University of Texas Health Science Center at San Antonio, San Antonio, Texas
Surgeon and Pathologist, The Hematolymphoid System

Leon Barnes, M.D.
Professor of Pathology and Otolaryngology, University of Pittsburgh School of Medicine; Director of Anatomic Pathology, Presbyterian University Hospital, Pittsburgh, Pennsylvania
The Head and Neck

David G. Bostwick, M.D.
Professor of Pathology, Mayo Medical School; Consultant in Laboratory Medicine and Pathology, Mayo Clinic, Rochester, Minnesota
The Urologic and Male Reproductive Systems

R. Jean Campbell, M.B., Ch.B.
Professor of Pathology, Mayo Medical School; Consultant, Division of Pathology and Department of Ophthalmology, Mayo Clinic and Mayo Foundation, Rochester, Minnesota
The Eye and Ocular Adnexa

Thomas V. Colby, M.D.
Professor of Pathology, Mayo Medical School, Rochester, Minnesota; Consultant in Surgical Pathology, Mayo Clinic Scottsdale, Scottsdale, Arizona
The Lung and Pleura

Louis P. Dehner, M.D.
Professor of Pathology and Professor of Pathology in Pediatrics, Washington University School of Medicine; Director of Anatomic Pathology and Surgical Pathology, Surgical Pathologist-in-Chief, Barnes Hospital; Pathologist-in-Chief, St. Louis Children's Hospital, St. Louis, Missouri
Special Considerations for the Pediatric Patient

Claude Deschamps, M.D.
Assistant Professor of Surgery, Department of Surgery, Mayo Medical School; Consultant, Section of General Thoracic Surgery, Mayo Clinic and Mayo Foundation, Rochester, Minnesota
The Lung and Pleura

Jesse E. Edwards, M.D.
Clinical Professor, Laboratory Medicine and Pathology, University of Minnesota, Minneapolis; Senior Consultant, Registry of Cardiovascular Disease, United Hospital, St. Paul, Minnesota
The Cardiovascular System

William J. Frable, M.D.
Professor of Pathology, and Director, Division of Surgical Pathology, Virginia Commonwealth University, Medical College of Virginia, Richmond, Virginia
Fine Needle Aspiration Biopsy

James A. Garrity, M.D.
Associate Professor of Ophthalmology, Mayo Medical School; Consultant, Department of Ophthalmology, Mayo Clinic and Mayo Foundation, Rochester, Minnesota
The Eye and Ocular Adnexa

Nancy Lee Harris, M.D.
Professor of Pathology, Harvard Medical School; Associate Pathologist, Massachusetts General Hospital, Boston, Massachusetts
The Mediastinum

Ralph H. Hruban, M.D.
Associate Professor of Pathology and Associate Professor of Oncology, Johns Hopkins University School of Medicine, Baltimore, Maryland
Endocrine Pathology

Jonas T. Johnson, M.D.
Professor of Otolaryngology and Radiation Oncology, Vice Chairman, Department of Otolaryngology, and Director, Division of Head and Neck Oncology and Immunology, University of Pittsburgh School of Medicine; Director, Division of Head and Neck Oncology and Immunology, The Eye and Ear Institute, Presbyterian University Hospital, Pittsburgh, Pennsylvania
The Head and Neck

William G. Kraybill, M.D.
Associate Professor of Surgery, State University of New York at Buffalo; Chief, Soft Tissue-Melanoma-Bone Service, Department of Surgery, Roswell Park Cancer Institute, Buffalo, New York
Surgeon and Pathologist, The Skin, Soft Tissue Tumors

Jeffrey Y. Lin, M.D.
Assistant Professor, Department of Obstetrics and Gynecology; Director, Division of Gynecologic Oncology, The George Washington University Medical Center, Washington, D.C.
Obstetric and Gynecologic Pathology

M. Beatriz S. Lopes, M.D.
Assistant Professor of Pathology (Neuropathology), University of Virginia Health Sciences Center, Charlottesville, Virginia
The Nervous System

Elizabeth A. Montgomery, M.D.
Assistant Professor of Pathology, Department of Pathology, Georgetown University Medical Center, Washington, D.C.
Soft Tissue Tumors

Michael A. Nalesnik, M.D.
Associate Professor of Pathology, University of Pittsburgh Medical Center, Department of Pathology/Division of Transplantation Pathology, Pittsburgh, Pennsylvania
Transplantation Pathology

Demetre M. Nicoloff, M.D., Ph.D.
Cardiothoracic Surgeon, Minneapolis Heart Institute, Minneapolis, and St. Paul Heart and Lung Center, St. Paul, Minnesota
The Cardiovascular System

Joseph E. Oesterling, M.D.
Professor and Urologist-in-Chief, The University of Michigan Medical Center; Director, The Michigan Prostate Institute, Ann Arbor, Michigan
The Urologic and Male Reproductive Systems

Carey P. Page, M.D.
Professor of Surgery, The University of Texas Health Science Center at San Antonio; Chief, General Surgery Section, Audie L. Murphy Memorial Veterans Hospital, San Antonio, Texas
The Hematolymphoid System

David G. Piepgras, M.D.
Professor of Neurosurgery, Mayo Medical School; Chairman, Department of Neurosurgery, Mayo Clinic, Rochester, Minnesota
The Nervous System

Donald R. Pulitzer, M.D.
Associate Professor of Pathology, Department of Pathology, The University of Texas Health Science Center at San Antonio; Director of Surgical Pathology and Dermatopathology, University Hospital, San Antonio, Texas
The Skin

Hector C. Ramos, M.D.
Associate Professor of Surgery, University of New Mexico School of Medicine; Chief, Division of Transplantation; Director of Transplant Services, Department of Surgery, University of New Mexico Health Sciences Center, Albuquerque, New Mexico
Transplantation Pathology

Michael G. Rock, M.D., F.R.C.S.
Professor of Orthopedic Surgery, Mayo Clinic and Mayo Foundation, Rochester, Minnesota
Tumors and Tumorlike Conditions of Bones and Joints

Bernd W. Scheithauer, M.D.
Professor of Pathology, Mayo Medical School; Consultant in Laboratory Medicine and Pathology, Mayo Clinic, Rochester, Minnesota
The Nervous System

Charles H. Scudamore, M.D.
Associate Professor of Surgery, Department of Surgery, University of British Columbia, Vancouver, British Columbia, Canada
The Gastrointestinal Tract

Donald Serafin, M.D.
Professor and Chief, Division of Plastic, Reconstructive, Maxillofacial and Oral Surgery, Duke University Medical Center, Durham, North Carolina
The Skin

Steven G. Silverberg, M.D.
Professor of Pathology and Director of Anatomic Pathology, The George Washington University Medical Center, Washington, D.C.
Obstetric and Gynecologic Pathology

Jean F. Simpson, M.D.
Attending Pathologist, Division of Pathology, City of Hope National Medical Center, Duarte, California
The Breast

Thomas J. Smith, M.D.
Chairman, Department of Surgery, Morristown Memorial Hospital, Morristown, New Jersey
The Breast

William H. Snyder III, M.D.
Professor of Surgery, Department of Surgery, University of Texas Southwestern Medical School; Active Attending Staff, Parkland Memorial Hospital; Zale Lipshy University Hospital, Dallas, Texas
The Liver, Biliary Tract, and Pancreas

Jack L. Titus, M.D., Ph.D.
Clinical Professor, Laboratory Medicine and Pathology, University of Minnesota, Minneapolis; Director, Registry of Cardiovascular Disease, United Hospital, St. Paul, Minnesota
The Cardiovascular System

Krishnan K. Unni, B.S., M.B.
Professor of Pathology, Mayo Medical School; Consultant in Laboratory Medicine and Pathology, Mayo Clinic and Mayo Foundation, Rochester, Minnesota
Tumors and Tumorlike Conditions of Bones and Joints

Sharon W. Weiss, M.D.
A. James French Professsor of Diagnostic Pathology and Director of Anatomic Pathology, The University of Michigan Medical Center, Ann Arbor, Michigan
Soft Tissue Tumors

Mark R. Wick, M.D.
Professor of Pathology, Washington University School of Medicine; Director of Surgical Pathology, Washington University Medical Center, St. Louis, Missouri
Special Techniques in Surgical Pathology

Earle W. Wilkins, Jr., M.D.
Clinical Professor of Surgery, Emeritus, Harvard Medical School; Senior Surgeon, Massachusetts General Hospital, Boston, Massachusetts
The Mediastinum

Robert A. Wolber, M.D.
Clinical Instructor, Department of Pathology, University of British Columbia, Vancouver, British Columbia, Canada
The Gastrointestinal Tract

Martha A. Zeiger, M.D.
Assistant Professor of Surgery, Johns Hopkins University School of Medicine, Baltimore, Maryland
Endocrine Pathology

Foreword

Since the fundamental discoveries of Rudolf Virchow at the famed Charité Hospital and the University of Berlin in the mid 19th century, the basic concepts of pathology shifted from an *organ* to a *cellular* basis. In his now famous textbook *Cellularpathologie*, Virchow described the *histologic* characteristics of many disorders in stained microscopic sections. Since that time, surgeons and pathologists alike have recognized the necessity to establish pathological diagnoses at the cellular level.

In addition to microscopic sections, contemporary surgical pathology now encompasses many innovative techniques, which have greatly expanded the ability to establish a firm diagnosis. Special tests also serve as reliable prognostic indicators. The profession is much indebted to Dr. Peter M. Banks, Professor and Director of Anatomic Pathology at the University of Texas Health Science Center at San Antonio, for editing this remarkable text, which thoroughly updates the field and includes the most recent diagnostic methods. With 40 contributors, the editor has created an unabridged text consisting of 21 chapters with authoritative reviews and illustrative data. It is a thoroughly reliable resource for surgeons and pathologists alike in a rapidly advancing field.

The initial chapter entitled the *Surgeon and Pathologist* is written by Dr. Peter M. Banks and a surgeon, Dr. William G. Kraybill. They emphasize that it was recognized quite early that rapid intraoperative diagnosis was necessary and cited the work of Thomas Cullen at Johns Hopkins at the turn of the century in developing techniques for frozen sections. It is interesting that such techniques were slow in being accepted, having been used in only a few selected centers, whereas today they are the *sine qua non* of the field. Drs. Banks and Kraybill also present classic cases illustrative of significant points with review of the interplay between the surgeon and surgical pathologist in solving some of the more difficult and unusual clinical problems. At the conclusion of the chapter, emphasis is placed upon the necessity for both the surgeon and the surgical pathologist to be thoroughly familiar with the patient and when possible to create a preoperative, an intraoperative, and a postoperative plan of communication to ensure that the patient's best interests can be uniformly served. As in other chapters of the text, fascinating sections on *pitfalls for the surgeon* and *pitfalls for the pathologist* emphasize ways to prevent problems, and indeed catastrophes, which might otherwise occur.

A quite timely chapter on *Special Techniques in Surgical Pathology* is contributed by Professor Mark R. Wick of Washington University. He emphasizes the role and significance of the newer tests, many of which have become essential to establishing a thorough surgical pathologic diagnosis. Detailed discussions of immunostains, electron microscopy, flow cytometry, cytogenetics, cell enzyme analysis, and molecular probe analysis are concisely reviewed. Individual case histories are cited to illustrate the role of these special techniques and their significance in obtaining an accurate diagnosis for proper therapy.

The importance of *fine needle aspiration biopsy* and its many ramifications are carefully presented and assessed. Current techniques, pitfalls encountered, and necessity for interactive discussions are thoroughly reviewed. Carefully prepared chapters follow on the surgical pathology of the skin, the breast, and the head and neck. This is a very thorough text with further sections on endocrine pathology, the mediastinum, and the lungs and pleura. Considerable attention is directed toward the gastrointestinal tract with emphasis upon the liver, biliary tract, and pancreas. Obstetric and gynecologic pathology is presented as well as that of the urologic and male reproductive systems. Especially significant are specific assays including the prostate specific antigen (ie, PSA) and other biochemical markers for neoplastic disease.

The importance of the cardiovascular system is presented in an excellent review as is the hematolymphoid system. Other chapters encompass soft tissue tumors as well as tumors and tumorlike conditions of bones and joints. Transplantation pathology and selected considerations for the pediatric patient then follow, maintaining the high standard of excellence achieved throughout the text.

It has been a special privilege to review this work and to note the carefully selected illustrations that are an important part of each chapter. In summary, this text is a *masterwork* and predictably a classic that will be widely used in daily practice and cited in future literature.

DAVID C. SABISTON, JR., M.D.

Preface

The purpose of this book is to assist surgeons in the successful utilization of pathology. Until the 1970s, surgeons and pathologists had contact early in their training together. Every surgeon individually received enough experience in pathology to understand its appropriate application in surgical practice. Most pathologists were trained initially in a clinical internship, which enabled them to empathize and successfully communicate with surgeons, in particular during the stress of intraoperative decision making. Today, the pressures for specialty and subspecialty training have robbed the newest generation of surgeons and pathologists of these common backgrounds. In deference to the requirements for training in increasingly sophisticated techniques, both surgical and diagnostic, the basic principles for productive interactive practice have often been lost. In the first chapter of this text, we have listed and analyzed these principles. Clinical case examples—with both favorable and unfavorable outcomes—are presented to illustrate the power of these principles for patient management.

Forty contributors, surgeons and pathologists, have contributed the following 21 chapters, all in uniform format. The emphasis in each is practical. Each chapter begins with a topical definition, each proceeds to common surgical disease entities, and each emphasizes areas where problems are likely to arise. Every chapter concludes with listings of major pitfalls, for the surgeon and for the pathologist.

Coordinating the assembly of such uniformly formatted chapters was an educational experience for the editors. Early in the effort, it became apparent that surgeons and pathologists approach their disciplines differently. Pathologists think principally about the *nature* of the disease process, its causes, mechanisms, and behavior. Surgeons think principally in terms of *action*—what should be *done* and, conversely, what should be *avoided*.

The uniform theme throughout this book is the complementary relationship of these two disciplines—surgery and pathology. In order to overcome differences in backgrounds and thought processes, the key to success for such specialists is a free and frequent communication in a common language—the language of *surgical pathology*. Only in this manner can mutual respect and confidence be developed. Surgeons must appreciate the pathophysiology of disease processes, and pathologists must recognize the needs of surgeons in relation to patient care decisions. Our inspiration for assembling this book derives largely from the many positive experiences we have had—as a pathologist working with exemplary surgeons and as a surgeon working with exemplary pathologists.

Practicing surgeons and pathologists will find this book a useful means to become updated. It will also guide surgical trainees in relation to the patient's particular disease process. During specialty rotations, related topics are concentrated in respective chapters.

PETER M. BANKS, M.D.
WILLIAM G. KRAYBILL, M.D.

Acknowledgments

Dr. Deborah Douglas generously contributed much time and applied her highly developed writing abilities to this book's manuscript preparation.

The word processing keyboard of Linda Streckfus was the final common pathway for all the manuscripts.

Contents

1

Surgeon and Pathologist

Peter M. Banks and William G. Kraybill

Definition

Drawing a geologic analogy, it can be said that the unending rearrangement of medicine's tectonic plates has accelerated in recent decades, heaving up mountains of information and creating countless formations of specialty practice. The resultant landscape is complex and exciting, but its vastness defies mastery. For this reason, most physicians concentrate on one or, at most, two mountain ranges. In doing so they lose sight of other landforms. Surgeons and pathologists can ill afford to be uninformed about one another's territories.

This book seeks to assist the surgeon in exploring pathology as a resource for patient management. The following chapters describe special techniques or anatomically or functionally defined topics in surgical pathology. Attempts to narrow the rift between surgeons and pathologists that has grown out of specialization are predicated on four principles: mutual professional respect; dedication to proper patient management; effective communication pre-, intra-, and postoperatively; and the curiosity to comprehend the disease processes that underlie clinical manifestations and guide surgical management. Stated another way, both specialties must want to know the lay of the land.

Unfortunately, there has been a decline among surgeons in the understanding and application of surgical pathology. Likewise, pathologists have lost some insight into the problems faced by surgeons in the care of their patients. An explanation for these sequelae of specialization can be gained from a historical perspective.

Historical Analysis

During the 19th century, rapid progress was made in the field of pathology; however, this surge derived almost exclusively from autopsy findings. Pathologists were absorbed in the development of the new science of histopathology and were regarded more as scientists than as physicians (see Chap. 2). It was not a pathologist but a surgeon, Sir James Paget, who was applying lessons learned from observations in pathology to improve operative practices.[1] Nineteenth-century surgeons usually confronted diseases in advanced stages and were thus able to serve as their own pathologists. Therapeutic decisions were based on physical examination and gross operative findings. Most surgeons of the time intuitively assumed that the delay inherent in conventional microscopy methods allowed dissemination of disease. So entrenched were these ideas that one surgeon paid for his independent thought by being ridiculed when he sent biopsies to German pathologists for interpretation.[2]

In the latter 19th century, the development of general anesthesia permitted longer operative procedures. This served as an impetus for the development of a rapid intraoperative method for surgical specimen microscopy. The first claims of success came from Thomas S. Cullen in 1895 at Johns Hopkins Hospital.[3] Conventional microscopic slide preparations required one or two days to fix, dehydrate, and infiltrate the tissue blocks sequentially with melted wax. When allowed to solidify, the wax blocks were thinly sectioned for staining and mounting on the slides. In contrast, Cullen's new method allowed sections to be produced within minutes by freezing unfixed tissue blocks. Like solid wax, the frozen tissue was hard enough to section. The frozen sections of tissue were applied to glass slides and, because they were thin, fixation and staining were achieved rapidly. Ironically, this rapid method was slow to gain popularity, even at Cullen's own institution. It was there that the prominent surgeon Joseph Colt Bloodgood declared in 1908: "Up to the present time, a stained frozen section has never been of aid in making the diagnosis when we have been unable to come to a conclusion from the fresh appearance of the tissue.''[4]

By contrast, the Mayo brothers and their surgical colleagues in Minnesota were more enthusiastic about the technique. In 1905 Louis B. Wilson, a pathologist recruited from the University of Minnesota, published a supravital staining method for intraoperative frozen sections. The following year William Carpenter MacCarty, a young American physician trained both in surgery at Johns Hopkins and in pathology in Germany, became the second pathologist to join the Mayo staff, which then totaled 14![5] In 1917 MacCarty and Albert Broders published a study of 1,800 surgical cases of breast disease. Intraoperative frozen section technique was used for 933 cases in the series. Of these, 211 cases, or 22%, were diagnosed intraoperatively as carcinoma, when combined physical examination and gross operative evaluation alone had suggested breast disease of benign or uncertain nature. Intraoperative histology had avoided a 22% false-negative rate; similarly, the technique had eliminated a 5% false-positive rate.[6] In the face of these data and those from subsequent studies, even skeptics such as Bloodgood eventually capitulated. Improved public health education allowed evaluation of patients at earlier stages of disease. In 1927 Bloodgood published a brief editorial entitled ''When cancer becomes a microscopic disease, there must be tissue diagnosis in the operating room.''[7] In retrospect, this was a defining moment for surgical pathology.

Bloodgood's newfound zeal converted him into a public proponent of intraoperative surgical pathology. He raised the issue of the lack of facilities for frozen section in hospitals as a deficiency warranting consideration by the American College of Surgeons.[7]

Until the middle of the 20th century, the American College of Surgeons was the sole hospital accrediting authority in the United States. Initially this role stemmed from the organization's own needs to review hospital records to assess the practice performance of surgeons applying for membership. This role soon burgeoned to include delineation of comprehensive standards of patient care. As early as 1918, hospitals were required to provide ''chemical, bacteriological, serological, and pathological services . . . under competent medical supervision.''[8] With the backing of prominent surgeons such as Bloodgood, the Board of Regents of the American College of Surgeons voted in 1929 ''to undertake the promotion of better cancer service throughout the continent and entrusted to the Committee on the Treatment of Malignant Disease the task of perfecting the details by which this can be accomplished.''[9] This committee was the forerunner of today's Commission on Cancer; in subsequent years it recommended frozen section as a standard procedure for intraoperative diagnosis.[9]

Clearly, surgical pathology evolved in response to the needs of surgeons. In fact, many of the pioneers in this field, such as Authur Purdy Stout of Columbia University in New York, developed their careers within departments of surgery.[10]

Recent decades have seen an explosion of the knowledge base of both surgery and pathology. The development of sophisticated operative techniques has demanded subspecialization in surgical training. A glance at a typical list of divisions within academic departments of surgery confirms this—critical care and trauma; cardiothoracic, vascular, plastic, gastrointestinal, endocrine, transplantation, oncologic surgery; and so on. Individual faculty members carry this a step further when they become ''superspecialists,'' with practices confined to breast or pancreatic-hepatobiliary or other anatomically circumscribed targets.

The trend toward subspecialization in surgery has been accompanied by a decline in surgeons' training and participation in pathology. Thirty years ago a typical trainee spent 6 months or more in pathology and developed not only familiarity with pathology but also proficiency in it. Today, a pathology rotation is no longer required for surgical board eligibility; in most programs, pathology is dashed through in a 1-month scramble or is left entirely optional.

Surgery is not alone in its march toward subspecialization. Pathology has kept pace. In academic programs, the demand for scholarly productivity and research requires skills in sophisticated study methods such as immunology and molecular biology. Only a small percentage of pathology trainees participate in a clinical internship before beginning their pathology residency. The untoward result is a new generation of pathologists that is unfamiliar with the complexities of surgical management. Furthermore, in many university departments and even in larger private practice groups, cases are routinely triaged according to subspecialty expertise for diagnosis. This is particularly true for complicated disciplines such as renal pathology, neuropathology, and dermatopathology. Only a minority of cases are left to the ''undifferentiated'' surgical pathologist.

This trend toward tunnel vision undermines the clinical practice setting. As surgeons and pathologists have lost their common educational moorings, so too have they lost their ability to communicate and to strengthen each other's role in patient care. This phenomenon is ironic. Scientific progress has refined diagnostic resolution in pathology, and this could serve as a powerful resource in the surgeon's armamentarium—but only if properly recruited. As shown in some of the following case examples, inadequate communication and limited awareness of these resources can hinder optimal patient management.

Case Examples

Lessons can be learned from individual case examples, presented here in an analytic format. Most of these paradigms illustrate either extremely positive or extremely negative clinical outcomes resulting from interactions (or lack thereof) between surgeons and pathologists.

Case 1–1. Metastatic Renal Adenocarcinoma Simulating Inflammatory Pseudotumor of Lung

HISTORY. Two years previously, a 44-year-old woman underwent radical nephrectomy for a renal cortical adenocarcinoma. She had been without evidence of relapse until vague pleuritic symptoms occasioned chest x-rays showing a solitary peripheral density about 4 cm in greatest dimension in the left lateral lung field. Thorough medical evaluation revealed no evidence of disease elsewhere, and she was scheduled for thoracotomy. On the operating room schedule the day of surgery, her case was listed as "peripheral lung tumor, resection."

SURGEON'S ACTIONS. At thoracotomy, a firm, subpleural, sharply defined mass was identified in the lateral aspect of the left upper lobe. The pleura was not puckered by this, nor was there any roughening of the overlying pleural surface. A segmental resection was performed and the specimen was sent to the pathology laboratory with a requisition slip stating "lung tumor, left upper lobe."

PATHOLOGIST'S ACTIONS. After measuring and examining the intact specimen, the pathologist made a sweeping knife cut from the pleural surface through the palpable mass, revealing a tumor of 4 × 3 × 3 cm that was mottled yellow and gray and sharply demarcated. Scrape-smear cytology preparations and a frozen section were produced. Microscopically, the frozen section showed pulmonary parenchyma replaced by a spindling proliferation with areas of plump foam cells (Fig. 1–1*A*). These appearances suggested an inflammatory process featuring fibroblasts and histiocytes, i.e., so-called inflammatory pseudotumor or plasma cell granuloma of the lung (see Chap. 11). The pathologist communicated this impression to the surgeon over the intercom.

SURGEON'S ACTIONS. The surgeon asked the pathologist if this was then not consistent with metastatic renal carcinoma, as had been diagnosed 2 years earlier.

PATHOLOGIST'S ACTIONS. The pathologist expressed surprise at this suggestion, not having been previously informed of the history, and told the surgeon that a review of the findings was in order with this in mind. The frozen section was studied again with the same observations. However, review of the cytology preparation allowed recognition of definite nuclear atypia among some of the plump foamy cells, as distinct from associated benign macrophages (Fig. 1–1*B*). The pathologist reviewed the patient's chart and in it found the pathology report from 2 years previously. This described the renal tumor as of mixed low- and high-grade composition, with areas featuring a sarcomatoid spindling growth pattern. Based on this past description, the pathologist's impression changed to metastatic carcinoma consistent with renal cortical origin. This impression was conveyed verbally to the surgeon over the intercom and documented in an intraoperative pathology report placed in the patient's chart.

SURGEON'S ACTIONS. Careful examination of the left lung revealed one additional small, suspicious subpleural nodule in the left middle lobe. This was removed in its entirety in another segmental resection.

PATHOLOGIST'S ACTIONS. The following day, permanent sections of both resected pulmonary nodules showed an overtly malignant process with a mixture of plump clear-cell epithelial features and malignant spindle cells (Fig. 1–1*C*). Comparison with the original renal tumor showed similar features (Figs. 1–1*D* and 1–1*E*).

OUTCOME. The patient was told that a second small nodule of tumor had been found in the left lung but that the likelihood of further problems with tumor spread was uncertain. After 10 months without evidence of disease, there was progression of localized headaches, and a large cerebral metastasis was resected. The patient remains alive without further evidence of disease progression 4 months later.

COMMENTS. The pathologist's first erroneous interpretation would have been avoided if the operating room listing or pathology requisition slip had alluded to the past history of a renal carcinoma. Well-differentiated clear-cell adenocarcinomas can mimic benign foamy macrophages microscopically, so that the unwary surgeon, operating without benefit of clinical history, may accept an intraoperative diagnosis of "lipid pneumonia" or "inflammatory pseudotumor." In this case the spindling growth pattern of the sarcomatoid elements of the tumor, together with the inflammatory response in surrounding pulmonary parenchyma, gave the false impression of an inflammatory tumefactive process—i.e., so-called inflammatory pseudotumor. Because the surgeon communicated well with the pathologist, the correct diagnosis was established intraoperatively, permitting identification of a second, radiologically inapparent metastasis. Had the pulmonary process actually been an inflammatory one, there would have been no indication for searching for additional tumors.

Renal cortical adenocarcinoma is capricious in behavior. Although in this case there was subsequent metastatic disease in other organs, there are many cases with long-sustained disease-free intervals after resection of one or even several metastases.

Case 1–2. Alveolar Rhabdomyosarcoma Eluding Diagnosis Due to Tumor Necrosis in Biopsies

HISTORY. A 58-year-old woman suffered progressive nasal "stuffiness," leading to biopsy of the nasal vestibule; this was interpreted as "poorly differentiated carcinoma." The patient avoided further medical care for 8 weeks, at which time she was evaluated in a university outpatient clinic for unilateral proptosis and a large maxillary soft tissue mass (Fig. 1–2*A*). Review of the original nasal biopsy slides by a university pathologist revealed a high-grade, largely necrotic neoplasm of uncertain nature. The head-and-neck surgeon was consulted for a new biopsy sampling.

SURGEON'S ACTIONS. Direct examination of the nasal cavity showed an exophytic mass filling the right nasal vestibule. This was curetted; about 3 cm² of tissue was submitted in formalin to pathology.

PATHOLOGIST'S ACTIONS. Although there was a ghostlike pattern of tumor cellularity, all sections were necrotic, with no intact cellularity for diagnosis (Fig. 1–2*B*). The surgeon was told that the sample was nondiagnostic and a rebiopsy with intraprocedural pathology monitoring for adequacy of tissue was recommended.

SURGEON'S ACTIONS. Additional curettings were obtained from the right nasal vestibule and a pathologist was called for intraoperative assessment. The first two samples were interpreted as "necrotic tissue only." The third was inter-

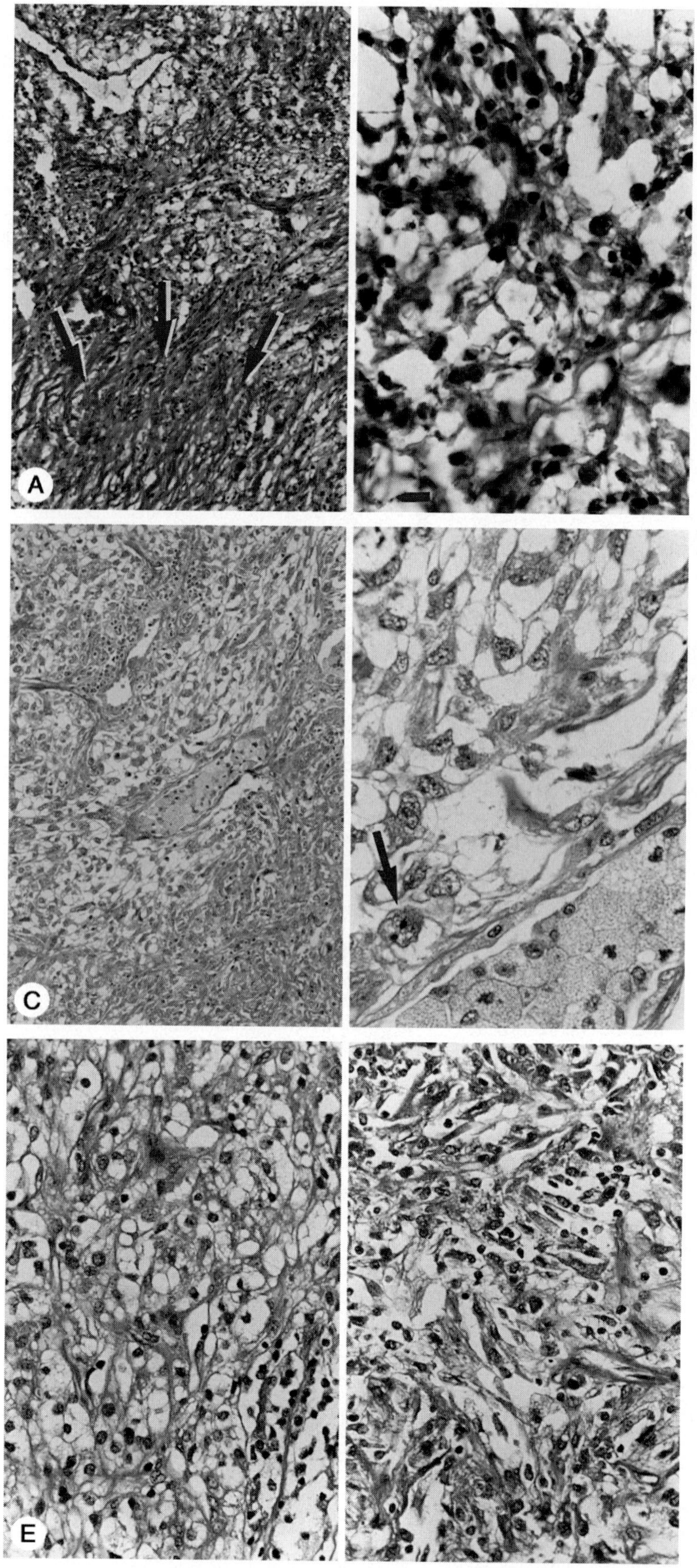

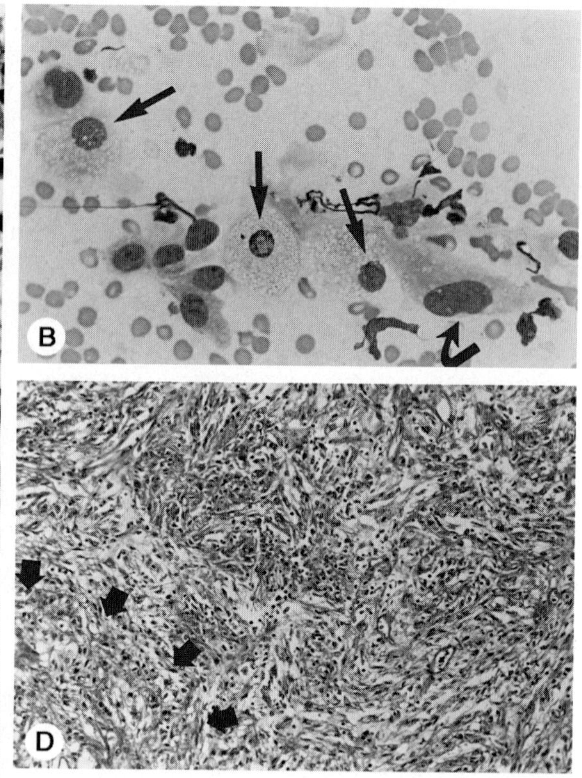

Figure 1–1. *A,* Frozen sections from pulmonary nodule exhibit microscopic features initially interpreted as benign inflammatory pseudotumor. Low magnification *(left)* shows zones of hypocellular fibrosis *(arrows);* high magnification *(right)* reveals a mixture of spindle cells, thought to be fibroblasts, and plump cells, taken to be histiocytes.

B, Air-dried scrape-smear cytology preparation from the nodule was rapidly stained with Diff-Quik method and studied carefully after the surgeon mentioned history of renal cortical carcinoma. In this preparation nuclei of benign foamy histiocytes appear small *(straight arrows)* in comparison to large, atypical nucleus of spindle cell *(curved arrow).* On the basis of this finding and history, the intraoperative diagnosis was changed to metastatic carcinoma, consistent with renal origin.

C, Permanent sections the following day confirmed the intraoperative interpretation. Low magnification *(left)* shows whorls of spindling clear cells. At high magnification *(right),* there are anaplastic cellular features indicative of malignancy, including large, vesicular nuclei with prominent nucleoli *(arrow).* Such cellular features of malignancy stand in striking contrast to those of the benign foamy histiocytes along the inferior margin of this field.

D, Reviews of sections from the renal tumor 2 years previously showed microscopic features similar to those of the metastasis. In this low-magnification field, a spindling cellular growth pattern is manifest in most areas; however, in the lower left is a zone of plump epithelial tumor cells *(arrows).*

E, Higher magnification allows comparison of variation in cellular appearances within this renal cortical adenocarcinoma. An epithelioid area *(left)* consists of plump, foamy, clear tumor cells typical of hypernephroma. An area of spindle tumor cells *(right)* produces a sarcomatoid appearance. Metastases with such features can be mistaken for primary or secondary sarcomas or, intraoperatively, as in this case, for benign fibroblastic processes.

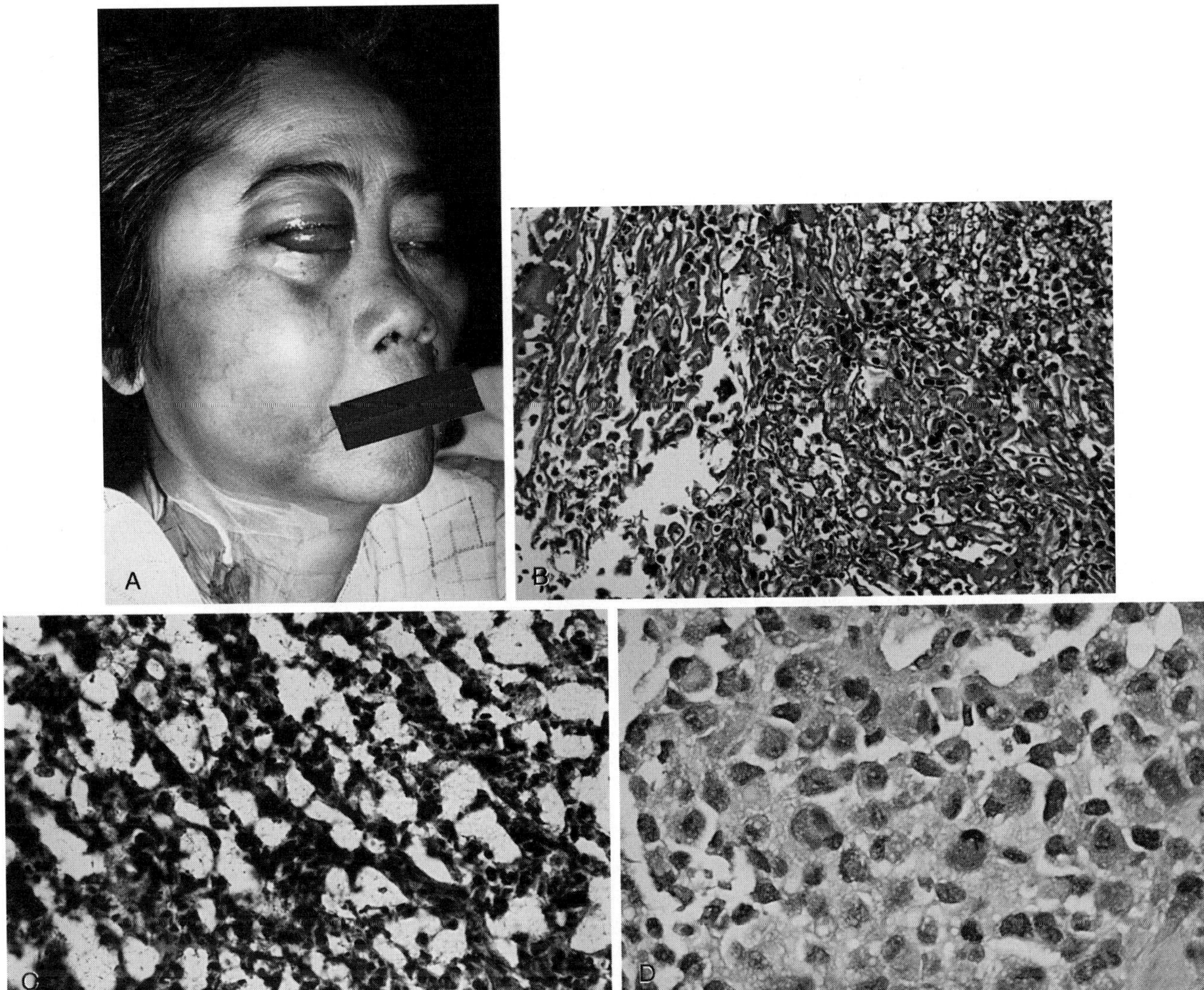

Figure 1–2. *A,* An alveolar rhabdomyosarcoma arising in the nasal sinuses has rapidly spread to involve soft tissues and orbit of the right maxillary region in this 58-year-old woman (Case 1–2). Despite easy access for biopsy, the first two samples were nondiagnostic due to necrosis.

B, Tumor cells are uniformly shrunken, with dark, small nuclei due to early necrosis in this biopsy from the nasal vestibule, which was carried out without pathologic monitoring *(intermediate magnification).*

C, Intraoperative frozen section of the third biopsy shows dark appearance due to high nuclear:cytoplasmic ratio of intact tumor cells. The surgeon was told that this was an area of intact tumor; sampling was adequate *(high magnification).*

D, Permanent section reveals features diagnostic for alveolar rhabdomyosarcoma. Blastic tumor cells exhibit abundant (pink) cytoplasm and eccentric nuclei. Cellular detail is vastly superior to frozen section (compare Fig. 1–2*C*) *(high magnification).*

preted as "intact tumor present, defer to permanents for classification, sample adequate" (Fig. 1–2*C*).

PATHOLOGIST'S ACTIONS. The day following biopsy, permanent sections showed a few foci of intact tumor cellularity with features diagnostic for alveolar rhabdomyosarcoma (Fig. 1–2*D*). Because of the unusual clinical presentation and difference in diagnosis from the original biopsy, immunostains were carried out to confirm the diagnosis of rhabdomyosarcoma.

OUTCOME. Staging evaluation disclosed bone marrow involvement by tumor. The patient was begun on an intensive regimen of polychemotherapy.

COMMENTS. Even relatively large tumor biopsies can prove inadequate. This is a significant risk when the tumor is high-grade and necrotic or when there is extensive fibrosis of the tumor, as is sometimes encountered in tumors of the mediastinum or retroperitoneum. Intraoperative pathology monitoring with frozen section or cytology smear preparations avoids this problem. It also gives the pathologist an early microscopic differential diagnosis to use in assigning priority to allocations of tissue for special study methods (see Chap. 2). When large, open procedures are used for tumor biopsy (abdominal, retroperitoneal, intrathoracic), it is critical that the sampled tissue be monitored for diagnostic adequacy *before closing* the incision.

Case 1–3. Mediastinal Lymphoma Resected as Thymoma

HISTORY. A 35-year-old woman presented with shortness of breath. Chest radiographs and computed tomography (CT) revealed a slightly lobate tumor of the superior anterior mediastinum (Figs. 1–3*A*, *B*, and *C*).

SURGEON'S ACTIONS. Mediastinoscopy was performed and yielded several biopsy samples interpreted as "neoplasm, of uncertain nature, obscured by crush artifact." The patient's condition worsened over the ensuing 2 days and a median sternotomy procedure was carried out. The surgeon encountered a large, firm, fixed tumor that was largely confined to the mediastinum with focal infiltration of the pleura. A 2-cm wedge biopsy was taken from the anterior aspect of the tumor and submitted for intraoperative frozen section. "?Thymoma" was on the requisition slip.

PATHOLOGIST'S ACTIONS. The biopsy specimen was divided and a portion examined by frozen section. A diffuse expanse of monomorphic tumor cells was seen in association with recognizable thymus (Figs. 1–3*D* and *E*). A diagnosis of "thymoma" was communicated to the surgeon.

SURGEON'S ACTIONS. The entire tumor was resected, including an involved portion of right-lower-lobe pleura.

OUTCOME. In permanent sections, tumor cells were complex and pleomorphic; paraffin immunostains showed reactivity for leukocyte common antigen but not for cytokeratin, confirming the diagnosis of malignant lymphoma of diffuse large-cell type. The patient had paralysis of the right hemidiaphragm after postoperative recovery. She received 6 months of combined radiation therapy and chemotherapy and was free of disease 3 years after diagnosis.

COMMENTS. Even in retrospect, this case is complex and deficiency in management is debatable. If a tumor is known to be lymphoma, attempted resection is generally contraindicated, since most lymphomas are sensitive to nonsurgical treatment modalities. On the other hand, debulking of large lymphomas can be beneficial by reducing posttherapy fibrosis and can even enhance the efficacy of radiation therapy and chemotherapy. In retrospect, the surgeon's decision to sample the anterior surface of the "tumor" was unlucky, since this included residual thymus and fooled the pathologist into interpreting the process as thymoma in frozen section. Correct management of thymoma is indeed resection. Even in permanent sections, the distinction of thymoma from lymphoma can be difficult and may require immunoperoxidase studies, as this case did.

The outcome was so favorable, despite loss of hemidiaphragm function, that the management of this patient must be considered ultimately favorable.

Case 1–4. Early, Well-Differentiated Carcinoma of the Breast Identified with Avoidance of Intraoperative Frozen Section

HISTORY. Two years previously, a 53-year-old woman underwent modified radical mastectomy for carcinoma of the right breast. Follow-up examination revealed no evidence of recurrent carcinoma; however, a subtle, ill-defined nodularity was palpable in the left (contralateral) breast, and mammography was interpreted as suspicious for malignancy.

SURGEON'S ACTIONS. A large, open biopsy of the suspicious quadrant was carried out. Intraoperative pathology consultation was requested.

PATHOLOGIST'S ACTIONS. The specimen measured 6.5 × 3.5 × 2.0 cm, and careful palpation revealed numerous small nodules 0.5 cm in maximum dimension. Specimen radiographs showed corresponding zones of soft tissue density. India ink was blotted over the external surface of the specimen to indicate resection planes. Sectioning of the specimen at 0.5-cm intervals revealed no single lesion that was grossly suspicious for carcinoma. The surgeon was informed that frozen section was contraindicated because of the absence of a grossly definable lesion; that margins appeared adequate, with fatty tissue enclosing all firm nodular tissue; and that microscopy would be deferred to permanent sections.

SURGEON'S ACTIONS. Convinced that the entire tissue region considered suspicious for malignancy had been excised, the surgeon closed the wound and told the patient that preliminary findings were all favorable but a careful examination would take several days. The patient was scheduled for a clinic visit 5 days later.

PATHOLOGIST'S ACTIONS. After fixation, the pathologist sampled all firm areas and submitted 12 tissue blocks. The following day, permanent sections revealed widespread proliferative breast disease with several foci of atypical ductal hyperplasia. A single 0.3-cm focus of well-differentiated tubular carcinoma was identified (Figs. 1–4*A* and *B*); this process did not encroach upon the inked resection

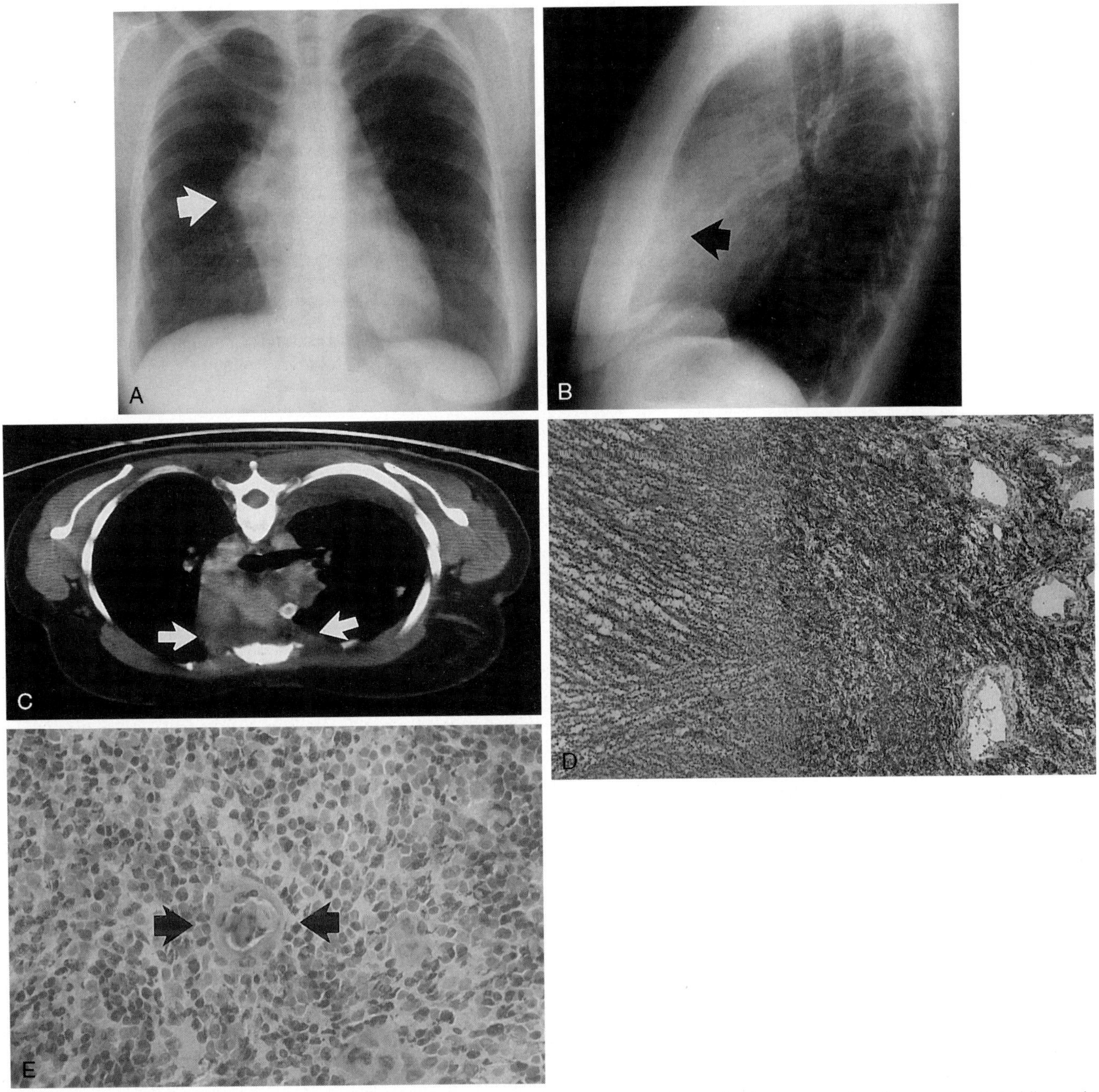

Figure 1–3. *A* and *B,* Chest radiographs of a 35-year-old woman show a large anterior mediastinal mass extending into the right hilar region *(arrow);* from Case 1–3 *(A, posteroanterior; B, lateral).*

C, Computed tomography shows soft tissue density in anterior mediastinum *(arrows).*

D, Low magnification of intraoperative frozen section shows pale neoplasm at left, residual darker thymus at right.

E, High magnification of intraoperative frozen section shows an intact thymic epithelial nest—i.e., a Hassall's corpuscle *(arrows)* surrounded by uniform tumor cells. The presence of this structural marker was interpreted as evidence of thymoma; however, subsequent paraffin section immunostains demonstrated the tumor to be a lymphoma that had infiltrated the thymus.

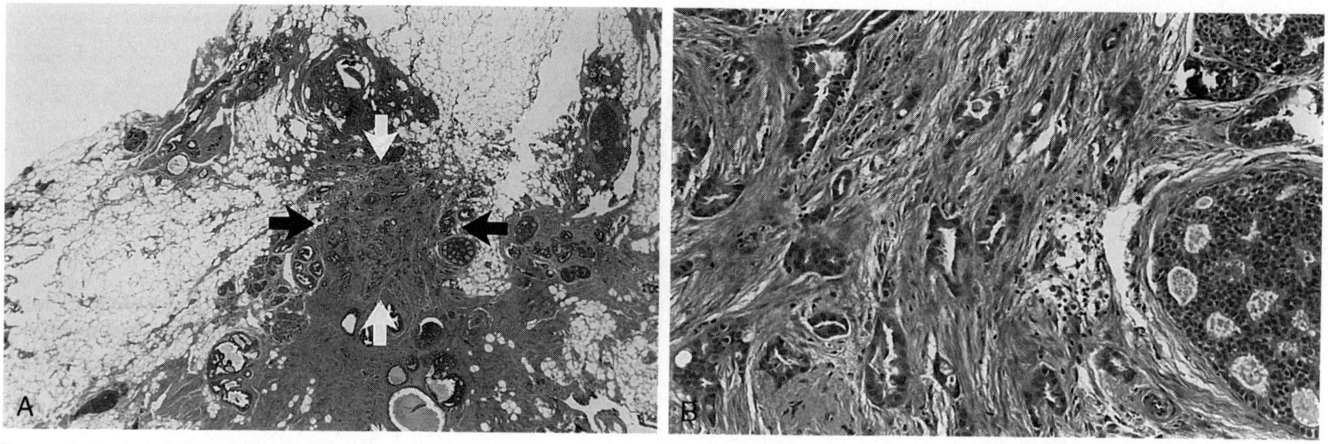

Figure 1–4. *A,* Low magnification shows a small focus of well-differentiated tubular carcinoma *(arrows)* arising in the setting of profuse ductal hyperplasia and fibrosis (Case 1–4).

B, Intermediate magnification reveals atypical tubules of well-differentiated carcinoma within proliferative fibrosis. Such a lesion could not be diagnosed if freezing artifact had been introduced with intraoperative frozen section preparation. In the right portion of the field are ducts showing atypical hyperplasia.

surfaces. The surgeon was contacted by phone with the diagnosis.

SURGEON'S ACTIONS. The patient was advised that a small focus of malignancy had been successfully removed but that there were changes of premalignancy throughout the quadrant, which carried a significant risk for subsequent malignancy. In anticipation of continued freedom from recurrence from the earlier right-sided cancer, subcutaneous mastectomy was advised and carried out. Pathologic examination revealed proliferative disease with atypical ductal hyperplasia.

COMMENTS. Because small, well-differentiated tubular carcinomas are difficult to distinguish from benign sclerosing lesions, the final diagnosis would have been jeopardized by freezing artifact if the pathologist had done intraoperative frozen sections (see Chap. 5). When no grossly recognizable tumor greater than 1.0 cm in diameter is present, frozen sections should be avoided.[11]

Case 1–5. Sclerosing Adenosis Mimicking Malignancy in Intraoperative Frozen Sections

HISTORY. A 57-year-old woman came to the surgical outpatient clinic after noting a "lump" in her left breast during regular self-examination. Mammography confirmed a suspicious soft tissue density about 0.8 cm in maximum dimension (Fig. 1–5*A*).

SURGEON'S ACTIONS. After wire-loop localization in radiology, the patient underwent excisional biopsy with local anesthesia. The specimen was submitted to radiology to confirm the presence of the suspicious lesion within the excised tissue (Fig. 1–5*B*). A pathology consultation was requested.

PATHOLOGIST'S ACTIONS. By comparing the tissue specimen and the specimen radiograph, the suspicious lesion was palpated. Parallel knife slices revealed a sharply demarcated, soft, uniform-appearing tumor surrounded on all sides by at least 1 cm of normal fatty breast. A portion of tumor was examined by the frozen section method. The process was highly cellular and composed of uniform spindle cells (Figs. 1–5*C* and *D*). Although these findings were worrisome for malignancy, the lesion was not recognizable as a typical breast carcinoma. Diagnostic considerations included a myoepithelial lesion, sarcoma, and metastasis from another site. Because of this uncertainty, the surgeon was told that excisional margins were adequate by gross inspection, that a tumor of uncertain nature was present, and that tumor typing would be deferred to permanent section review. This information was communicated by telephone rather than by intercom so as to spare the patient additional anxiety. A portion of the tumor was sent for estrogen receptor assay; other portions were snap-frozen and stored at −70°C for other potential special studies.

SURGEON'S ACTIONS. The surgeon informed the patient that the nodule was indeed found to be a tumor but that its nature, whether benign or malignant, could not be determined until detailed laboratory studies were performed. The incision was closed and the patient was scheduled for a clinic appointment 5 days later.

PATHOLOGIST'S ACTIONS. Paraffin sections the following day revealed features of an exceptionally large, cellular focus of sclerosing adenosis (Figs. 1–5*E* and *F*). The spindling appearance resulted from compression of adjacent small ductal structures, which showed characteristic peripheral dilation with luminal distention. There was a sharply defined rim of fibrosis. Tiny microcalcifications were found within the lumen of many ducts. The surgeon was contacted by telephone and given the results.

SURGEON'S ACTIONS. At the clinic visit, the patient was reassured that the tumor was benign. She was commended for her regular breast self-examination, warned that similar lumps might appear, and urged to return to the clinic should that occur.

COMMENTS. Intraoperative breast pathology can be extremely difficult; the guiding principle among pathologists is to avoid a false-positive diagnosis of malignancy. Even though this lesion was cellular and suggestive of malignancy, the wary pathologist was reluctant to diagnose the

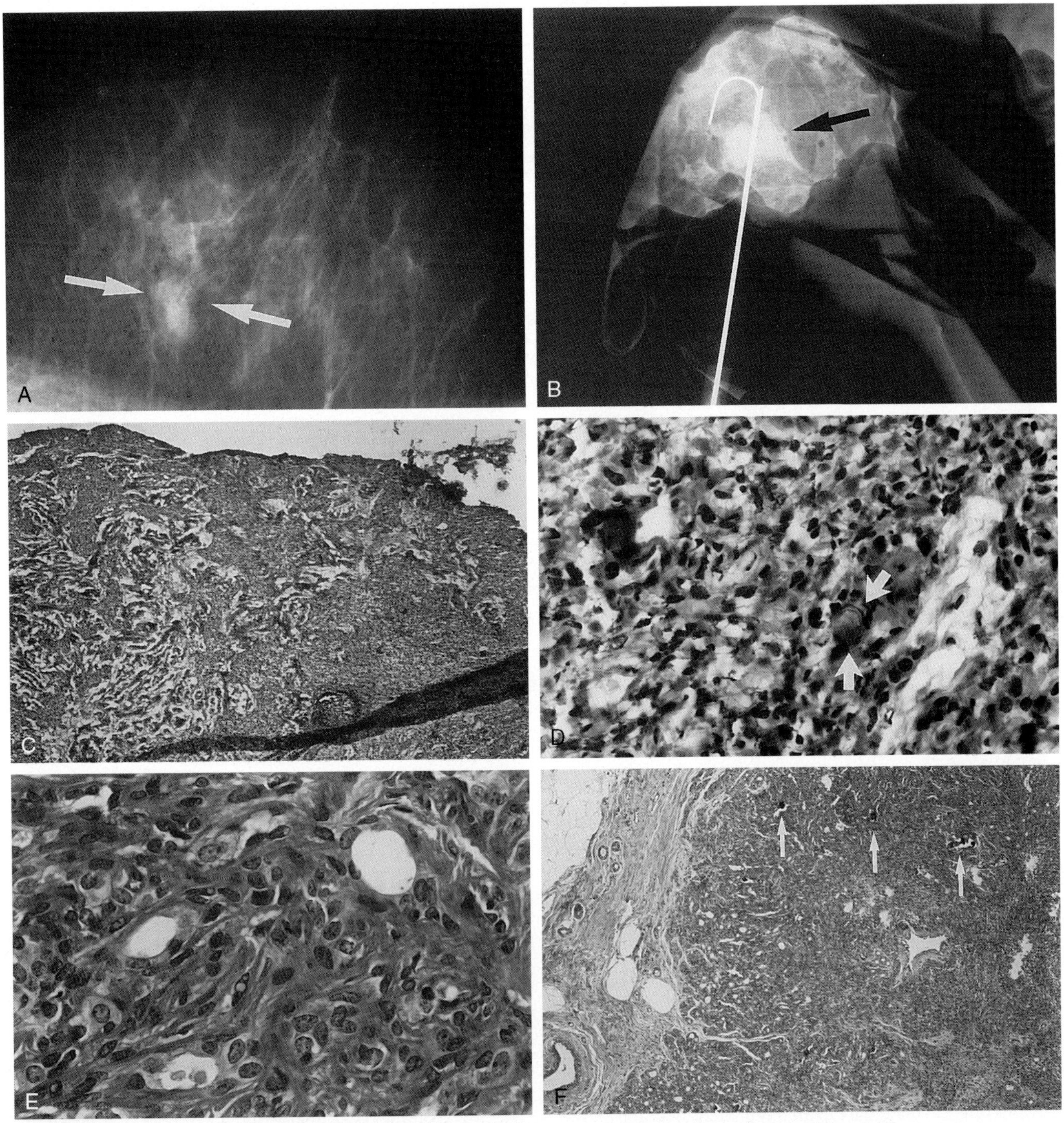

Figure 1–5. *A,* Mammogram of left breast shows soft tissue density *(arrows)* suspicious for malignancy (Case 1–5).

B, Radiograph of excisional biopsy specimen confirms the presence of the suspicious density within the wire loop *(arrow).*

C, Frozen section of 0.7-cm nodular breast lesion shows a dark, dense cellular appearance *(low magnification).*

D, High magnification of frozen section reveals an atypical spindle-cell appearance of uncertain significance. Note subtle laminated microcalcification, appearing somewhat refractile *(arrow).*

E, Permanent section at high magnification shows uniform, delicate spindle cells without atypia or mitotic figures of malignancy.

F, At low magnification, permanent section shows features recognizable as a large focus of sclerosing adenosis. There is uniform dilation of tubules peripherally with an associated dense fibrosis along the edge. Microcalcifications appear as tiny dark dots along the upper portion of the field *(arrows).*

tumor as carcinoma because there were atypical features. Nevertheless, tumor tissues were appropriately allocated for special studies in the event that carcinoma was indeed present.

Not until the 1930s was the distinction between sclerosing adenosis and carcinoma well defined.[12]

Case 1–6. Primary Malignant Lymphoma of Bone Simulating Sarcoma

HISTORY. After 6 months of progressive discomfort while walking, a 32-year-old male prison inmate was seen in an outpatient clinic. His complaints were initially dismissed as spurious, being seen as an attempt to avoid physical labor. However, radiographs showed a large area of medullary and cortical bone destruction in the distal right femur (Fig. 1–6*A*), and magnetic resonance imaging (MRI) studies revealed soft tissue extension. The patient was afebrile, denied fever or night sweats, and laboratory studies did not suggest an infectious process. Further evaluation, including skeletal survey and body CT, was negative for additional tumor foci. There was, however, palpable enlargement of the right (ipsilateral) inguinal lymph nodes, to about 3 cm in greatest dimension. These nodes were nontender and freely movable within surrounding fat.

SURGEON'S ACTIONS. Using general anesthesia and a lateral approach to avoid the posterior neurovascular compartment, about 2 cm^2 of soft tumor tissue was curetted from the bone and surrounding soft tissues and submitted for intraoperative pathology consultation. A portion of the tissue was retained in a sterile container for potential microbial cultures.

PATHOLOGIST'S ACTIONS. Two of the six curettings were processed for immediate frozen section study. Tissue imprints were stained with the rapid Romanowsky-type method—Diff-Quik stain (see Chap. 3). Frozen sections revealed a uniform cellular neoplasm without matrix (osteoid or cartilage) production (Figs. 1–6*B* and *C*). Tumor nuclei were moderately pleomorphic. Imprint cytology preparations showed tumor nuclei to be delicate and complexly irregular, with scant cytoplasm (Fig. 1–6*D*). These features were considered diagnostic for malignancy; however, the features were not specific for any particular bony sarcoma—e.g., osteosarcoma, Ewing's sarcoma, fibrosarcoma, and so on (see Chap. 19). The surgeon was told that there was no evidence of infection and that this was a malignancy of uncertain nature. Sampling was adequate to allow definitive diagnosis with permanent sections. Portions of fresh, intact tumor were snap-frozen for storage at −70°C and the remaining tissue was processed routinely.

SURGEON'S ACTIONS. The surgeon wisely anticipated that examination of the ipsilateral inguinal lymph nodes might be crucial for tumor staging. Several nodes were excised and submitted to pathology in formalin, as was the remaining bony sampling, which had initially been kept in a sealed sterile container for the option of microbial cultures.

PATHOLOGIST'S ACTIONS. Permanent sections were available the following afternoon. These confirmed the frozen section impression of a poorly differentiated tumor with a diffuse growth pattern (Fig. 1–6*E*). Features were most consistent with a large-cell malignant lymphoma—an impression confirmed by focal involvement of germinal center regions in the sampled inguinal lymph nodes. Paraffin immunostains of the tumor showed reactivity for B-cell lymphoid antigens.

The surgeon was called, given the diagnosis, and congratulated on the forethought demonstrated in the sampling of the lymph nodes.

OUTCOME. Hematology-oncology consultants performed bilateral iliac crest bone marrow biopsies that were negative for lymphoma. The lymphoma was considered stage IIE. Six months later, after he had completed six cycles of polychemotherapy, the patient's femur showed moderate bony repair in the original distribution of the lesion and the patient's gait had improved markedly. There was no evidence of disease elsewhere.

COMMENTS. Whenever the clinical presentation and radiologic findings are atypical for a primary sarcoma of bone, intraoperative diagnosis for definitive resection is ill advised. In this case, the pathologist diagnosed the process as malignancy, not infection, and concluded that the features did not suggest common types of primary bone sarcoma. Because lymphomas are treated with radiation and/or chemotherapy, limb-sparing resection or amputation would have been inappropriate. The surgeon was wise to excise the regional lymph nodes within the single anesthetic period. If the pathologist had considered lymphoma during the intraoperative evaluation, the surgeon could have included the iliac crest biopsy in the same anesthetic procedure as well (see Chap. 17). The pathologist's use of imprint preparations provided cytologic detail better than that in frozen sections for the intraoperative interpretation.

Case 1–7. Gastric Adenomyoma and Coincidental Adrenal Cortical Adenoma Simulating Carcinoma

HISTORY. A 54-year-old woman had a 3-month history of weight loss, night sweats, nausea and vomiting, and epigastric pain associated with a 30-lb weight loss. Computed tomography revealed an 8-cm mass within the gastric lumen and a 2-cm left adrenal mass (Figs. 1–7*A* and *B*). Laboratory studies revealed no electrolyte imbalance and serum cortisol levels were within normal limits. Screen for urine catecholamines was negative. There was anemia, presumed to be due to associated blood loss.

SURGEON'S ACTIONS. After celiotomy exposure, the stomach was examined externally and a discrete 7-cm mass was found within the anterior wall of the distal fundus. A firm 0.5-cm lymph node in the gastrocolic ligament was sent for frozen section interpretation. When this was reported as "negative for tumor," a partial gastrectomy was performed and pathology consultation requested.

PATHOLOGIST'S ACTIONS. The partial gastrectomy specimen measured 21 cm along the greater curvature. It was opened along the greater curvature, revealing a sessile, ulcerated tumor 6.0 × 6.0 × 2.0 cm in size on the superior-anterior aspect. Frozen sections (Figs. 1–7*C* and *D*) showed well-differentiated, dilated glands extending

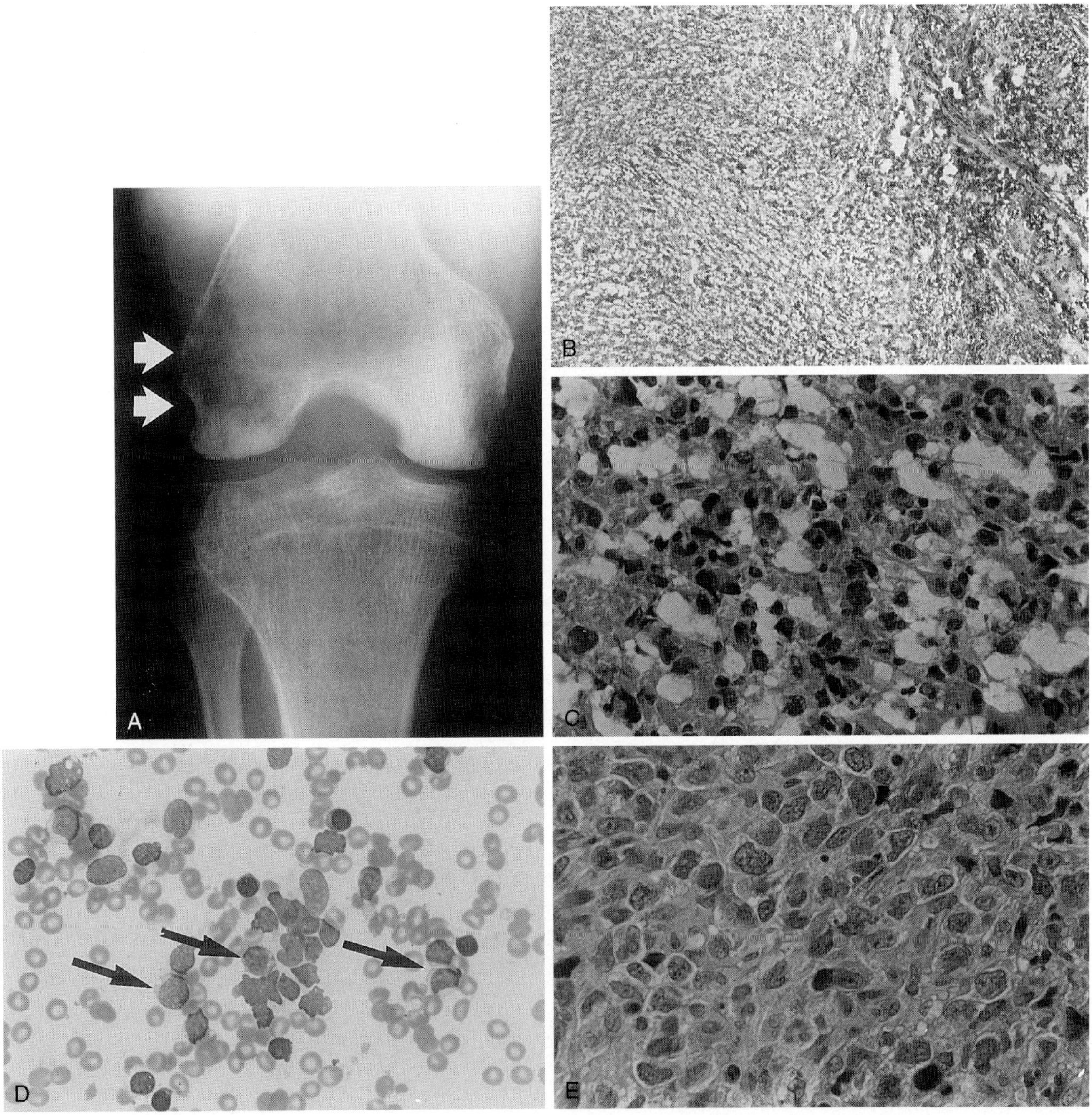

Figure 1–6. *A,* Radiograph of right knee shows a large, irregular, poorly defined zone of bony destruction in the lateral distal femur *(arrows).* There is cortical destruction, and magnetic resonance imaging demonstrated extension of the process into adjacent soft tissue (Case 1–6).

B and *C,* Frozen section at low magnification reveals a cellular tumor with a diffuse growth pattern devoid of any matrix such as osteoid or chondroid substance. High magnification *(C)* shows pleomorphic tumor nuclei; no neutrophils or plasma cells are present to suggest osteomyelitis.

D, Diff-Quik–stained, air-dried imprint preparation used for intraoperative interpretation shows delicate tumor cell chromatin and scant cytoplasm *(arrows).* This was not consistent with osteosarcoma, chondrosarcoma, or fibrosarcoma. Therefore, intraoperative diagnosis of sarcoma was withheld *(high magnification).*

E, Permanent paraffin section at high magnification shows features typical for large-cell lymphoma: irregular, complex vesicular nuclei and scant, pale-staining cytoplasm. Although granulocytic/monocytic sarcomas (i.e., solid manifestations of myeloid leukemia) can simulate lymphoma morphologically, in this case both the microscopic finding of early lymph nodal involvement and immunostains showing a B-cell lymphoid phenotype ruled out such a possibility.

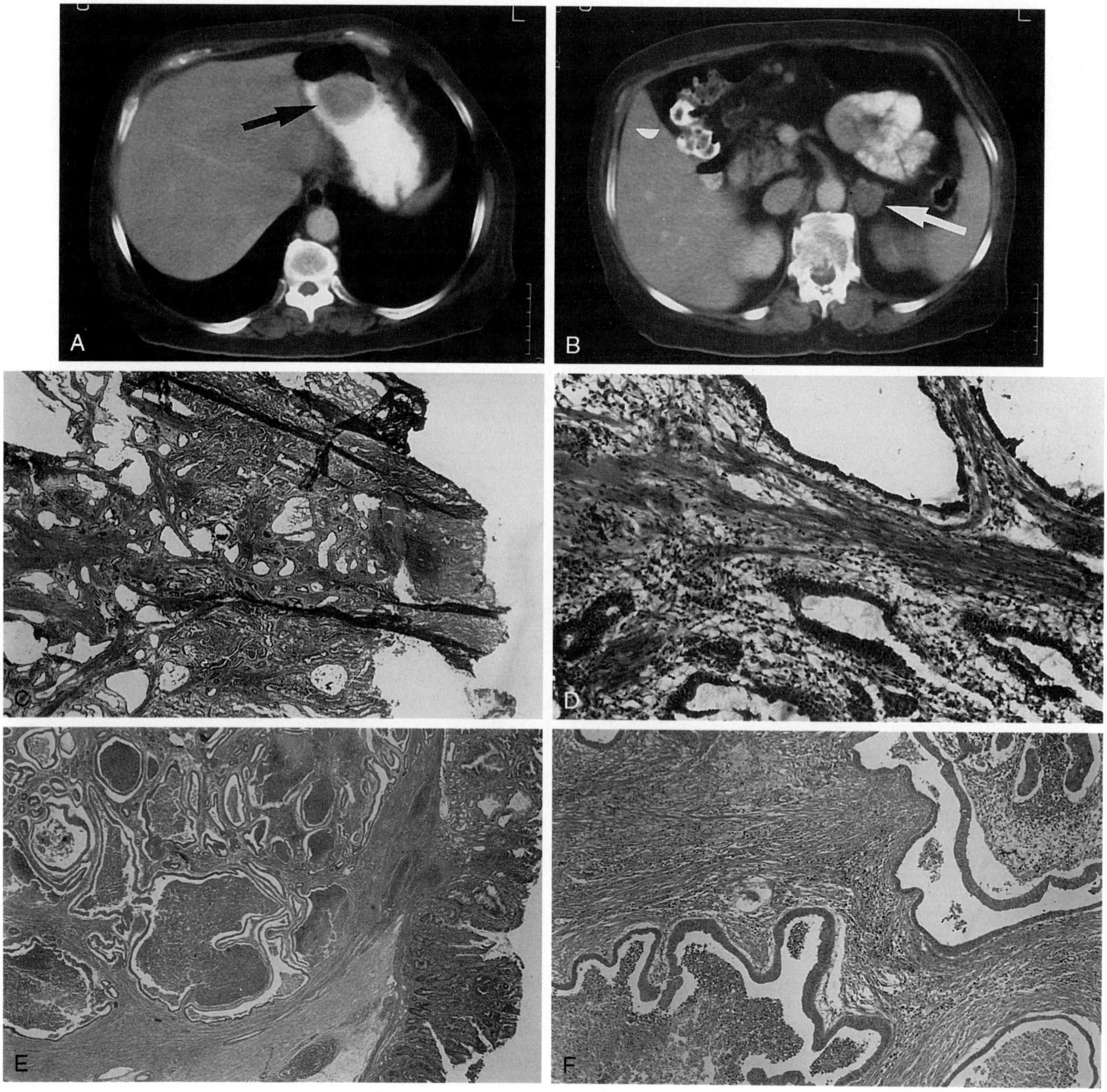

Figure 1–7. *A* and *B*, In Case 1–7, computed tomography with both oral and intravenous contrast markers reveals a large soft tissue mass in the stomach *(black arrow in A, superior level)* and an adrenal mass on the left side *(white arrow in B, inferior plane)*.

C and *D*, Frozen section of the gastric mass shows large gland spaces extending into and massively expanding submucosa *(C, low magnification)*. Intermediate magnification *(D)* shows well-differentiated epithelium lining the gland spaces. This process was interpreted as a "well-differentiated adenocarcinoma."

E and *F*, Permanent sections provide better detail than frozen sections; however, the features are similar. *E* shows intact mucosa at low magnification *(right side of field)* overlying a profusion of complex and dilated glands. At intermediate magnification *(F)*, the expanses of smooth muscle and fibrous tissue separating glands can be appreciated. These features led an expert pathology consultant to interpret the process as an adenomyoma, a rare mimicker of gastric carcinoma.

into submucosa associated with fibrosis. This was interpreted as a "well-differentiated adenocarcinoma." Because it extended to within 0.8 cm of the proximal line of resection, 2.5 cm of additional proximal stomach was submitted; this was grossly and microscopically free of tumor.

SURGEON'S ACTIONS. Prompted by the intraoperative diagnosis of gastric adenocarcinoma, the surgeon then resected the left adrenal. It weighed 33 g and, on cut section, a bright yellow cortical nodule measuring 2.2 × 2.0 × 2.0 cm was found.

PATHOLOGIST'S ACTIONS. After the gastrectomy specimen was fixed in formalin overnight, numerous tissue blocks were submitted to demonstrate the tumor and associated gastric wall.

Microscopic examination of the gastric tumor showed features unusual for carcinoma (Figs. 1–7*E* and *F*). The large glands in the submucosa were extremely well differentiated and were surrounded by a proliferation of bland fibrous tissue and smooth muscle. All pathologists in the department reviewed the case but no consensus was reached.

Gastric planes of resection and lymph nodes were all free of tumor. The adrenal tumor was an adenoma, composed of essentially normal-appearing cortical cellularity.

The surgeon was told that there was no evidence of metastatic disease and that resection margins were adequate, but that the tumor was exceptionally well differentiated. A report was issued indicating the "indeterminate" nature of the tumor, with a notation that consultative assistance was being sought. Six days later, a telephone call was received, soon followed by a telefacsimile report, from a gastrointestinal pathology specialist, who interpreted the lesion as "gastric adenomyoma with low-grade dysplasia of epithelium."

OUTCOME. The patient did well over the ensuing 3 years, with only the expected postgastrectomy restrictions in eating habits.

COMMENTS. Occasional cases are virtually impossible to diagnose preoperatively and intraoperatively. Adenomyomas of the stomach are rare and usually occur in the pylorus rather than the fundus. If the nature of this tumor had been known, a less extensive partial gastrectomy would have been indicated. But, even in retrospect, preoperative identification of the tumor as an adenomyoma was impossible. Endoscopic biopsies are of little value in these tumors because of their size and superficiality. Even permanent sections of the resected specimen initially proved problematic for the departmental pathologists.

Likewise, the adrenal mass was suspected to represent metastatic disease preoperatively. Fine needle aspiration biopsies would have shown normal-appearing adrenal cortex (deriving from the adenoma). Sampling adequacy would have been considered questionable, and metastatic tumor could not have been excluded. Of course, in isolation, without the associated gastric tumor, such a small, nonfunctioning "incidentaloma" would not be an indication for surgery (Chap. 9).

This case illustrates that rare and unlikely biologic events will sometimes necessitate radical surgical intervention. Ultimately, this patient was well served by undergoing a "cancer operation" even though no cancer was actually present.

Case 1–8. Popliteal Soft Tissue Sarcoma Clinically Misinterpreted as "Baker's Cyst"

HISTORY. A 57-year-old man developed progressive pain in the back of his right knee beginning 4 months prior to evaluation. Examination revealed tenderness and expansion of the right popliteal soft tissue compartment. Surgical intervention was delayed for a month by an episode of deep vein thrombosis in the right (ipsilateral) calf, which required anticoagulant therapy.

SURGEON'S ACTIONS. The preoperative clinical impression was popliteal synovial cyst; no radiologic imaging studies were performed prior to surgery. An incisional exposure was carried out; by verbal report only, the popliteal nerve was observed in this procedure. No cystic lesion was identified; instead, abnormal soft tissue was encountered and was sampled and submitted in formalin to pathology.

PATHOLOGIST'S ACTIONS. Permanent sections revealed a pleomorphic spindle-cell malignancy with numerous mitotic figures (Fig. 1–8*A*). A diagnosis of grade 2 malignant fibrous histiocytoma was rendered.

SURGEON'S ACTIONS. The patient was referred to a surgical specialist experienced with soft tissue tumors. Radiologic imaging studies were done (Fig. 1–8*B*). However, because of the recent open biopsy, it was unclear whether tumor infiltrated the neuromuscular bundle or whether hemorrhage and edema only gave the appearance of "invasion." Thorough evaluation for metastatic disease proved negative. The choice of limb-sparing surgery versus amputation was explained to the patient, including the fact that chances for a limb-sparing approach were suboptimal because of possible tumorous involvement of the neurovascular bundle. On the basis of this negative admonition, the patient opted for amputation and an above-the-knee procedure was done. Intraoperative pathology consultation indicated adequate margins of resection.

PATHOLOGIST'S ACTIONS. Gross examination of sequential cross sections of the specimen revealed a circumscribed 6-cm tumor with zones of hemorrhage and edema (Fig. 1–8*C*). The tumor was unattached to bone but was adherent to adventitial tissues of the neurovascular bundle.

OUTCOME. The patient is alive without evidence of disease 5 years after amputation.

COMMENT. Although this patient has done well, with apparent surgical cure of a soft tissue sarcoma, it is possible that a limb-sparing procedure would have offered a similar outcome had the surgeon initially considered neoplasm rather than only synovial cyst. Prebiopsy imaging studies would have demonstrated the status of the neurovascular bundle. After incisional biopsy, which exposed the neurovascular bundle, imaging studies could no longer resolve this issue owing to the resulting hemorrhage and edema. Furthermore, previous surgical exposure would represent a significant risk for tumorous contamination of planes of resection.

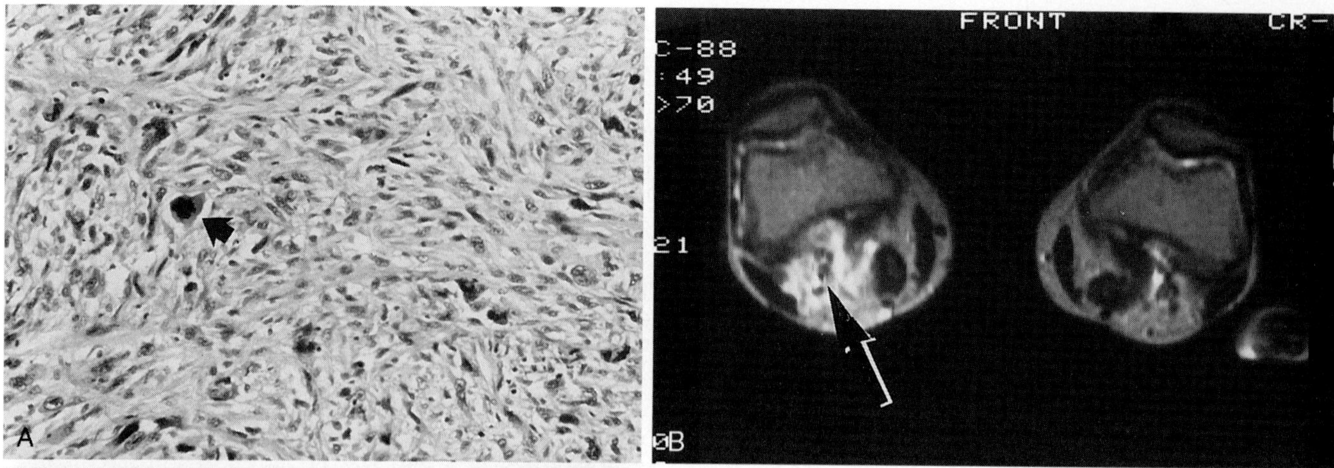

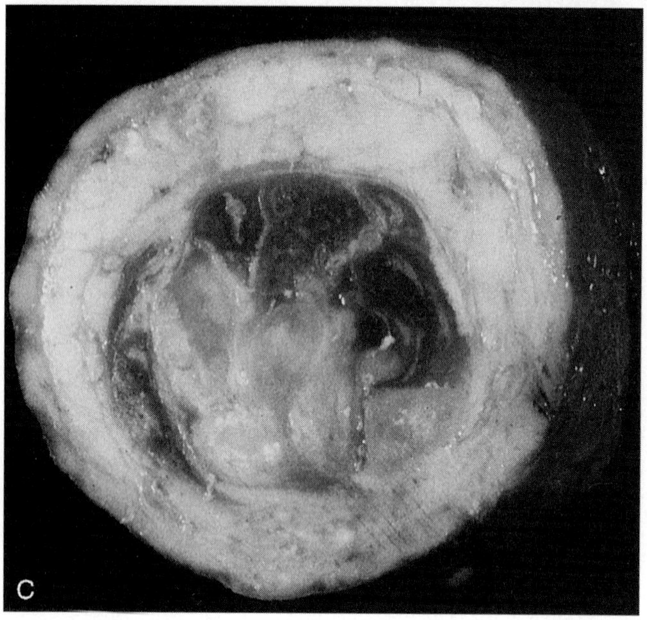

Figure 1–8. *A,* Incisional biopsy of a popliteal mass reveals a pleomorphic spindling sarcoma (malignant fibrous histiocytoma, from Case 1–8). This high-magnification microscopic field shows a mitotic figure in a bizarre large cell *(arrow).*

B, Imaging study from Case 1–8 reveals an ill-defined area of increased signal intensity in the right popliteal space, which surrounds blood vessels *(dark spots, arrow).* This MRI study was performed about 1 week after incisional biopsy, so that the effects of hemorrhage and edema cannot be distinguished from the neoplasm itself.

C, Gross section of soft tissue tumor shows a surprisingly sharply circumscribed mass with areas of hemorrhage *(dark zones).* Tumor was adherent to but not invading the neurovascular bundle.

Because soft tissue tumors are rare, they are often omitted from the initial differential diagnosis (see Chap. 18).

Case 1–9. Low-Grade Liposarcoma Evaluated for Muscle Group Resection

HISTORY. Nontender gradual enlargement of the right thigh had been noticed over the preceding several months by a 58-year-old man. On examination, a bulky, soft mass was identified in the medial-posterior region. Magnetic resonance imaging (MRI) studies revealed a sharply delimited mass of fatty density within the adductor muscle group measuring 21 × 12 × 8 cm (Figs. 1–9*A* and *B*).

SURGEON'S ACTIONS. The patient's private general surgeon performed a small incisional biopsy along the posterior aspect of the tumor, avoiding the anterior-medial neurovascular bundle.

PATHOLOGIST'S ACTIONS. Permanent section microscopy revealed mature-appearing adipose tissue with slight variation in nuclear size of the adipocytes. Partly because of the size and depth of the tumor, the diagnosis of low-grade liposarcoma was reached.

SURGEON'S ACTIONS. The surgeon referred the patient to a specialist in soft tissue tumor surgery, who asked pathologists at the referral center to review the biopsy slides. After considerable discussion and review of the slides, the pathologists interpreted the biopsy as "most consistent with infiltrating (intramuscular) lipoma." Because radiologic review of the MRI studies revealed a zone of varying density, a repeat incisional biopsy was performed at the posterior aspect of the lesion distal to the earlier biopsy site. Permanent section pathology interpretation was again "intramuscular lipoma." Discussion of the case with the pathologist focused on the difficulty of distinguishing histologically between well-differentiated liposarcoma and infiltrating lipoma.

Because of the size and sharp delineation of the tumor, the adductor muscle group was resected in continuity with both previous cutaneous biopsy tracts.

PATHOLOGIST'S ACTIONS. Examination of the resected specimen revealed no evidence of fatty tumor extending to any surgical plane. Successive fresh cross sections con-

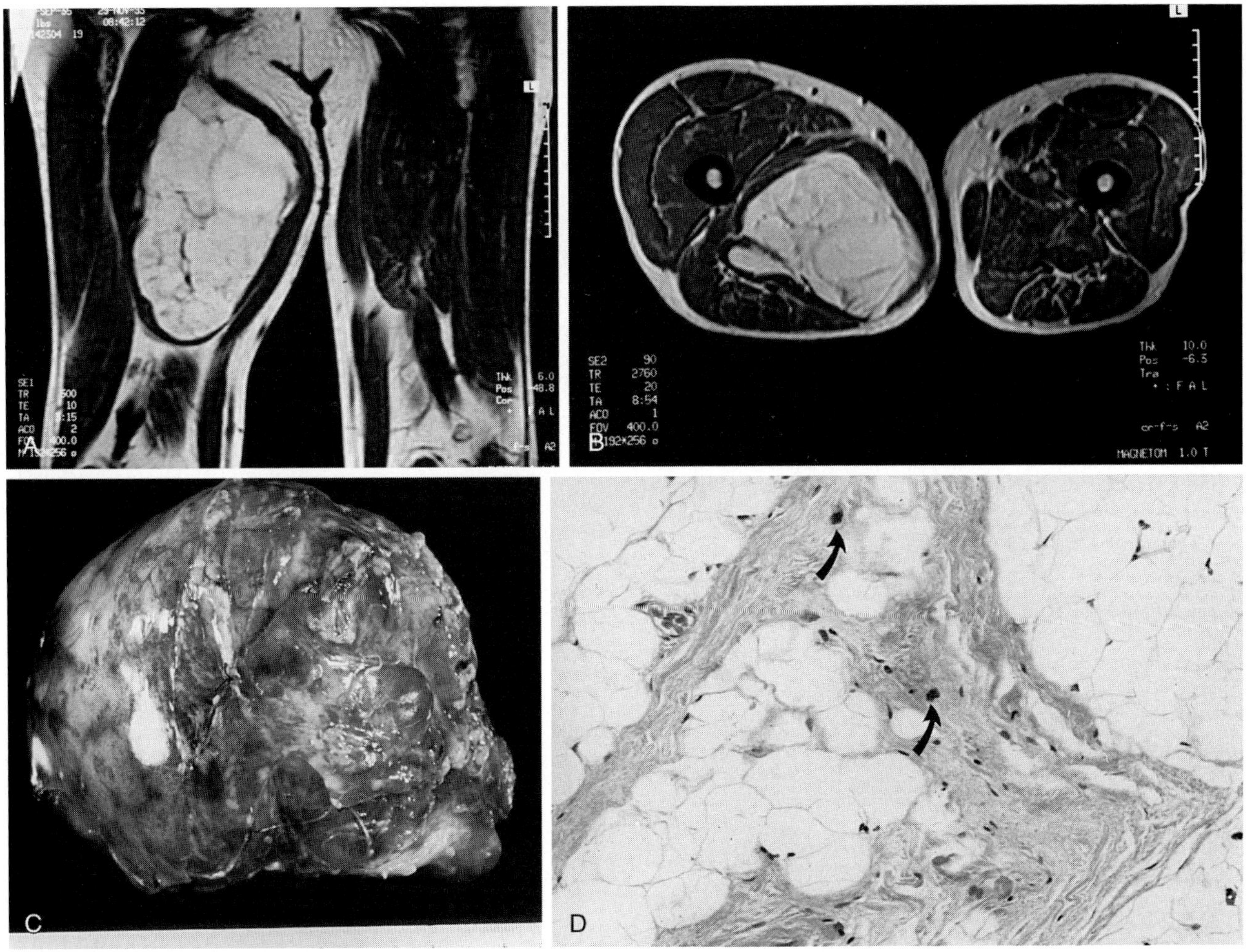

Figure 1–9. *A* and *B,* Magnetic resonance imaging studies of Case 1–9 reveal a large, well-demarcated tumor identical in density to subcutaneous fat. This distends surrounding muscles of the adductor group *(A, coronal plane; B, transverse plane).*

C, Resected specimen shows glistening surface of muscular fascia with adherent fatty tissues. No tumor could be identified, grossly or microscopically, extending to the plane of resection.

D, Microscopic features of the fatty tumor are intermediate between benign (infiltrating) lipoma and well-differentiated liposarcoma. Rare cells resembling lipoblasts were identified in more cellular regions *(arrows).* This finding, together with the tumor's size and history of recent growth, was incorporated into the final diagnosis of a low-grade liposarcoma *(high magnification).*

firmed a rim of benign muscle and/or fascia along all surfaces (Fig. 1–9*C*). The surgeon was informed that margins appeared adequate and that frozen sections were not needed. (At this juncture, it is appropriate to point out that fatty tissue is virtually impossible to freeze, so that frozen section monitoring of such processes should not be expected.) On permanent section, the tumor consisted of well-differentiated adipose tissue. However, in some areas, cellularity was increased and occasional atypical lipocytes, some resembling lipoblasts, were identified (Fig. 1–9*D*). A diagnosis of low-grade liposarcoma was rendered.

OUTCOME. The patient received short-term physical therapy and tolerated the loss of unilateral adductor function well. At 6 months there was no evidence of tumor recurrence.

COMMENTS. Even though the initial biopsy was performed by a non-specialized surgeon, preprocedure imaging studies and a proper surgical approach away from neurovascular compartments permitted subsequent resection with minimal functional or anatomic loss. In a few situations, histologic features are not independent predictors of tumor behavior. This was thoroughly discussed by the referral center's surgeon and pathologists. Because so-called intramuscular lipomas and low-grade liposarcomas have similar biologic potential,[13] the surgeon planned a procedure appropriate for either diagnosis. Careful gross examination of the specimen was the only intraoperative information the pathologist could offer, since fatty tissue resists frozen section evaluation. The final diagnosis of (low-grade) malignancy presented no problem, since this possibility had been anticipated and surgical management was appropriate.

Recommendations for Practice

It is, of course, impossible to anticipate every clinical situation that will be encountered by the surgeon-pathologist team; however, the following general guidelines offer ways to avoid mishaps.

Know the Patient

Even when a patient is a referral case and has been evaluated by another physician, independent chart review, patient interview and examination, and incorporation of radiologic and laboratory data are crucial in the independent assessment for surgical management.

Know the Pathology

An understanding of each anatomic or functional organ system's susceptibility to disease allows the surgeon to predict accurately which diseases are more likely to be encountered. Such an understanding lends insights into adequate tissue sampling for pathologic diagnosis and has implications for the ideal surgical approach.

Create a Differential Diagnosis

By developing a differential diagnosis on each case, the surgeon avoids an incomplete evaluation. In more complex cases, a written differential diagnosis assists the surgeon in analyzing, reformulating, and considering likely diagnostic possibilities.

Preoperative Communication with the Pathologist

The surgeon should alert the pathologist when a particular case is likely to be challenging, when special questions are anticipated, and when there are previous, relevant pathologic specimens (Fig. 1–10). Therapeutic decisions should never rest on pathology reports from outside institutions. To perform surgery based on such information is equivalent to extending hospital privileges to pathologists in other hospitals. Furthermore, if the previous pathology materials are available for comparison, they may be valuable to the pathologist for interpreting current samplings (even intraoperative frozen sections). By enlisting preoperative consultation from the pathologist, the surgeon assures informed involvement intraoperatively and postoperatively.

It is sometimes appropriate to discuss an anticipated surgical case with the pathologist even when no previous pathology interpretation exists. For instance, if the surgeon has doubts about the type of sample that is ideal for documenting a particular disease process, a preoperative discussion with the pathologist is useful. A "detailed" conversation with the pathologist is necessary if a patient's circumstances (bleeding disorders and so on) will limit the sampling technique.

Intraoperative Communication with the Pathologist

Intraoperative decision making requires a clear line of communication between the surgeon and the pathologist and may affect the overall success of the surgical procedure (see Fig. 1–10). Widespread confusion exists about the distinction between communication, consultation, and diagnosis in the team's interactions. Communication with and consultation from the pathologist should be maximized during a complex case. If unexpected appearances of tissues or organs are described to the pathologist (over the telephone or intercom), this may elicit some useful differential diagnostic insights. Likewise, careful descriptions of operative findings and labeling of numerous operative specimens safeguard pathologic interpretation of such specimens. On the other hand, requesting a specimen interpretation (diagnosis) intraoperatively is justified only when there is potential impact on operative decision making or when appropriate tissue allocation can be secured by such means. Intraoperative diagnoses should not be requested simply to satisfy the surgeon's curiosity. Tissue that has been used for frozen sections suffers severe morphologic artifact (see Cases 1–2, 1–3, and 1–5). In a case with limited tissue sampling, such as in nonpalpable, mammographically detected breast cancer, accurate final diagnosis can be jeopardized by insistence on a frozen section interpretation.[11]

Good examples of intraoperative communication with the pathologist include demonstration of the specimen in situ in the operating room for orientation and allocation of fresh tissue specimens for fastidious special study techniques (see Chap. 2). Good reasons for requesting intraoperative diagnosis include decision making regarding radical resections (benign versus malignant neoplasm), assessment of adequacy of resection margins, and assessment of adequacy of biopsy sampling for final diagnostic purposes.

It is essential that communication between surgeon and pathologist be unencumbered during the operation. If either has questions, these should be expressed during (not after) the operation. For example, if the pathologist is unsure of the anatomic source of a particular biopsy or the orientation of a resection specimen, the confusion should be resolved then and there. Correspondingly, if the pathologist's intraoperative interpretation seems complex or ambiguous to the surgeon, the surgeon should ask for clarification. It is the pathologist's responsibility to render straightforward, succinct intraoperative interpretations that leave no doubt as to whether a definitive diagnosis has been rendered or whether it has been deferred.

Postoperative Communication with the Pathologist

There are three overlapping stages in the postoperative period that may call for interaction between surgeon and pathologist: immediately after surgery, before the case has been signed out, and after the case has been signed out (see Fig. 1–10).

In the immediate postoperative stage, unexpected intraoperative findings should be communicated to the pathologist as soon as possible. This may allow special handling of the tissues for some special study purposes before they are irretrievably lost. If gross photographs are desired, this must be requested before the specimen is dissected. The pathologist should contact the surgeon directly if specimen identification or orientation is unclear.

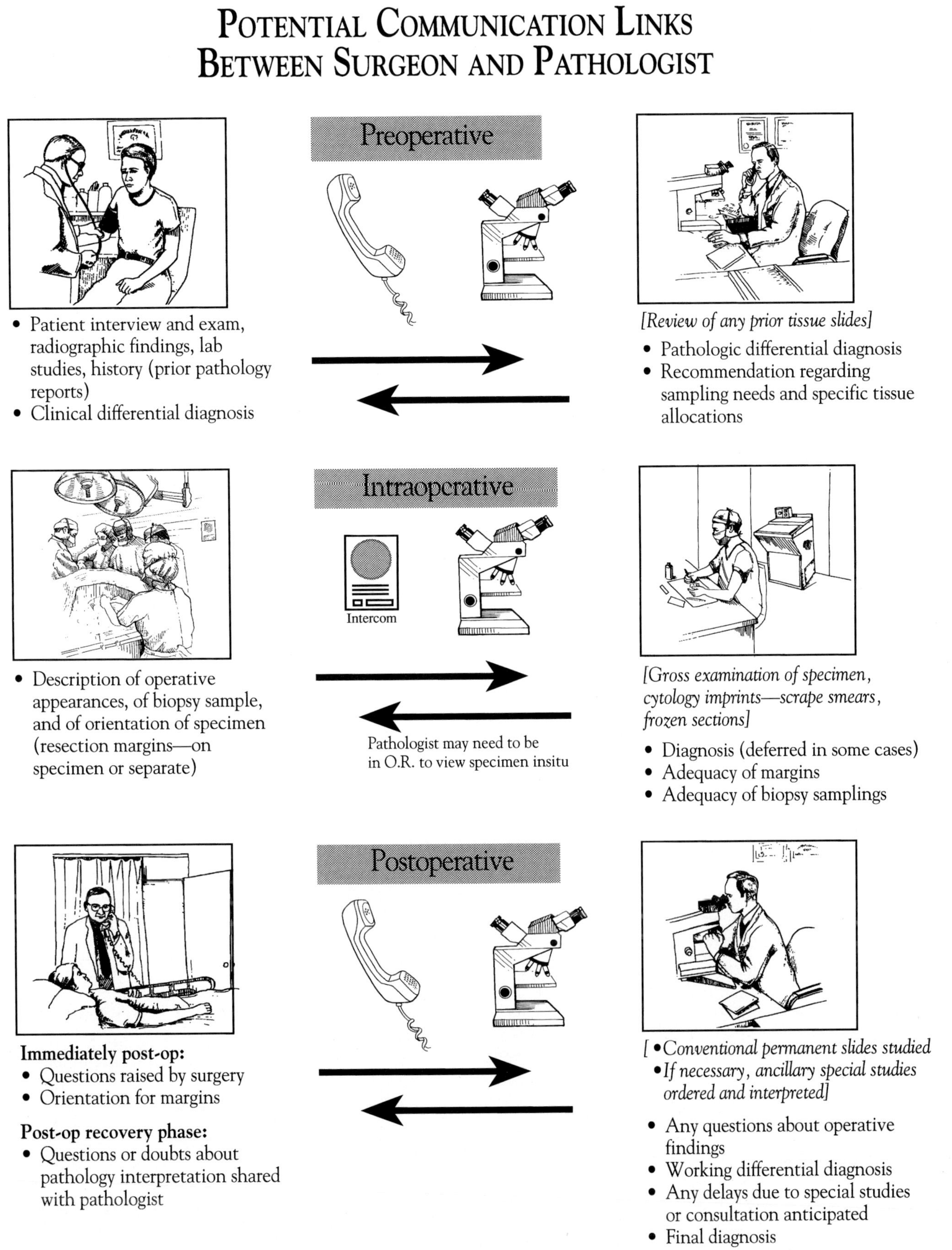

Figure 1–10. Diagrammatic representation of potential communication opportunities between surgeon and pathologist at the three stops of patient management: pre-, intra-, and postoperative.

In the stage before final sign-out, both surgeon and pathologist should feel free to contact one another if questions arise. For example, the surgeon may want to share concerns about the appearance and texture of the liver in a patient who has undergone cholecystectomy and in whom needle and wedge biopsies were performed for this reason, despite the lack of preoperative clinical history suggesting cirrhosis. Additionally, this time period is an opportunity for the surgeon to update the pathologist about changes in the patient's clinical condition that may have a bearing upon the nature of the disease process. When the surgeon goes to the trouble of informing the pathologist about such special concerns, it generates greater interest and enthusiasm toward the case on the part of the pathologist. It is an unusual pathologist who would not welcome clinical information in the interpretative approach to any particular case. Likewise, when the initial microscopic review reveals features unexpected on the basis of the original preoperative differential diagnosis, the pathologist should contact the surgeon before rendering such a final diagnosis. For example, in a uterine or colonic resection specimen, if a segment of what appears to be ureter is identified, it would be important to ''compare notes'' with the surgeon before sending out a final written diagnosis. If a case requires time-consuming special studies that will delay the final diagnosis for several days, the surgeon should be forewarned of this.

If final diagnoses raise doubts or create confusion, the surgeon should not hesitate to contact the pathologist directly. Often, other pathologists will be recruited into the effort on a particularly difficult or controversial case. Occasionally, extramural consultations from subspecialty experts are required to resolve a case. Referral of cases to such specialists does not imply incompetence on the part of the pathologist. Even renowned experts at the most prestigious medical centers encounter cases that are diagnostically problematic, and they must seek the opinions of other renowned experts! It is far better to raise questions about a diagnosis than to withhold comment and risk persisting error.

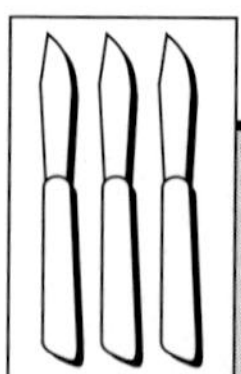

PITFALLS FOR THE SURGEON

1. Operating without sufficient information from pathology.
2. Failure to supply the pathologist with adequate information for accurate pre-, intra-, or postoperative diagnosis.
3. Inadequate operative sampling to allow a definitive diagnosis—e.g., no intraoperative pathology monitoring of biopsy samples from a large, open procedure.
4. Insisting on intraoperative frozen sections when they are contraindicated—e.g., early, small breast lesions of less than 1 cm.
5. Failure to orient a specimen clearly for the pathologist.

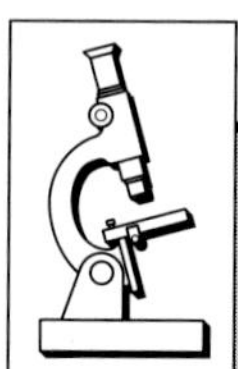

PITFALLS FOR THE PATHOLOGIST

1. Rendering a diagnosis with insufficient clinical information.
2. Failure to inform the surgeon intraoperatively that sampling is or may be inadequate to allow definitive diagnosis.
3. Failure to provide a direct, comprehensible intraoperative consultation in response to the surgeon's needs.
4. Failure to share difficult diagnostic cases with other pathologists, intramural or extramural.
5. Accepting a specimen that has been inadequately oriented anatomically.

FURTHER READING

Nochomovitz L, Sidawy M, Silverberg S, et al. *Intraoperative Consultation.* Chicago: ASCP Press; 1989.

Oneson RH, Minke JA, Silverberg SG. Intraoperative pathologic consultation: An audit of 1,000 recent consecutive cases. *Am J Surg Pathol.* 1989;13:237–243.

Rosai J, Ackerman LV. The pathology of tumors (in four parts). *CA* 28:331–342, 1978; *CA.* 29:22–39, 66–77, 130–143, 1979.

Silva EG, Kraemer BB. *Intraoperative Pathologic Diagnosis.* Baltimore: Williams & Wilkins; 1987.

REFERENCES

1. Shenoy BV, Scheithauer BW. Paget's perspectives in pathology. *Mayo Clin Proc.* 1988;63:184–192.
2. Wright JR. The development of frozen section technique, the evolution of surgical biopsy, and the origins of surgical pathology. *Bull Hist Med.* 1985;59:295–326.
3. Cullen TS. A rapid method of making permanent specimens from frozen sections by the use of formalin. *Johns Hopkins Hosp Bull.* 1895:67.
4. Bloodgood JC. The clinical and pathological differential diagnosis of diseases of the female breast. *Am J Med Sci.* 1908;135:157–168.

5. Clapesaddle H. The surgeons' club. In: *The Doctors Mayo.* New York: Simon & Schuster; 1941:295.
6. MacCarty WC, Broders AC. Studies in clinico-pathologic standardization and efficiency: I. Legitimate actual error in diagnosis of mammary conditions. *Surg Gynecol Obstet.* 1917;25:666–673.
7. Bloodgood JC. When cancer becomes a microscopic disease, there must be tissue diagnosis in the operating room. *JAMA.* 1927;88:1022–1023.
8. American College of Surgeons. *Thirteenth Yearbook.* Chicago: American College of Surgeons; 1926:33–46.
9. Committee on the Treatment of Malignant Diseases (American College of Surgeons). Organization of service for the diagnosis and treatment of cancer. *Surg Gynecol Obstet.* 1930;51:570–574.
10. Azar HA. Arthur Purdy Stout (1885–1967). The man and the surgical pathologist. *Am J Surg Pathol.* 1984;8:301–307.
11. Fechner R. Immediate management of mammographically detected breast lesions. *Am J Clin Pathol.* 1993;100:92–93.
12. McDivitt RW, Stewart FW, Berg JW. Benign breast lesions—sclerosing adenosis. In: *Atlas of Tumor Pathology.* Second series. Fascicle 2. *Tumors of the Breast.* Washington, DC: Armed Forces Institute of Pathology; 1968:113.
13. Evans HL, Soule EH, Winkelmann RK. Atypical lipoma, atypical intramuscular lipoma, and well differentiated retroperitoneal liposarcoma: A reappraisal of 30 cases formerly classified as well differentiated liposarcoma. *Cancer.* 1979;43:574–584.

2

Special Techniques in Surgical Pathology

Mark R. Wick

Definition

The definition of a ''special'' procedure in surgical pathology is, of course, relative to the practice patterns of the laboratory and the surgeons in any given hospital. However, there are certainly many more ''menu choices'' provided by current technology than one might have encountered even 10 years ago, and the details of new assays represent complicated information for both clinicians and pathologists.

This chapter is devoted to an overview of those adjunctive techniques that can be applied to human biopsy specimens and resected tissues for the purposes of securing more definitive diagnostic information or providing data of prognostic import. Inherent in this discussion is a consideration of whether or not such procedures should or must be performed as well as elaboration and illustration of how they can be done.

Historical Perspectives

The advent and rapid progress of technology in surgical pathology are placed in proper perspective by a brief review of the history of this subspecialty. Up until a century ago, pathologists confined their activities and attention to studying the changes caused by disease as seen at the autopsy table. Accordingly, *surgical* pathology was considered to be a contradiction in terms![1]

This situation stemmed largely from the opinions of prominent surgeons and their feelings that even the need to use a microscope was the mark of an inferior macroscopic diagnostician. In particular, Bloodgood—a pioneering breast surgeon—committed his unequivocally negative impressions of pathology to print in the early part of this century. In 1908, he wrote:

> *For the last three years I have made immediate frozen sections of fresh tissue received in the pathology laboratory, but up to the present time a stained frozen section has never been of aid in making the diagnosis when we have been unable to come to a conclusion from the fresh appearance of the tissue, nor, up to the present time, have I ever depended upon a frozen section to influence the operative procedure.*[2]

An unfortunate and widely publicized single case incident from 20 years previous may well have contributed to this negativism. It concerned Kaiser Frederick III, the ruler of Germany, who had developed symptoms and signs of a laryngeal tumor in the mid-1880s. Sir Morell Mackenzie, an eminent British surgeon, was engaged to consult in the case; he subsequently obtained biopsies of a laryngeal mass that were sent for histologic examination.[3] Despite the fact that Professor Rudolph Virchow of Berlin was widely regarded as the ''father'' of cellular pathology and a giant in his field, his experience was nil in ''surgical'' pathology. However, in deference to his national fame, he was asked to provide the diagnosis of the Kaiser's lesion.[4] Predictably, the tumor was misinterpreted as benign; there then followed a rapidly fatal progression of manifest laryngeal carcinoma. As a consequence of this notorious mishap, the ''biopsy''—from the Greek *bios* (living tissue) and *opsis* (appearance)—was, thereafter, generally considered by Europeans to be an inherently unreliable method of diagnosis.

Fortunately, these skeptical stances on the ''special'' techniques of frozen section and microscopic examination were countered strongly by the announced experiences of the surgeons and pathologists of the Mayo Clinic, where, as early as 1905, histopathology had become firmly entrenched as a diagnostic procedure.[5] Subsequent studies based on cumulative patient outcome and the interpretations of experienced observers provided irrefutable evidence as to the merit of histopathologic diagnosis; even Bloodgood, in his later years, underwent ''conversion'' to become a proponent of the method[1] (see Chap. 1).

In the first half of the 20th century, the technology inherent in tissue fixation, embedding procedures, microscopic discrimination, and staining methods progressed steadily. Knowledge of biochemistry was first applied in histopathology to produce histochemical techniques that provided insights into the chemical composition of the microscopic subject of study. Such now familiar stains as the periodic acid–Schiff procedure to detect sugar residues; the Masson trichrome technique for differential labeling of various mesenchymal tissues; the Rio de Ortega, Cajal, and Bodian silver stains for neural fiber impregnation; and similar methods for recognition of matrix materials and microorganisms were added to the pathologist's armamentarium.[6] Immunostaining was initiated in 1941 by Coons et al., with the application of fluoresceinated antibodies as diagnostic reagents.[7] However, only with the development of enzyme-driven techniques (i.e., immunohistochemistry) in the 1970s and the availability of highly specific monoclonal antibodies in the 1980s was this method to gain its modern foothold in diagnostics. Practical electron microscopes were generally made available for the recognition of subcellular elements in human tissues in the late 1960s.[8]

With the discovery of nucleic acids—deoxyribonucleic acid (DNA) and ribonucleic acid (RNA)—and their role in biology in the early 1950s,[9] the stage was set for the present ''revolution'' in molecular diagnosis. Our current ability to recreate DNA and RNA sequences synthetically and to label them with chromogenic or radioactive compounds has yielded the new diagnostic discipline of in situ hybridization.[10] Fragments of ''unknown'' nucleic acids can be compared in electrophoretic gels with previously characterized marker fragments in order to size and identify them in the ''Southern'' and ''Northern'' blot procedures.[11] ''Primer'' nucleic acid pieces and nucleotide ''building blocks'' can be exposed to nucleic acid polymerases in the polymerase chain reaction (PCR) to amplify a sequence of interest so powerfully that only a minuscule cellular sample is needed.[12]

These many methods give modern pathologists the ability to probe human diseases for more and more sophisticated information. We are presently engaged in a frenetic attempt to place these new data in proper order and to use them sensibly in the diagnosis and management of clinical disorders. However, such developments also carry the obligation for physicians to be thoroughly educated as to which facts and observations are independently important and worthy of pursuit and which, instead, constitute superfluous esoterica. The purpose of this chapter is to provide the surgeon with useful insights into how modern pathology may best contribute to the care of his or her patients and how pitfalls may be avoided that would preclude the use of current laboratory techniques.

What Is a "Good" Test in Surgical Pathology?

The foregoing material serves, then, to introduce a question that is extremely pertinent to this discussion; that is, what constitutes a ''good'' test in surgical pathology? As one might expect, there is no simple answer to this query. Instead, attention must be paid to the context in which a test is used, what its statistical performance is in that specific setting, which alternative assays are available, how long the procedure will take, and how much the evaluation will cost. In some contexts, even a slow, expensive laboratory technique may be preferable to its principal alternative. For example, the PCR can be used to evaluate the presence of cellular monotypism (monoclonality) for light chain immunoglobulins or T-cell receptor genes in extremely small samples of lymphoid proliferations[13]; in the correct clinical and histologic setting, this effectively equates with the presence of malignancy. This assay—which is expensive and requires sophisticated equipment to perform—would, however, certainly be preferred over procurement of additional surgical biopsies in the event that the brain were the site of the lesion! However, in other anatomic sites, a repeated biopsy may indeed be the least expensive and the most expeditious course of action.

If a test is to be used to provide a simple yes-or-no answer, the main considerations can be reduced to those of sensitivity and specificity.[14] Nevertheless, extensive data must be obtained through formal clinical studies (usually of at least several hundred cases) in order to ensure validity. This caveat has more than passing importance, because the clinical medical literature is sullied with anecdotal reports that make vastly exaggerated claims of significance. It would be patently ridiculous to claim that test ''X'' was ready for large-scale clinical application—even in the event that it appeared to show perfect discrimination—if this decision were based on a preliminary assessment of only 50 cases.

Another category of specialized testing—that relating to ''prognostic'' markers in neoplasia—is a much more complicated one to analyze. Here, one is not seeking a simple dichotomous result in doing the assay. Instead, such assessments have been proposed to produce probability-associated strata that relate to relative prognosis. Several admonitions must be heeded in evaluating such tests. First, it is essential that clinical data bases be derived from identical treatment protocols within each study group, which must be composed of patients with similar demographic makeup and similar stage of disease. This is necessary because patient gender, age, extent of disease, and differing therapies all have the potential to significantly affect outcome, and each of these variables may have an independent impact. Here again, the medical literature has not, in aggregate, adhered to these principles, and the resulting abundance of disparate publications has been misleading and confusing.

These comments make it evident that all physicians must acquire the ability to read and digest scientific literature in a discerning fashion. As a cardinal rule, it should be remembered that ''new is not always better, or even necessary.'' Translated into practical terms, the surgeon should not request a particular method of tissue study simply because a recent paper has appeared that recommends it; similarly, the pathologist should not implement new assays in unquestioning deference to the opinions of others. Rather, efforts should be directed at helping to analyze such newly published observations cooperatively, to ascertain whether implementation of the test in question is indeed justified.

Table 2–1. Representative Turnaround Times for Special Procedures in Surgical Pathology

Procedure	Expected Turnaround Time (Range)
Fine needle aspiration	Less than 1 hour to 1 day
Immunohistology	1 to 3 days
In situ hybridization	2 to 14 days
Electron microscopy	3 to 5 days
Polymerase chain reaction	Less than 1 day to 2 days
Flow cytometry	Less than 1 day to 2 days
Cytogenetic analysis	3 to 14 days
Cellular enzymatic analysis	7 to 21 days

Interactions Between Surgeons and Surgical Pathologists: Philosophical Considerations and General Information

It is essential that surgeons and pathologists take time to communicate meaningfully with one another, both inside and outside the operating room (see Chap. 1). Indeed, both of these locales have essential importance in the development of a good interactive working relationship. In particular, a surgeon will seldom decide to request a special procedure while in the middle of a surgical procedure, although the pathologist will certainly be asked to help with other important judgments of a more immediate nature in that setting. Adjunctive pathologic studies are usually selected after initial examination of a diagnostically difficult pathologic specimen has occurred, or, alternatively, it may be obvious that such studies are necessary (based on clinical data) before the patient is ever taken to the operating theater. In this context, the to-and-fro interchange of information between pathologist and surgeon cannot be stressed too strongly. Under optimal circumstances, each party knows the other well enough, both professionally and personally, that the conjoint goal of excellence in patient care needs no verbalization and needed communication will proceed in an unimpeded way.

An important aspect of this interchange is the development of a reasonable timeline over which test results will be expected. Whereas some adjunctive special tests can be done rapidly, others may require up to several weeks for results to be available. Examples of the latter include Southern blot molecular probe techniques for the establishment of lymphoid clonality and certain microbial culture methods. It is certainly understandable that patients, their families, and attending physicians will become anxious for definitive answers in challenging cases. Nonetheless, if realistic expectations are initially engendered, based on established turnaround times that can be guaranteed by the laboratory, emotional stress can usually be reduced or avoided. To assist with such matters, representative time requirements for several special laboratory studies are provided in Table 2–1.

Another critical issue concerns anticipating the need for special tissue allocations for the performance of certain ancillary pathologic studies. Unfortunately, even today, many tissues are inappropriately submitted in formalin, having been placed routinely (by habit) in this fixative by a surgeon who is unacquainted with the fastidious requirements of some special analyses. Many technical advances over the past decade have been pursued specifically to allow pathologists to perform an ever-wider array of tests on such ''routine'' specimens, but there are still exceptions. For example, selected immunohistologic procedures for the diagnosis of malignant lymphoma still require submission of fresh tissue.[15] In addition, the ability to perform cytogenetic analyses not only mandates receipt of unfixed specimens, but also these should be kept sterile and placed in specific nutrient media that maximize the viability of the excised tissues during transport to the laboratory and preparation for the procedure. This important facet of specimen processing is summarized in Table 2–2, which outlines optimal, acceptable, and contraindicated submission protocols for designated adjunctive studies. To reiterate a point made earlier, such information underscores the benefits of open communications between the operating theater and the laboratory before, during, and after any given surgical procedure.

Applications of Special Techniques: Case Studies

Rather than simply cataloguing special studies for surgical pathology—and how they may improve or even hinder patient care—a series of case studies is provided in the following categorical sections. These were chosen in order to make specific points—both pro and con—and are accompanied by brief introductions and commentaries. Obviously, such discussions make no pretense of representing an encyclopedic treatment of the material at hand; rather, they are offered in order to emphasize important concepts.

IMMUNOSTAINING

Immunostaining procedures allow for the immunologic recognition of antigens within the microscopic field. Over the past decade, monoclonal (hybridoma) antibodies have become commercially available as standardized reagents for the recognition of intracellular molecular moieties with

Table 2–2. Recommended Submission Protocols for Specimens Intended for Special Tests in Surgical Pathology

	Protocols		
Procedure	***Best***	***First Alternative***	***Unacceptable***
Fine needle aspiration	Fresh[a]	Air-dried or alcohol-fixed smears[b]	Fixed in solutions other than alcohol
Immunohistology	Fresh	Formalin-fixed or alcohol-fixed[c]	GLUT-fixed
Flow cytometry	Fresh	Formalin-fixed	Fixed in solutions other than formalin
Electron microscopy	GLUT[d,e]	Formalin-fixed	Fresh or fixed in solutions other than GLUT or formalin
Polymerase chain reaction	Fresh	Formalin-fixed	Fixed in solutions other than formalin
In situ hybridization	Fresh	Formalin-fixed	Fixed in solutions other than formalin
Cytogenetic analysis	Fresh and in sterile nutrient medium	None	Any fixative
Cellular enzymatic analysis	Fresh in nutrient medium	None	Any fixative

[a]If pathologist performs procedure.
[b]If clinicians do procedure.
[c]Not suitable for lymphoid tumors.
[d]Tissue must be minced into 1-mm cubes.
[e]GLUT = buffered glutaraldehyde.

enormous clinical utility. These antibodies are numerous and varied and include not only human targets but microbial determinants as well. The binding of these ''primary'' antibodies is detected by using ''secondary'' antibodies with species-specificity for the first (e.g., rabbit primary and mouse antirabbit secondary) that are tagged with a chromogenic enzyme or fluorescent label.[16] Binding of the primary antibody to the tissue (indicating the presence of the antigen in question in the sample) is therefore visualized indirectly with these color markers.

Immunohistochemical procedures have largely supplanted immunofluorescence methods, because the former permit the simultaneous comparison of cellular morphology with antigen distribution in permanent slides with nuclear counterstains; this allows simultaneous evaluation of morphology and of antigen distribution.[17] These procedures are widely employed in surgical pathology and represent perhaps the most diversified of the special procedures in this field. The applications of immunohistology include the differential diagnosis of ''undifferentiated'' malignant tumors (encompassing carcinomas, hematopoietic proliferations, melanomas, and selected sarcomas)[18]; prediction of anatomic origins for metastatic carcinomas[19–22]; determination of cellular lineage for morphologically indeterminate sarcomas[23]; distinction of benign from malignant B-lymphocytic proliferations[15]; assignment of specific lineage for hematopoietic malignancies[24]; and rapid identification of selected infectious agents in human tissues.[25]

Algorithms for the application of immunostains can be devised that depict their utility in logical progression, in the context of the pathologist's differential diagnoses. One of these is exemplified by Figure 2–1. The starting point is determined by the particular microscopic features of the tumors under study; the one illustrated in Figure 2–1 is designed for pleomorphic neoplasms. This is only one of many morphologic starting points. For example, an entirely different differential diagnostic grouping of neoplasms would be included in an algorithm for ''small round-cell tumors'' of childhood. In other words, many diagnostic entities in the latter group would only be included in the ''small-cell tumor algorithm''; likewise, Kaposi's sarcoma would only be included in the ''spindle-cell tumor algorithm,'' and so on. It is a general truism that no single antibody has absolute positive or negative predictive power in diagnostic settings, and these markers are therefore best utilized in groups or panels that are chosen by the pathologist based on the particular details of the case being evaluated.

In some cases, immunostaining requires that fresh tissue be available in order for proper results to be obtained. The best example of the latter applications is that of determining light chain immunoglobulin (LCI) monoclonality in lymphoid lesions. In many types of lymphoid cells, the small amounts of LCI found on the surfaces of B cells are effectively chemically degraded by formalin or other fixatives.[26] Hence, they are no longer detectable immunohistochemically. The practical solution to this problem is obvious. If malignant lymphoma constitutes one of the potential differential diagnoses in any given clinical situation, the surgeon should be certain to alert the pathologist to this fact and to submit biopsy specimens in saline or another transport medium that maintains the integrity of lymphocyte membranes completely. This provision is also necessary for optimal immunodetection of estrogen/progesterone receptors in mammary carcinomas, inasmuch as fixation may mask or otherwise damage these proteins.[26] When maximal preservation of antigens is required, as in these instances, the pathologist freezes the fresh tissues and immunostaining can then be performed on frozen sections, in which antigenic expression remains effectively 100%.

Case 2–1

A 67-year-old woman noted a ''lump'' under her left arm while bathing and consulted her physician because of this abnormality; she was otherwise well with no major past medical problems. Her internist confirmed the pres-

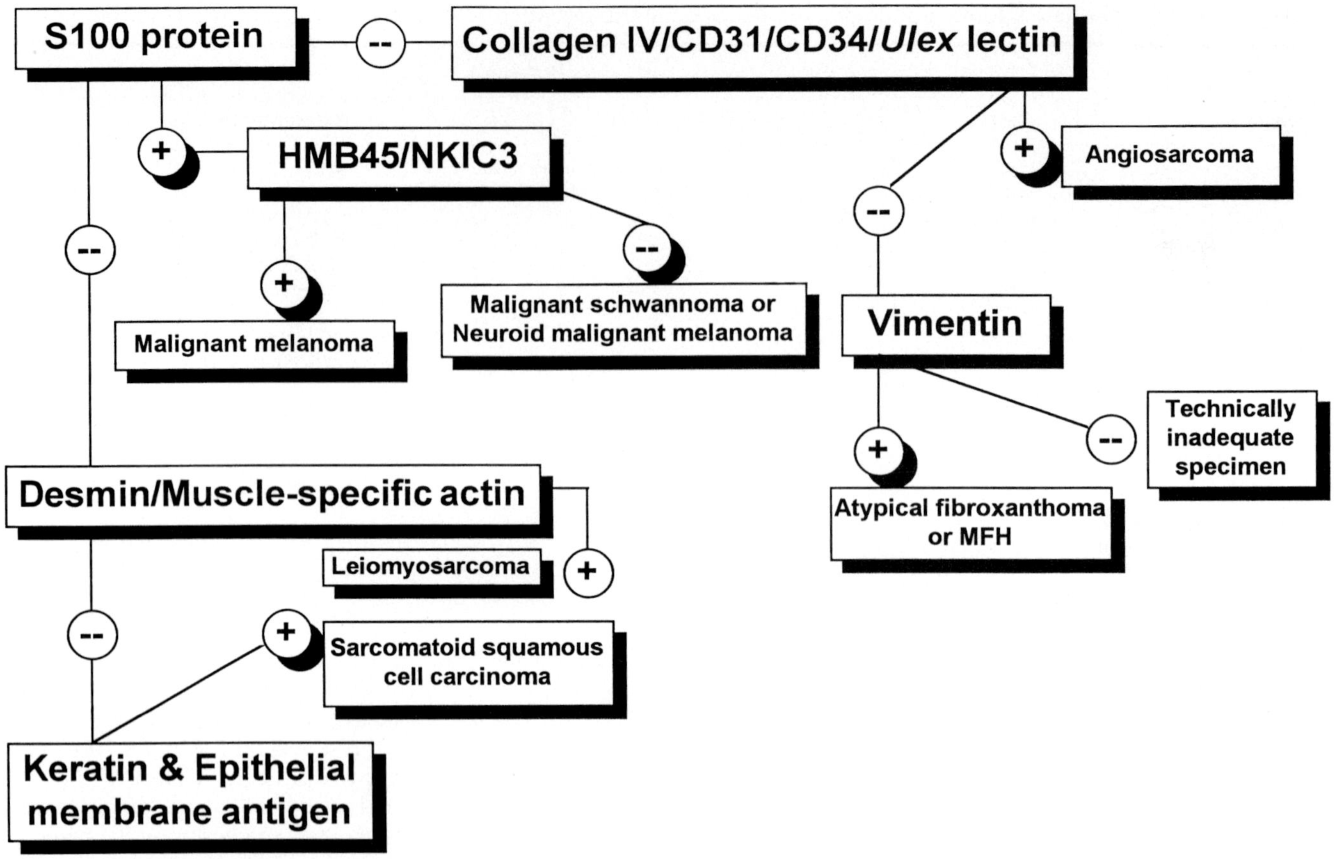

Figure 2–1. Algorithm for immunohistochemical diagnosis of pleomorphic undifferentiated neoplasms.

ence of an enlarged, firm, 4-cm lymph node in the axilla and referred the patient for an excisional biopsy. Examination by the surgeon showed no palpable breast masses or lymphadenopathy outside of the axilla, and results of a hemogram, mammograms, and chest radiographs were likewise normal. Histologic examination of the excised node showed an undifferentiated malignant polygonal-cell tumor, the differential diagnosis of which included metastatic carcinoma (potentially from the breast or lung), malignant melanoma, and large-cell non-Hodgkin's lymphoma (Fig. 2–2). An initial panel of immunostains was obtained for keratin, CD45 (leukocyte common antigen), vimentin, and S100 protein, showing reactivity only for the latter two determinants (Fig. 2–3). Because these findings indicated a diagnosis of melanoma in the absence of any cutaneous or mucosal lesions, two additional confirmatory antibodies with specificity for melanocytes (HMB-45 and NK1/C3) were also applied to the specimen, with similarly positive results. The final diagnosis was therefore that of metastatic melanoma of unknown anatomic origin (possibly a regressed lesion).

Case 2–2

A 75-year-old man complained of sharp pain in his left anterior chest, which had worsened progressively over 3 months. He reported point tenderness of his chest wall as well. Evaluation by the patient's internist confirmed the presence of palpation-induced pain over the midpoint of the left sixth rib. There were no other abnormalities on physical examination. Radiographs of the chest demonstrated a blastic destructive lesion in the left sixth rib, suggestive of metastatic carcinoma. Based on this finding, biochemical tests were obtained that showed elevation of

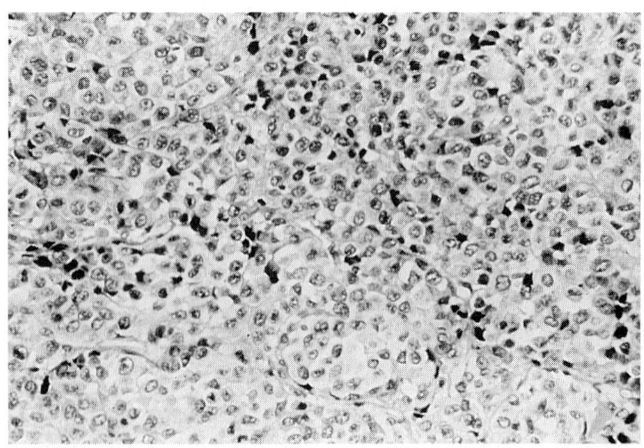

Figure 2–2. Malignant large-cell neoplasm in an excised axillary lymph node in a 67-year-old woman with no other abnormalities. The tumor is morphologically indeterminate on conventional staining with hematoxylin and eosin; it could be interpreted as a carcinoma, a lymphoma, or a melanoma.

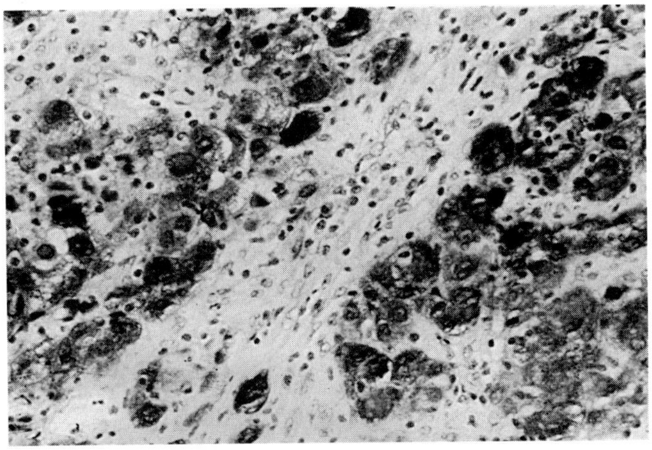

Figure 2–3. Immunostaining of the tumor in Figure 2–2 for S100 protein shows combined nuclear and cytoplasmic reactivity, as demonstrated in this photograph. Other stains for keratin and CD45 were negative. This constellation of findings establishes the diagnosis of metastatic malignant melanoma, which was further substantiated by the results of other immunohistochemical studies (see text).

the serum alkaline phosphatase and prostate-specific antigen levels; however, repeated digital and ultrasonographic examination of the prostate gland failed to reveal a mass. A closed needle biopsy of the left sixth rib was obtained, showing metastatic, poorly differentiated adenocarcinoma (Fig. 2–4). Immunostains on this specimen were reactive for keratin, prostate-specific antigen, and prostatic acid phosphatase (Fig. 2–5), confirming a prostatic origin for the tumor.

Case 2–3

A 56-year-old woman had undergone left modified radical mastectomy in 6 years previously for a grade III infiltrating ductal carcinoma. She was found to have a stage I tumor with uninvolved axillary lymph nodes; results of

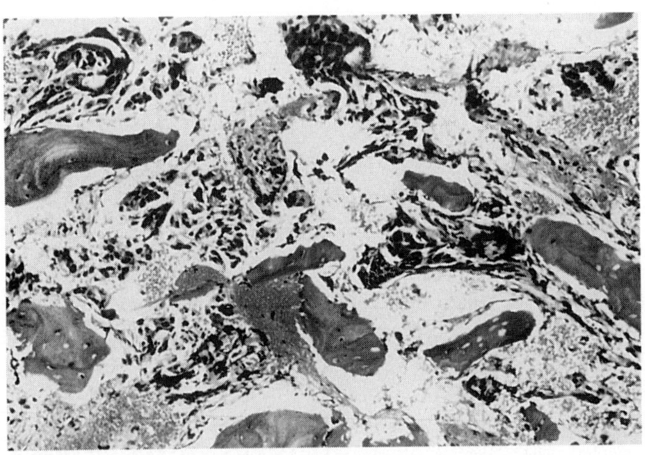

Figure 2–4. Closed needle biopsy of a blastic lesion of the left sixth rib in a patient with elevated serum prostate-specific antigen. Between the irregular geographic shapes of bony trabeculae are distorted clusters of foreign polygonal cells, representing a metastatic, poorly differentiated nonhematopoietic neoplasm.

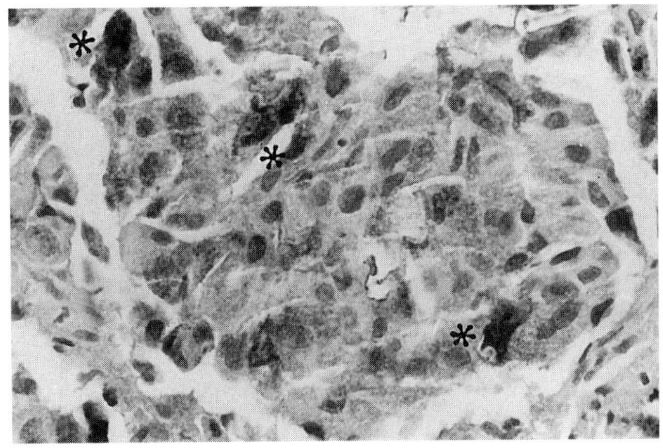

Figure 2–5. Multifocal immunoreactivity for prostate-specific antigen *(asterisks)* is evident in the specimen shown in Figure 2–4, confirming a diagnosis of metastatic prostatic adenocarcinoma.

radionuclide scans of the viscera and bones were likewise negative. Biochemical analysis of fresh tumor tissue showed that it was positive for estrogen- and progesterone-receptor proteins (ERP/PRP). The patient was treated with daily oral tamoxifen with no evidence of disease activity until almost 3 years later. At that time, an enlarged left supraclavicular lymph node was detected on follow-up physical examination. It was subjected to fine needle aspiration, showing metastatic adenocarcinoma that was identical morphologically to the primary tumor (Fig. 2–6). Immunocytochemical stains for ERP/PRP were performed on the fine needle aspiration biopsy (FNAB) specimen, showing that these markers were now absent in the tumor cells. Accordingly, the patient was begun on conventional cytotoxic chemotherapy.

The foregoing cases are merely illustrations of common diagnostic or management problems that may be addressed

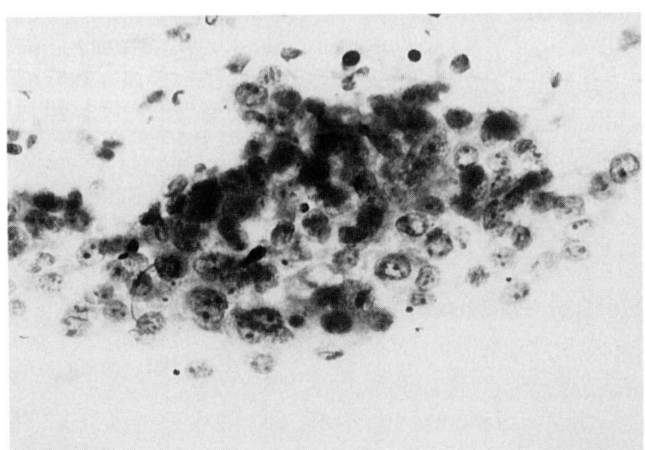

Figure 2–6. Fine needle aspiration biopsy (FNAB) of left supraclavicular lymph node, showing a three-dimensional grouping of relatively homogeneous polygonal cells with discernible nucleoli consistent with metastatic mammary adenocarcinoma. Other slides prepared during the FNAB were used for immunostaining to detect estrogen and progesterone receptor proteins in the tumor, both of which were absent.

through immunohistology. Although formal cost-effectiveness analyses have not as yet been performed on these procedures, it is very likely that they provide as much or more information per health care dollar as any other investigation in clinical medicine. For example, even an extensive battery of immunostains currently costs considerably less than computed tomography of the abdomen or chest, or endoscopic procedures such as esophagogastroscopy or cystoscopy in the assessment of malignant tumors. These special stains are not a panacea, however. Used in other than the appropriate contexts, they can actually *create* confusion; thus, it is critical that such results always be *integrated* with other clinicopathologic data by the pathologist and the clinician.

Another application of immunohistochemistry that has come into vogue is in detecting "prognostic" cellular protein products or other markers that can be used to monitor the course of therapy. In breast cancer (see Case 2–3), ERP and PRP are the best known of these,[28] but other examples are numerous. They include oncoplacentofetal determinants such as alpha-fetoprotein, human placental lactogen, beta-chorionic gonadotropin, and ferritin in human germ-cell tumors[29]; various neuropeptides in neuroendocrine neoplasms[30]; carcinoembryonic antigen (CEA) in malignancies of the gut[22, 29]; blood group antigens (BGA) in tumors of the urothelial tract[31]; "proliferation markers" such as Ki-67 and proliferating cell nuclear antigen[32]; growth factors and their receptors (e.g., epidermal growth factor receptor in squamous carcinomas of the head and neck or carcinomas of the bladder)[31, 33]; a legion of oncogene products, including the p21 *ras* protein, Her-2/*neu* (c-*erb*B-2) oncopeptide, *fes* and *fms* oncoproteins, and others[34]; "antioncoproteins" such as the retinoblastoma gene product (RB-1) and the p53 protein[35]; antiapoptotic (anti-programmed cell death) products such as *bcl*-2 protein[36]; and cellular enzymes that may play a role in tumor invasion and metastasis (e.g., selected metalloproteinases; collagenase type IV).[37, 38]

Among these, the oncoplacentofetal markers, CEA, BGA, ERP, and PRP can be considered to have definite utility in the surveillance or planning of antineoplastic therapy in predefined settings. However, it is the author's firm opinion that the other determinants listed above must be considered as investigational and of unproven independent value in the prognostication or management of human malignancies.[39] Hence, their use in clinical settings is considered to be unjustified at the present time.

Electron Microscopy

Electron microscopy (EM) can best be performed only after tissue has been prospectively processed by the pathologist in a specific fixative (buffered glutaraldehyde), which optimizes the preservation of submicroscopic cellular organelles. Because EM is an expensive procedure that necessitates 3 to 4 days to accomplish, specimens are currently not submitted for this modality of study on a routine basis. Thus, if the surgeon is aware of the possibility of a disease that is well delineated by ultrastructural analysis[40] (Table 2–3), it is important that the pathologist be alerted and that tissue be directed to his or her immediate attention and submitted fresh or partly in glutaraldehyde.

Table 2–3. Diseases in Which Electron Microscopy Is Helpful Diagnostically in Surgical Pathology

Nonneoplastic Diseases

—Bullous dermatoses (e.g., pemphigus, pemphigoid)
—Medical pulmonary diseases (especially pneumoconioses)
—Medical renal diseases
—Metabolic storage diseases

Neoplastic Diseases

—Undifferentiated malignant tumors
—Metastatic carcinomas of unknown anatomic origin
—Soft tissue sarcomas of round-cell, spindle-cell, and pleomorphic types
—Malignant mesothelioma versus adenocarcinoma of serosal surfaces
—Histiocytosis X (Langerhans' cell disease)
—Neuroendocrine tumors (e.g., carcinoids; pancreatic endocrine tumors, etc.)

Case 2–4

A 25-year-old woman had suffered three episodes of spontaneous pneumothorax over a 2-year period. Chest radiographs and computed tomograms of the chest done after the most recent occurrence of this problem showed reticulonodular interstitial infiltrates in the upper lobes of both lungs, along with small parenchymal pulmonary cysts. After bronchoscopy and transbronchial biopsy failed to yield diagnostic pathologic material, an open-lung biopsy was performed. At the time of the latter procedure, the surgeon informed the pathologist that the two favored clinical diagnoses were those of Langerhans' cell disease ("eosinophilic granuloma") and lymphangioleiomyomatosis of the lung (see Chap. 11). In light of this information, a portion of the specimen was fixed in glutaraldehyde and submitted for electron microscopy. Histologic study demonstrated a cellular interstitial pulmonary infiltrate with the general characteristics of eosinophilic granuloma (Fig. 2–7). The latter diagnosis was confirmed by the finding of characteristic cytoplasmic Birbeck granules in the proliferating cells (Fig. 2–8) using the electron microscope.

Case 2–5

A 24-year-old man had a 5-year history of progressive renal insufficiency due to documented dense-deposit disease (DDD) or type 2 membranoproliferative glomerulonephritis, ultimately culminating in the need for chronic peritoneal dialysis and placement of the patient on the prospective renal transplantation roster. Two years after dialysis was instituted, he received a cadaveric allogeneic renal transplant. This functioned well for 12 months, at which time an episode of moderate cellular rejection was documented by allograft biopsy (Fig. 2–9) and treated with augmentation of immunosuppressive medication. Ten

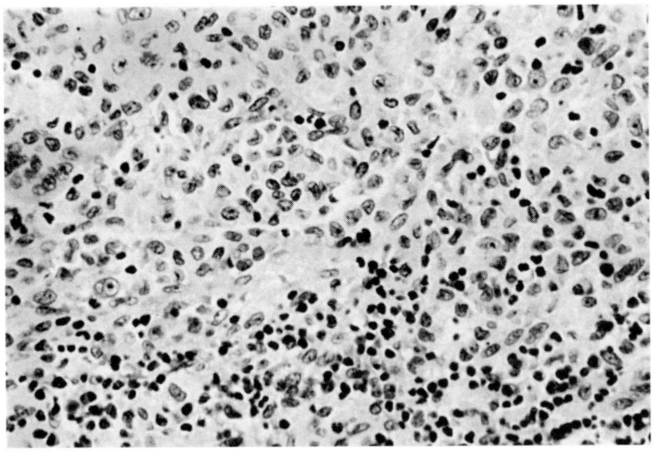

Figure 2–7. Interstitial infiltrate in the lung of a 25-year-old woman as seen in an open lung biopsy specimen. It shows numerous large histiocytelike cells *(top of figure)* in admixture with eosinophils and lymphocytes; this appearance is suggestive of Langerhans' cell disease (histiocytosis X).

months later, massive proteinuria and rising serum creatinine levels appeared. These were presumed to reflect another episode of cellular rejection, and this assumption was so portrayed in communications with the pathologist when another transplant biopsy was obtained. However, the latter specimen showed no evidence of cellular infiltrates and instead demonstrated thickened glomerular capillary basement membranes, suggesting recurrent DDD. However, because of the clinical impressions, no material had been submitted for special studies and disease recurrence could not be confirmed. Another biopsy was therefore necessary, which, on the basis of EM study, did indeed secure an interpretation of DDD (Fig. 2–10).

The expense of ultrastructural analysis is justified when the method is reserved for situations in which it can provide

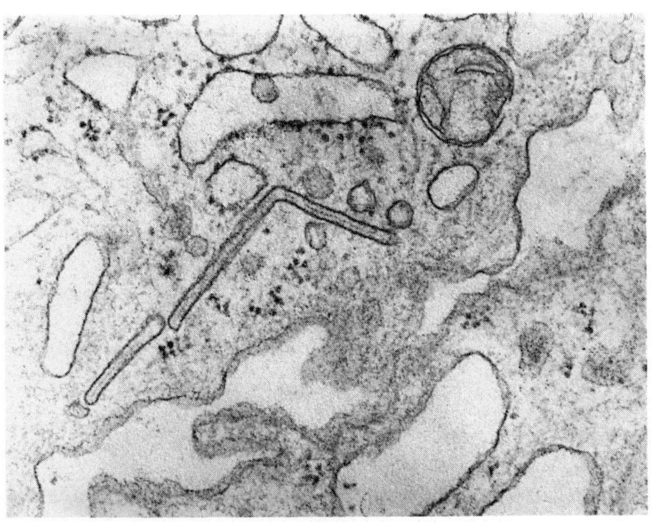

Figure 2–8. This electron micrograph of the tissue shown in Figure 2–7 discloses the presence of diagnostic Birbeck granules *(center of figure)*. These are linear or curvilinear membranous inclusions that secure a diagnosis of Langerhans' cell disease.

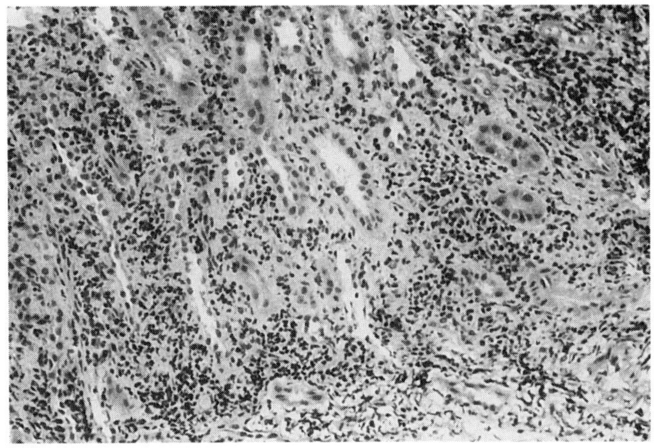

Figure 2–9. Tubulointerstitial renal rejection grade 3, typified by multifocal areas of tubulitis and confluent stromal aggregates of activated lymphocytes.

the definitive diagnosis, as in these two cases. Many soft tissue sarcomas, metastatic carcinomas of unknown origin, selected hematopoietic proliferations, medical renal disorders, and several metabolic diseases (e.g., mucopolysaccharidoses, sphingolipidoses, ceroid lipofuscinosis) show characteristic findings using this technique.[41] Moreover, properly prepared ultrastructural specimens can also be studied using x-ray diffraction analysis to localize and quantitate minerals of medicolegal or epidemiologic interest (e.g., silica, beryllium) in human tissues.[42]

It cannot be emphasized too strongly how important it is for samples to be selected *prospectively* for EM. Cellular degeneration begins as soon as tissue is removed from the body, potentially compromising the visualization of ultrastructural details and necessitating procurement of more tissue if special studies are indispensable (as in Case 2–5). Pathologists have attempted to devise methods for the retrospective retrieval of suitable EM material from routinely processed specimens, but this is almost universally of compromised quality, allowing for recognition of

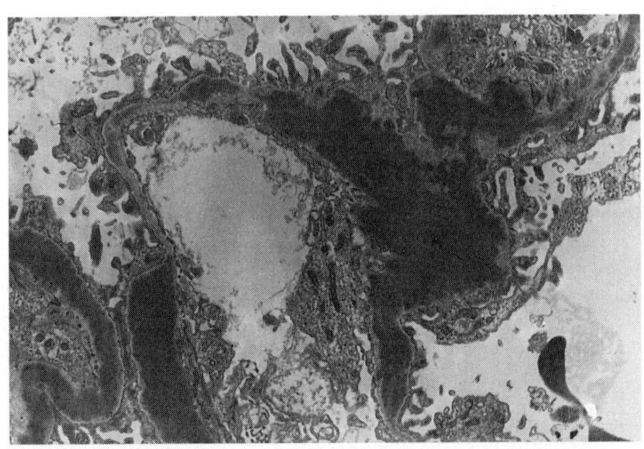

Figure 2–10. Electron micrograph of a subsequent biopsy specimen from the renal allograft in the same case as that portrayed in Figure 2–9, showing recurrent dense-deposit disease (type II membranoproliferative glomerulonephritis). Large, dark, linear deposits of immune complexes are seen in the capillary walls of the glomeruli.

only a few of the most resilient and coarsest cellular organelles. Last, this is a procedure that cannot be rushed. Although it may seem strange that up to 96 hours may elapse before the pathologist can provide an ultrastructural interpretation, this requirement relates mainly to the need for intricate embedding procedures using epoxy resin, careful sectioning of the specimen at a thickness of less than 1 μm with an ultramicrotome, and painstaking staining techniques.

FLOW CYTOMETRY

Flow cytometry (FCM) involves the passage of a disaggregated suspension of cells or cell components through the aperture of an electronic instrument. It can be programmed to ''see'' only those cells or components that are in a certain size range or possess other specialized characteristics. Various antibodies labeled with differing fluorescent tags may be allowed to simultaneously react with the cell suspension before analysis in the cytometer, permitting multiparameter analysis—an attribute not usually achieved with immunohistology.[43]

The main aims of FCM are, therefore, twofold. One is to segregate and antigenically characterize mixed cell groupings in a sampled human tissue rapidly. The other is to measure the density of selected cellular components—such as DNA—in a predefined cellular population. The first of these applications has basically the same aims as those of immunohistology, but FCM can be accomplished much more quickly than the latter procedure. The second use of FCM relates to the knowledge that certain human tumors show distinct strata of clinical behavior based on their *ploidy*—that is, their individual cellular content of DNA.

One may often be able to obtain acceptable but limited results in FCM studies using routinely processed (formalinized) specimens.[44] However, the best and most reliable substrate for this technique is that of unfixed tissue. Hence, preoperative consultation with the pathologist is highly advisable if it is anticipated that FCM may be necessary in analyzing a specimen from any given case. If it is mutually agreed that this procedure is indicated, the tissue should be sent immediately to the laboratory in a fresh state.

Case 2–6

A 44-year-old man had a known history of diffuse large B-cell non-Hodgkin's lymphoma, which had first become manifest with left supraclavicular lymphadenopathy and night sweats 10 months previously. He underwent several cycles of multiagent chemotherapy and entered an apparent remission. However, a mass had recently become evident in the belly of the left biceps muscle, accompanied by renewed night sweats. Because of the likelihood that this represented a soft tissue focus of recurrent disease, FNAB of the lesion was performed and a portion of the specimen that was procured was sent immediately for FCM. This confirmed the clinical diagnosis, showing a population of cells that were larger than reactive lymphocytes and labeled by antibodies to CD5, CD19, CD20, HLA-DR, and CD45 (i.e., showing an aberrant B-lymphocytic immunophenotype) as analyzed with the flow cytometer. Because of the rapidity of FCM, the oncologist was provided with this interpretation the same day that FNAB had been performed.

Case 2–7

A 2-year-old boy was found to have an upper abdominal mass by his mother while she was bathing the child. Examination by the family pediatrician confirmed this finding but showed no other physical abnormalities. A computed tomogram of the abdomen disclosed an 8-cm mass at the right superior renal pole, probably centered in the adrenal gland. Laparotomy confirmed this conclusion, and a frozen section of the excised mass showed a small round-cell tumor that was consistent in appearance with classic neuroblastoma. In light of this diagnosis, fresh tissue was sent for FCM analysis. This procedure revealed that the neoplasm was DNA-diploid, with a DNA index of 1.0. Accordingly, after examination of permanent sections confirmed the diagnosis of neuroblastoma, an intensified regimen of chemotherapy was planned.

Case 2–6 illustrates the integration of several specialized pathologic techniques—FNAB, ploidy FCM, and immunophenotyping FCM methods—in order to obtain a quick, reliable, and sophisticated diagnosis. Case 2–7 shows the manner in which certain FCM observations have influenced current therapy. In that example, a DNA-diploid neuroblastoma was presented; this tumor is known to pursue a more aggressive clinical course than its microscopically identical but DNA-aneuploid counterparts.[45] Case 2–7 also shows that one must apply FCM results in very specific contexts, because many other childhood malignancies would be expected to pursue a *favorable* course if they were DNA-diploid.

CYTOGENETICS AND CELLULAR ENZYME ANALYSIS

Until a few years ago, the analysis of human chromosomes was primarily of interest only to clinical geneticists, hematologists, and hematopathologists. Certain heritable disorders that are related to chromosomal aberrations are diagnosed by such means; in addition, many hematologic dyscrasias and malignancies and a growing number of solid tumors show characteristic karyotypic abnormalities as well.[46, 47] On the other hand, a multitude of enzymopathies with systemic consequences are genetic but not chromosomal in causation.[48, 49] These can be recognized by analyzing the relative concentrations of responsible enzymes in affected tissues.

The means whereby such diseases are characterized definitively is by explant cell culture and biochemical evaluation (for enzymopathies) or preparation of quinacrine-banding arrays of cellular chromosomes (for chromosomal anomalies). Both techniques require the availability of fresh tissue, and, in the former circumstance, it is furthermore preferred that this tissue be submitted in nutrient medium. As one might expect, the technology involved in this area is meticulous and therefore results typically require several days—or even weeks—for availability (see Table 2–1).

Case 2–8

A 25-year-old man complained of a slowly enlarging mass in the deep tissues of his right foot, which had been present for at least 1 year. It had recently reached such a size that it made wearing his usual-size shoe uncomfortable. Examination by his internist showed a vague fullness in the deep soft plantar tissues of the right foot, and this area was slightly tender to vigorous palpation. A plain film radiograph of the foot showed a definite mass effect in the soft tissue, with a "scalloping" deformity of the cortex of the third metatarsal bone. Because of these findings, the patient was referred to an orthopedic oncologist. He underwent an incisional biopsy of the mass, at which time the specimen was sent fresh to the pathology laboratory. Because a diagnosis of synovial sarcoma was favored on the basis of aggregate clinical observations, a portion of the tissue was sent for karyotypic analysis. Histologic examination did indeed show a densely cellular spindle-cell neoplasm that was consistent with synovial sarcoma (Fig. 2–11), and its immunoreactivity for epithelial membrane antigen also supported that interpretation. The characteristic X;18 chromosomal translocation of synovial sarcoma[50] (inset) was documented karyotypically, further confirming the diagnosis.

Case 2–9

A 48-year-old man presented to his internist with complaints of worsening fatigue and shortness of breath on exertion, which had been present for 6 months. Physical examination disclosed pallor of the mucous membranes and nail beds, a resting heart rate of 105/min, an ejection-type cardiac murmur at the left sternal border, and moderate hepatosplenomegaly. A hemogram showed moderate to severe pancytopenia. Because of these abnormalities, a bone marrow aspiration was obtained, showing focal infiltration of the marrow by large, foamy histiocytes. Their cytologic appearance raised the question of adult-onset (type I) Gaucher's disease.[51] A radioactive chromium–tagged erythrocyte survival study was undertaken to assess the possibility of hypersplenism, with positive results. Therefore, the patient was taken to the operating room for elective splenectomy. Having been apprised of the probable diagnosis, the pathologist immediately sent fresh splenic tissue (in tissue-culture medium) for enzymatic analysis. This study demonstrated the lack of detectable glucocerebrosidase in the spleen, confirming the histologic diagnosis of adult Gaucher's disease (Fig. 2–12).

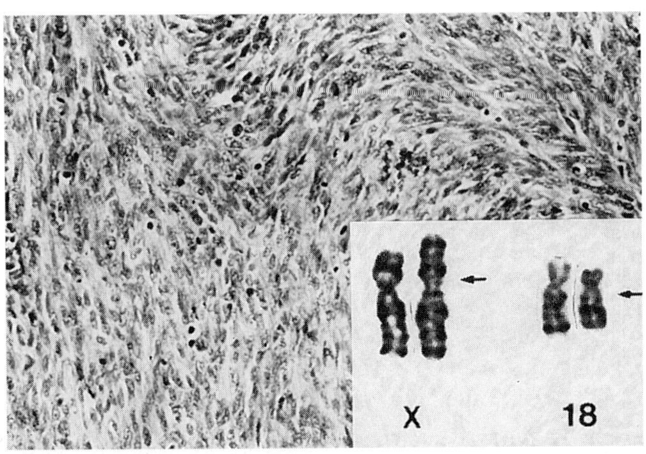

Figure 2–11. Malignant spindle-cell neoplasm of the foot in a 25-year-old man, which is histologically indeterminate. Synovial sarcoma, leiomyosarcoma, fibrosarcoma, and malignant peripheral nerve sheath tumor are all diagnostic possibilities based on conventional morphological study. Chromosomal analysis of fresh tissue *(inset)* from the tumor shown in the larger portion of this figure. This evaluation showed the characteristic X;18 translocation of synovial sarcoma. (Reprinted with permission from Fletcher JA. Cytogenetic aberrations in malignant soft tissue tumors. *Adv Pathol Lab Med.* 1991;4:235–246.)

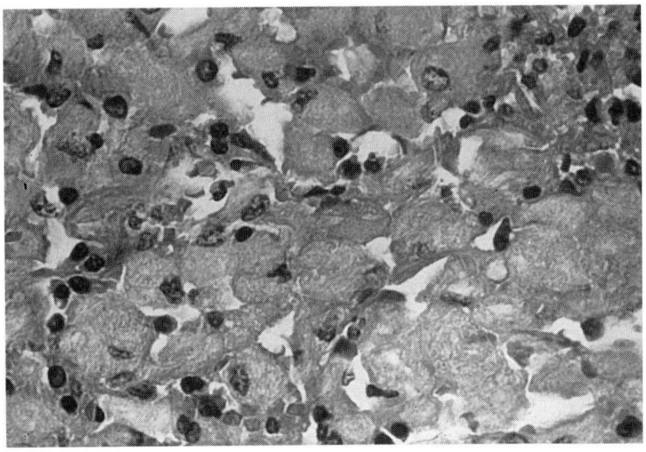

Figure 2–12. Section of splenectomy specimen from a 48-year-old man with pancytopenia and splenomegaly, showing expanses in the red pulp that are filled by large histiocytes with abundant pale cytoplasm. This finding suggested a diagnosis of Gaucher's disease, which was confirmed by biochemical analyses of cultured tissue.

At the risk of redundancy, the importance of making fresh tissue available for cytogenetic or enzymatic analysis cannot be overstressed. Given current technologic constraints, there is little or nothing that laboratory physicians can do with routinely processed specimens for the purposes of this type of study.

Molecular Genetic Analysis: In Situ Hybridization and Polymerase Chain Reaction–Based Assays

Within the past decade, it has become feasible to probe directly into the nucleic acid constituency of human cells, using the in situ hybridization (ISH) and PCR methods.[52, 53] Both of these techniques are more "pure" than immunohistology from a mechanistic standpoint, because they assess the templates for protein synthesis rather than the protein products themselves. This is done by annealing labeled nucleic acid probes to DNA or RNA in the target tissue (ISH) or by multiplying tissue DNA sequences thousands of times with predetermined ''primers'' (PCR). At present, the greatest utility for either ISH or PCR is in the rapid diagnosis of infectious diseases that would otherwise require several days or even weeks for confirmation via more traditional laboratory methods. Fresh tissue is preferred for both assays, but routinely fixed and processed specimens can sometimes be used as well.

Case 2–10

A 57-year-old woman with a 35-pack-year cigarette smoking history presented with hemoptysis. On physical examination, she was febrile, with audible rales and rhonchi over the right superoposterior thorax; right supraclavicular lymphadenopathy was also detected. The patient was generally thin and appeared chronically ill. Radiographs of the chest showed a perihilar mass in the right upper lobe, with apparent pneumonitis in the adjacent parenchyma. Bronchoscopy showed no specific abnormalities; cytologic specimens obtained from this procedure were negative for malignancy, and all cultures were negative after 1 week. Because of these findings, a diagnostic supraclavicular lymph node biopsy was performed. Histologic examination demonstrated numerous noncaseating granulomas (Fig. 2–13), one of which contained a single mycobacterial organism with the Ziehl-Neelsen stain. In light of these observations, additional tissue was cut from the paraffin block of the node and analyzed by PCR with DNA primers that are specific for *Mycobacterium tuberculosis*. This analysis yielded positive results 1 day thereafter, allowing initiation of antituberculous drug therapy.

The speed with which diagnoses of selected viral, fungal, and mycobacterial diseases can now be made with PCR is remarkable.[54, 55] However, this method is exceedingly demanding from technical and quality-assurance standpoints, and therefore few diagnostic laboratories currently offer it. On the other hand, ISH is easier to perform but has a relatively high risk of false negativity.

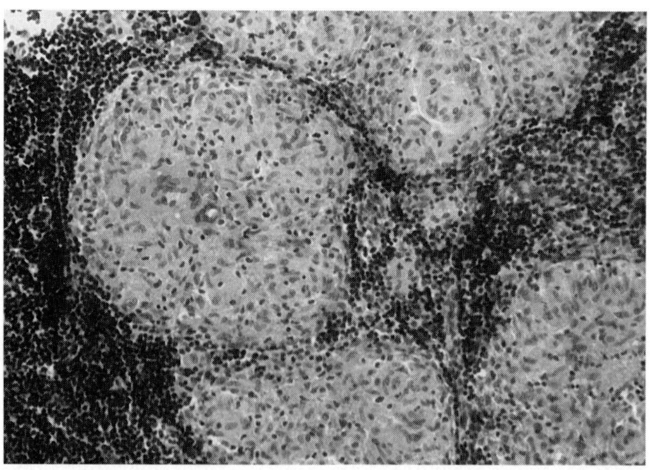

Figure 2–13. Supraclavicular lymph node specimen showing multiple noncaseating granulomas in a 57-year-old patient with hemoptysis and an abnormal chest x-ray. The node was found to contain *Mycobacterium tuberculosis* by polymerase chain reaction assay.

Practical and Economic Considerations

In selecting which special studies *must* be done and assessing those that *could* be done, the surgeon and the pathologist must together decide how the need for prompt and definitive diagnosis is balanced by fiscal realities. It is, perhaps, a commentary on the last few decades of medical practice in the United States that many physicians today will select a test ''because it is there'' or ''just to be absolutely sure.'' Patients' expectations of ever greater technology and increasing medicolegal pressures have contributed to this scenario as well.

In addressing the problem of rising costs for special analyses, all physicians must ask themselves two questions: (1) Is this test crucial to the diagnosis and management process, or is it an ''extra''? and (2) Has the technology concerned been *proved* sufficiently that the patient (or the health insurer) can—in good conscience—be charged for the test? If the answers to both queries are yes, the evaluation can proceed. If one or the other elicits a negative response, serious reservations over the utility of the test should arise. The great challenges to surgeons and pathologists over the coming decades will be to prove the validity of clinical practice patterns in all of their many details; to provide outcome data on the application of current and emerging tests and procedures; and, at the same time, to restrain the growth of health care spending. Only by informed and collegial interaction can these goals be realized.

Summary

The major groupings of special diagnostic techniques, with indications for their use, are as follows:

Immunostaining

- Determination of lineage for poorly differentiated neoplasms
- Detection of clonality in lymphoid proliferations (immunoglobulin light chain restriction)
- Rapid demonstration of selected microorganisms in tissue
- Detection of steroid receptor proteins in tissue sections
- Qualitative analysis of selected "prognostic" cell markers

Electron Microscopy

- Determination of lineage for poorly differentiated neoplasms
- Confirmation of neuroendocrine tumor differentiation
- Differential diagnosis of adenocarcinoma versus mesothelioma
- Detection of intracellular viral inclusions
- Elucidation of possible etiology in medical renal, pulmonary, and cutaneous diseases

Flow Cytometry

Aids in delineation of clonality of lymphoid proliferations
Contributes to determination of B-cell or T-cell lineage in evaluations of malignant lymphomas
Measurement of DNA content in neoplastic cells (of possible prognostic significance)

Cytogenetics

Detection of diagnostic or prognostic karyotypic aberrations in hematologic diseases
Diagnosis of selected heritable diseases
Delineation of diagnostic chromosomal abnormalities in selected malignant "solid" tumors (especially sarcomas)

Cellular Enzyme Analysis

Definitive diagnosis of diseases characterized by intracellular enzymopathies (e.g., lysosomal storage diseases)
Characterization of selected immunologic diseases featuring enzyme-related effector-cell deficiencies (e.g., chronic granulomatous disease of childhood)

Molecular Probe Analysis (Including In Situ Hybridization/PCR)

Rapid diagnosis of selected infectious diseases
Detection of clonality in lymphoid proliferations
Detection of certain cellular products (e.g., oncoproteins) with putative prognostic significance

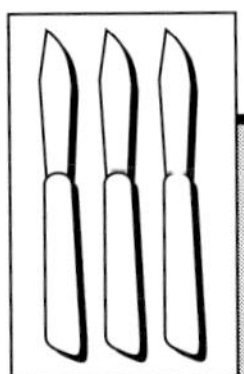

PITFALLS FOR THE SURGEON

1. Failure to communicate concerns to the pathologist regarding selected diagnostic categories that require special handling of tissue (e.g., possible lymphomas; possible inborn errors of metabolism; certain medical diseases of the lung, skin, liver, and kidney).
2. Submission of all tissues to pathology in formalin or other fixatives, or, conversely, failure to submit tissue in a timely fashion after excision, allowing cellular autolysis (degradative changes) to occur.
3. Failure to confirm claims made for new tests by reviewing independent medical literature.

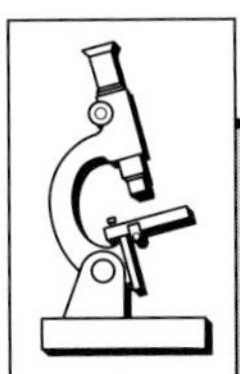

PITFALLS FOR THE PATHOLOGIST

1. Failure to make note of pertinent clinical information provided on cases that will require ancillary investigation.
2. Failure to assure adequate quality-control measures in laboratory performance of special procedures.
3. Failure to maintain submitted tissues under necessary conditions for needed evaluations (e.g., failure to freeze fresh tissue suspected of representing malignant lymphoma).
4. Failure to confirm claims made for new tests by reviewing independent medical literature.

FURTHER READING

Bauer KD, Duque RE, Shankey TV. *Clinical Flow Cytometry.* Baltimore: Williams & Wilkins: 1993.
Dickersin GR. *Diagnostic Electron Microscopy: A Text Atlas.* New York: Igaku-Shoin, 1988.
Elias J. *Immunohistopathology: A Practical Approach to Diagnosis.* Chicago: ASCP Press; 1990.
Farkas DH, ed. *Molecular Biology and Pathology.* San Diego, CA: Academic Press; 1993.
Rosai J, ed. *Ackerman's Surgical Pathology,* 7th ed. St. Louis: Mosby; 1989.
Sternberg SS, ed. *Diagnostic Surgical Pathology,* 2nd ed. New York: Raven Press; 1994.

REFERENCES

1. Underwood JCE: *Introduction to Biopsy Interpretation and Surgical Pathology,* 2nd ed. London: Springer-Verlag; 1987:1–16.
2. Bloodgood JC: The clinical and pathologic differential diagnosis of diseases of the female breast. *Am J Med Sci.* 1908;135:157–168.
3. Ober WB. The case of the Kaiser's cancer. *Pathol Annu.* 1970;5:207–216.
4. Virchow R. Professor Virchow's report on the portion of growth removed from the larynx of H.I.H. the Crown Prince of Germany by Dr. M. MacKenzie on June 28th. *Br Med J.* 1887;2:199.
5. Wilson LB. A method for the rapid preparation of fresh tissues for the microscope. *JAMA.* 1905;45:1737.
6. Wright JR. The development of the frozen section technique, the evolution of surgical biopsy, and the origins of surgical pathology. *Bull Med Histol.* 1985;59:295–326.
7. Coons AH, Creech JH, Jones RN: Immunological properties of an antibody containing a fluorescent group. *Proc Soc Exp Biol Med.* 1941;47:200–202.
8. Pease DC. *Histological Techniques for Electron Microscopy.* New York: Academic Press; 1964.
9. Watson JD, Crick FHC. Genetical implications of the structure of deoxyribonucleic acid. *Nature.* 1953;171:964–970.

10. Hofler H, DeLellis RA, Wolfe HJ. In situ hybridization and immunohistochemistry. In: DeLellis RA, ed. *Advances in Immunohistochemistry.* New York: Raven Press; 1988:47–66.
11. Towbin JA. Introduction to the techniques of molecular biology. *Herz* 1993;18:213–221.
12. Belak S, Ballagi-Pordany A. Experience on the application of the polymerase chain reaction in a diagnostic laboratory. *Mol Cell Probes.* 1993;7:241–248.
13. Inghirami G, Szabolcs MJ, Yee HT, et al. Detection of immunoglobulin gene rearrangement of B cell non-Hodgkin's lymphomas and leukemias in fresh, unfixed, and formalin-fixed, paraffin-embedded tissue by polymerase chain reaction. *Lab Invest.* 1993;68:746–757.
14. Galen RS. Interpretation of laboratory tests. *N Engl J Med.* 1975;292:433–438.
15. Warnke RA, Rouse RV. Limitations encountered in the application of tissue section immunodiagnosis to the study of lymphomas and related disorders. *Hum Pathol.* 1985;16:326–331.
16. Swanson PE. Foundations of immunohistochemistry: A practical review. *Am J Clin Pathol.* 1988;90:333–339.
17. Falini B, Taylor CR. New developments in immunoperoxidase techniques and their application. *Arch Pathol Lab Med.* 1983;107:105–110.
18. Gatter KC, Alcock C, Heryet A, Mason DY. Clinical importance of analysing malignant tumours of uncertain origin with immunohistological techniques. *Lancet.* 1985;1:1302–1305.
19. Nadji M, Tabei SZ, Castro A, et al. Prostatic origin of tumors: An immunohistochemical study. *Am J Clin Pathol.* 1980;73:735–739.
20. Permanetter W, Nathrath WBJ, Lohrs U. Immunohistochemical analysis of thyroglobulin and keratin in benign and malignant thyroid tumors. *Virchows Arch A.* 1982;398:221–232.
21. Wick MR, Lillemoe TJ, Copland GT, et al. Gross cystic disease fluid protein-15 as a marker for breast cancer. *Hum Pathol.* 1989;20:281–287.
22. Wick MR. Monoclonal antibodies to carcinoembryonic antigen in diagnostic immunohistochemistry. In: Wick MR, Siegal GP, eds. *Monoclonal Antibodies in Diagnostic Immunohistochemistry.* New York: Marcel Dekker; 1988:539–567.
23. Wick MR, Swanson PE, Manivel JC. Immunohistochemical analysis of soft tissue sarcomas: Comparisons with electron microscopy. *Appl Pathol.* 1988;6:169–196.
24. Perkins SL, Kjeldsberg CR. Immunophenotyping of lymphomas and leukemias in paraffin-embedded tissues. *Am J Clin Pathol.* 1993;99:362–373.
25. Kaye VN. Monoclonal antibodies to microbial antigens in diagnostic pathology. In: Wick MR, Siegal GP, eds. *Monoclonal Antibodies in Diagnostic Immunohistochemistry.* New York: Marcel Dekker; 1988:623–630.
26. Warnke RA. Alteration of immunoglobulin-bearing lymphoma cells by fixation. *J Histochem Cytochem.* 1979;27:1195–1196.
27. Shintaku IP, Said JW. Detection of estrogen receptors with monoclonal antibodies in routinely processed formalin-fixed paraffin sections of breast carcinoma: Use of DNAse pretreatment to enhance sensitivity of the reaction. *Am J Clin Pathol.* 1987;87:161–167.
28. Press MF. Estrogen and progesterone receptors in breast cancer. *Adv Pathol Lab Med.* 1993;6:117–148.
29. Schwartz MK. Serologic tests for cancer. *Adv Pathol Lab Med.* 1993;6:103–116.
30. Schumann G, Raeth U, Wiedenmann B, et al. Serum chromogranin-A in the diagnosis and follow-up of neuroendocrine tumors of the gastroenteropancreatic tract. *World J Surg.* 1992;16:697–701.
31. Wick MR, Swanson PE. Potential immunological and oncogenetic prognostic factors in carcinoma of the urinary bladder. *Adv Pathol Lab Med.* 1992;5:75–100.
32. Linden MD, Torres FX, Kubus J, Zarbo RJ. Clinical application of morphologic and immunocytochemical assessments of cell proliferation. *Am J Clin Pathol.* 1992;97(suppl 1):S4–S13.
33. Rikimaru K, Takokoro K, Yamamoto T, et al. Gene amplification and overexpression of epidermal growth factor receptor in squamous cell carcinoma of the head and neck. *Head Neck.* 1992;14:8–13.
34. Spandidos DA, Liloglou T, Field JK. Prognostic significance of oncogenes and tumor suppressor genes in human malignancy. *Stem Cells.* 1993;11:194–198.
35. Carbone DP, Minna JD. Antioncogenes and human cancer. *Annu Rev Med.* 1993;44:451–464.
36. Pezzella F, Turley H, Kuzu I, et al. Bcl-2 protein in non-small-cell lung carcinoma. *N Engl J Med.* 1993;329:690–694.
37. Kusukawa J, Sasaguri Y, Shima I, et al. Expression of matrix metalloproteinase-2 related to lymph node metastasis of oral squamous cell carcinoma: A clinicopathologic study. *Am J Clin Pathol.* 1993;99:18–23.
38. Levy AT, Cioce V, Sobel ME, et al. Increased expression of the Mr 72,000 type IV collagenase in human colonic adenocarcinoma. *Cancer Res.* 1991;51:439–444.
39. Wick MR. Oncogene analysis in diagnostic pathology: A current perspective. *Am J Clin Pathol.* 1992;97(suppl 1):S1–S3.
40. Gyorkey F, Min KW, Krisko I. The usefulness of electron microscopy in the diagnosis of human tumors. *Hum Pathol.* 1975;6:421–441.
41. Olsen TS, Racusen LC, Solez K. Ultrastructural investigation of renal biopsies. *J Electron Microsc Technol.* 1988;9:283–291.
42. Gibbs AE, Pooley FD, Griffiths DM, et al. Talc pneumoconiosis: A pathologic and mineralogic study. *Hum Pathol.* 1992;23:1344–1354.
43. Willman CL, Stewart CC. General principles of multiparameter flow cytometric analysis: Applications of flow cytometry in the diagnostic pathology laboratory. *Semin Diagn Pathol.* 1989;6:3–12.
44. Hedley DW. DNA analysis from paraffin-embedded blocks. *Methods Cell Biol.* 1990;33:139–147.
45. Nakazawa M. The prognostic significance of DNA ploidy for neuroblastoma. *Surg Today.* 1993;23:215–219.
46. Nowell PC. Chromosomal approaches to hematopoietic oncogenesis. *Stem Cells.* 1993;11:9–19.
47. Elias AD. Advances in the diagnosis and management of sarcomas. *Curr Opin Oncol.* 1992;4:681–688.
48. Arey JB. The lipidoses. *J Clin Lab Sci.* 1975;5:475–490.
49. Dorfman A, Matalon R. The mucopolysaccharidoses (review). *Proc Natl Acad Sci USA.* 1976;73:630–642.
50. Dal-Cin P, Rao U, Jani-Sait S, et al. Chromosomes in the diagnosis of soft tissue tumors: I. Synovial sarcoma. *Mod Pathol.* 1992;5:357–362.
51. Lee RE. Histiocytic diseases of bone marrow. *Hematol Oncol Clin North Am.* 1988;2:657–667.
52. DeLellis RA, Wolfe HJ. New techniques in gene product analysis. *Arch Pathol Lab Med.* 1987;111:620–626.
53. Grody WW, Gatti RA, Naeim F. Diagnostic molecular pathology. *Mod Pathol.* 1989;2:553–568.
54. Patou G, Pillay D, Myint S, Pattison J. Characterization of a nested polymerase chain reaction assay for detection of parvovirus B19. *J Clin Microbiol.* 1993;31:540–546.
55. Rattan A. Diagnosis of tuberculosis by polymerase chain reaction. *Indian J Pediatr.* 1990;57:673–677.

3

Fine Needle Aspiration Biopsy

William J. Frable

Definition

Thin or "fine" needle aspiration (FNA) biopsy is a simple, quick, and inexpensive method to biopsy superficial masses, usually in the office or clinic setting. It causes minimal trauma to the patient. The FNA biopsy technique carries virtually no risk of complications except in transthoracic and, rarely, transabdominal aspiration. Even abdominal masses that are easily palpable may be sampled directly by this method. Aspiration biopsy involves the use of thin needles of external diameter 0.6 to 1.0 mm, (22-, 23-gauge and higher) to sample masses for diagnosis based on cytologic features.

History of Fine Needle Aspiration

Dr. Hayes Martin, an American surgeon and radiotherapist, first published in 1930 on the needle aspiration method, using an 18-gauge needle.[1] Sixty cases from a variety of body sites—including breast, lung, and head and neck organs (lymph nodes, thyroid and salivary glands)—were described in his original series. Martin worked in close collaboration with Dr. Fred Stewart, attending pathologist and successor to James Ewing as director of pathology at Memorial Sloan Kettering Cancer Center in New York. Dr. Stewart became proficient in interpreting both aspiration smears and histologic sections of the very small core fragments of tissue that were procured with the 18-gauge needle. Stewart's 1933 publication on diagnosis by the aspiration method is still one of the largest personal series ever reported.[2]

The development of the thin needle method, using even smaller-diameter needles, occurred in Europe after World War II: in the Netherlands at Leiden; at the Karolinska Institute in Stockholm, Sweden; and in Lund, also in Sweden.[3–5] With one exception, the physicians at these centers were not pathologists but instead had trained in hematology. Like Martin, they wished to have a quick bedside diagnostic method for palpable tumors and were capable of both obtaining and interpreting their own aspiration smears. They adapted the Romanowsky staining methods (May-Grunwald-Giemsa, Giemsa alone, and Wright's stain) for the interpretation of epithelial lesions and hematologic processes. They found that use of thin needles, rather than the larger 18-gauge needles, allowed rapid and good cytologic sampling with little or no discomfort to the patient and was virtually free of complication. In the late sixties and early seventies, a few American pathologists and some clinicians were exposed to the work of the group at the Karolinska Institute in Stockholm.[6] This kindled a revival of aspiration biopsy using fine needle techniques in the United States. Interest was subsequently fueled by radiologists when diagnostic imaging became available.

Examples of Clinical Applications

Some brief clinical examples demonstrate where aspiration biopsy is of value.

Case 3–1

A 50-year-old male was seen in the medical clinic for evaluation of an enlarged supraclavicular lymph node. Aspiration demonstrated a pleomorphic malignant epithelial tumor with giant cells (Fig. 3–1). The smear pattern was

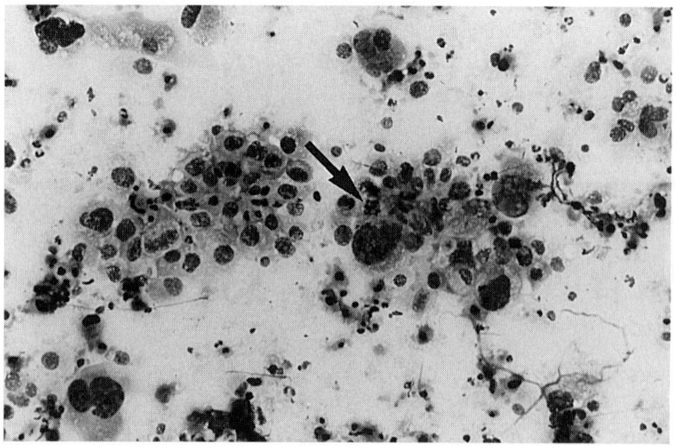

Figure 3–1. Aspiration smear of supraclavicular lymph node from Case 3–1, with irregular sheets of malignant tumor cells containing large, bizarre, and sometimes multinucleated tumor giant cells. Note phagocytosis of polymorphonuclear leukocytes within tumor cells *(arrow)*, a feature of giant-cell carcinoma of the lung. Diff-Quik stain, ×250.

that of giant-cell carcinoma. A chest film was advised, and this confirmed the presence of a lung mass highly suspicious for carcinoma. Sputum cytology demonstrated similar malignant cells. The patient was treated for advanced lung cancer with radiation and chemotherapy. The entire evaluation for therapeutic intervention was handled on an outpatient basis.

Case 3–2

A 32-year-old patient was seen in endocrinology clinic for a thyroid mass of several months' duration. Examination revealed a firm, circumscribed mass in the upper pole of the left lobe of the thyroid. Aspiration biopsy was cellular, with clusters having overlapping, elongated nuclei. There were nuclear grooves and some intranuclear inclusions (Fig. 3–2). A diagnosis of papillary carcinoma of the thyroid was given. The patient was advised of the diagnosis and its implications for therapy, and the extent of anticipated surgery was discussed ahead of time.

Case 3–3

A 70-year-old female presented with a breast mass of several months' duration. The mass had not changed in size since it was first noted by the patient. Clinical examination showed a firm but very circumscribed mass in the upper outer quadrant of the right breast. Aspiration was reported as "colloid" or mucinous carcinoma of the breast (Fig. 3–3). The treatment options for this favorable variant of breast cancer were discussed fully with the patient.

Case 3–4

A 32-year-old male was seen in the medical clinic for enlarged cervical lymph nodes of several weeks' duration. The patient had lost weight and felt generally unwell. There had not been any documented fever. Aspiration revealed numerous organisms with morphologic features of *Cryptococcus* (Fig. 3–4). Subsequent evaluation indicated the patient suffered from acquired immunodeficiency syndrome (AIDS) with disseminated cryptococcosis.

Case 3–5

A 65-year-old male was admitted for evaluation of painless jaundice. Computed tomography (CT) demonstrated a mass in the head of the pancreas. No evidence of metastatic disease was found and the patient underwent surgical exploration. Intraoperative FNA biopsy of the pancreatic mass was immediately reported as adenocarcinoma (Fig. 3–5). No local metastatic spread was detected intraoperatively, allowing a Whipple procedure to be performed.

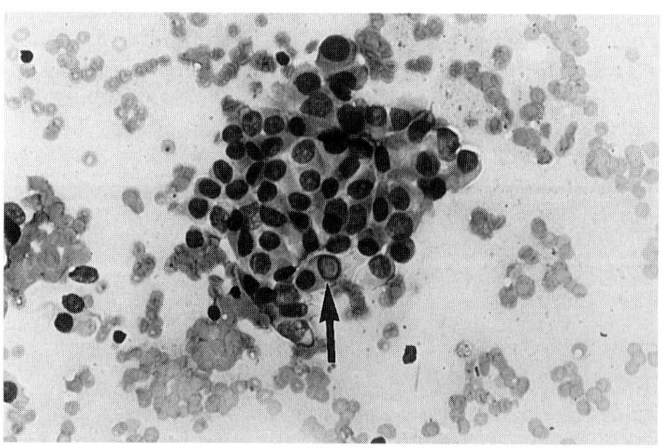

Figure 3–2. Clusters of cells with nuclear overlap from a cellular aspiration of a thyroid mass from Case 3–2. Within this cluster of thyroid cells, there are nuclei with sharply defined intranuclear inclusions *(arrow)* and also examples of nuclei with linear grooves. These are two of several features that support the diagnosis of papillary carcinoma of the thyroid. Diff-Quik stain, ×400.

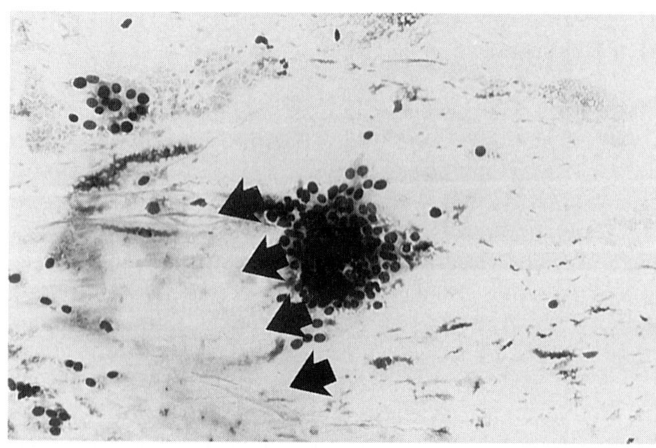

Figure 3–3. Cluster of monotonous-appearing cells seen in a background of metachromatic mucinous material *(arrows)* in FNA biopsy of breast from Case 3–3. Cytologic atypia may be minimal in colloid carcinoma of the breast. The diagnosis is based on the pattern of the smear, which mimics the tissue pattern of this type of breast cancer. Diff-Quik stain, ×250.

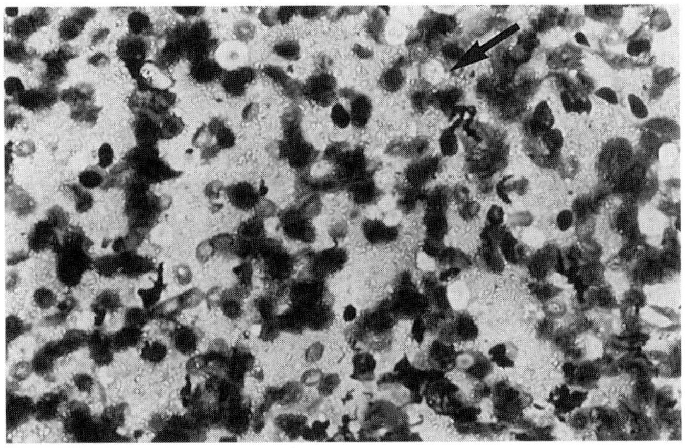

Figure 3–4. Clear round-to-oval structures with a slightly gray center can be found scattered throughout this smear, otherwise composed of lymphocytes and red blood cells from Case 3–4. Some of these structures appear to be budding *(arrow)*. They represent *Cryptococcus neoformans*, in this case a disseminated infection in a patient suffering from AIDS. Diff-Quik stain, ×600.

Planning for Implementation of Fine Needle Aspiration Biopsy in a Surgical Practice

WHO PERFORMS THE ASPIRATION?

Either the surgeon or the cytopathologist can perform the aspiration biopsy. If the surgeon wishes to perform the aspiration, it is very important to work closely with the pathologist who will process and interpret the biopsy. Stewart's admonition of 60 years ago still holds today: "Aspiration biopsy is as good as the combined intelligence of the clinician and pathologist makes it."[2]

LEARNING THE ASPIRATION METHOD

As with any biopsy procedure, the patient should be informed about what to expect. The author has used the analogy of drawing blood. That is, the procedure will take no longer to perform or be more uncomfortable than a successful venipuncture. A patient brochure that reviews the FNA biopsy procedure can be provided to the patient for the initial visit. This should include the general indications for FNA biopsy, what it is intended to accomplish, and a summary of the few potential complications. This can be sent ahead with an appointment letter in the case of referrals to the cytopathologist or be left available to be read in the waiting room (see Appendix 3–1).

Some may choose to have the patient sign a standard informed consent form. The author has not usually obtained written consent for the aspiration of superficial masses except from parents in the case of a child's biopsy. Informed consent should be obtained for any deep aspiration biopsy, with or without imaging, particularly in the case of biopsy of the chest, abdomen, or pelvis.

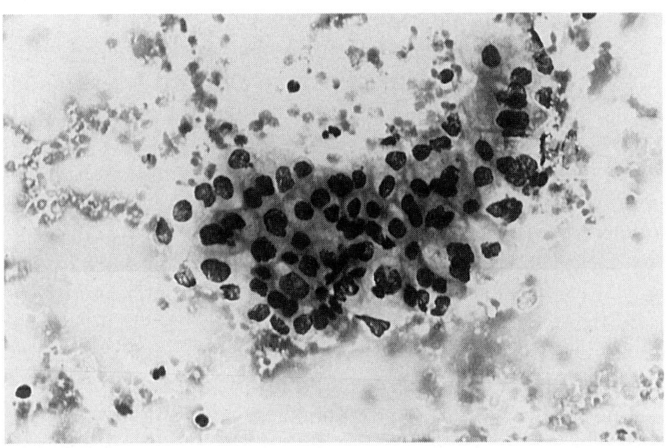

Figure 3–5. Clusters of cells from adenocarcinoma of pancreatic duct type, Case 3–5. The cells are large, with abundant clear to very slightly metachromatic cytoplasm. The nuclei are variable in size and shape, with coarse chromatin and irregular nuclear edges. Diff-Quik stain, ×400.

COMMUNICATION AND COLLABORATION WITH THE PATHOLOGIST

To achieve success with aspiration biopsy, a close working relationship must be established between the responsible clinician and the cytopathologist. This is particularly critical if the surgeon is the one performing the aspiration biopsy in that the cytopathologist does not have an opportunity to examine the patient or to review the clinical problem first-hand.

A detailed description of the location of the mass for biopsy, its consistency upon aspiration, the clinical history of the patient, and the clinician's differential diagnosis must be either clearly recorded in the report form by the aspirator or directly communicated verbally to the cytopathologist. The cytopathologist must render a report meaningful to the clinician—a report that makes sense within the framework of the clinical presentation. The quality of the aspirate obtained must be reported as well. No attempt should be made to develop a definitive interpretation on inadequate material or even on a good aspirate with incomplete clinical information. Also, when the initial cytologic diagnosis does not fit the clinical situation, caution is advised in terms of making major therapeutic decisions on the basis of cytologic findings alone.

Because critical diagnoses are based upon such small cellular or tissue samples in FNA biopsy cytology, experience and mutual trust between surgeon and pathologist are essential. The extent to which the cytopathologist can commit to definite diagnoses on the basis of FNA biopsy alone is predicated not only on specimen adequacy but also on past experience and implicit confidence in the clinical information furnished. Likewise, the surgeon's belief in FNA biopsy diagnoses depends on cumulative experience—individual and institutional—with a particular pathologist or group of pathologists. A "comfort index" on the part of surgeon and pathologist is achieved over months and years of handling cases together.

TECHNICAL ASPECTS OF FINE NEEDLE ASPIRATION

The basic equipment required for performance of aspiration biopsy is as follows (see Appendix 3–2):

1. Cameco Syringe Pistol, Aspir-Gun, or other type of aspiration handle.
2. 10.0- or 20.0-mL disposable plastic syringe with Luer-Lok tip depending on size of aspiration gun handle.
3. 22- to 23-gauge, 0.6- to 1.0-mm external diameter disposable needles, 3.8, 8.8, 15, and 20 cm long, with or without stylus.
4. Alcohol prep sponges and antiseptic sponges for deeper, transabdominal aspirations (transthoracic, bone, or deep soft tissue).
5. Sterile gauze pads.
6. Microscopic glass slides with frosted ends.
7. Small vial of balanced salt solution or RPMI tissue culture transport medium.
8. Suitable alcohol spray fixatives for immediate fixation of wet smears.
9. Vial of local anesthetic (e.g., 1 to 2% lidocaine) is optional. Topical spray anesthesia is useful for aspirates in children or intraoral aspirates.
10. Small vial of buffered glutaraldehyde for fixing aspirate for electron microscopy, if required.

A small plastic tray easily holds all the equipment. Local anesthetic is required for FNA biopsy of transthoracic or transabdominal masses and for oral mucosal masses but is rarely necessary for other clinically palpable lumps. Aspiration may be repeated in one procedure enough times to procure amounts of cellular material sufficient for conventional diagnostic purposes and for special tests such as flow cytometry, immunohistochemistry for tumor antigen markers, and electron microscopy (see Chap. 2).

Performance of the Aspiration

The steps in aspiration biopsy are listed next. Figure 3–6 illustrates the procedure for an enlarged cervical lymph node.

1. By palpation, attempt to determine the location of the lesion to be biopsied in relation to surrounding structures. Estimate its depth. Assess the optimal direction for approach to accomplish the aspiration biopsy.
2. Place the patient in a comfortable position for the procedure but with the mass readily palpable and easily grasped during the aspiration biopsy.
3. Grasp the lesion with one hand, usually between two fingers, or push it into a position where it seems fixed and stable.
4. Prepare the skin with an alcohol sponge, as for venipuncture.
5. Lay the syringe pistol with attached needle against the skin at the determined puncture site and angle.
6. With a quick motion, insert the needle through the skin.
7. Advance the needle into the mass.
8. Puncture of the target may be tested by differences in resistance, feeling that a capsule was penetrated, or by moving the syringe pistol very slightly laterally and detecting a corresponding movement of the mass beneath the fingers.
9. Apply suction to the aspirating syringe, usually about one-third the length of the syringe barrel.
10. Move the needle back and forth within the tumor with short, quick strokes and in *slightly* different directions.
11. *Note at all times the junction of the needle and the hub of the syringe for the appearance of any specimen.*
12. *At the first appearance of any sample at the junction of the syringe and the needle, release the trigger of the syringe pistol to let the vacuum in the syringe equate to normal.*
13. With air pressure in the syringe equalized, withdraw the needle from the mass.
14. Apply gentle pressure to the puncture site with a sterile gauze pad. The patient, a nurse, or an assistant may apply pressure to the puncture site while the aspirator turns to smear preparation and appropriate fixation.

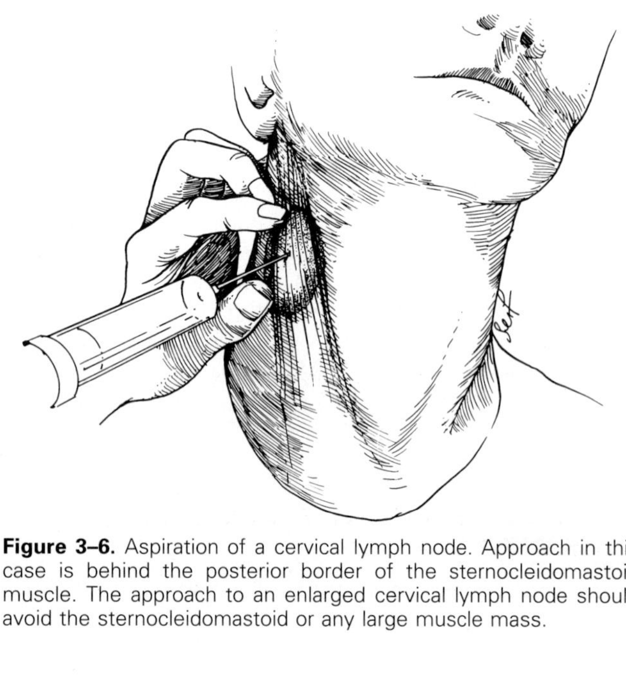

Figure 3–6. Aspiration of a cervical lymph node. Approach in this case is behind the posterior border of the sternocleidomastoid muscle. The approach to an enlarged cervical lymph node should avoid the sternocleidomastoid or any large muscle mass.

Deeply seated masses are usually best approached directly and perpendicularly to the skin surface. Superficial and very small tumors are best approached by penetrating the skin at a nearly horizontal plane, subsequently probing for the mass with the tip of the needle.

Step 2 is most important for head and neck aspiration biopsy, where the prominence of an enlarged lymph node, or lump, may depend on whether the patient is lying down or sitting up. The sternocleidomastoid muscle, with its relationship to the cervical lymph nodes, mandates positioning the patient so that a minimum of soft tissue is traversed before reaching the target. Aspirating through any large muscle mass should be avoided, as such tissue may fill the needle and be mistaken for a good sample.

When aspirating thyroid lesions, place a small pillow under the patient's upper back, extend the neck, and tilt the head back. The sternocleidomastoid muscle forms the lateral border of a groove bounded medially by the trachea, within which nodules of the thyroid can be isolated and immobilized (Fig. 3–7). Aspirating in a perpendicular plane along that groove can be done with no fear of puncturing the carotid artery or plugging up the needle with muscle tissue. The transverse vertebral process may act as a refer-

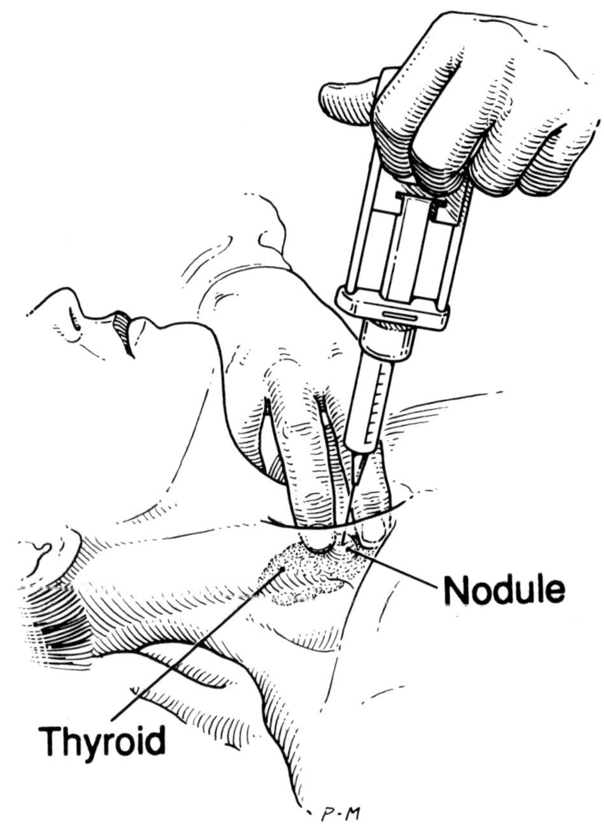

Figure 3–7. Technique of thyroid aspiration directing the needle in a perpendicular plane in the groove between the medial border of the sternocleidomastoid muscle and the lateral border of the trachea. For nodules that are in the deep part of the lobe, the transverse process of the vertebra is a reference point indicating that the thyroid has been completely penetrated. No important structures other than the thyroid are within this groove in a perpendicular plane.

ence point for deep-lying thyroid nodules. Inadvertently puncturing the trachea with a small needle is of no consequence. The patient may cough and it will be readily apparent that the trachea has been entered when vacuum is applied to the syringe.

The amount of suction should be modified in accordance with the type of target. For example, in the thyroid, minimal or no suction is often sufficient to obtain a biopsy, as the thyroid is generally quite vascular, exceptions being some tumors and chronic forms of thyroiditis. Reactive lymph nodes and some cases of chronic sialadenitis also produce excessive blood if too much suction is applied.

Aspiration is usually most effective when one describes with the needle a small cone, with the apex at the point where the needle penetrates the skin. If the target is large, multiple separate aspirates are indicated, describing overlapping cones. It is critical to successful aspiration to keep the material within the needle and not to aspirate excessive blood or fluid, which dilutes the cellular composition of the specimen (see step 12). Therefore the aspiration itself should be of very short duration in most instances.

Never withdraw the needle from the mass with any vacuum in the syringe pistol. With residual vacuum, the small aspirate biopsy will be pulled into the syringe, where

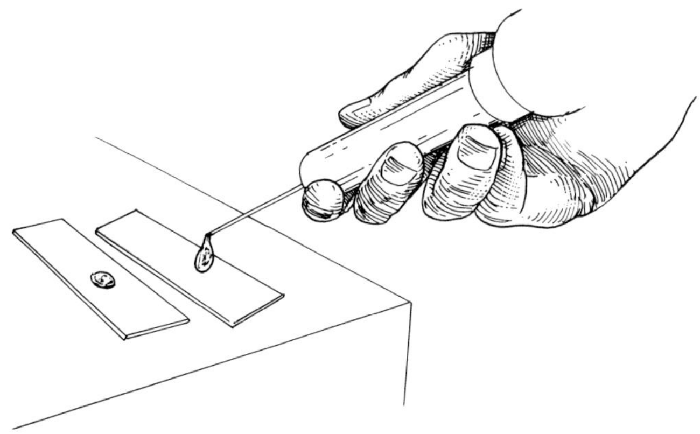

Figure 3–8. Aspirate is expressed as a 2- to 4-mm drop on the center of a plain glass slide. When expressing the drop, place the needle, bevel side down, on the surface of the glass slide to avoid splattering the drop, with resultant excessive air-drying before the smears can be prepared.

it is difficult to recover and where it begins to dry immediately. In such manner, the critical part of the specimen can be irretrievably lost.

If a cyst is detected, particularly in FNA biopsy of the breast, it should be evacuated as completely as possible. After evacuation of a cyst, *it is essential that any residual mass detected by subsequent palpation be reaspirated.* Remember that inclusion of additional blood and fluid is not better for aspiration biopsy but rather dilutes what tissue fragments and cells are present.

Becoming adept at FNA biopsy takes practice. This is possible using both cadavers and surgical specimens. Practice enables one to acquire skills in the technical aspects of FNA biopsy as well as the preparation of smears.

There are excellent instructional videos now available that emphasize the points above. The simple mechanics of aspiration can also be practiced using an apple or orange.

Making Aspiration Smears

The steps in making good aspiration biopsy smears are listed as follows (Figs. 3–8 through 3–10):

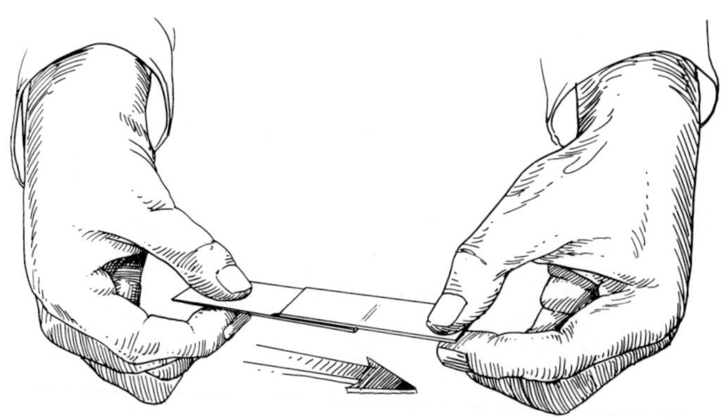

Figure 3–9. Smear prepared by pulling the slides apart horizontally as the drop of aspirate begins to spread. The weight of the glass slide is sufficient pressure on the aspirate to make an even smear. Alternatively, the slides may be pulled apart vertically as the drop of aspirate begins to spread, creating a relatively compact circular smear.

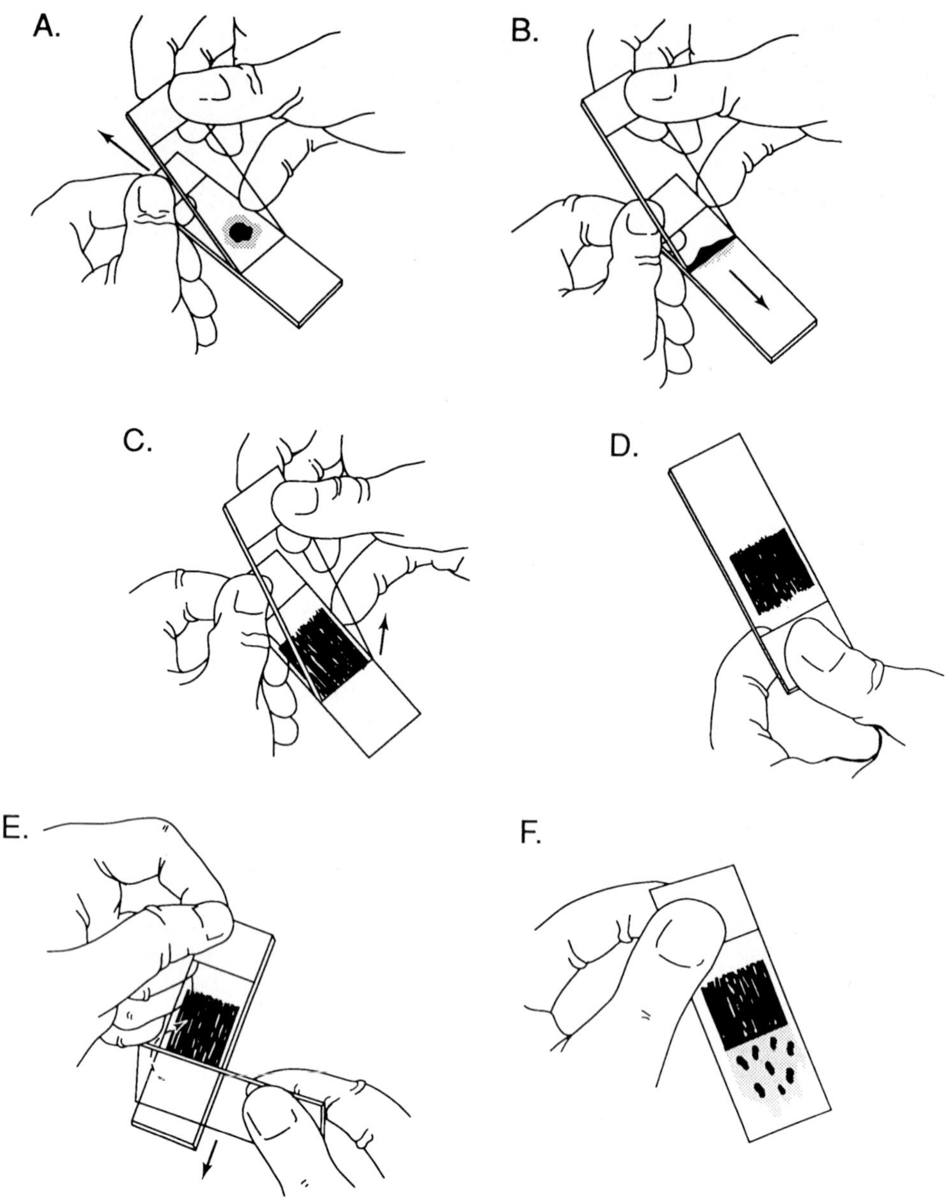

Figure 3–10. Steps in preparing aspiration smears from bloody samples. Steps A and B attempt to separate the blood from cellular material present by using the edge of the slide in the manner of making a blood smear and then lifting this slide clear of the smear and tilting the smear slide so that the blood runs away from the leading edge. Steps C and D take a clean slide to make the smear from the edge where cellular material may be more concentrated (E). Final smear shown in F, with cellular material, if present, concentrated in one area of the slide.

1. *Immediately* following completion of the aspiration, detach the needle from the syringe and fill the syringe with air.
2. Reattach the needle and place the needle in the center and *on the surface of a plain glass slide.*
3. Advance the plunger of the syringe to express a small drop of aspirate, 2 to 3 mm in diameter onto the slide (Fig. 3–8).
4. Carry out this procedure over a series of slides as quickly as possible.
5. Invert a second plain glass slide over the drop and, as it spreads, gently pull the two slides apart horizontally (Fig. 3–9).
6. Alternatively, as the drop spreads, pull the two slides apart vertically.
7. Repeat this procedure for all slides, immediately fixing those to be stained by *other* than Romanowsky (Diff-Quik, May-Grunwald-Giemsa, and so on) methods with 95% alcohol. Simply drop the slide into a suitable container of alcohol as for a conventional cervical Pap smear, or use a pump sprayer with alcohol (several are commercially available; see Appendix 3–2) to spray the material on the slides.
8. Allow unfixed smears to air-dry.

Care must be taken to place the bevel of the needle against the slide while expressing the biopsy, so that there is no intervening air gap. This prevents splattering or excessive air-drying prior to fixation in alcohol. With sufficient practice, it is possible to place all the aspirated material, normally four or five drops within a 3.8-cm (1½-in) needle, on a series of slides and then to begin actual smear preparation without encountering significant drying artifacts in those smears, which are then wet-fixed.

The important point is that the final smears should occupy only a small area of the slide. This creates a tissuelike pattern in the smears and reduces the area of the smears that must be screened for diagnostic features. Compressing smears (and pulling the slides apart vertically) and also consistently confines the smear to a small area of the slide. When preparing smears by pulling the slides apart horizontally, do it only once. *Do not scrub the sample back and forth, because this ruptures cells individually and ruins any tissuelike pattern.*

The method of smear preparation from bloody or other fluid aspirates is as follows (Fig. 3–10*A* to *F*):

1. Place the drop of biopsy material on slide A, as described previously, usually 5 to 10 mm in diameter.
2. Hold slide A with the drop of biopsy in the left hand.
3. Hold a second slide, B, with the right hand and bring the edge of slide B up to the drop.
4. The drop will spread along the edge of slide B. As it does, push the edge of slide B toward the end farthest from the drop of bloody aspirate in the manner of making a blood smear and about halfway down slide A.
5. At that point, lift slide B straight up.
6. Immediately tilt slide A away from the leading edge of the smear, so that the blood runs back toward the original point of the placement of the biopsy sample.
7. Continue smear preparation by rotating slide B 90°, so that there is a clean edge. Use this edge of slide B to make a smear from the leading edge of slide A.

Aspiration biopsies that are diluted by fluid or blood do not provide optimal smears. They cover large areas of the slide and are very dilute in relation to any cellular material present.

There is the mistaken belief that aspiration of large bloody samples is of value. This is not true. Blood pulled into the syringe should be placed entirely in a small container of 10% buffered formalin to be processed as a cell block.

Smears should be made only from the sample left within the needle. Large volumes of blood, even a few milliliters, will result in quick clotting. This greatly interferes with good smear preparation. Cells become entrapped within the clotted blood, distorting the picture of the smear and resulting in heavy and uneven staining. It is important to learn to be quick and sure with the mechanics of the aspiration procedure and smear preparation.

Franseen-style needles (with a notched tip) have a tendency to provide microcores. Such contents usually need to be dislodged by inserting the stylus into the needle and pushing them out onto a plain glass slide. *One should not attempt to smear these small cores.* If an immediate diagnosis is needed, they can be rolled gently over a small area of the slide to make an imprint, but the core should then quickly be placed in fixative for small biopsy tissue processing. These cores are particularly valuable in problem cases, as they give a tissue pattern more familiar to the surgical pathologists and they can be used for special stains including immunocytochemistry.

For specimens that are largely fluid (e.g., breast and thyroid cysts), place the sample into a clean container with an equal volume of *50%* alcohol in order to provide initial fixation, and transport to the pathology laboratory. Do not use concentrations of alcohol higher than 50%. Depending upon the laboratory's preferred method for examining cyst fluids cytologically, it may be preferred that fluids be submitted fresh and unfixed. This is best accomplished by placing the fluid into a clean container with an equal volume of balanced salt solution, refrigerating (but not freezing) the sample until transport to the laboratory. If refrigerated, fluids can retain good cellular preservation in balanced salt solution for up to 48 hours or even longer. It is important to check with the laboratory that handles your specimens in regard to how they wish to receive aspiration biopsies and fluids and to work closely with that laboratory to ensure optimal samples for interpretation.

SPECIAL PROBLEMS WITH SPECIMENS INCLUDING CYSTS

The author believes that fluid from breast cysts that is clear and yellow in color does not need to be examined cytologically and can be discarded. Any other gross type of fluid from breast aspirates and cyst fluid from all other sites aspirated should be sent for cytological examination. In the case of cysts, reexamination for any residual mass after cyst evacuation is much more important than submitting the clear yellow fluid for cytologic examination. When aspirating masses in and around the thyroid, the surgeon may encounter a cyst with water-clear fluid. This is essentially diagnostic of a parathyroid cyst. The fluid or a portion thereof may be submitted for determination of parathormone levels, which are usually highly elevated.

A rare lesion, and one that is difficult to recognize, is cystic papillary carcinoma of the thyroid. Clinical clues to this condition are fresh blood in a thyroid cyst fluid, a residual mass after aspiration of a thyroid cyst, or a cyst that immediately refills after aspiration. In the author's experience, the vast majority of thyroid cysts that do reaccumulate fluid are cystic nonneoplastic goiters. The reaccumulation takes place slowly over weeks, months, or even years. Use of thyroid suppression may keep this process in check. A good policy is to aspirate the cyst two or three times. If, on suppression therapy, the cyst refills again, surgical excision should be considered. Occasionally such a case will be cystic degeneration of a follicular adenoma.

STAINING, INITIAL EVALUATION, AND PROVISIONAL DIAGNOSIS

Air-dried smears are stained by the Romanowsky methods. Smears that have been spray-fixed with 95% ethyl, methyl, or isopropyl alcohol or that have been submerged in these fixatives are suitable for Papanicolaou staining. If the laboratory prefers staining by rapid hematoxylin and eosin, the smears will benefit from immersion for a few seconds in equal parts of 50% ethyl alcohol and 10% neutral buffered formalin. The quality of the aspirate and the smear can be checked. The use of rapid stains can allow diagnosis in some cases immediately following the aspiration biopsy. Repeat aspirates, if necessary, can then be obtained for both conventional preparations and special studies.

I have used a rapid (90 seconds) Pap stain to stain some aspiration biopsy smears.[9] This rapid stain, developed by

Yang and Alvarez, has several advantages over other Pap stains that take several minutes. All smears may be air dried—an advantage to clinicians—since they do not have to be concerned about improper or delayed fixation. The smears are rehydrated briefly in normal saline, which hemolyzes the red blood cells—a second advantage with bloody smears. Comparable cellularity of smears to those stained by Romanowsky methods is maintained, which is another advantage. Using this rapid Pap method, the cytoplasm of squamous epithelial cells may be less differentially stained as seen with the conventional Pap stain, but this has not proven to be of any disadvantage.

SPECIAL PREPARATION METHODS FOR ANCILLARY STUDIES

Immunocytochemistry and/or electron microscopy may be needed in selected cases to establish a diagnosis precisely. Common differential problems include large-cell lymphoma versus anaplastic carcinoma versus sarcoma, the differential diagnosis of small round-cell tumors in children, and identification of small numbers of tumor cells in necrotic metastatic tumor in lymph nodes. Evaluation of the initial rapidly stained smears may indicate the need for these types of ancillary studies. For immunocytochemistry, cell block material is the most valuable. A separate aspiration should be taken for these studies. Material for cell block can be placed directly into buffered 10% formaldehyde or other conventional fixative.

Interpretation of the Report

On the report form for FNA biopsy, the aspirator, either clinician or pathologist, supplies demographics, history, and the procedure performed. The microscopic findings and diagnosis are the responsibility of the cytopathologist. The diagnosis should include the site as well as the morphology—for example ''squamous-cell carcinoma, keratinizing, metastatic to right cervical lymph node following same from tongue.'' These cytologic diagnoses are rendered in the same manner as standard surgical pathology diagnoses. They are complete diagnoses. If the cytopathologist is unsure or feels that a definitive diagnosis cannot be made, this must be explicitly stated. Examples of uncertainty are ''atypical cells of undetermined type or significance, from aspirate of right cervical lymph node,'' and ''nondiagnostic aspirate of left breast mass.'' Recommendations for appropriate additional studies are indicated, including a possible request for repeat aspiration biopsy. A recommendation for an open biopsy may be made in some cases, depending on the degree of certainty of the cytopathologist in the reporting of the aspiration biopsy. An intraoperative frozen section should be specifically suggested in some cases after aspiration biopsy if the cytopathologist cannot make a definitive diagnosis of malignancy, and immediate major surgery would be indicated were such a diagnosis rendered. In view of the current legal climate in the United States, it may be advisable to confirm a diagnosis of malignant aspiration biopsy by intraoperative frozen section, particularly if the contemplated surgery is extensive. Even with this caveat, the aspiration biopsy is still quite useful because, among patients with suspected malignant tumors, it distinguishes between those that definitely require immediate surgery and those that do not.

Complications and Liability

Most ''lumps and bumps'' considered for FNA biopsy are superficially located or at least in such a position that they are not closely related to anatomic structures hazardous for biopsy. Complications from FNA biopsy of superficial masses are few and of little consequence. These include some minor discomfort in the area of the aspiration, usually lasting no more than a few hours, some bruising and discoloration of the aspiration site, and, rarely, small hematomas. Complications are directly related to needle size and have been less than 0.03% in a review of published series when needles of gauge 20 or finer have been used.[7] Needle tract seeding of tumors has been reported only rarely with this size needle; most such cases are poorly documented. The author has observed no cases of needle tract seeding in either superficial or deep aspirations in performing or assisting in this procedure since 1972.

With superficial aspiration biopsy, particularly in the area of the head and neck, some patients may experience light-headedness or actual syncope. Most of these patients have had similar vasovagal responses to needle puncture in the past. A history of such a tendency can usually be elicited prior to biopsy, allowing suitable precautions to be taken. Another very rare complication with breast aspiration, and occasionally with sampling of a supraclavicular or high axillary lymph node, is pneumothorax. For breast aspirations in patients with small breasts or with a mass deeply placed at the margin of the breast, care should be taken to angle the aspiration needle away from the chest wall so as to avoid this complication.

There are three areas of vulnerability to legal action following FNA biopsy. These are false-negative diagnosis of malignancy, a false-positive diagnosis of malignancy, and complications of the needle aspiration procedure itself.

A false-negative diagnosis may arise in diverse ways: failure to find or recognize malignant cells that are present; inadequate or poorly prepared samples; missing the actual tumor by aspiration; and characteristics intrinsic to some tumors, such as sclerosis, which render them poorly suited to the FNA biopsy approach. Avoiding the first problem, that of failure to recognize malignant cells, is fully the responsibility of the cytopathologist, while most of the remaining problems are those of the aspirator. They reflect the importance of attention to details in all aspects of the FNA biopsy method.

Aspiration of the breast presents the potential problem of false-negative results. Patients are often referred for FNA biopsy due to vague ''thickenings'' of the breast that do not constitute a defined mass and are not suspicious for malignancy. The entire breast is often ''lumpy.'' With a benign FNA biopsy report and a benign appearance of the mammogram, the risk of a breast cancer's being overlooked is quite small. Most such patients can be followed safely at regular intervals both with physical examination scrutiny for any changes, or the development of a definite mass, and with serial mammography. If a clear-cut plan of follow-up is established and is understood by the patient, the rare small carcinoma that may be missed for a time in this type of situation should not adversely affect prognosis. Emphasis must be placed on a precise plan for follow-up for this group of patients with negative FNA biopsy in order to avoid the potential adverse effect of an unrealistically long-term sense of security from a false-negative result. As Stewart concluded, the surgeon and the pathologist must function as an intelligent team. Ultimately, the surgeon must decide in each case, on the combined basis of clinical features, the likelihood of the FNA biopsy being representative, and the confidence in the FNA biopsy interpretation whether to accept a diagnosis of "negative for malignancy" as a final step in the patient's evaluation.

False-positive results are invariably the result of overreading atypical-appearing cells, usually few in number. If a malignant diagnosis from FNA biopsy does not fit the clinical picture, the surgeon is wise to ask for a review of the slides specifically with this question in mind. Good sampling is important for accurate diagnosis, because masses that consistently yield few cells despite the performance of a technically good FNA biopsy, regardless of suspicion of abnormality, are nearly always benign. The notable exception is in the breast, where both fibroadenomas and benign phyllodes tumors often contain large numbers of atypical cells in aspiration biopsy. Such cells may even appear to infiltrate fat that is found in the smears, thus simulating the pattern of invasive carcinoma. Although myoepithelial cells are often present in such cases, usually in large numbers, in this way indicating a benign lesion, they may be few in number and easily overlooked by the cytopathologist.

PITFALLS FOR THE SURGEON

The most common pitfall for the surgeon is failure to procure a good specimen from aspiration biopsy. This should be judged not on the total volume of sample but rather on the numbers of cells obtained and their distribution upon the slide. More sample is not necessarily better if most of it is only blood or cyst fluid. There is no substitute for proper technique. The target for aspiration must be clearly and completely identified and a clinical differential diagnosis should be transmitted to the pathologist. "What are the indications for this aspiration biopsy?" and "What do I wish to learn to influence my management of this patient?" are the two fundamental questions that the surgeon should always have in mind and effectively communicate when using aspiration biopsy.[8]

PITFALLS FOR THE PATHOLOGIST

The pathologist's most obvious pitfall is trying to read too much into limited material, particularly with inadequate clinical information. The seven "golden rules" of aspiration biopsy are listed below.[8] They are worth remembering at all times.

1. Be aware of the limitations of FNA biopsy for the body site being sampled.
2. Obtain cellular samples that are adequate and well prepared.
3. Be aware of the diagnostic pitfalls for each body site sampled.
4. Correlate cytologic impressions with the patient's history and physical findings.
5. Live within your experience and limitations.
6. Compare the cytology of FNA biopsy with tissue samples whenever they are available.
7. Maintain good lines of communication among clinician, cytopathologist, and patient.

FURTHER READING

Abele JS, Miller TR. Implementation of an outpatient needle aspiration biopsy service and clinic: A personal perspective. In: *Cytopathology Annual,* Baltimore: Williams & Wilkins; 1993:43–71.

Frable WJ. Thin needle aspiration biopsy. In: Bennington J, ed. *Major Problems in Pathology.* Vol 14. Philadelphia: Saunders; 1983.

Koss LG, Woyke S, Olszewski W: *Aspiration Biopsy: Cytologic Interpretation and Histologic Bases,* 2nd ed. New York: Igaku-Shoin; 1993.

Orell SR, Sterrett GF, Walters Max N-I, et al: *Manual and Atlas of Fine Needle Aspiration Cytology,* 2nd ed. New York: Churchill Livingstone; 1992.

REFERENCES

1. Martin HE, Ellis EB. Biopsy by needle puncture and aspiration. *Ann Surg.* 1930;92:169–181.

2. Stewart FW. The diagnosis of tumors by aspiration biopsy. *Am J Pathol.* 1933;9:801–812.
3. Lopes Cardozo P. *Clinical Cytology.* Leiden: Stafleu, 1954.
4. Zajicek J. Aspiration biopsy cytology: Part I. Cytology of Supradiaphragmatic Organs. *Monographs in Clinical Cytology.* Vol 4. New York: Karger; 1974:1–15, 20–26.
5. Soderstrom N. *Fine Needle Aspiration Biopsy.* Stockholm: Almqvist & Wiksell; 1966:13–18.
6. Linsk JA, Franzen S. *Clinical Aspiration Cytology,* 2nd ed. New York: Lippincott; 1989.
7. Powers CN. *Cytopathology Annual.* 1995. In press.
8. Stanley MW, Lowhagen T. *Fine Needle Aspiration of Palpable Masses.* Boston: Butterworth-Heinemann; 1993.
9. Yang GCH, Alvarez II. Ultrafast Papanicolaou stain. An alternative preparation for fine needle aspiration cytology. *Acta Cytol.* 1995;39:55–60.

Sample Patient Brochures for Fine Needle Aspiration Biopsy

accurate diagnosis upon which to begin treatment. When this happens, the doctor will often order a surgical biopsy or other tests. It is important to find out exactly what the lump is.

HOW LONG DOES IT TAKE TO OBTAIN THE RESULTS OF THE FINE NEEDLE ASPIRATION BIOPSY?

The material obtained by aspiration biopsy is immediately examined under the microscope by a physician experienced in cytopathology to make a *preliminary* diagnosis of your problem and to assure that a sufficient amount of tissue is present for final study and special tests if they are indicated. We will notify your doctor of the preliminary findings, who will make them known to you upon request. If you have been referred by a physician outside of The Medical College of Virginia, the physicians directing the aspiration biopsy service may make the preliminary results of your biopsy known to you upon request.

Your doctor is notified of the ***final*** results of your biopsy only after all the tissue obtained is thoroughly examined. In most cases this process takes from 24-48 hours. However, you may have to wait an extra day or two if special tests are required on your aspiration biopsy sample.

ANY MORE QUESTIONS?
PLEASE WRITE THEM DOWN BELOW.

The Aspiration Biopsy Service is available to answer questions from 8:00 A.M. to 4:30 P.M. weekdays at the following numbers, 786-9743, 786-9738.

MEDIA PRODUCTION DEPARTMENT

FINE NEEDLE ASPIRATION BIOPSY

Your Appointment for an Aspiration Biopsy

Division of Surgical and Cytopathology
Medical College of Virginia
Virginia Commonwealth University

Your doctor has recently found that you have a lump and has scheduled you for or requested a **fine needle aspiration biopsy.** This procedure is a good way to find out what this lump might be because it is fast, safe and reliable and will cause you only minimal discomfort. Fine needle aspiration biopsy is not new being invented in the United States over 60 years ago. FNAB has been in continuous use at MCV for over 20 years. Fine needle aspiration biopsy is also a procedure quite useful for determining the nature of lumps found in children. This pamphlet will explain what **fine needle aspiration biopsy** is and will answer some of your questions. Please read it carefully. If you have other questions write them down in the space on the back of this pamphlet or ask the doctors who will perform the aspiration biopsy (when you come for your appointment). All of your questions will be answered before the biopsy is done.

WHY DO I NEED A BIOPSY?

A lump may result from several different causes including infection, excessive normal tissue growth or fluid collection, a benign tumor, or a malignancy (cancer). Most lumps are not malignant but your doctor's treatment of the lump will depend upon its exact nature. **Fine needle aspiration** is a simple test that often tells the doctor how to proceed with your treatment.

ARE THERE ALTERNATIVES?

Until recently, the usual method of obtaining a tissue diagnosis was a minor operation called a surgical biopsy. Surgical biopsy is highly reliable, but can involve some discomfort, is usually more expensive and has several risks, such as bleeding, infection and scar tissue formation. Fine needle aspiration can, in most cases, accurately determine the nature of the lump more safely and comfortably than surgical biopsy.

HOW IS THE ASPIRATION BIOPSY PERFORMED?

After cleansing the skin overlying the lump, a very small needle is passed through the skin and into the mass. The needle is less than one millimeter in diameter. It is smaller than the needles used in most laboratories to draw blood from your arm. During the procedure you may briefly feel some discomfort like that encountered when a laboratory technician draws blood from your arm. The aspiration biopsy takes only a few seconds to perform. One to three separate biopsies of the lump are taken during your visit.

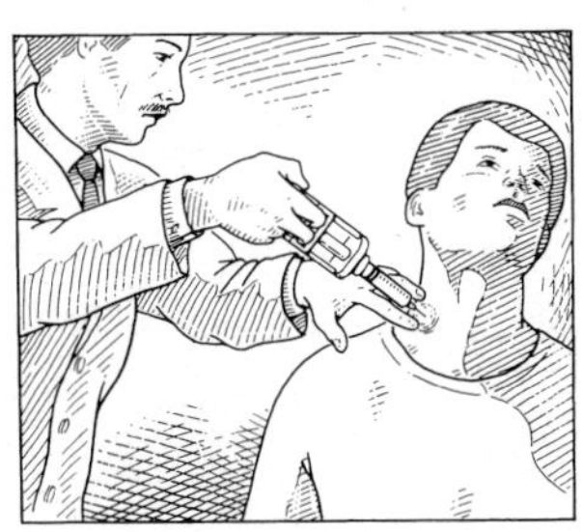

After the aspiration biopsy, you will be able to drive, return to work, or perform any other activity that you normally do. Continue taking any medicine your doctor has given you as directed since the biopsy does not affect medication schedules.

WHAT ARE THE RISKS ASSOCIATED WITH FINE NEEDLE ASPIRATION BIOPSY?

Fine needle aspiration poses no significant risk to you. Some patients report a mild, dull, throbbing sensation in the area of the biopsy, which usually subsides within 30 to 60 minutes. This minor discomfort does not bother most patients and requires no medication. A small bruise or tenderness may occur at the aspiration site. If you experience any unusual discomfort or swelling, please call your doctor. Some patients have experienced lightheadedness as may also occur with the giving of a sample of blood. This is quite rare with aspiration biopsy. Please inform the doctor taking the biopsy if you have experienced this problem in the past when a blood sample was taken.

Some patients have expressed concern that passage of a needle through a tumor might cause the tumor to spread. This concern has been examined by scientists at several universities and is considered to be highly unlikely.

Finally, the risk of infection exists any time the skin is penetrated. However several thousand biopsies have been done by the aspiration biopsy service without a single case of infection having been reported to date.

WHAT RESULT CAN I EXPECT FROM THIS BIOPSY?

About 85-90% of the time, the biopsy result can tell the doctor the exact nature of the lump so that correct treatment can be determined. About 5 percent of the time the biopsy can tell something about the lump, but will not give the doctor all the information that may be needed to determine your treatment. In the remaining 5-10 percent of cases, it is not possible to obtain enough tissue from a particular lump for an aspiration biopsy, write them below. Your doctor will be happy to answer them. You can also call MCV's Fine Needle Aspiration Biopsy Service at (804) 786-9743 or (804) 786-9738. (Ask for the supervisor of cytology, who can direct your call to the right person.)

1. ______________________________

2. ______________________________

3. ______________________________

4. ______________________________

WHAT YOU NEED TO KNOW ABOUT FINE NEEDLE ASPIRATION BIOPSY

Department of Pathology
Medical College of Virginia
Virginia Commonwealth University

MEDIA PRODUCTION DEPARTMENT

WHY DO I NEED A FINE NEEDLE ASPIRATION BIOPSY?

Your doctor has recently found that you have a lump. Whenever a doctor finds a lump in a person's body, it is important to find out what kind of lump it is. Sometimes a lump is only a cyst, but sometimes it can be a cancerous growth.

Fine needle aspiration biopsy is a good way to find out more about a lump. Fine needle aspiration biopsy is also safe, quick and dependable.

This brochure explains what fine needle aspiration biopsy is. (Your doctor or nurse may also call it an "FNA biopsy.") It also lets you know what you can expect when you have a fine needle aspiration biopsy. If you have any questions after you read this brochure, please write them in the space on the back page. Your doctor will be happy to answer your questions.

WHAT IS FINE NEEDLE ASPIRATION BIOPSY?

Most of the time, a lump is nothing to worry about. Lumps can be caused by an infection, a cyst or scar tissue. But some lumps can be caused by cancerous growths.

To find out more about a lump, a doctor needs samples of the lump to look at under a microscope. Fine needle aspiration biopsy lets a doctor collect these tiny samples.

Fine needle aspiration biopsy is a lot like giving blood. The good news is, the needle used in fine needle aspiration biopsy is even smaller than the needle used when you give blood. And the needle goes into your lump, not into your vein. The whole process takes only a few seconds.

WHAT DOES A FINE NEEDLE ASPIRATION BIOPSY FEEL LIKE?

Fine needle aspiration biopsy feels like giving blood (or getting a shot). Sometimes doctors want more than one sample of your lump, so you may have two or three fine needle aspiration biopsies during your office visit.

Some patients say they feel a mild pain during or just after the fine needle aspiration biopsy. (The pain usually goes away within an hour). If you notice any redness or swelling in the area where you had your biopsy, call your doctor. (Sometimes the place where the needle entered your body can become infected, but this is very rare). Also call your doctor if the area continues to be painful.

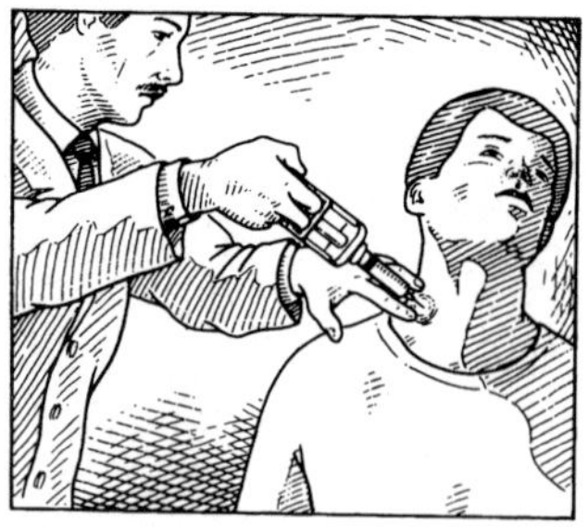

Let your doctor know if you are a person who feels lightheaded when you give blood. Some patients say they feel lightheaded after fine needle aspiration biopsy, but this does not happen very often.

After the fine needle aspiration biopsy, you should be able to drive home or return to work. Unless your doctor tells you differently, after the biopsy you can do whatever you usually do. (**Reminder:** Fine needle aspiration biopsy does **not** affect medications. You should stay on your normal medication schedule.)

WHEN WILL I GET THE RESULTS OF MY FINE NEEDLE ASPIRATION BIOPSY?

You should get the results of your biopsy within two days. Sometimes you may have to wait an extra day or two if the doctor needs to run more tests on your samples.

Most of the time, your fine needle aspiration biopsy will tell your doctor everything he or she needs to know about your lump. If more samples from your lump are needed, your doctor may order a surgical biopsy or other tests.

To protect your privacy, the MCV staff will not give out test results over the phone. Only your doctor can tell you the results of your fine needle aspiration biopsy.

DO YOU HAVE ANY QUESTIONS ABOUT FINE NEEDLE ASPIRATION BIOPSY?

If you have questions about fine needle

APPENDIX 3–2

Equipment for Fine Needle Aspiration Biopsy

1. Cameco Syringe Pistol. 20.0- and 10.0-mL size. Available from Precision Dynamics Corporation, 13880 Del Sur St., San Fernando, CA 91340–3490. Tel: 1-800-847-0670.
2. Aspir-Gun. Available from Everst Company, 5 Sherman Street, Linden, NJ 07036.
3. Inrad Aspiration Biopsy Syringe Gun. Available from INRAD Inc., 620 Watson S.W., Grand Rapids, MI 49504. Tel: 1-800-253-1540.
4. 20.0- and 10.0-mL disposable plastic syringe with Luer-Lok tip. Available from Becton Dickinson, Division of Becton Dickinson & Company, Rutherford, NJ 07070.
5. 22-, 23-, and 25-gauge 0.6- to 1.0-mm external diameter disposable needles 3.8 and 8.8 cm long, with or without mandrin. (Used for most aspirations of palpable lumps.) Available from Becton Dickinson, Division of Becton Dickinson & Company, Rutherford, NJ 07070.
6. Aspiration biopsy needles 15 and 20 cm (6 and 7 in) long, 21- and 22-gauge, with or without mandrin. (For biopsy of lung, transabdominal use, pelvic masses, and prostate.) Available from Cook Co. Inc., P.O. Box 227, Spencer, IN 47460. Both Chiba-style and Franseen-type needles are available from Cook Co. Inc.
7. Franseen-style needle, 22-gauge, 3½ in, with mandrin, available from Manan Mfg. Co., Inc., Skokie, IL 60076. Distributed by First Medical Supply Inc., P.O. Box 634, Baltimore, MD 21203. Tel: 1-301-377-1519.

4

The Skin

Donald R. Pulitzer, Donald Serafin,
and William G. Kraybill

The skin may be viewed as the organ of interface, serving as a boundary and medium through which we communicate with our environment. Although it is our most familiar organ, its functions, complexities, and perhaps its very importance are often poorly understood or overlooked. The skin is an organ through which many diseases are revealed, yet it often serves as a barrier to the diagnosis and management of such processes. Indeed, for the surgeon, the adage "Never let the skin get between you and the diagnosis," may be a daily reality. Despite major advances in radiologic imaging and laboratory sciences over the past decades, for disease processes requiring surgical and nonsurgical management, a microscopic tissue diagnosis remains an essential prerequisite.

Functions of the Skin

The skin is an effective barrier to harmful agents in the environment, including noxious chemicals, microorganisms, and ultraviolet light. In addition, the skin is a cushion with limited, yet important, capabilities in reducing the effects of mechanical trauma. Sensory input supplies vital information that allows us to successfully respond to our immediate environment. The skin also performs important metabolic functions, notably vitamin D metabolism and melanin production. Lastly, the skin's important role in the immune system has been defined in recent decades.

For the surgeon, the skin presents both challenges and opportunities. Many skin conditions are associated with underlying abnormalities. Examples include pyoderma gangrenosum in patients with inflammatory bowel disease and cutaneous metastases in patients with visceral malignancies. Either directly by the patient or through consultation, the surgeon may be asked to participate in the diagnosis (biopsy) or management of skin conditions. Large burns, for example, are usually managed by surgeons, who may eventually perform skin grafts and reconstructive procedures. Some skin diseases are encountered by the surgeon while treating patients with nondermatologic conditions.

Histology

The skin has three basic layers: epidermis, dermis, and subcutaneous tissue (subcutis) (Fig. 4–1). The epidermis serves as a barrier and is comprised predominantly of cells whose primary function is keratin production: *keratinocytes*. The keratinocytes are arranged in successively designated layers, from the *basal layer* (germinative layer) to the *keratin layer* (stratum corneum), where the cells are flat and anucleate. In addition to keratinocytes, the epidermis contains melanin-producing cells, *melanocytes*. The epidermis also contains *Langerhans cells*, specialized histocytes that process foreign antigens for presentation to other components of the immune system. Small numbers of *Merkel cells*, which are believed to function as mechanoreceptors, are also present within the epidermis. Microscopically, melanocytes appear as clear cells within the basal layer of the epidermis. Langerhans cells appear as clear cells in more superficial layers of the epidermis. Merkel cells are not recognizable by conventional light microscopy.

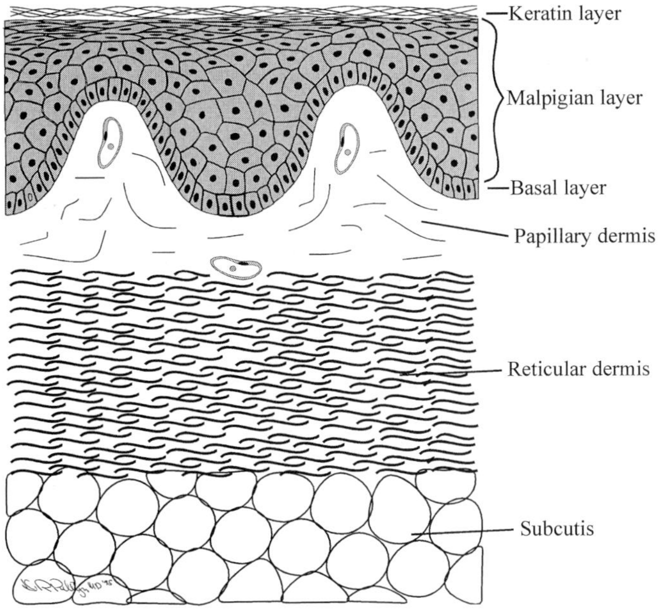

Figure 4–1. Basic histology of the skin.

The dermis is divided into two zones: the *papillary dermis* and the *reticular dermis*. The former is richly vascular and serves primarily a nutritive role for the avascular epidermis and skin appendages (*adventitial dermis*). The reticular dermis consists primarily of thick collagen bundles; its primary function is presumed to be mechanical support. The skin appendages, eccrine and apocrine sweat glands, sebaceous glands, hair follicles, and nails, are derived from the epidermis to which they connect. In conditions in which the epidermis is destroyed, it is regenerated primarily by the proliferation of cells from the skin appendages. The dermis also contains numerous blood vessels and nerves as well as arrector pili muscles for hair erection.

Embryologically, the skin is derived from ectoderm, mesoderm, and neuroectoderm. The epidermis and skin appendages are of ectodermal origin. Arrector pili muscles, blood vessels, and connective tissues are derived from mesoderm. Nerves, melanocytes, and special sensory organs are of neuroectodermal origin.

The Surgical Approach to Pathologic Conditions of the Skin

Patients may come to the attention of the surgeon through a number of channels. Patients will often consult a surgeon directly when they think that a skin lesion needs to be removed. In other instances, patients are referred to a surgeon for purposes of diagnosis (incisional biopsy) or definitive treatment (excision) of a lesion. Lastly, a skin lesion may be noticed coincidentally by the surgeon while evaluating the patient for another condition.

If the diagnosis is in doubt after examination, a surgical biopsy should be considered. If the lesion is solitary and small, an excisional biopsy is the best approach. If, however, the lesion is large or if it occurs in multiple areas, a punch or an incisional biopsy is appropriate. The surgeon must weigh the aesthetic consequences of a biopsy. If the biopsy site would cause an unsightly scar or depression, a shave biopsy is an option. When alternatives remain unclear, particularly for larger lesions, a plastic surgery consultation is indicated (Table 4–1).

PUNCH BIOPSY

Ideally, a punch biopsy is obtained from a nonexposed site. Biopsy punches range in size from 2 to 6 mm in diameter. In general, the larger the biopsy, the happier the pathologist. Subtle conditions may be difficult or even missed if the biopsy specimen is small. If material is required for concomitant bacterial and fungal culture, a relatively large biopsy (4 mm or more) is preferable so that the specimen can be bisected to serve two purposes. A punch biopsy should be full thickness and include epidermis, dermis, and subcutis. Ideally, biopsy samples should include an adjacent portion of uninvolved skin. This may be difficult to achieve with small punch biopsies. For this reason, in cases in which uninvolved adjacent skin is critical for diagnosis, an incisional biopsy should be considered. The surgical technique of punch biopsy is a simple office procedure. The area is infiltrated with local anesthetic, which usually contains epinephrine for hemostasis. The biopsy is performed without tissue orientation and submitted to the pathologist for permanent sectioning. The punch biopsy site is usually left to heal by secondary intention. This technique is efficient and relatively inexpensive.

INCISIONAL BIOPSY

An incisional biopsy is indicated when (1) the lesion is large or multiple; (2) a significant portion of uninvolved

Table 4–1. Recommended Therapy for Common Neoplasms of the Skin

Epidermal Neoplasms	
Keratoacanthoma	Complete excision
Superficial basal-cell CA	Cryotherapy
Basal-cell carcinoma	Complete excision
Sclerosing basal-cell carcinoma	Complete excision
Squamous-cell carcinoma	Complete excision
Skin appendage tumors	Complete excision
Dermal Neoplasms	
Kaposi's sarcoma	Excision/radiation/chemotherapy
Atypical fibroxanthoma	Complete excision
Dermatofibrosarcoma protuberans	Complete excision
Melanocytic Lesions	
Atypical nevus	Complete excision
"Melanoma in situ"	Complete excision with 0.5-cm margin
Lentigo maligna	Complete excision with 0.5-cm margin
Melanoma (1 mm thick or less)	Complete excision with 1.0-cm margin
Melanoma (1–4 mm thick)	Complete excision with 2.0-cm margin

tissue surrounding a small lesion needs to be included with the biopsy specimen; (3) a lesion is deeply situated and inaccessible by punch biopsy; and (4) a surgical approximation of the wound edges is a consideration. Incisional biopsy is more complicated than punch biopsy. Unlike punch biopsy, the wound must be closed following partial excision of the lesion. Consequently, a setup for surgery is required for sterile technique and instrumentation. Incisional biopsy specimens are submitted to the pathologist in the fresh state for intraprocedural frozen section evaluation or in formalin for permanent sectioning. If indicated, the specimen is marked with a suture for orientation. The precise anatomic site, e.g., "left forearm, dorsum," must be specified for the pathologist to correctly orient the specimen.

EXCISIONAL BIOPSY

An excisional biopsy is useful when (1) the lesion is small and can be easily excised, avoiding an additional future surgical procedure (if dictated by the nature of the lesion); (2) the diagnosis is suspected on clinical grounds and total removal of the lesion is required for appropriate treatment; and (3) following removal the aesthetic consequences dictate the selection of this technique. Pigmented lesions should be removed by excisional biopsy whenever possible. Other types of biopsy may compromise the ability to accurately discern thickness in malignant melanomas. Large pigmented lesions of the face may best be evaluated with punch or incisional biopsies of the thickest portion of the lesion followed by therapeutic excision as indicated. Like an incisional biopsy, operating facilities must be available to ensure an optimal result.

SHAVE BIOPSY

A shave biopsy is a useful technique when (1) the superficial layer of the epidermis and dermis would be expected to provide accurate diagnosis and (2) when a benign diagnosis is anticipated and the consequences of incisional or excisional biopsy would be undesirable (e.g., nevi in the head and neck region). The deep dermal elements, including epithelial appendages, are spared in this biopsy procedure, allowing the wound to reepithelialize and heal with minimal scarring. This technique is performed as an office procedure requiring infiltration with local lidocaine solution with epinephrine. The superficial shave is done with a modified razor blade or scalpel. This is a rapid and cost-effective diagnostic method with satisfactory aesthetic results. However, shave biopsy is not considered appropriate if malignant melanoma is in the clinical differential diagnosis.

SHAVE EXCISION

Many dermatologists use the shave excision technique to treat benign, premalignant, and minimally invasive squamous cell carcinomas and basal cell carcinomas. The technique is similar to that of a shave biopsy; however, the central specimen often extends to the deep (reticular) dermis. To control hemostasis and ensure extirpation of the malignant lesion, the base and periphery of the lesion are electrodesiccated. This technique leaves an open wound, which, when small, heals by wound contraction and reepithelization. However, scarring is often unacceptable and conspicuous if the lesion occurs in an exposed area such as the face.

CRYOTHERAPY

Certain benign, premalignant, and malignant tumors are treated by cryotherapy, which involves the application of liquid nitrogen over a varying period of time. Depending on the duration of application, this results in a superficial or deeper burn. Certain benign lesions, such as seborrheic keratoses, and premalignant lesions, such as actinic keratoses, are effectively treated with this method. Cryotherapy is a rapid and safe procedure that is easily performed in the office. Local anesthetic is unnecessary because the technique causes only minor discomfort. Another advantage is that minimal scarring results if only the superficial layers of the skin are burned. This technique may be indirectly diagnostic as well as curative. For example, if the lesion is thought to be a seborrheic keratosis, and responds to cryotherapy, no further treatment is indicated. If, however, there is any reasonable doubt about the clinical diagnosis, biopsy is imperative: cryotherapy of a malignant melanoma, for example, proves disastrous, therapeutically and medicolegally. Furthermore, if a lesion recurs after cryotherapy, biopsy is indicated. Cryotherapy is most useful for the treatment of verruca vulgaris and lesions occurring on glabrous skin where scarring is undesirable, or in cases in which nail growth may be affected or altered by more invasive techniques.

Pathologic Evaluation of Skin Lesions

When obtaining a diagnosis is not urgent, evaluating permanent sections of the specimen is preferable. This involves fixation of the specimen in formaldehyde solution, with subsequent processing and sectioning by a histology laboratory (see Chapter 1). Final interpretation is usually available within 2 to 4 days. If the specimen is an excisional biopsy, orientation with sutures or a diagram should be furnished. The pathologist may then evaluate the margins and inform the clinician about adequacy of excision. If margins are inadequate, consideration of reexcision is in order. In certain instances, depending on the nature of the lesion and the degree of involvement of the positive margin, close observation alone is acceptable. For example, if the excisional biopsy reveals a small focus of basal cell carcinoma extending to one surgical margin, observation, rather than immediate reexcision, is an option.[1]

FROZEN SECTION

Intraprocedural frozen section is a useful tool if the diagnosis will influence the surgeon's intraoperative management. Frozen section examination is important in cases in which complete, yet conservative, removal of a malignant lesion is necessary. Basal cell carcinoma of the face is one example in which frozen section alone is useful in establishing the extent of a clinically indistinct lesion. Frozen section margins of lesions requiring wide excision, such as dermatofibroma protuberans or melanoma in noncritical sites, are seldom necessary, since gross examination itself is usually sufficient. The pathologist is the best judge of this situation and should be asked to initially evaluate specimens grossly when necessary, as long as there is no exceptional threat, such as proximity to suture lines of the skull.

The main limitation in evaluating the specimen by frozen section is loss of cellular detail (see Chapter 1). This is particularly true in cases of malignant melanoma in which accurate diagnosis can be critically compromised by freezing artifact.

MOHS MICROGRAPHIC SURGERY

This process involves the intraprocedural frozen section evaluation of the surgical margins of a lesion by the surgeon—usually a dermatologist who has had special training in this procedure. It involves tissue fixation, careful and accurate mapping of the lesion, and staged surgical removal of any involved margins. The success of this technique in effecting complete removal of a cutaneous lesion is said to exceed that of conventional means. Most often, Mohs surgery is used for treatment of basal cell carcinomas with irregular or ill-defined margins, i.e., morpheaform (sclerosing) basal cell carcinoma. The process is also employed in certain cases of minimally invasive well-differentiated squamous cell carcinoma. It should not be used for treatment of malignant melanoma. Following the Mohs micrographic removal of a lesion, a defect of varying size is apparent. Small defects may be left to heal secondarily; larger defects are best treated by plastic surgical procedures employed in wound closure. Larger wounds left to secondary healing may yield poor cosmetic results. This is an important consideration if the lesion involves the face. Furthermore, large wounds require a prolonged period of time for secondary healing. The inconvenience of daily dressing changes is required for proper wound management.

Nonneoplastic Conditions of the Skin

Nonneoplastic skin diseases are classified by clinical type of lesion: *pigmentary disorders* (such as vitiligo and melasma), *papular eruptions* (such as psoriasis and lichen planus), or *vesicular processes* (such as pemphigus and dermatitis herpetiformis). Nonneoplastic skin diseases (such as granuloma faciale and pseudolymphoma) can also simulate tumors. The converse also applies, i.e., neoplasms may occasionally mimic either papular inflammatory conditions (cutaneous T-cell lymphoma) or pigmentary disorders (Kaposi's sarcoma).

Management of most nonneoplastic skin disorders requires accurate clinical diagnosis; however, biopsy is unnecessary in the majority of these conditions. Indeed, biopsy of a clinically straightforward lesion is a disservice to the patient. Empiric treatment (i.e., with topical steroids or antifungal agents) without informed clinical or pathologic diagnosis is also poor medical practice. For this reason, consultation should be sought whenever there is doubt about the clinical diagnosis or, more specifically, the indications for biopsy.

For most nonneoplastic skin conditions punch biopsy is sufficient for diagnosis. The biopsy should be from a nontraumatized lesion and include a rim of uninvolved skin. For cosmetic purposes, it is preferable to biopsy a lesion in an unexposed site if such is available. The presumed disease process and the anatomic site dictate the size of the biopsy.

Neoplasms of the Skin

Neoplasms of the skin may be classified in the following manner: tumors of the epidermis (benign, malignant, and premalignant), tumors of the dermis (benign and malignant), melanocytic lesions (benign, premalignant, and malignant), and noncutaneous processes present in the skin. As with nonneoplastic conditions, an informed clinical differential diagnosis is necessary to ensure that surgical intervention is appropriate. A summary of treatment indications and options for selected common neoplasms is provided in Table 4–1.

EPITHELIAL LESIONS

Epidermal Inclusion Cyst

Epidermal inclusion cysts (''sebaceous cysts'') are common lesions. They occur most frequently on the trunk, face, and neck.[2] Rarely, they are seen in non-hair-bearing sites, such as palms and soles. Lesions range in size from 1 to 3 cm, but larger examples (5 cm or more) are occasionally encountered. They appear as circumscribed, rubbery nodules beneath the skin surface; in many instances, a small pore resembling a comedo overlies the lesion. Histologically, epidermal inclusion cysts are lined by flattened squamous epithelium (resembling epidermis), with a central lumen containing laminated, keratinous debris. If the lesion has been traumatized or has ruptured, the lining may be partially absent, associated with a foreign body giant cell reaction (to keratin) in the surrounding dermis with corresponding clinical evidence of intense inflammation. *Trichilemmal cyst* (pilar cyst) is a variant of epidermal inclusion cyst and occurs primarily on the scalp. This cyst is lined by epithelium with trichilemmal (hair-forming) patterns of keratinization. The keratin product is not laminated.[2, 3] Multiple epidermal inclusion cysts may be seen in patients with Gardner's syndrome.[4]

An epidermal inclusion cyst may also occur in glabrous skin. A history of previous trauma (including surgical excision, laceration, or puncture wound) is often obtained. Surgical treatment of an epidermal inclusion cyst consists of excisional biopsy. In nonglabrous skin, clinical diagnosis is often supported by the small dimplelike pore that is evident upon manipulating the lesion. In glabrous areas the location of a previous puncture wound or scar is often useful in diagnosis. Excisional biopsy should include complete removal of the lesion. If a portion of the lining is left behind, recurrence is likely. A variety of skin neoplasms may be mistaken clinically for epidermal inclusion cysts.

Verruca Vulgaris

The common wart or verruca vulgaris is caused by human papillomavirus infection and occurs most commonly on the hands and soles of the feet (*plantar verruca*).[5] It may be multiple and generalized in immunocompromised patients.[6] Clinically, common warts appear as circumscribed, exophytic, firm, nontender nodules. Plantar warts are firm, deep seated, and exquisitely tender. Histologically, verrucae show regular, upward projections of the epidermis (papillomatosis), which appear to radiate outward. Parakeratosis is usually present at the tips of these projections. In active lesions, many of the cells are vacuolated with irregularly shaped nuclei (koilocytosis); cells near the surface often have large, irregularly shaped keratohyalin granules. Plantar verrucae are histologically identical, but appear to arise within a downward projection of the epidermis.

Cryotherapy is the treatment of choice for all verruca vulgaris lesions. Because hyperkeratosis is always present, the surface of the lesion is shaved prior to the application of the cryotherapy. Excisional biopsy and electrodesiccation are discouraged because painful scars can result in glabrous skin.

Seborrheic Keratosis

Seborrheic keratoses are common lesions. They occur most often on the face and trunk of middle-aged and older individuals. Clinically, they are tan to dark brown, raised lesions that are frequently described as having a ''stuck-on'' appearance.[7] Histologically, they are comprised of small, polygonal keratinocytes, often arranged in elongated, interconnected cords. Small cysts containing laminated keratin (*horn cysts*) are usually present within expanses of the proliferating cells.

As indicated previously, seborrheic keratoses are best treated with cryotherapy. Treatment with this modality is both diagnostic and curative. If a lesion does not respond to cryotherapy, an excisional or incisional biopsy can be performed. Pigmented basal cell carcinomas and malignant melanomas can mimic seborrheic keratoses.

Actinic Keratosis

As the name implies, actinic (solar) keratoses are caused by prolonged sun exposure. They occur exclusively in sun-exposed sites: face, neck, forearms, and hands. Clinically, they appear as hyperkeratotic, usually crusted papules. Histologically, the hallmark of the actinic keratosis is dysplasia of keratinocytes.[8] The epidermis is often thinned, and the basal layers of cells are disorderly and show variability in nuclear size and staining quality (dysplasia). The keratin layer is often parakeratotic. Because cellular atypia may be subtle, it is helpful to examine the periphery, where an abrupt transition between the clonal proliferation and surrounding normal skin is seen. Over time, actinic keratoses may give rise to squamous cell carcinoma.

Actinic keratosis must be distinguished from basal cell carcinoma (usually the superficial type) and squamous cell carcinoma. If the lesions are few or solitary, initial treatment is with cryotherapy. However, when the lesions are multiple and extensive, topical 5-fluorouracil (5-FU) is used. Regression of the lesions must be carefully monitored. If certain areas remain refractory to such treatment, incisional or excisional biopsy should be employed.

Keratoacanthoma

Keratoacanthomas are distinctive lesions characterized by rapid onset (6 to 8 weeks), large size (1 to 5 cm), and spontaneous involution (approximately 6 months). They are usually solitary lesions that occur in sun-damaged skin of elderly individuals; however, they can also be multiple and not associated with solar damage. Grossly, the lesions are dome shaped with a central crater containing keratinized debris. Histologically, the lesions show columns of pale-staining, histologically bland keratinocytes that ''flood'' the dermis (Fig. 4–2).[9] The lesions are roughly symmetric and the central crater observed grossly is also recognizable and distinctive microscopically. Unlike squamous cell carcinomas, cellular atypicality is usually mild and limited to the deep, lateral aspects of the lesions. Chronic inflammatory cells accumulate in the dermis as the lesion regresses; as the lesion approaches complete regression it becomes thin, and the dermis shows fibrosis (scar).

It is often extremely difficult, if not impossible, to distinguish between keratoacanthoma and well-differentiated squamous cell carcinoma clinically. The history of rapid growth and proliferation should alert the clinician that the lesion is more likely a keratoacanthoma. If the patient is immunocompromised, however, a squamous cell carcinoma is likely. Treatment involves an excisional biopsy, providing the pathologist with optimal tissue for diagnosis.

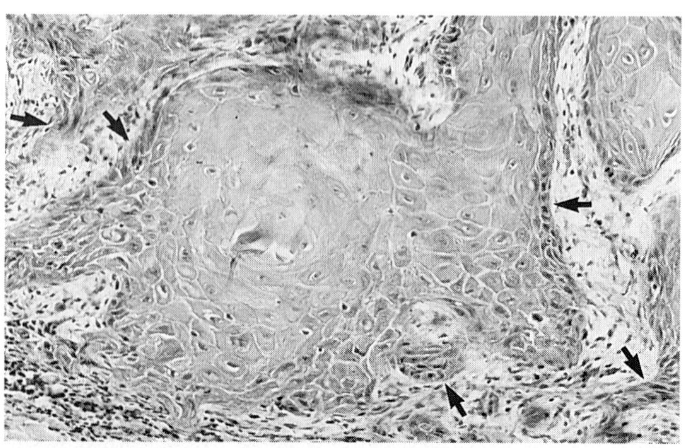

Figure 4–2. Keratoacanthoma. The lesion consists of pale-staining keratinocytes with abundant eosinophilic cytoplasm. There is only mild cytologic atypia, which is most prominent along the advancing margins of the lesion *(arrows)*.

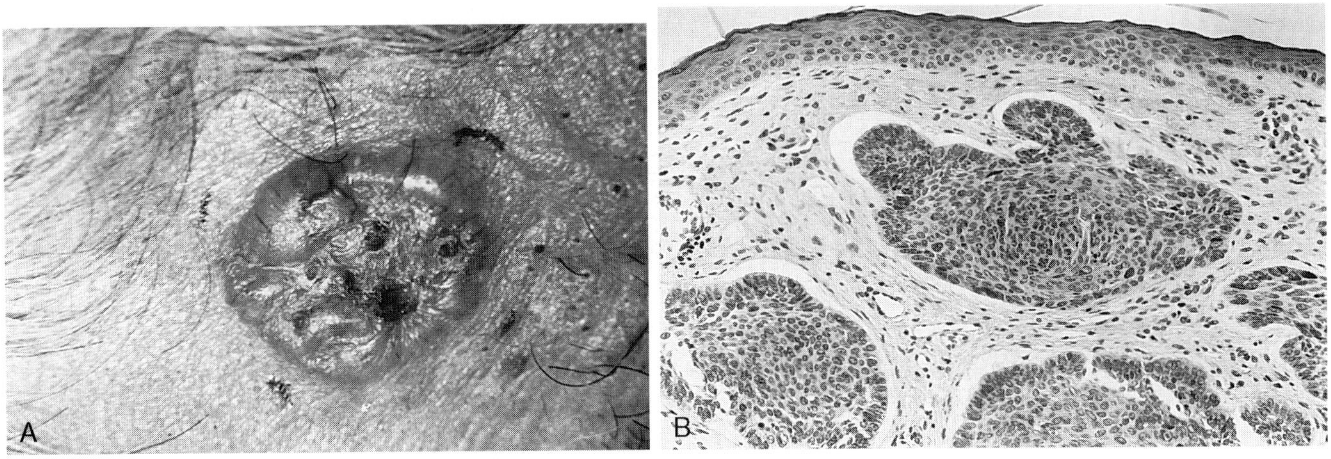

Figure 4–3. Basal cell carcinoma. *A*, Clinically, the lesions occur on sun-exposed areas and manifest as pearly plaques or nodules, with "rolled" borders and a central zone of ulceration. (Courtesy of Drs. Wayne Fagan and Brent Paulger, Department of Dermatology, The University of Texas Health Science Center, San Antonio.) *B*, Microscopically, the lesions consist of nests of basophilic tumor cells with "palisading" of nuclei at the periphery; the cleftlike spaces surrounding the nests contain extracellular mucin.

The adequacy of the margins can also be ascertained. If a definite diagnosis is made, incomplete excision is not a problem. However, a shave biopsy may leave behind the diagnostic deep portion of the lesion. The pathologist is therefore forced to issue a disclaimer that "squamous cell carcinoma cannot be ruled out," obligating the surgeon to excise the remainder of the lesion. Although some pathologists consider keratoacanthomas to be "self-healing" variants of squamous cell carcinomas, the distinctive histologic and clinical differences do not support their position.

Basal Cell Carcinoma

Basal cell carcinomas are the most common malignant neoplasms of the skin. Although they are potentially locally aggressive, they almost never metastasize. Sun-exposed areas, usually of the head and neck, are the most common sites of occurrence.[10] Grossly, they are pearly plaques or nodules, with "rolled" borders and a small central ulcer (Fig. 4–3*A*). The most subtle and aggressive histologic type, the *sclerosing variant*, is characterized by a plaque-like zone of apparent atrophy, hence the alternate designation, *morpheaform variant*.[11] Microscopically, basal cell carcinomas are comprised of cells resembling those in the basal layer of the epidermis. Nests of these atypical basophilic cells extend from the epidermis into the dermis. There are two distinctive histologic features: "palisading" of nuclei at the periphery of nests of tumor cells and mucin-filled clefts separating tumor from the surrounding dermis (Fig. 4–3*B*). Cells may form rounded nests, cords, and sheets. Occasionally, cells surround collagen deposits or pools of mucin, resulting in a glandlike (adenoid) pattern. *Superficial basal cell carcinoma* resembles conventional basal cell carcinoma histologically, but cell nests are confined to the epidermis. These nest-like buds are discontinuous and therefore appear multifocal.[12] The *morpheaform (sclerosing) basal cell carcinoma* presents clinically as a localized zone of cutaneous atrophy (Fig. 4–4*A*). Histologically, it consists of slender nests and cords of cells in a cellular, fibrotic matrix (Fig. 4–4*B*). This variant is frequently quite aggressive locally, and the extent of the lesion is often difficult to appreciate clinically.

The goal in the treatment of basal cell carcinoma is complete extirpation. If the lesion is well defined (i.e., of nodular type), then excisional biopsy should be done. If the borders are less well defined and the lesion is large, Mohs micrographic excision followed by reconstruction may be employed. Local excision with careful evaluation of the microscopic margin may also be used quite effectively in this situation. Cost is much less using simple local excision with careful review of the margin. If the lesion is recurrent and in an anatomically "tight" area, the Mohs micrographic technique with reconstruction is the preferred treatment. Whether wide excision or Mohs surgery is used, it is crucial that careful histologic evaluation of a properly oriented specimen be done. As previously indicated, shave excision with electrodesiccation of the margins and bed of the wound often leave unacceptable scars with subsequent distortion of adjacent anatomy. Healing is secondary and often prolonged. If the lesion is in an unexposed area of the body, shave excision with electrodesiccation is acceptable. This approach has the advantages of being rapid and cost effective, since it requires a minimal operating facility and instrumentation.

Squamous Cell Carcinoma

Despite the prevalence of its main precursor lesion, actinic keratosis, squamous cell carcinoma of the skin is relatively uncommon. It occurs most often in sun-exposed sites: head, neck, and extremities.[13] Occasionally, squamous cell carcinoma arises in burn scars and in chronic ulcers of the skin.[14, 15] Less than 1% of sun-induced lesions metastasize; those due to other causes and those occurring in certain anatomic sites (such as the genitals and perioral area) metastasize much more frequently. Grossly, the lesions are often ulcerated with a wide, firm, raised border. If untreated, they may become large and locally destructive (Fig. 4–5*A*). Histologically, they consist of nests of atypical keratinizing squamous cells that originate from the epider-

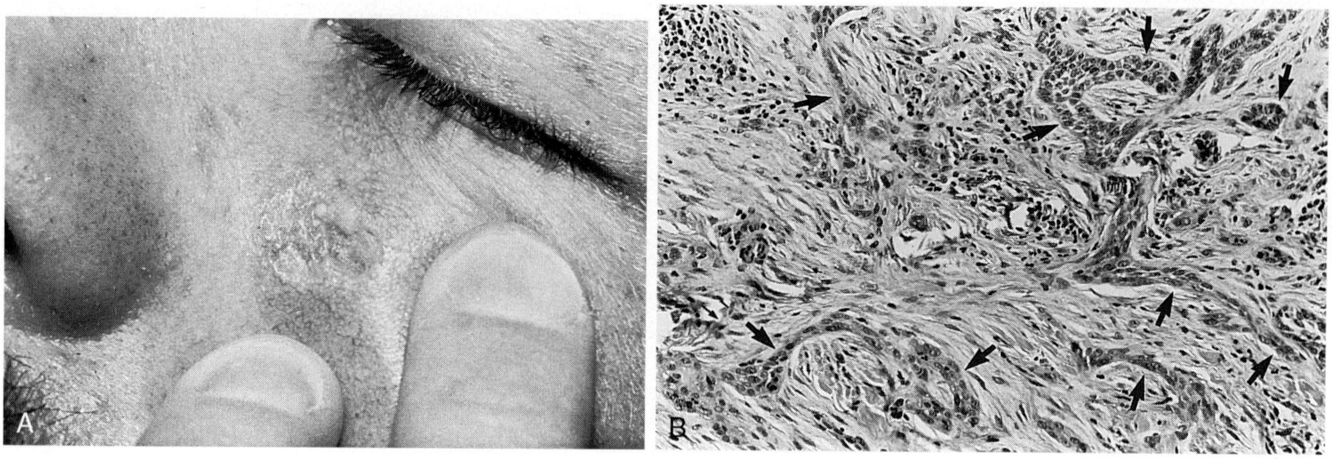

Figure 4–4. Morpheaform (sclerosing) basal cell carcinoma. *A*, Clinically, the lesions present as ill-defined zones of cutaneous atrophy. (Courtesy of Drs. Wayne Fagan and Brent Paulger, Department of Dermatology, The University of Texas Health Science Center, San Antonio.) *B*, Histologically, the lesions consist of slender nests and cords of tumor cells *(arrows)* in a cellular, fibrotic matrix.

mis and infiltrate the dermis (Fig. 4–5*B*). The surrounding tissue is inflamed and fibrotic. Unlike keratoacanthomas, most of these lesions are uniformly atypical and often arise from dysplastic epidermis. Nevertheless, some squamous cell carcinomas may be nodular and cup shaped with a central keratin-filled crater, closely resembling keratoacanthomas.

The treatment of squamous cell carcinoma depends on the site, grade, and stage of the tumor. There is an extensive experience managing patients with very small tumor burdens with ablation (cryosurgery and electrosurgery).[16] These methods of treatment are used more often with basal cell cancers and should be used for squamous cell carcinomas only in favorable situations. For the most part, squamous cell cancers of the skin should be removed and assessed for adequacy of margin. Depending on the extent of the tumor, this may involve only a simple excisional biopsy or a more extensive removal with reconstruction. Although there is no uniform recommendation for the size of margins, many surgeons excise small, well-defined lesions with margins of 3 to 5 mm. Margins of at least 1 cm are required for larger, more aggressive lesions. Careful microscopic evaluation, usually with inked surfaces, is important. Many squamous cancers occur on the face in sun-exposed areas. Recurrence because of inadequate excision or an overlooked positive margin may require more extensive reexcision with cosmetically less acceptable results. Although the Mohs micrographic surgical approach has been used in patients with extensive or poorly defined morpheaform basal cell carcinomas, it has also been used for squamous cell carcinoma. The indications with these tumors seem less clear. While metastases from squamous cancers are uncommon, they may result from more advanced lesions. More advanced and higher-grade tumors that are greater than 4 cm in diameter are usually ulcerated and can also spread hematogenously, through the lymphatic system or directly with ''satellitosis'' through the interstitial compartment.[16] Neglected squamous cancers of the extremities may require radical surgical intervention including lymph node dissection and even limb amputation.[17, 18] Such aggressive surgical procedures can be life saving and should be considered in appropriately selected patients.

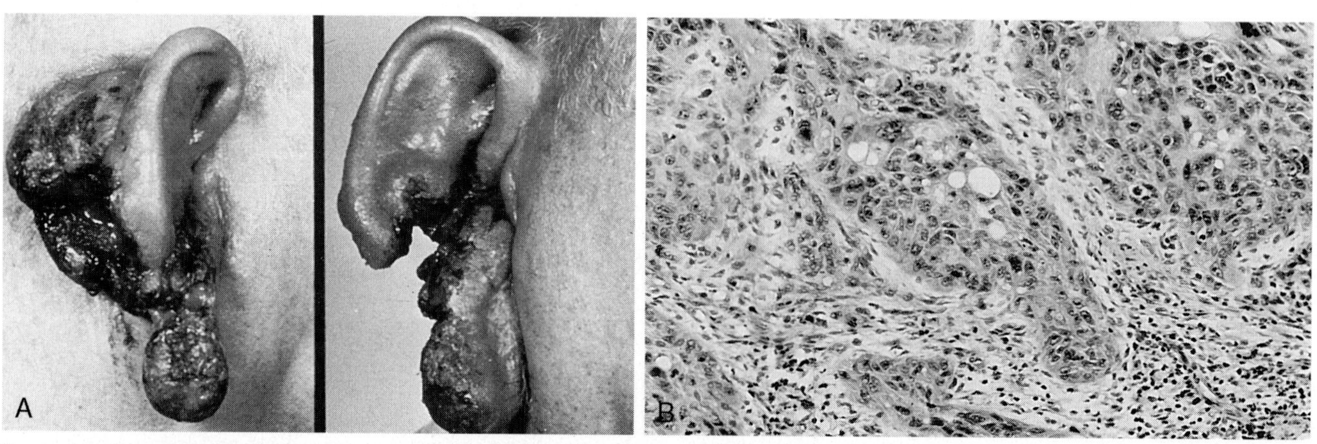

Figure 4–5. Squamous cell carcinoma. *A*, This large, fungating, lesion has partially destroyed the pinna of the ear. (Courtesy of Drs. Wayne Fagan and Brent Paulger, Department of Dermatology, The University of Texas Health Science Center, San Antonio.) *B*, Histologically, the lesion consists of nests of markedly atypical keratinocytes that invade the surrounding dermis (compare to Figure 4–2).

Close consultation between surgeon and pathologist is imperative for squamous cell carcinomas of the skin. The surgeon should properly orient the specimen by suture placement. If margins are positive, extended margins should be resected to achieve a free margin of at least 5 mm. In patients with high-risk lesions, regional lymph nodes should be carefully assessed. If there is any suspicion that the regional lymph nodes may harbor metastases, then lymph node dissection should be performed. Radiation therapy may be an effective adjuvant modality in such cases.

Skin Appendage Tumors

Skin appendage tumors are defined as neoplasms arising from epidermal appendages (hair follicles, sweat glands, sebaceous glands) or as neoplasms with differentiation that recapitulates that of a skin appendage. A detailed discussion of the skin appendage tumors is beyond the scope of this book; however, an abridged list is provided (Table 4–2).

Except for those lesions designated as either "malignant" or as "carcinoma," skin appendage tumors as a group are regarded as benign. Nonetheless, because some of the lesions may recur or be locally aggressive, it is advisable to totally excise them. Some have advocated that skin appendage tumors be regarded as similar to basal cell carcinoma in biologic potential and be treated accordingly. Histologically, benign skin appendage tumors can mimic malignant neoplasms, particularly basal cell carcinoma and squamous cell carcinoma (Fig. 4–6). Larger skin appendage lesions, especially those designated as malignant or carcinoma, require more aggressive therapy. Indeed, the comments made above concerning high-risk squamous cell cancer of the skin apply here.

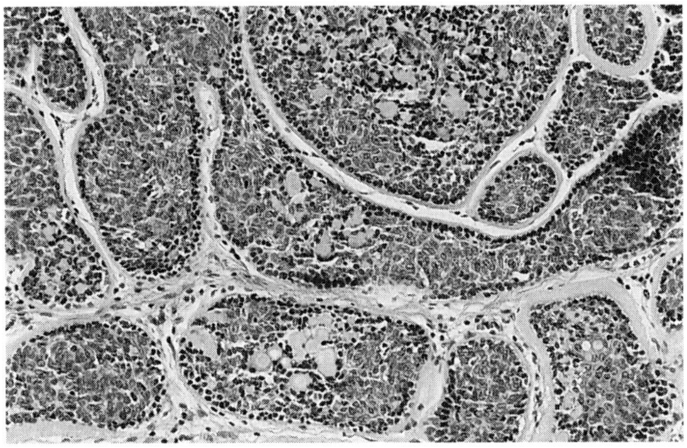

Figure 4–6. Cutaneous cylindroma (dermal eccrine cylindroma). This benign skin appendage tumor most commonly occurs on the scalp. Histologically, it consists of basaloid tumor cells, and the pattern may closely mimic that of basal cell carcinoma (Figure 4–3*B*). The lesion lacks significant cytologic atypia and is biologically indolent.

MESENCHYMAL LESIONS

Keloid

Keloids invariably arise at a site of prior injury and are thought to represent an exaggeration of the healing process.[19] Clinically, they resemble hypertrophic scars; however, the latter slowly resolve, whereas keloids persist or even continue to increase in size. They may even spread beyond the site of injury. Occasionally, the patient does not recall a cutaneous injury at the site. The most common sites of occurrence are the presternal area and the earlobes (often as a consequence of pierced ears). Grossly, the lesions are nodular with a smooth surface and rockhard consistency. The histologic hallmark of keloids is irregularly arranged, broad (up to ten times normal width) collagen bundles in a myxoid matrix.

Keloids may be treated by the intralesional injection of corticosteroids. The undesirable sequelae of such treatment should first be made known to the patient. These include pigmentary alteration and subcutaneous atrophy. Injection may also be quite painful. Surgical excision should be approached cautiously because recurrence rates are high. In patients in whom excision has failed, external beam irradiation may be considered. On the day of surgery and the day after, 500 rads are administered. Finally, there may be a role for the prolonged application of Silastic sheeting and pressure to the wound margins. If the patient has multiple pedunculated keloids, serious consideration should be given to conservative management (patient tolerance) with avoidance of further surgical procedures.

Table 4–2. Common Skin Appendage Tumors

Sweat Duct Origin	Hair Follicle Origin
Syringoma	Trichilemmoma
Poroma/hydroacanthoma simplex/ dermal duct tumor/acrospiroma	Trichoepithelioma
Spiradenoma	Pilomatrixoma
Mixed tumor (chondroid syringoma)	Proliferating pilar tumor
Cylindroma	**Sebaceous Gland Origin**
Microcystic adnexal carcinoma	Sebaceous hyperplasia
Adenoid cystic carcinoma	Sebaceous adenoma
Porocarcinoma	Sebaceous epithelioma
Malignant eccrine acrospiroma	Sebaceous carcinoma
Extramammary Paget's disease	

Dermatofibroma (Fibrous Histiocytoma)

Dermatofibromas are localized fibroblastic proliferative lesions that typically occur in the extremities of adults.[20] Clinically, the overlying skin is slightly raised and hyperpigmented; the lesions are firm and nodular and range in size from 0.3 to over 2 cm. Sometimes they clinically simulate melanocytic lesions because of their pigmentation or epidermal cysts because of their nodularity. Histologically, dermatofibromas consist of slender spindle-shaped cells in a fibrotic matrix. Blood vessels are regularly spaced within the lesions. The cells surrounding these vessels are characteristically arranged in a starburst or storiform pattern. A variety of elements, including foamy histiocytes, multinucleated giant cells, and hemosiderin-laden cells, may be present. The lesions are usually confined to the dermis but may extend a short distance into the subcutis.

Mitotic figures may be present in moderate number. The epidermis overlying the lesions is invariably hyperplastic, with elongation of rete ridges and hyperpigmentation. This finding contrasts to the epidermal atrophy overlying dermal scars.

Dermatofibromas are benign. Indications for removal are cosmetic purposes and uncertain clinical diagnoses. Simple excision is curative.

Neurofibroma

Neurofibromas are tumoral dysplasias of cutaneous nerves. They may be solitary or multiple, the latter sometimes manifesting von Recklinghausen's disease.[21] The lesions are typically soft and pedunculated, with normal-appearing overlying skin. Histologically, neurofibromas consist of delicate, often wavy, fascicles of spindle cells in a fibrous to myxoid matrix. Mast cells may be numerous. Special stains for S-100 protein are usually strongly positive. In von Recklinghausen's disease, neurofibromas may diffusely infiltrate the dermis or be plexiform. The *plexiform neurofibroma* is considered pathognomonic for neurofibromatosis. Only rarely do superficial plexiform neurofibromas undergo malignant transformation.

Neurofibromas are removed by simple excision, primarily for cosmetic reasons. Local denervation is a predictable consequence of excision.

Dermatofibrosarcoma Protuberans

Dermatofibrosarcoma protuberans is a slowly growing, low-grade sarcoma that arises in the dermis. The most common site is the trunk, followed by the extremities.[22] Grossly, the lesions are nodular to multinodular and, as the name implies, protuberant. Histologically, they are composed of slender spindle cells with oval nuclei that vary little in size or staining quality. The characteristic histologic pattern is storiform, with diffuse involvement of the dermis and extension into the subcutis. At their periphery the lesions characteristically grow in plaquelike fashion in the dermis with extension along septa of the subcutis. Because there may be extension some distance from the main portion of the lesion, wide surgical excision is advised. Recurrence is a common phenomenon; metastasis is rare.

Selection of the treatment modality is determined by the location, size, and extent of the lesion as well as the resultant deformity. Frozen section interpretation is notoriously difficult, especially in recurrent lesions in relation to distinction from scarring.

In patients with large tumors in anatomically "tight" areas, Mohs micrographic removal may be considered and will help ensure removal with negative margins. However, in most patients, simple excision with split thickness skin graft or flap reconstruction provides excellent treatment at much less expense.

Atypical Fibroxanthoma

Some controversy still exists about the nature of the so-called atypical fibroxanthoma, although it is generally accepted that these lesions are superficial variants of the soft tissue tumor *malignant fibrous histiocytoma*.[23] As is the case for patients with other soft tissue neoplasms, the relatively good prognosis is related to the comparatively small size (1 to 3 cm) and superficial location. Only rarely do such lesions metastasize. Grossly, they are circumscribed nodular lesions, often occurring in the head and neck area of elderly individuals. Microscopically, they are composed of plump spindle cells with pleomorphic nuclei and numerous mitotic figures (Fig. 4–7). Bizarre multinucleated giant cells are an aid in diagnosis. The histologic differential diagnosis for atypical fibroxanthoma includes spindle-cell melanoma and spindle-cell squamous carcinoma. Immunoperoxidase stain markers that are sensitive for these lesions (S-100 protein and HMB-45 for melanoma; cytokeratin in carcinoma) are negative in atypical fibroxanthoma. The lesions usually involve the dermis and often the superficial subcutis. Complete surgical excision is the treatment of choice.

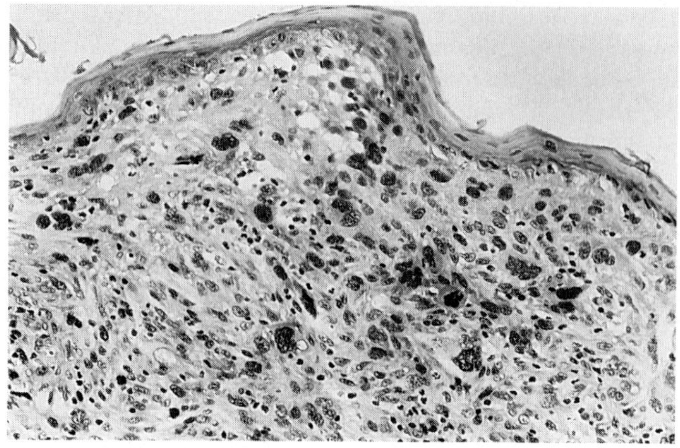

Figure 4–7. Atypical fibroxanthoma. These polypoid lesions commonly occur in sun-exposed skin in elderly patients. Histologically, they are composed of plump spindle cells with pleomorphic nuclei and numerous mitotic figures. Bizarre multinucleated giant cells are often present.

Kaposi's Sarcoma

Kaposi's sarcoma is a relatively common lesion in immunocompromised individuals. Prior to the era of the acquired immunodeficiency syndrome (AIDS) such lesions were rare, occurring most often as small, indolent nodules on the lower extremities of elderly individuals of Mediterranean descent.[24, 25] They are still perhaps most common on the legs, but they may occur on the skin and in the lymph nodes, oral cavity, and viscera. Grossly, the lesions are red or purple and range from a plaquelike to nodular configuration. Histologically, Kaposi's sarcomas consist of closely aggregated spindle cells with large oval nuclei. In plaquelike lesions, cells extend between dermal collagen bundles to produce slitlike spaces. There is some nuclear variability, and mitotic figures are present in moderate numbers. Hemorrhage and hemosiderin deposition are common within the lesions. Some of the cells have cytoplasmic vacuoles containing red blood cells. This tumor is of endothelial derivation. Kaposi's sarcoma associated with

AIDS most frequently appears as an aggressive, widely disseminated neoplasm.

While treatment of classic non-AIDS-associated Kaposi's sarcoma may consist of local excision of these tumors, possibly in combination with radiation or chemotherapy, treatment in patients with AIDS is considered palliative. In the latter instance, local irradiation or other therapies may be appropriate. Systemic chemotherapy and lymphokines have been used with some success. Response and longevity are usually related to the extent of disease and the blood CD4 lymphocyte count.

MELANOCYTIC LESIONS

Early in embryonic life melanocytes migrate from the neural crest to the skin. There they reside among keratinocytes in the basal portion of the epidermis where they produce melanin, which is distributed among surrounding keratinocytes. Melanin is primarily responsible for skin coloration and is presumed be an adaptive mechanism for the prevention of damage by ultraviolet radiation from the sun.

When melanocytes proliferate, they may do so either as individual cells spreading along the dermal-epidermal interface (*lentiginous* pattern) or as nests (*theques*).

Nevocellular Nevus

The earliest phase in the development of a melanocytic nevus is thought to be a lentiginous proliferation of melanocytes. From such proliferations, theques appear at the dermal-epidermal junction, a pattern referred to as *junctional nevus*. Junctional nevi and their precursors are most commonly observed in younger individuals. As the lesions age, nests of nevus cells migrate into the dermis. In so doing, the property of melanogenesis is usually lost. A lesion consisting of theques of melanocytes in both the epidermis and dermis is referred to as a *compound nevus*.[26] By adulthood, most nevi consist entirely of nevus cells within the dermis (*intradermal nevus*). Grossly, nevi range from slightly raised papules to pedunculated nodules. In general, flat lesions are more frequently pigmented and are more apt to have a junctional component histologically. Polypoid lesions are often lightly pigmented and the intradermal pattern predominates.

As the name implies, *congenital nevi* are present at birth or very early in life. Occasionally, such nevi cover large expanses of the body (''bathing trunk nevus'' or ''giant hairy nevus'').[27] Histologically, congenital nevi are distinguished from ''acquired'' nevi by the extension of individual nevus cells into the reticular dermis, often along skin appendages. However, similar patterns may also be observed in nevi that are not known to be congenital.

For practical purposes, nevocellular nevi are benign. It is estimated that the average adult has 15 to 50 such lesions. In rare instances, melanoma may also arise within the dermal component of an acquired nevus. Ordinary nevi are removed primarily for cosmetic reasons. Melanoma may arise in congenital nevi. The risk of this occurrence is roughly proportional to the number of nevus cells present (i.e., size of the lesion).

Other Nevi

The *blue nevus* derives its name from its somewhat bluish clinical appearance. Histologically, blue nevi consist of slender dendritic pigmented melanocytes that grow in a wedge-shaped pattern within the reticular dermis.[28] They are benign and are removed for cosmetic reasons.

The *Spitz nevus* primarily affects children and young adults.[29] Before its characterization as a benign entity, it was considered to be a ''juvenile melanoma.''[30] Clinically, such lesions are dome shaped and tan or red. They are often mistaken clinically for vascular neoplasms rather than melanocytic lesions. Microscopically, they are composed of fascicles of plump, spindle-shaped, or epithelioid cells, with oval nuclei and prominent nucleoli. Nests of cells are usually present within the epidermis and dermis. They may extend deeply and grow along skin appendages, nerves, and blood vessels. They vary considerably in nuclear size, and occasionally mitotic figures are observed. A key to their benign nature is the symmetric pattern of growth. Simple excision is curative.

The *combined nevus* is a lesion comprised of two or more histologically different melanocytic nevus cell types, including nevocellular, blue, Spitz, and others.[31] These lesions are of importance because they may simulate malignant melanoma, both clinically and pathologically. Excision is curative.

The treatment selected for benign melanocytic lesions is influenced by several factors. If the lesion is clinically benign and in an exposed area in the head and neck region, either a shave or an excisional biopsy is appropriate. However, if the diagnosis is uncertain and differentiation must be made between a benign melanocytic lesion and malignant melanoma, an excisional biopsy with permanent section histologic evaluation is mandatory. (Frozen section evaluation is discouraged for the reasons previously mentioned.) At times immunohistochemical staining techniques are useful for the pathologist. Adults with a prior biopsy diagnosis of melanocytic dysplasia should be examined at regular intervals for newly appearing atypical lesions. Some of these patients are at a significantly higher risk for the development of malignant melanoma, and indeed there may be a family history of melanoma. In such kindred congenital nevi should be excised because of the risk of malignant transformation of the lesions. Surgical excision should be accomplished at a young age, particularly if staged excision is part of the treatment plan. Skin grafting of soft tissue defects following excision of larger lesions may be necessary. In unusual instances the nevus is so extensive that surgical resection is not possible.

Malignant Melanoma

Malignant melanoma is one of the most aggressive and capricious neoplasms.[32] Lesions as small as 5 mm in diameter and 1 mm thick may result in metastasis and death. Grossly, most melanomas arise as plaquelike or nodular elevations within an irregularly shaped zone of pigmentation. The background pigmentary changes are referred to as the *radial growth phase*, the early phase in which the lesion is noninvasive and incapable of metastasis. The appearance of a nodule or thickened plaque within such a lesion is known as the *vertical growth phase*. When a lesion progresses to vertical growth, it is considered malignant. The single factor that correlates best with prognosis is lesion thickness.[33] A lesion that is in vertical growth from its inception is referred to as *nodular melanoma* (de novo melanoma).

Superficial spreading melanoma occurs most commonly on the trunk, neck, and lower extremities. The radial growth phase is usually present for 1 to 5 years prior to the onset of vertical growth (Fig. 4–8*A*).[34] *Lentigo maligna melanoma* occurs primarily on the head and neck area of elderly individuals. The precursor lesion, *lentigo maligna* (Hutchinson's freckle), is perhaps the best example of radial growth phase melanoma.[35] Lentigo maligna is usually present for 5 to 20 years before the vertical growth phase supervenes. *Acral lentiginous melanoma* arises on the soles and palms; it usually occurs in dark-skinned races.[36] A radial growth phase is often present for several years prior to vertical growth.

Histologically, all melanomas share certain features.[37] The radial growth phase is characterized by nests of atypical melanocytes confined primarily to the dermal-epidermal interface. The underlying dermis contains infiltrates of lymphoid cells and shows fibrosis—presumably reflecting an immunologic host response to a clone of abnormal cells. For lentiginous melanomas (acral lentiginous and lentigo maligna melanoma) the distribution of melanocytes in radial growth is primarily lentiginous (individual cells along the dermal-epidermal interface). In superficial spreading melanoma the radial growth phase is characterized by nests of melanocytes within the epidermis, along with individual atypical cells at all levels of the epidermis (Pagetoid growth pattern) (Fig. 4–8*B*). Once vertical growth proceeds, all melanomas are similar. They show nests of atypical epithelioid to spindle-shaped cells within the dermis. Individual cells have large oval nuclei with prominent nucleoli. There is variability in nuclear outline and chromatin density. Mitotic figures are conspicuous. There are often delicate, "powdery" cytoplasmic melanin granules. Lesions lacking pigment both grossly and microscopically are referred to as *amelanotic melanoma*.

Treatment for malignant melanoma should consist of wide surgical resection. Randomized prospective trials have demonstrated that adequate margins for primary tumors measuring up to 1 mm thick are adequate as narrow as 1 cm.[38] Tumors that are between 1 and 4 mm thick have been shown to be adequately treated with 2-cm margins.[39] There are no randomized data to instruct us with regard to tumors greater than 4 mm thick. However, these tumors are expected to have a greater risk of local recurrence and probably should be managed with wider margins. Management of lymph nodes draining the primary site is controversial, although most workers do not recommend prophylactic lymph node dissection. The intergroup melanoma trial that assessed resection margins also assessed prophylactic lymph node dissection for melanomas of intermediate thickness (1 to 4 mm). The results from this trial are pending.

Another development regarding lymph node dissection for melanoma concerns the issue of "sentinel" lymph node biopsy. This technique was developed by Morton et al. as a means of detecting the lymph node most immediately draining a presumptive primary stage I melanoma, to identify patients who may benefit from lymph node dissections.[40] The procedure utilizes vital dyes that permit intraoperative identification of the lymph node on the direct drainage pathway from the primary lesion to the lymph node station; the node may then be biopsied and evaluated microscopically (both with conventional stains and with immunohistochemical stains for melanoma). Prospective evaluation of this technique resulted in a false-negative rate of only 1%. Gamma-probe-guided lymph node localization,

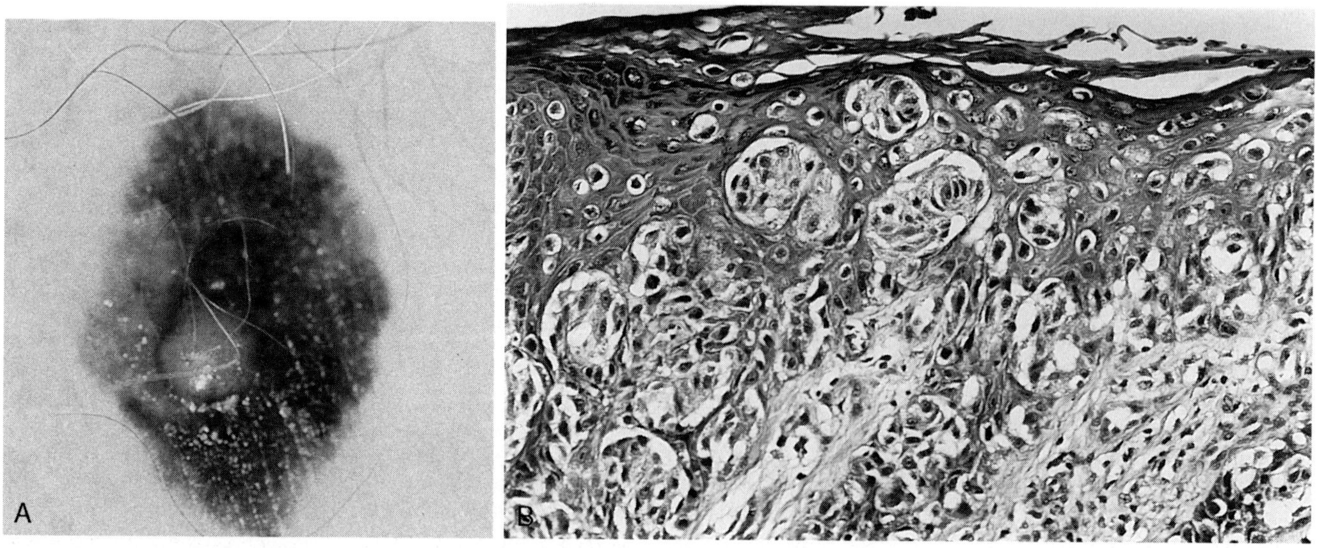

Figure 4–8. Superficial spreading malignant melanoma. *A*, Clinically the radial growth phase consists of irregularly shaped papule with mottled pigmentation. In time, one or more nodules may appear *(center)*, heralding the phase of vertical growth. (Courtesy of Drs. Wayne Fagan and Brent Paulger, Department of Dermatology, The University of Texas Health Science Center, San Antonio.) *B*, Microscopically, the radial growth phase is characterized by markedly atypical polygonal cells that are dispersed individually and in small nests within the epidermis—the typical "Pagetoid" pattern of growth.

used in combination with this dye technique, may enhance its efficacy even further.[41] If confirmed by ongoing studies, this new technology may allow the selection of patients with clinically inapparent lymph node metastasis for "therapeutic" lymph node dissection to lessen tumor burden. Whether patients will ultimately benefit from such intervention will require long-term prospective clinical trials.

Melanocytic Dysplasia

Of great interest and controversy are precursors to melanoma: melanocytic dysplasia. Some experts contend that precursors do not exist and that histologic features for distinguishing these lesions are unreliable. Although the term "dysplastic nevus" has been used for over 2 decades, one undeniable precursor of malignancy has been recognized for considerably longer: the phase of radial growth.

Clinically, atypical nevi exhibit features that are quite similar to those of the radial growth phase of melanoma: irregular outlines and mottled (brown, black, red, and white) pigmentation (Fig. 4–8*A*). Microscopically, the two lesions are similar. They both exhibit melanocytic atypia, dermal lymphoid infiltrates, and fibrosis of the papillary dermis.

The *dysplastic nevus syndrome* is a hereditary condition in which individuals have dozens to hundreds of clinically and histologically atypical nevi.[42] Such patients are at high risk for the development of melanoma. Atypical nevi may also occur *sporadically* in individuals with no apparent hereditary predisposition. In fact, some studies have estimated that a majority of white individuals have one or more of these lesions. The risk of developing melanoma in a single atypical nevus is small and proportional to the size of the lesion. That these lesions are so prevalent and that so very few progress to melanoma have caused some to challenge the premalignant nature of such melanocytic lesions.

OTHER NEOPLASMS OF THE SKIN

Cutaneous T-cell Lymphoma

Cutaneous T-cell lymphoma arises in the skin but eventually spreads to lymph nodes and viscera. For most of the life history of these lesions, the clinical and histologic picture is easily mistaken for an inflammatory dermatosis, rather than a neoplasm. In the early phases of the disease, a diffuse dermal infiltrate of slightly enlarged lymphocytes focally extends to involve the epidermis. Such epidermotropism is characteristic of cutaneous T-cell lymphoma but may be confused with a number of benign conditions. Late in the course of the disease tumors appear; histologically, large atypical lymphoid cells with convoluted nuclei diffusely infiltrate the dermis. At any stage of the disease, punch biopsy is used for diagnosis. The clinical term *mycosis fungoides* has traditionally been applied to cases with numerous patches, plaques, or distinct tumors. *Sézary's syndrome* is used for cases showing only diffuse erythroderma and blood involvement by the neoplastic lymphocytes.

Metastatic Carcinoma

Carcinoma metastatic to the skin is a relatively rare phenomenon, occurring in roughly 3% of patients who die of an internal malignancy. The prevalence of carcinoma metastatic to the skin is proportional to the incidence of the primary in a given population. In the United States, metastatic breast carcinoma is most common in women, while metastatic lung carcinoma predominates in men. Interestingly, renal cell carcinoma seems to feature cutaneous metastases at a rate proportionately higher than its prevalence.

Metastatic carcinoma is suspected when a large nodule arises in an unusual cutaneous site (e.g., non-sun exposed), or when more than one such unusual lesion occurs. A history of visceral malignancy is, of course, suggestive. When a diagnosis of either adenocarcinoma or "clear cell carcinoma" is rendered for a skin lesion, the surgeon should consider the possibility of a metastatic rather than primary process. Few primary skin lesions belong to either histologic category. If the pathology report does not indicate whether such a lesion is primary, this matter should be pursued with the pathologist. In some instances (e.g., prostatic and thyroid carcinoma), immunoperoxidase stains may be diagnostic. A metastatic nature should be considered for any skin carcinoma that is histologically puzzling.

Soft Tissue Tumors Appearing in the Skin

Soft tissue tumors, both benign and malignant, may appear in the skin. The approach to such lesions is covered in Chapter 18.

PITFALLS FOR THE SURGEON

1. Failing to properly orient specimen for the pathologist.
2. Failing to obtain intraprocedural frozen section evaluation of suspected surgical margins for large basal cell and squamous cell carcinomas.
3. Failing to appreciate that certain basal cell carcinomas may result in significant morbidity and even death if inadequately or inappropriately treated.
4. Failing to appreciate that some cutaneous squamous cell carcinomas may be life threatening if not appropriately treated and managed.
5. Performing biopsy of pigmented lesions in a manner that may hamper the pathologist's ability to assess thickness and/or level of invasion if the process is malignant melanoma.
6. Failing to seek clinical consultation when the need for biopsy/excision is questionable.

PITFALLS FOR THE PATHOLOGIST

1. Failing to recognize that the anatomic orientation of a specimen has not been fully or adequately described.
2. Misinterpreting portions of a hair follicle as basal cell carcinoma on frozen section.
3. Failing to identify a morpheaform (sclerosing) component in a basal cell carcinoma.
4. Failing to adequately (completely) sample a suspicious pigmented (melanocytic) lesion.
5. Misdiagnosing a skin appendage tumor as squamous or basal cell carcinoma.

FURTHER READING

1. Farmer ER, Hood AF, eds. *Pathology of the Skin*. Norwalk, CT: Appleton & Lange; 1990.
2. Lever WJ, Schaumburg-Lever G. *Histopathology of the Skin*. Philadelphia: Lippincott Co.; 1990.
3. Rosai J. *Ackerman's Surgical Pathology*. St. Louis: Mosby; 1989.
4. Silverberg SG, ed. *Principles and Practice of Surgical Pathology*. New York: John Wiley & Sons; 1983.
5. Sternberg SJ, ed. *Diagnostic Surgical Pathology*. New York: Raven Press; 1989.

REFERENCES

1. Gooding CA, White G, Yatsuhashi M. The significance of marginal extension in excised basal cell carcinoma. *N Engl J Med*. 1965;273:923–924.
2. McGavran MH, Ninnington B. Keratinous cysts of the skin. *Arch Dermatol*. 1966;94:499–508.
3. Leppard BJ, Sanderson KV. The natural history of trichilemmal cysts. *Br J Dermatol*. 1976;94:379–390.
4. Weary PE, Linthicum A, Cawley EP, et al. Gardner's syndrome. *Arch Dermatol*. 1964;90:20–30.
5. Cornelius CE, Witkowski JA, Wood MG. Viral verruca, human papova virus infection. *Arch Dermatol*. 1968;98:377–384.
6. Barnett N, Mark H, Winkelstein JA. Extensive verrucosis in primary immunodeficiency diseases. *Arch Dermatol*. 1983;119:5–7.
7. Sanderson KF. The structure of seborrheic keratoses. *Br J Dermatol*. 1968;80:588–593.
8. Ackerman AB, Reed RJ. Epidermolytic variant of solar keratosis. *Arch Dermatol*. 1973;107:104–106.
9. Lawrence N, Reed RJ. Actinic keratoacanthoma. Speculations on the nature of the lesion and the role of cellular immunity in its evolution. *Am J Dermatopathol*. 1990;12:517–533.
10. Smith OD, Swerdlow MA. Histogenesis of basal-cell epithelioma. *Arch Dermatol*. 1956;74:286–292.
11. Caro MR, Howell JB. Morphea-like epithelioma. *Arch Dermatol Syph*. 1952;63:471–476.
12. Madsen A. The histogenesis of superficial basal-cell epithelioma. *Arch Dermatol*. 1955;72:29–30.
13. Broders AC. Squamous-cell epithelioma of the skin. *Ann Surg*. 1921;73:141–160.
14. Arons MS, Lynch JB, Lewis SR, et al. Scar tissue carcinoma. I. A clinical study with special reference to burn scar carcinoma. *Ann Surg*. 1965;161:170–188.
15. Barr LH, Menard JW. Marjolin's ulcer. *Cancer*. 1983;52:173–175.
16. Preston DS, Stern RS. Non-melanoma cancers of the skin. *N Engl J Med*. 1992;327:1649–1662.
17. Glass RL, Spratt JS, Perez-Mesa C. Epidermoid carcinomas of lower extremities: an analysis of 35 cases. *Arch Surg*. 1964;80:955–960.
18. Schiavon M, Mazzoleni F, Chiarelli A, Matano P. Squamous cell carcinoma of the hand: fifty-five case reports. *J Hand Surg Am Vol*. 1988;13:401–404.
19. Murray JC, Pollock SV, Pinnel SR. Keloids: a review. *J Am Acad Dermatol*. 1981;4:461–470.
20. Villanova JR, Flint A. The morphological variations of fibrous histiocytoma. *J Cutan Pathol*. 1974;1:155–164.
21. Reed RJ. Cutaneous manifestations of neural crest disorders (neurocristopathies). *Int J Dermatol*. 1977;16:807–826.
22. Taylor HB, Helwig EB. Dermatofibrosarcoma protuberans. *Cancer*. 1961;15:717–725.
23. Enzinger FM. Atypical fibroxanthoma and malignant fibrous histiocytoma. *Am J Dermatopathol*. 1979;1:185.
24. Safai B, Johnson KG, Myskowski PL, et al. The natural history of Kaposi's sarcoma in the acquired immunodeficiency syndrome. *Ann Intern Med*. 1983;103:744–750.
25. Cox FH, Helwig EB. Kaposi's sarcoma (review). *Cancer*. 1959;12:289–298.
26. Rhodes AR, Silverman RA, Harrist TJ, et al. A histologic comparison of congenital and acquired nevomelanocytic nevi. *Arch Dermatol*. 1985;121:1266–1273.
27. Reed WB, Becker WS Jr, Becker WS Sr, et al. Giant pigmented nevi, melanoma, and leptomeningeal melanocytosis. *Arch Dermatol*. 1965;91:100–199.
28. Leopold JG, Richards DB. The interrelationship of blue and common nevi. *J Pathol*. 1968;95:37–43.
29. Paniago-Pereira C, Maize JC, Ackerman AB. Nevus of large spindle and/or epithelioid cells (Spitz nevus). *Arch Dermatol*. 1978;2114:1811–1923.
30. Allen AC. Juvenile melanomas of children and adults and melanocarcinomas of children. *Arch Dermatol*. 1960;82:325–335.
31. Pulitzer DR, Martin PC, Cohen AP, Reed RJ. Histologic classification of the combined nevus: an analysis of the variable expression of melanocytic nevi. (Clinicopathologic study of 95 cases.) *Am J Surg Pathol*. 1991;15:1111–1122.
32. McGovern VJ. The classification of melanoma and its relationship with prognosis. *Pathology*. 1970;2:85–98.
33. Breslow A. Thickness, cross-sectional areas and depth of invasion in the prognosis of cutaneous melanoma. *Ann Surg*. 1970;172:902–908.
34. Clark WH Jr, Elder DE, Guerry D IV, et al. A study of tumor progression. The precursor lesions of superficial spreading and nodular melanoma. *Hum Pathol*. 1984;15:1147–1165.
35. Clark WH Jr, Mihm MC Jr. Lentigo maligna and lentigo-maligna melanoma. *Am J Pathol*. 1969;55:39–67.
36. Arrington Jr III, Reed RJ, Ichinose H, et al. Plantar lentiginous melanoma. *Am J Surg Pathol*. 1977;1:131–143.
37. Clark WJ Jr. A classification of malignant melanoma in man correlated with histogenesis and biologic behavior. In Montagna W, Hu F, eds. *Advances in Biology of Skin*, Vol 8. New York: Permagon Press;1966:621.
38. Veronesi U, Cascinelli N. Narrow excision (1-cm margin): a safe procedure for thin cutaneous melanoma. *Arch Surg*. 1991;126:438–441.
39. Balch CM, Urist MM, Karakousis CP, et al. Efficacy of 2-cm surgical margins for intermediate-thickness melanomas (1 to 4 mm). *Ann Surg*. 1993;218:262–269.
40. Morton DL, Wen DR, Wong JH, et al. Technical details of intraoperative lymphatic mapping for early stage melanoma. *Arch Surg*. 1992;127:392–399.
41. Alex JC, Weaver DL, Fairbank JT, Rankin BS, Krag DN. Gamma-probe-guided lymph node localization in malignant melanoma. *Surg Oncol*. 1993;2:303–308.
42. Elder DE, Goldman LI, Goldman SC, et al. Dysplastic nevus syndrome. *Cancer*. 1980;46:1787–1794.

5

The Breast

Jean F. Simpson and Thomas J. Smith

Breast cancer diagnosis and management have changed dramatically during the past 20 years. The widespread use of mammography, the implementation of conservative surgical approaches, and the introduction of radiation and chemotherapy in an adjuvant setting have produced management issues that were nonexistent a few years ago. These advances in diagnostic and therapeutic modalities have greatly expanded the responsibilities of the surgical pathologist to include (1) recognizing a borderline group of lesions that are not malignant, but indicate an increased risk of later cancer development, (2) subclassifying noninvasive carcinoma that currently represents up to 20% of newly detected cases, and (3) predicting behavior of malignant lesions. One of the most important roles of the surgical pathologist is to identify groups of patients who may be treated conservatively both surgically and medically. The surgeon too must understand the implications of these various categories of breast disease, to plan with the patient appropriate treatment and follow-up. Increased understanding of the biology of breast cancer has allowed less radical surgery in particular situations. Likewise, identification of cancer patients with high likelihood of long-term survival allows conservative medical approaches to management. This chapter delineates the role of pathology in the multidisciplinary approach to the diagnosis and management of breast disease.

Microscopic Anatomy of the Breast

The normal human female breast is composed of milk-producing lobular units that are drained by coalescing ducts that terminate at the nipple. These branching ducts are arranged in a segmental fashion radiating outward from the nipple. This radial arrangement is not sharply defined and there is frequent overlap between adjacent ''segments''; nonetheless, this configuration can be used to plan the surgical approach for certain segmental diseases. The normal lobular unit (Fig. 5–1) consists of acini (or terminal ductules) embedded in a loose specialized connective tissue, which is itself frequently altered in disease states. The acini empty into intralobular terminal ducts, which in turn emerge from the lobular unit as extralobular terminal ducts. The terminal duct-lobular unit is the site of origin of most proliferative breast lesions, including most carcinomas.[1]

Proliferative Breast Disease and Risk Assessment

For many years, benign conditions of the breast had an implied (but imprecisely defined) risk of subsequent carcinoma development. For rational management of benign conditions of the breast, the *magnitude* of risk is critical. Long-term follow-up studies of women who have undergone benign breast biopsy have defined risk levels based on specific histopathologic patterns.[2, 3] The magnitude of risk (Table 5–1) is based on comparisons with age-matched control women and therefore defines risks *relative* to this control group.[2] The practical consideration of such risk assessments is that they describe probabilities and not an individual patient's risk. The magnitude of risk decreases 10 to 15 years after the biopsy in patients with

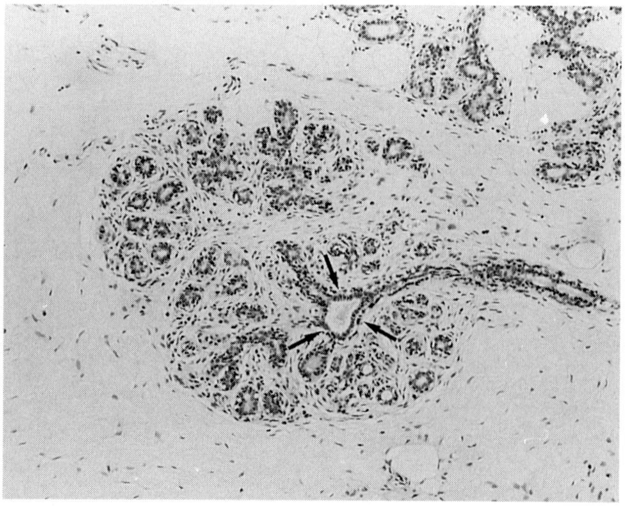

Figure 5–1. Normal lobular unit from a nonlactating woman. Terminal ductules (acini) surround an intralobular terminal duct *(arrows)* that exits the lobular unit as an extralobular duct *(right)*.

microscopically defined risk factors. For those women who do not develop an invasive cancer during this interval, their risk approaches age-matched controls.[6] These risk assessments are designed to compare *groups* of subjects and should *not* be confused with a woman's lifetime risk of developing cancer (one in nine in North America).

The following discussion highlights a stratified approach to benign breast disease, based on subsequent breast cancer risk. Most of the conditions have been grouped together in the past as "fibrocystic disease." Although this term has clinical utility for describing women with lumpy and even painful breasts, it lacks utility for stratification of risk and thwarts understanding of the biologic process. Many clinicians now use the preferred term "fibrocystic changes" to describe the constellation of symptoms and physical findings that are found in up to 50% of perimenopausal women in certain North American groups.[7]

Table 5–1. Relative Risk for Subsequent Development of Invasive Carcinoma Based on Pathologic Examination of Benign Breast Tissue[2, 4]

Not at increased risk[a]	
Adenosis	Cysts, macro, and/or micro[b]
Apocrine metaplasia	Mastitis
Mild hyperplasia	Duct ectasia
Slightly increased risk (1.5–2.0 times)[a]	
Hyperplasia, moderate or florid	Fibroadenoma[c]
Papilloma	Sclerosing adenosis, well developed[d]
Moderately increased risk (4–5 times)[a]	
Atypical ductal hyperplasia	
Atypical lobular hyperplasia	

[a]Risk of implication of developing invasive carcinoma for women with these changes in a biopsy compared with women who have had no breast biopsy.

[b]Although there is a suggestion that women with cysts (palpable) and a family history have a slightly greater risk than identified by family history alone, this has not been controlled for the simultaneous presence of hyperplastic lesions.

[c]From a large epidemiologic study, fibroadenomas indicate a slight risk.[5]

[d]At the time of the consensus meeting,[4] all forms of adenosis were accepted as not increasing cancer risk. Since that time, well-developed examples of sclerosing adenosis[20] indicate a slightly increased risk.

CYSTS AND APOCRINE CHANGE

Breast cysts are extremely common, especially in perimenopausal women. Although the stimulus is unknown, cyst formation is thought to occur as lobular units unfold and coalesce, with loss of specialized connective tissue (Fig. 5–2).[1] The cells that line cysts are often enlarged with abundant cytoplasm (apocrine cells). In fact, the presence of these cells assures the diagnosis of cystic change when found in a fine needle aspirate (see Chap. 3). Cysts may reach several centimeters in diameter and may reexpand after incomplete drainage by fine needle aspiration. Some consider women with breast cysts at increased risk for developing cancer;[8] however, with no other proliferative components (see the following) and no family history of breast cancer, cysts *alone* do *not* indicate an increased risk.[2, 9, 10] There is, however, an interaction between cysts and positive family history, resulting in a slightly increased risk.[2]

EPITHELIAL PROLIFERATIVE BREAST DISEASE

The normal terminal ductule (acinus) has a two-cell lining; any increase in the number of cells above the basement membrane is termed *hyperplasia.* Epithelial hyperplasia represents a spectrum of changes, ranging from mild and clinically insignificant to severe, resembling carcinoma in situ (CIS). Hyperplasia embodies quantitative and qualitative changes that frequently do not develop concomitantly. Specific histologic criteria allow stratification of the hyperplasias, considering architectural and cytologic features.[11] This combined approach explains how a florid example of hyperplasia, resulting in enlarged, distorted lobular units, can nevertheless indicate only a slight increase in cancer risk.

In the past, the terms *papillomatosis* and *epitheliosis*

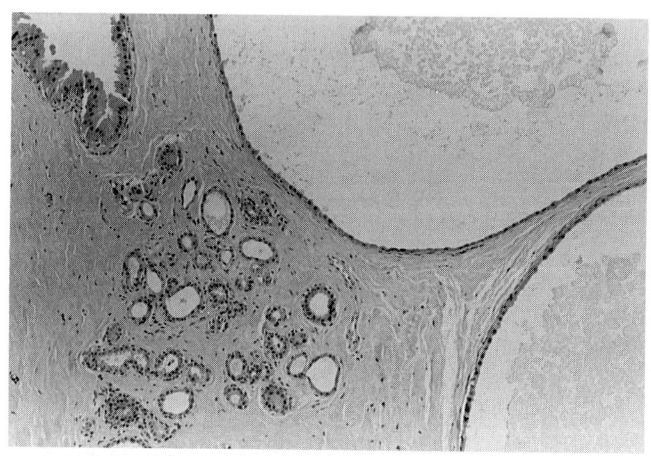

Figure 5–2. Cysts with heaped up apocrine epithelium *(upper left)* and flattened lining *(right)*. Note that the adjacent lobular unit *(left of center)* is lined by similar epithelium.

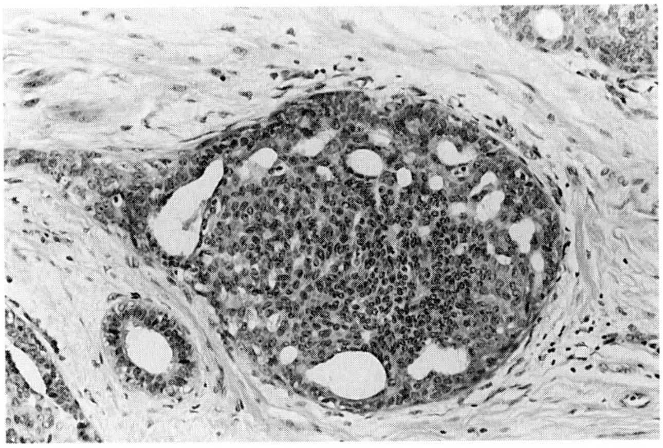

Figure 5–3. Florid ductal hyperplasia without atypia. Note irregularly shaped, peripheral spaces, mild nuclear variation, and nuclear overlap.

were used to describe the common proliferative lesions of the breast. Unfortunately, these terms are nonspecific, potentially confusing, and inexact. In contrast, *hyperplasia* is graded in this chapter to describe extent of changes (i.e., mild, moderate, florid, or atypical), with consequent specific risk implications.[12] A specific pattern of hyperplasia is termed *lobular* when it clearly involves lobular units and may be found in association with invasive *lobular* carcinoma (atypical lobular hyperplasia, described with lobular carcinoma in situ, LCIS, which follows). The most common form of hyperplasia is often termed "ductal" or "intraductal" and is different, biologically and histologically, from the lobular pattern. This terminology persists despite lack of evidence to prove that these lesions actually develop from ductal cells. Following the terminology that has been developed for invasive carcinoma, these common patterns of hyperplasia are designated *ordinary hyperplasia* or *hyperplasia of the usual type.*[12]

These usual patterns of hyperplasia range from *mild,* consisting of spaces lined by only three or four cells to *florid,* with proliferating cellular masses distending and distorting involved spaces. The key microscopic features of these ordinary patterns are *variability* and *irregularity* (Fig. 5–3). Thus, the proliferating cells have nuclei that vary in size, shape, and placement, with frequent nuclear overlap. The resultant cellular masses are irregularly arranged, usually with most cells centrally placed and secondary spaces remaining peripherally.

There is no increased risk associated with the mild form of hyperplasia. About 20% of benign biopsy samples contain hyperplasia of moderate or florid degree with a subsequent slight increase in risk—about twice that of age-matched controls (see Table 5–1).[2] This level of increased risk is similar to that observed for some epidemiologic, nonmicroscopic risk factors such as early menarche, late menopause, and positive family history.[13]

A small percentage of biopsies does not fit the previous description of usual pattern hyperplasia. This group (4% in a large series[2] of biopsies performed in the premammographic era) is considered a borderline category, sharing some features of in situ carcinoma but displaying features that are clearly benign. Although the introduction of a borderline category (termed *atypical hyperplasia*) seems to imply diagnostic uncertainty, it in fact reinforces the diagnoses at the extremes, i.e., usual pattern hyperplasia and CIS.[14] Thus, atypical ductal hyperplasia (ADH) is diagnosed when either architectural or cytologic features suggest ductal carcinoma in situ (DCIS), but malignant features are not completely developed. Although usual patterns of hyperplasia are variable, ADH contains evenly placed cells that do not vary and that proliferate in a manner that outlines rigid, regular secondary spaces. These features suggest DCIS; however, within the involved spaces there is a second population of cells, and some of the secondary spaces may be irregular, assuring the diagnosis of ADH (Fig. 5–4). Criteria for distinguishing among the different forms of proliferative lesions are given in Table 5–2.[11]

As expected, the risk of carcinoma development in ADH falls between that predicted for usual pattern hyperplasia and DCIS. During a 15-year follow-up period, women whose biopsy findings contained ADH developed invasive cancer 4 times as often as controls.[2] In terms of absolute risk, about 10% of women, average age of 45 to 50 and having ADH, will develop invasive cancer. Both breasts are at risk, not just the biopsied breast. Note that this level of risk is equivalent to that for the contralateral breast after an invasive carcinoma has been effectively treated.

A positive family history increases the risk associated with ADH. The presence of a first-degree relative (mother, sister, daughter) with breast cancer doubles the relative risk to eight or nine times that of the general population.[2] This risk level is similar to that observed after a diagnosis of LCIS.[15]

Microscopically defined risk factors are invariably discovered incidentally, although their incidence is increased in mammographically directed biopsies.[16] Uncommonly, the epithelial proliferation itself contains microcalcifications.

The histopathologic evaluation of epithelial hyperplasias is based on clearly defined criteria, which consider growth

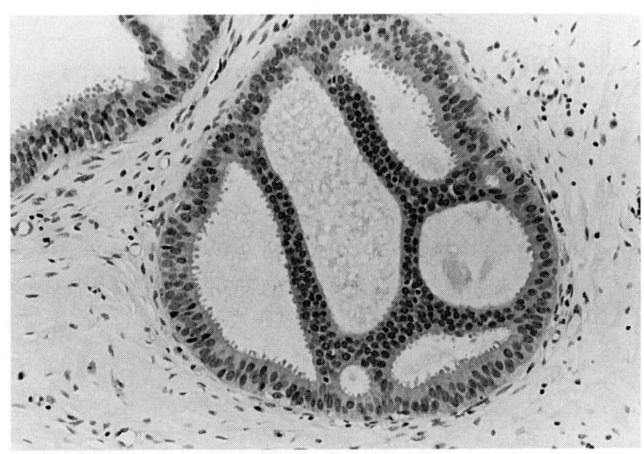

Figure 5–4. Atypical ductal hyperplasia. Sharp secondary spaces and rigid cellular bars suggest ductal carcinoma in situ, however, cells around the periphery of the space show a normal polar arrangement, a finding indicating atypical ductal hyperplasia rather than ductal carcinoma in situ.

Table 5–2. Criteria for Diagnosing Proliferative Breast Lesions[11]

Proliferative Lesion	Cytology	Pattern	Extent
PDWA[a]	Nuclear variability Nuclear overlap	Swirling cellular arrangement Slitlike secondary spaces	No minimum criterion
ADH[b]	Cellular monotony Evenly placed cells Hyperchromatic nuclei Second cell population present	Rigid cellular bars Round, regular secondary spaces	Involves less than two spaces[c]
DCIS (noncomedo)	Cellular monotony Evenly placed cells Hyperchromatic nuclei No secondary cell population	Rigid cellular bars Round, regular secondary spaces	Two or more spaces involved

[a]Proliferative disease without atypia.
[b]Atypical ductal hyperplasia.
[c]Basement membrane-bound space. The term "space" is used to avoid lobular versus ductal terminology.[11]

patterns, cytologic features, and extent of the lesions.[2, 11] Some workers emphasize the difficulty in diagnosing such lesions, citing lack of agreement among expert pathologists.[17] When diagnostic criteria are not in place, such lack of concordance is to be expected; however, when defining criteria[11] are agreed upon, reproducibility is strong.[18] Using these defined criteria, several epidemiologic studies have confirmed the risk implications of epithelial proliferative breast disease.[9, 10]

Hyperplasia refers to an increase in the cells' lining a ductule, whereas adenosis refers to an increase in the number of acini or ductules. Although they are increased in number, ductules are still lined by only two cells. *Sclerosing adenosis* refers to lobular units that have deformed, sclerotic glandular elements (Fig. 5–5). These lesions are often detected mammographically because of the frequent association of microcalcifications. Occasionally, aggregates of sclerosing adenosis can form a palpable mass, an *adenosis tumor* (see Chap. 1, Case 1–5).[19] The overriding concern regarding sclerosing adenosis is its mimicry, clinically and pathologically, of invasive carcinoma. It carries a risk for subsequent invasive cancer similar to that of ordinary pattern hyperplasia of moderate or florid degree.[20]

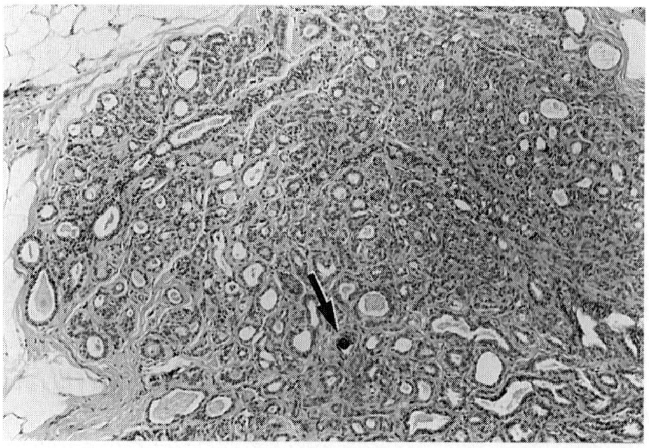

Figure 5–5. Sclerosing adenosis. This expanded lobular unit is composed of deformed glandular units and altered stroma. Microcalcification *(arrow)* is a frequent finding in sclerosing adenosis.

Carcinoma In Situ (Noninvasive Carcinoma)

In situ mammary carcinoma is defined histopathologically as malignant cells confined within existing ductal or lobular units. As straightforward as this definition may seem, CIS is a complex disease with heterogeneous biologic behavior.

The terminology for the two major types of CIS reflects their supposed relationship to the normal anatomic structures of the breast: ducts and the secreting cells of lobular units. With our current understanding of breast differentiation and our ability to detect markers of lactation in so-called ductal carcinomas, the term ductal should be understood to indicate *pattern* rather than site of origin or presentation.[21] Nevertheless, CIS can be subclassified, based on method of detection, histopathologic features, and prognosis.

DUCTAL CARCINOMA IN SITU

Ductal carcinoma in situ represents cases of noninvasive carcinoma in which the pattern of proliferation and the cytologic features are not those of LCIS (see subsequent discussion). This rationale (i.e., based on exclusion) parallels the designations applied to invasive lesions. Although LCIS is usually present in pure form, DCIS is heterogeneous, occurring as several different subtypes, frequently expressed within the same lesion.[22] Heterogeneity is also the hallmark of DCIS biologically, mammographically, and clinically.

Before mammography, noninvasive carcinoma was quite uncommon; however, with current early detection screening programs, DCIS represents about 20% of newly diagnosed breast cancers. Similarly, the size and types of DCIS currently diagnosed contrast with DCIS of the past, which often manifested as a palpable mass with nipple discharge. At that time, clinically evident DCIS was considered a single disease with a single therapeutic option. Our current understanding is that DCIS is a spectrum of disease: at one extreme is the tiny, mammographically detected lesion that can be treated by excision,[23, 24] whereas other DCIS lesions

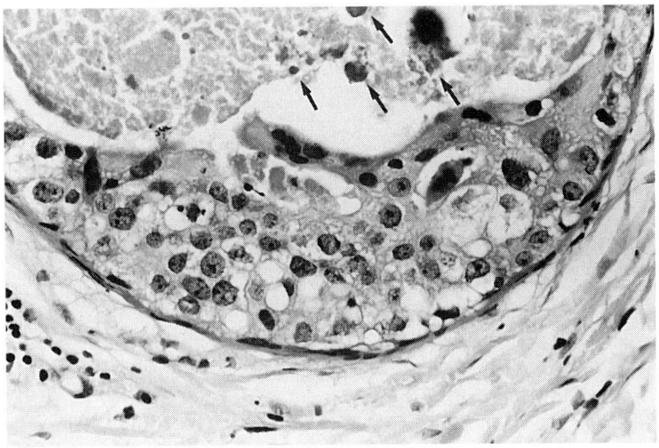

Figure 5–6. Ductal carcinoma in situ, comedo type. Pleomorphic, hyperchromatic nuclei line this space. Within the space *(top)* there are necrotic material and calcification *(arrows)*.

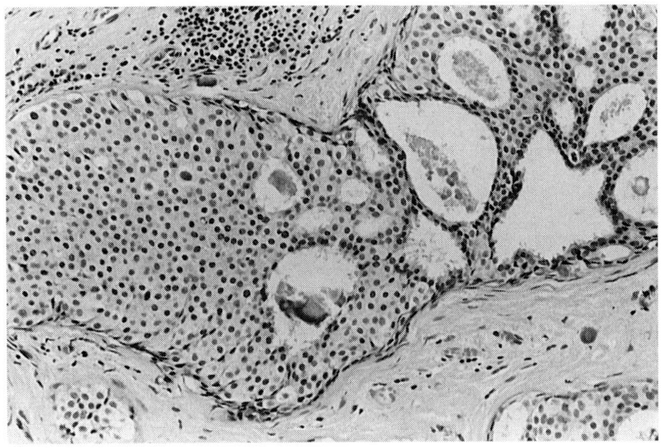

Figure 5–8. Ductal carcinoma in situ, solid *(left)* and cribriform *(right)* patterns. Solid DCIS is often seen adjacent to cribriform areas.

are widespread and thus not amenable to excision alone. The following discussion highlights the heterogeneity of DCIS.

Comedo DCIS

Comedo DCIS was originally defined by its gross appearance, characterized by caseous material dotting the cut surface of the breast, resembling a comedo. Microscopically, this finding corresponds to necrotic cellular debris present within ductal lumens. The necrotic debris frequently calcifies, with a resulting characteristic coarse, linear branching pattern of calcification seen on mammography. The lining cells that surround the intraluminal necrosis have no particular architectural pattern and are large and irregularly placed. Although some investigators have used the term comedo to describe any noninvasive carcinoma demonstrating central necrosis, clinical and biologic correlates underscore that *high nuclear grade* is essential for the diagnosis of comedo DCIS. Extensive, sheetlike necrosis and frequent mitotic figures reflect the high nuclear grade (Fig. 5–6). Although invasive carcinomas are frequently necrotic, the term comedo should be reserved only for *noninvasive* carcinoma.

Noncomedo DCIS

Several architecturally defined patterns of DCIS compose the noncomedo category, including cribriform, solid, and micropapillary types. *Cribriform* DCIS is diagnosed when a monomorphic, neoplastic population of cells proliferates within luminal structures, forming rigid cellular bars and secondary spaces (Fig. 5–7). *Solid* DCIS is uncommonly present in pure form, more often a component of the cribriform pattern (Fig. 5–8). The neoplastic population of *micropapillary* DCIS is arranged in bulbous fronds that extend into the lumen (Fig. 5–9).

Natural History and Clinical Implications

The natural history of DCIS lesions has been difficult to define because the standard treatment has been mastectomy. Two independent studies of incidental, initially undiagnosed DCIS found that about 30% of patients subsequently developed invasive carcinomas in the same area as the initial DCIS.[25, 26] Clinical experience with treatment

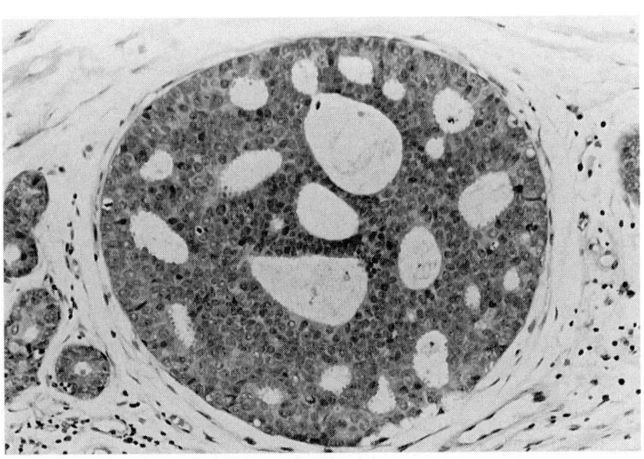

Figure 5–7. Ductal carcinoma in situ, cribriform pattern. The neoplastic cells are evenly spaced and outline sharply defined secondary spaces.

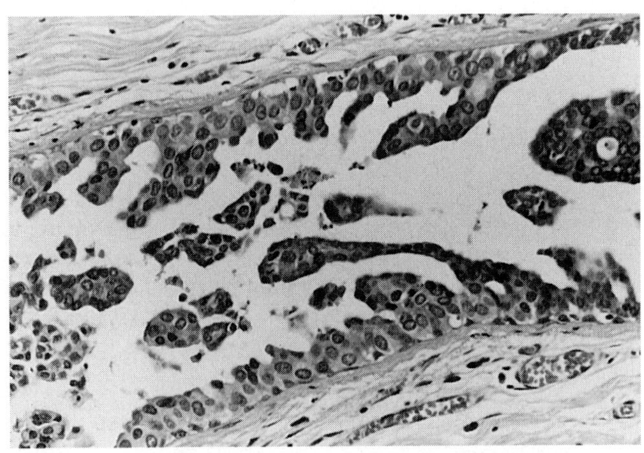

Figure 5–9. Micropapillary ductal carcinoma in situ. Neoplastic cells extend as bulbous projections into the center of the involved space.

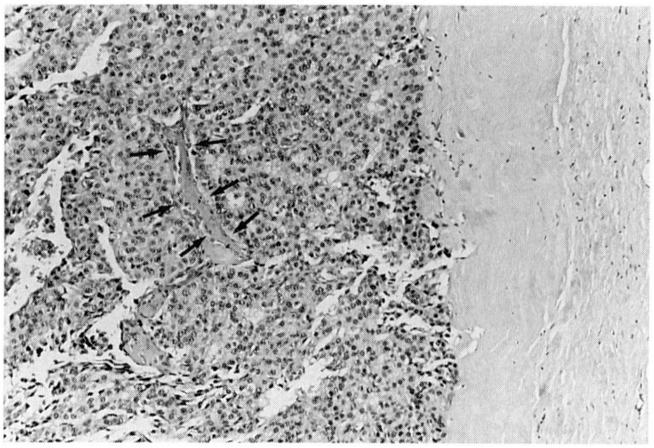

Figure 5–10. Noninvasive papillary carcinoma. A thick fibrous wall (right) surrounds this noninvasive carcinoma. This is a true papillary lesion, with neoplastic cells intimately associated with a fibrovascular core *(arrows)*.

options for DCIS (other than mastectomy) has been presented only lately. In a carefully selected group of patients with mammographically detected DCIS treated by local excision only, recurrences reflected the histologic subtype of DCIS. No recurrences were seen in low-grade DCIS, whereas 30% of high-grade (comedo) DCIS patients suffered recurrence.[23] Recurrences occurred in the same area as the initial biopsy and were evenly divided between noninvasive and small invasive carcinomas.[23] Recurrences *limited* to high-grade (comedo) DCIS have also been reported in patients treated by excision only[24, 27, 28] as well as in patients treated by lumpectomy and irradiation.[29]

Studies of conservative treatment of DCIS underscore the need to refine classification. The inadequacy of dichotomizing DCIS into comedo and noncomedo has been recognized, and an intermediate category has been proposed. This intermediate category allows for the presence of limited necrosis but lacks the high-grade nuclear features of comedo DCIS (so-called noncomedo with necrosis). A new classification scheme has been proposed, which is based primarily on cytonuclear differentiation and secondarily on architectural differentiation resulting in three similar strata.[30] Trials to determine reproducibility and clinical management implications are ongoing.

Breast-conserving treatment for mammographically detected DCIS requires close cooperation among surgeon, mammographer, and pathologist (see Considerations for Practice). Assuming a successful localization procedure, the pathologist is responsible for identifying the area that prompted the biopsy. This usually requires a second radiograph after the specimen has been serially sectioned, to identify the particular slice of tissue that contains the abnormality. A review of the mammographic abnormality with comparison to the specimen radiograph and the histopathologic findings should result in a diagnosis that establishes the nature of the lesion that was localized. Meticulous mammographic/pathologic correlation is required if extent of DCIS is to be accurately determined. Clear communication is also essential for assuring proper management of patients with mammographically detected lesions.

ENCYSTED PAPILLARY CARCINOMA

Encysted papillary carcinoma is a distinctive form of noninvasive carcinoma clinically and pathologically. In the past, the term *papillary* has had broad usage, including lesions that were invasive. This usage has compromised the term's specificity. Encysted papillary carcinoma is a *confined* (noninvasive) lesion consisting of proliferating neoplastic cells intimately associated with fibrovascular cores (Fig. 5–10). In this regard, these are true papillary lesions, as opposed to micropapillary DCIS in which the neoplastic cells form frondlike projections without a supporting fibrovascular core. The subclassification of noninvasive papillary carcinoma provided by Carter et al.[31] is particularly relevant, providing specific histopathologic definitions and long-term follow-up data. For women with no DCIS outside the delimited papillary lesion, local excision is curative.[31]

LOBULAR CARCINOMA IN SITU

Lobular carcinoma in situ has unique histologic and prognostic features. Described in 1941 by Foote and Stewart,[32] LCIS is characterized by a proliferation of a particular cell type within breast lobules. The proliferating cells are very round and regular, and, although they expand the involved acini, the cells often appear discohesive (Fig. 5–11). Lobular carcinoma in situ does not form a mass and is found incidentally in a biopsy performed for another reason.[33] Lobular carcinoma in situ is not detected by mammography, although there does appear to be an association with adjacent microcalcifications.[34] Because of its silent nature, the true incidence of LCIS is difficult to determine. Lobular carcinoma in situ also lacks a positive association with other indicators for biopsy. For this reason, we assume that the incidence of LCIS in the biopsied population reflects the incidence in the general population.[35] Several studies place the incidence at around 1% (Table 5–3). Lobular carcinoma in situ is frequently bilateral and multifocal, and there is a high likelihood that additional disease remains in the breast after biopsy.[40] Most examples remain clinically silent, however, since only about one quarter of patients subsequently develop an inva-

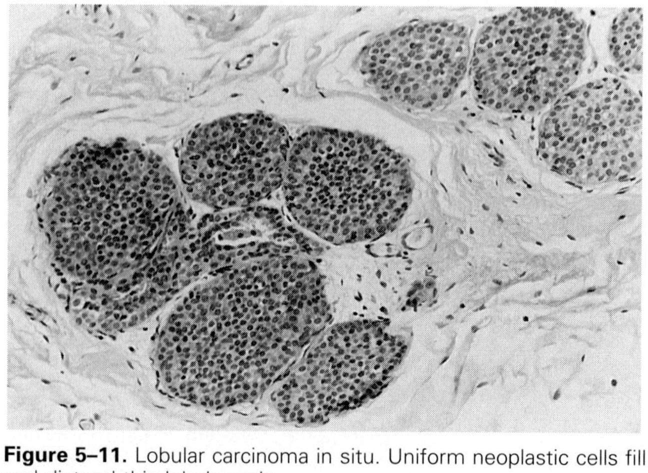

Figure 5–11. Lobular carcinoma in situ. Uniform neoplastic cells fill and distend this lobular unit.

Table 5–3. Reported Studies of Lobular Neoplasia with Outcomes

Study	Number of Cases	Average Age at Biopsy	% LCIS or LN	% IBC	Relative Risk
Page et al.[15]	44	45	0.5	23	9.0
Wheeler et al.[36]	32	44	0.8	12.5	
Rosen et al.[37]	99	45	1.3	36.4	9.0
Andersen[38]	47	46	1.5	21.3	12.0
Haagensen et al.[39]	211	46	3.8	17.0	7.2
Page et al.[3]	126	46	1.6	12.7	4.2

sive carcinoma (see subsequent discussion).[15] Because the majority of diagnoses of LCIS are in premenopausal women, it is thought that the disease may regress after menopause.[15]

Natural History and Clinical Implications

Lobular carcinoma in situ is an indicator for subsequent invasive carcinoma development. In 1978, two institutions reported their experience with patients having biopsy-proven LCIS who received no further treatment.[37, 39] Long-term follow-up showed that these patients were at an increased risk for invasive carcinoma. Since the first reports, several studies of the risk implications of this disease show an increased relative risk of about nine to ten times that of the general population (summarized in Table 5–3). This high risk is related to unequivocal well-developed examples of LCIS. Implementation of strict histopathologic criteria allows separation of a subgroup of women with a risk half that of LCIS.[3] The lesion found in this subgroup is termed *atypical lobular hyperplasia* (ALH); interestingly, the associated risk for subsequent development of carcinoma is similar to that for atypical *ductal* hyperplasia. The diagnosis of LCIS requires that (1) the involved acini are populated exclusively by the characteristic cells and (2) these cells fill, distend, and distort at least one half of the acini within the lobular unit (see Fig. 5–9). Atypical lobular hyperplasia is diagnosed when (1) fewer than half of the acini are expanded and distorted; (2) filling is incomplete, i.e., interspersed intercellular spaces remain; and (3) other cell types are intermixed (Fig. 5–12). Some have used the term lobular neoplasia to denote the full spectrum of disease, ranging from ALH through LCIS.[39] This term is appealing because of the absence of the word *carcinoma;* however, we prefer the specific designations LCIS and ALH. The former term is well established in the literature, and the latter term carries a lower risk for developing carcinoma.[15]

The risk of developing an invasive carcinoma after LCIS applies to *both* breasts, with a slight preponderance of subsequent carcinomas developing in the breast in which LCIS was diagnosed.[5, 36] The absolute risk for developing invasive carcinoma following a diagnosis of LCIS is approximately 1% per year at risk, amounting to 20 to 25% at 15 to 20 years after biopsy.[6] Clinically, LCIS is accepted as a definite risk indicator, although management varies. High-risk lesions such as LCIS offer an ideal situation for breast cancer prevention trials.[41]

Invasive Mammary Carcinoma

Invasive mammary carcinoma has a variety of histologic patterns, including specific types with separate prognostic implications. At one extreme are those carcinomas that pose no threat to life, including tubular and mucinous carcinomas, as well as microinvasive carcinoma. At the other extreme is a grouping of tumors with a dismal prognosis, consisting of large, high-grade carcinomas often with involved axillary lymph nodes at presentation. When all breast carcinomas were treated with radical mastectomy, subcategorization by histopathology was of limited consequence. With the development of more conservative alternative approaches, it has become vital to identify patients for whom more conservative therapy is appropriate. Adjuvant chemotherapy raises the issue of which patients will not benefit from such therapy, either because they already have excellent prognoses or because their prognoses are so grim that chemotherapy at high dose is indicated. Many therapeutic decisions are based on standard staging procedures (TNM system), which can recognize the extremes of the prognostic spectrum in many cases. However, additional prognostic resolution can be obtained by closer microscopic scrutiny. The two main approaches are related to the recognition of specific patterns (the so-called special type carcinomas) or the analysis of individual features (grading). We endorse a combination of these approaches, as described subsequently.

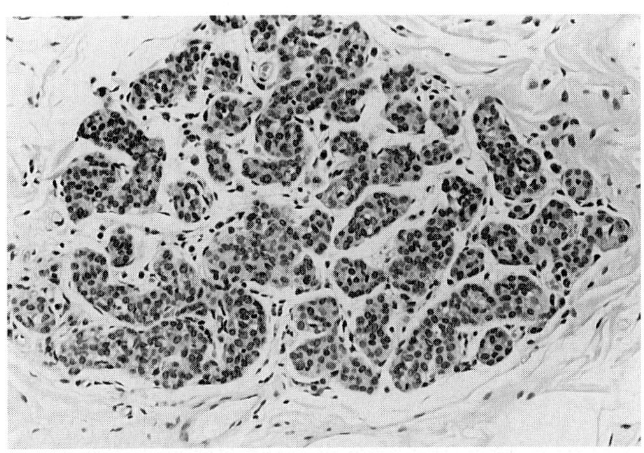

Figure 5–12. Atypical lobular hyperplasia. Some of the acini of this lobular unit contain the same cells found in LCIS (compare with Figure 5–11); however, none is completely filled and there is no distension; hence, the diagnosis of atypical lobular hyperplasia.

HISTOLOGIC TYPES OF INVASIVE CARCINOMA

Much of the terminology regarding breast lesions is dichotomized into *lobular* and *ductal* based largely on historical perspectives. Early histopathologic classification assigned the term *lobular* to those carcinomas that involved lobular units and presumably were the source of similar cells found infiltrating the stroma. By default, other lesions not of a lobular pattern went into the *ductal* classification because ducts are the other source of epithelium within the breast. In reality, the majority of breast lesions, benign and malignant, originate in the terminal ductule-lobular unit. The terms lobular and ductal remain deeply ingrained in clinical parlance, despite biologic evidence to the contrary.

About one quarter of breast carcinomas display specific histologic patterns that are readily spotted; these are the so-called special type carcinomas. Patients with these lesions have excellent prognoses, even though the lesions may attain a size that would suggest otherwise.[42] Criteria are well established for these special type carcinomas, and they require that the defining features be present homogeneously. By contrast, variant forms are recognized if the features are present in only 75 to 90% of the tumor. Although the prognosis is better than that when no special features are present, the reliability of prognosis of these variant forms is not as great as their pure (>90%) counterparts.[42] Despite some variation in terminology, there is concordance about the incidence of these special types within various series.[42–48] The special type carcinomas are prevalent in screening programs, being responsible for up to one third of carcinomas detected in this manner.[48]

The most important special type is *tubular carcinoma* and its variants.[49–51] When present in pure form, tubular carcinoma effectively has no distant metastatic potential (see Chap. 1). Histologically, angulated tubules, composed of cells with low-grade nuclei, compose at least 90% of the carcinoma (Fig. 5–13). Tubular carcinoma represents only about 3 to 5% of all invasive carcinomas. For this reason its significance may go unrecognized when cases are grouped and analyzed only by stage. The importance of tubular carcinoma lies with its therapeutic implication for *individual* patients. A review of surgical therapeutics indicates that pure tubular carcinoma with adequate margins does not require mastectomy, radiation, or axillary lymph node dissection.[52]

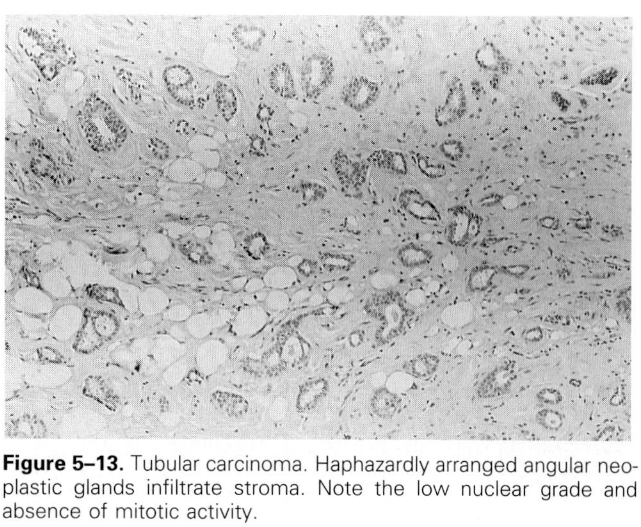

Figure 5–13. Tubular carcinoma. Haphazardly arranged angular neoplastic glands infiltrate stroma. Note the low nuclear grade and absence of mitotic activity.

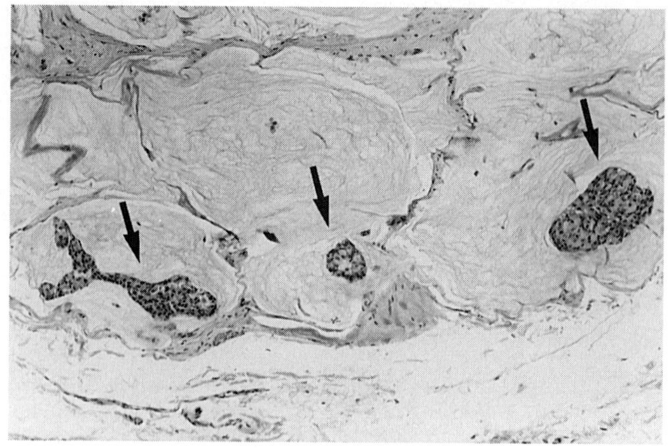

Figure 5–14. Mucinous carcinoma. Low-grade nests of tumor cells *(arrows)* appear suspended in surrounding pools of mucin.

Closely related to tubular carcinoma, histologically and biologically, is *invasive cribriform carcinoma.*[53, 54] Mixtures of tubular and cribriform patterns may be seen within the same carcinoma; the diagnosis is based on the predominant pattern. In studies of *pure* tubular[49] and invasive cribriform carcinoma,[53, 54] the presence of one or two positive low axillary lymph nodes did not adversely affect survival. The importance of pattern purity is emphasized, because the presence of *any* carcinoma *not* fulfilling these special-type criteria increases the likelihood of nodal involvement and decreased survival.[49, 53, 54]

Mucinous (colloid) carcinoma, when present in pure form, is also associated with an excellent prognosis. Its defining characteristic is the presence of extracellular pools of mucin in which low-grade tumor aggregates appear to be suspended (Fig. 5–14). When of pure mucinous form, 90% of patients with this lesion survive for more than 10 years.[55] Other studies confirm that patients with pure mucinous carcinomas have excellent prognoses.[56, 57]

These statements regarding the excellent prognosis of tubular, invasive cribriform, and mucinous carcinoma are predicated on two features: homogeneous pattern and low-grade nuclei. As the purity of pattern deteriorates, prognosis worsens, approaching that of stage-matched carcinomas of no special type (see subsequent discussion).[49, 55, 57] The second requirement is for the *entire* carcinoma, not just the area of pure pattern, to be low grade. Implicitly, this determination requires thorough pathologic sampling and microscopic study. Following these criteria, Dixon et al.[42] showed long-term survival for a group of patients having special type carcinomas. It is particularly impressive that these patients were treated over 30 years ago, and the average size of their tumor was 4 cm.[42]

Infiltrating lobular carcinoma (ILC) remains a useful subtype of invasive carcinoma, although disagreement remains regarding prognostic implications. This may be attributed to the inconstancy of histologic definition, as evidenced by the wide range of incidence, from less than 1%[58]

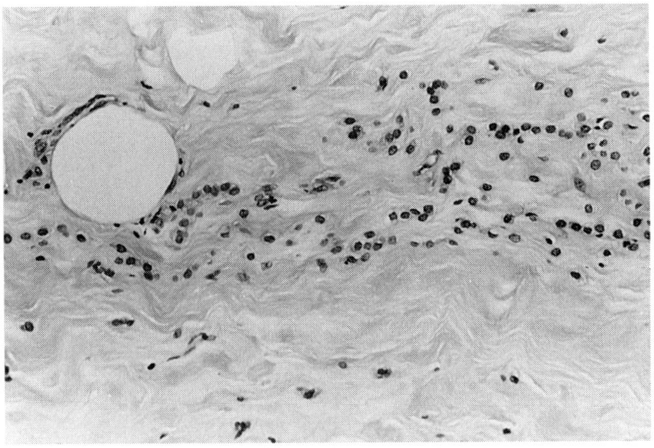

Figure 5–15. Infiltrating lobular carcinoma, classic type. Single-file growth pattern and bland nuclear features are essential for the diagnosis of classic ILC.

up to 20%.[59] Pure or classic ILC is characterized by two essential features, low-grade nuclei and single-file pattern of infiltration (Fig. 5–15). Subtypes of ILC have been described in which one but not the other feature is present.[46] When *restricted* to the pure or classic type of ILC, patient survival is improved in comparison with carcinomas of no special type, often called ductal carcinomas.[47, 60, 61] All types of ILC are associated with an increased incidence of bilaterality, but prognosis is affected only if the contralateral carcinoma is synchronous.[62] Because of its insidious growth pattern, the extent of ILC is difficult to ascertain by clinical, mammographic, and gross examination. In spite of this, when compared with stage-matched carcinomas of no special type, breast-conserving therapy for ILC does not result in a significantly higher rate of local recurrence.[63, 64]

Medullary carcinoma is a well-recognized entity with a characteristic gross appearance. The tumor is sharply circumscribed, with a soft and uniform consistency. The sharp circumscription seen mammographically and grossly corresponds microscopically to a rounded, pushing border rather than an infiltrative tumor edge. The other microscopic distinction is the presence of a dense lymphoid infiltrate. In contrast to the other special types of carcinoma, medullary carcinoma has high-grade nuclei.

Much has been written about the prognostic features of medullary carcinoma. The need for adherence to histologic guidelines is evident because this entity is currently overdiagnosed.[65, 66] Medullary carcinoma is more common in younger women[67] and may be increased in familial breast cancers.[67] The diagnostic significance of medullary carcinoma possibly lies in predicting a better prognosis than would be expected in comparable (high-grade) nonmedullary no special type (NST) carcinoma. Confirmatory studies are not yet available.

Approximately three quarters of invasive breast carcinomas do not have histopathologic features that allow their inclusion into the aforementioned categories. Based on the epithelial components normally found in breast parenchyma, these are referred to as *ductal* because they do not have the lobular pattern as described. Despite this common usage, these carcinomas are not proved to arise in ducts. In practice, they are diagnosed by exclusion because they do not fit into any of the special type categories. For these reasons, we support the terminology NST carcinoma, which is equivalent to the terminology of Fisher et al.[43] "ductal without special features or otherwise not specified type."

As the name would imply, there are no specific histopathologic features that are consistently found in infiltrating mammary carcinoma of NST. These NST carcinomas have a wide variety of patterns from solid to small, tightly cohesive nests, to single-cell infiltrative patterns (Fig. 5–16). Gland formation may be present, and frequently a mixture of these patterns will be found in an individual carcinoma. Moreover, any of the patterns described for special type carcinomas may be found but only focally.

Patients with these NST carcinomas have the worst prognoses. Unlike the special type carcinomas, limited prognostic information is obtained by identifying histologic patterns because these are quite variable. Instead, prognosis rests on tumor size and lymph node status (see Prognosis of Invasive Breast Carcinoma, below).

The preceding discussion of types of invasive carcinomas encompasses those frequently encountered. Rare types or those having descriptive terminology without prognostic implication (e.g., apocrine carcinoma) are not further considered. The lack of consistency in terminology in surgical pathology reporting of breast cancers is evident in an update from the National Cancer Institute, which listed over 20 histologic types of invasive carcinoma.[68] The source of these data, the Surveillance, Epidemiology, and End Results (SEER) program, is based on original pathology reports and not on a central microscopic slide review. Even based on such data, the 5-year survival for the special type carcinomas previously described was considerably better than for NST carcinomas.[68]

PROGNOSIS OF INVASIVE BREAST CARCINOMA

Predicting outcome for patients with breast carcinoma, especially for those whose axillary lymph node findings

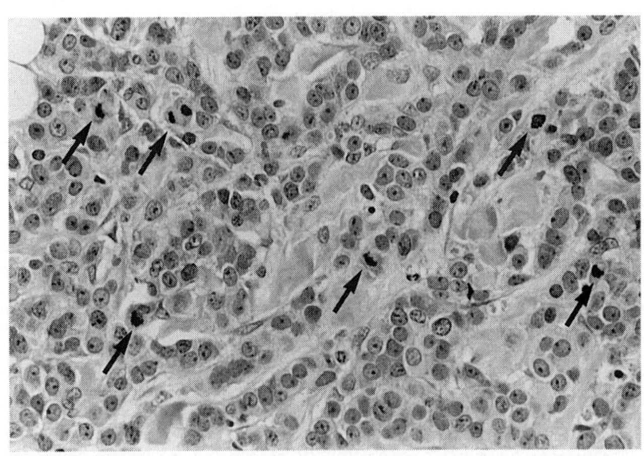

Figure 5–16. Small clusters of malignant cells are seen in this infiltrating mammary carcinoma of no special type. Note numerous mitotic figures *(arrows)*. Such evidence of high proliferative activity is a proven adverse prognostic indicator.

are negative, is of paramount importance. Advances in surgical, medical, and radiation oncology have resulted in therapeutic options that ideally should be individualized to derive maximum benefit with minimum morbidity. Enormous efforts have been exerted in searching for determinants of prognosis. Weighing the factors that give significant independent information is difficult. Available studies have evaluated different endpoints, patient groups, lengths of follow-up, and treatments. They are also hampered by inconsistent inclusion of known prognostic factors to test for independent significance in the final evaluation.[69–71] The following discussion emphasizes prognostic factors that have been widely used and shown, through outcome analysis, to be independent predictors of prognosis.

Tumor stage is the single most useful system for predicting survival. The TNM staging system[71] is the mainstay for prognostication for breast cancer and examines three variables: diameter of the primary tumor (T), lymph node metastasis (N), and distant metastasis (M). The primary tumor is categorized as T1 if less than 2 cm, T2 if greater than 2 but less than 5 cm, and T3 if 5 cm or greater in size. The size of the primary tumor and the status of axillary lymph nodes are independent and additive in predicting survival.[72] Both predictions reflect the tumor's ability to spread distantly.[72, 73] Staging is especially useful at the extremes of the scale. Clearly, the prognosis for a small carcinoma (1 cm) that does not involve axillary lymph nodes is so favorable that adjunctive measures are not indicated.[74, 75] In comparison, most would agree that a patient with a 3-cm carcinoma should receive adjuvant therapy. However, as previously discussed, patients with *pure special type carcinomas,* such as tubular and mucinous, have excellent long-term prognoses, even if the carcinomas attain such large size.[42] The challenge for surgical pathologists is to consistently apply the specific histologic criteria that allow recognition of pure special types so that their prognostic implications can be utilized.

Although the prognoses for patients having small or special type carcinomas are favorable, predicting outcome for the remainder of patients, particularly those with negative lymph node findings, is uncertain. *Histologic grading* of breast carcinomas may help stratify this group of patients. Unfortunately, careful grading of breast carcinoma has been inconsistent, despite the necessity of grading other malignancies (see Chap. 14). Grading systems may be based on architectural or cytologic features. We support the grading system of Scarff, Bloom, and Richardson (SBR), as modified by Elston.[76] This system, also known as the combined histologic grade, separately evaluates the degree of glandular formation, nuclear pleomorphism, and mitotic activity. Although the SBR system has been in place for many years, modifications by Elston and colleagues have clarified criteria, thereby strengthening its predictive ability and reproducibility. Since 1973, this group has graded over 2,000 cases of primary operable breast carcinoma in conjunction with various studies. Using this histologic grading system, a highly significant correlation has been demonstrated between the grade and the relapse-free interval and overall survival.[76] Of interest is the distribution of cases within the various grades: 19% were grade 1, 34% were grade 2, and 47% were grade 3. These findings are in contrast to other grading schemes that place approximately two thirds of cases in the poorly differentiated unfavorable category, thus reducing predictive utility.[77] Other workers have confirmed the value of grading as being second only to lymph node involvement as an independent prognostic factor.[78]

Although histologic grading of breast carcinoma in North America has not been as widely accepted as it has in Europe, there has been a trend for its greater use.[79] The reproducibility of histologic grading using the combined histologic grading system has been demonstrated.[80, 81]

Prognosis is gauged according to (1) tumor stage, (2) histologic recognition of special types of carcinomas, and (3) careful histologic grading. Surgical pathology reports are therefore incomplete without these considerations. Likewise, studies of new prognostic factors should include these proven factors in the final analysis of independent significance.

Other parameters are being examined to refine prognostication. Although these have not been as thoroughly studied as the aforementioned parameters, they are closely linked to them and may yet prove useful. Cellular proliferation is assessed in several ways, most practically by quantification of mitotic figures. This method is a powerful predictor of recurrence and survival.[82–84] Proliferation can also be analyzed through flow cytometric analysis of DNA, from which the percentage of cells in S-phase is calculated. Standardization of methodology as well as establishment of meaningful divisions of S-phase continue to be investigated.[85]

Another useful parameter is the presence or absence of estrogen receptor on tumor cells. Integral to most treatment plans, the presence of estrogen receptor is a well-established predictor of response to therapy. Biochemical determination of estrogen receptor has been linked to clinical outcome and is established as a prognostic factor.[86] Estrogen receptor may also be detected by immunohistochemical (IHC) methods. Unlike the biochemical method that uses a tissue homogenate, cellular relationships are maintained in IHC methods. This allows confirmation that the positive signal is localized in invasive carcinoma, not in adjacent normal epithelium. Several studies have shown close correlation between these two methods.[87] For cases that diverge, the IHC result is favored.[88] Biochemical methods may give false-positive results if normal tissue is included in analysis and false-negative results if an invasive carcinoma has low cellularity, e.g., invasive lobular carcinoma. Compared with the older biochemical method, however, fewer studies have yet been completed correlating IHC results and clinical outcome.

Some prognostic factors are useful within certain subsets of patients, such as the presence of the oncogene c-*erbB*-2 in node-positive patients.[89] Studies continue to clarify the utility of oncogenes and tumor suppressor genes, as well as to provide insight into the biologic processes involved in tumor progression.

Inclusion of the histopathologic parameters in the final assessment of new prognostic factors remains critical.[90] Many new markers show promise on initial examination through simple correlation with outcome; however, when compared with established predictors, many of these initially promising contenders are ousted by the veterans in the early rounds.

Special Prognostic Issues

MICROINVASIVE CARCINOMA

Invasive carcinoma detectable only microscopically has special treatment implications. These carcinomas are most often found with DCIS, frequently in a mammographically directed biopsy. Various terminology is used for describing the spectrum of limited invasive lesions: minimal breast cancer, minimal invasive cancer, and microinvasive carcinoma. Defining these terms is important but even more important is measurement of the extent of the invasive component. This should be reported in millimeters or fractions thereof. Invasion less than 5 mm in greatest dimension is rarely associated with lymph node involvement.[91] Microinvasive carcinoma should be diagnosed only when there is unequivocal evidence of invasion. Because scarring around an area of DCIS can mimic invasion (see Pitfalls for the Pathologist), the diagnosis of microinvasion requires the presence of malignant cells beyond the confines of the terminal ductule-lobular unit, i.e., in the nonspecialized connective tissue, which is measurable at 1 mm or larger. Among some pathologists there is a disturbing tendency toward the more malignant diagnosis as a hedge. This strategy is totally unacceptable because a diagnosis of microinvasive carcinoma will result in an axillary lymph node dissection or even adjuvant therapy—treatment modalities inappropriate for purely noninvasive carcinoma.

LOCAL RECURRENCE AFTER CONSERVATIVE THERAPY

Local treatment failure is an unfortunate consequence of conservative therapy of breast carcinoma. Predicting risk of local recurrence is the subject of considerable study. When evaluating risk factors, it is critical to distinguish those that indicate inherent disease aggression from those that reflect inadequate therapy initially. Histopathologic parameters associated with risk of local recurrence reflect residual tumor burden. Thus, margin involvement by carcinoma,[92–94] presence of lymphatic involvement,[92] and presence of an extensive intraductal component[73, 94, 95] are all associated with local recurrence. As with other predictors, interaction between risk factors is important. Thus, extensive intraductal component may be a negative indicator only if margins of resection are involved.[94]

The same caution applied to interpreting prognostic factors for survival in breast cancer should also be applied to evaluating risk of local recurrence. Hence, differences in histologic definitions, surgical approaches, and delivery of radiotherapy may complicate comparison of various series.

MULTICENTRICITY

Multicentricity refers to the occurrence of two or more foci of breast carcinoma physically separated from each other. Without three-dimensional reconstruction precise designations are difficult because apparently separate foci may be connected through the ductal system. In general, multicentricity is diagnosed if carcinoma is found discontinuously in different quadrants. Other criteria proposed have included radiographic, gross, and microscopic findings.[96] In addition to providing insight into pathogenesis, multicentricity of breast carcinoma has practical implications, especially in breast conservation.

Factors associated with a higher risk of multicentricity include (1) nipple or subareolar involvement,[97] (2) extensive intraductal component (EIC),[95] and (3) for some subsets of breast carcinoma, size.[98] Considering the radial arrangement of ducts emanating from the nipple, it is easy to understand how carcinoma involving the nipple may involve more than one quadrant by contiguous extension. Thus, multicentricity in this clinical setting may actually reflect extent of disease and not separate disease foci. For DCIS, multicentricity is more likely to be encountered with lesions over 25 mm.[98] Of the subtypes of DCIS, the micropapillary variety is more likely to be multicentric.[99] Among invasive carcinomas, ILC is more likely to be multicentric than other types. Invasive carcinomas with an extensive intraductal component predict residual DCIS up to 2 cm away from the primary tumor in one third of cases, compared with only 2% of cases without EIC.[100] These indicators of multicentricity therefore have important implications for predicting success of conservatively treated breast carcinoma.

Considerations for Practice

The contributions and potential limitations of pathology that are important to surgeons are highlighted in the following discussion. The information provided by pathologists is most useful if there is clear communication between the surgeon and pathologist.

The diagnostic approach depends on clinical impression, which in turn includes the patient's age, clinical history, and lesion characteristics. For palpable lesions, a fine needle aspirate (FNA), together with ultrasound or mammography, can support the clinical impression and guide follow-up strategy. Further evaluation is indicated in any setting if the clinical, mammographic, or cytologic interpretation is suspect for malignancy.

A stratified approach to reporting FNA results, rather than a simple "positive" versus "negative," produces the best use of information in the clinical setting.[101] Planning for treatment or follow-up is straightforward at the extremes of clinical suspicion, and it is in these areas that FNA is most beneficial. A confirmation of benignancy in a clinical setting of low suspicion reinforces the clinical diagnosis and obviates a more invasive procedure. At the other extreme, diagnosing malignancy by FNA allows for immediate initiation of counseling and exploration of treatment options (see Chap. 3).

Lesions that Require Excision. Several considerations are related to the handling of excised specimens. The specimen should arrive in the surgical pathology laboratory intact, either fresh from the operating room in a towel or in saline. Improper specimen handling introduces artifacts that compromise final histopathologic interpretation. The surgeon should orient the specimen, e.g., with short and long sutures; this allows the pathologist to pinpoint positive margins, so that additional surgery can be planned accordingly.

For palpable lesions or mammographically detected mass lesions that are suspicious looking and of sufficient size, intraoperative frozen section can be done. This procedure is performed for cases in which immediate mastectomy or axillary lymph node dissection is planned. In cases for which no further immediate surgery is an issue, handling of tissue depends on the type of specimen and indications for its excision. Frozen sections should not be done just to satisfy one's curiosity.

Palpable Lesions. If a palpable lesion is clinically suspected for carcinoma, and breast conservation is a consideration, the margins of the specimen should be inked by the pathologist for identification on permanent sections. Obviously, a specimen that has been sliced prior to arrival in the pathology laboratory cannot be accurately assessed for margin involvement. Performing frozen sections on grossly negative margins is almost always unnecessary.[102] For close margins, frozen section may aid in determining the need for immediate extension of the excision, thus sparing the patient additional surgery. For lesions greater than 1 cm, a small portion can be frozen to confirm that a carcinoma is present and a small piece allocated for ancillary studies (see subsequent discussion). For lesions less than 1 cm, frozen section should be avoided (see Chap. 1, Case 1–4).

Mammographically Detected Lesions. Communication among surgeon, pathologist, and radiologist is especially critical in this setting. Most biopsies are performed for microcalcifications or architectural distortions. The first step is specimen radiography, which confirms that the abnormality that occasioned the biopsy has indeed been excised. After the specimen is sectioned, a second specimen radiograph serves as a guide for submitting histologic sections, thus allowing correlation of the histopathologic and mammographic findings. For some needle-directed biopsies performed for architectural distortion, ex vivo radiography may not yield the same contrast densities that are recognizable in vivo.

Occasionally, microscopic sections do not disclose the microcalcifications noted on specimen x-ray. Histologic detection of calcification depends on its chemical composition. Calcium oxalate and calcium phosphate are indistinguishable mammographically, but differ microscopically. Calcium oxalate may be invisible by conventional microscopic examination but can be revealed by polarized light. If none is found, x-raying the paraffin block may demonstrate calcifications that are deeper in the tissue and can thus be identified on deeper levels.

The use of frozen sections to examine needle-localization specimens is contraindicated.[102, 103] These lesions are usually small and often focal. In addition, artifacts inherent to the freezing procedure may render certain lesions essentially undiagnosable.

Margin Assessment. In addition to establishing the diagnosis, the pathologist also assesses adequacy of excision. This may not be as straightforward as it seems. If margin involvement is identified by specimen radiography, wider excision should be performed, although a negative margin by specimen radiography is not entirely reliable.[104] Palpation may identify subtle density due to carcinoma that is not visible grossly or by specimen radiography.

If carcinoma is present at the inked margin of resection, all would agree that the plane of resection is positive. What constitutes a negative margin is not as well defined. Some argue that a single collagen fiber between ink and malignant cellularity constitutes a ''technically'' negative margin.[105] Although this definition does not consider the distribution of lesions within the breast, it may have some practical merit in some cases if this is only a solitary focus of tumor.[94] Others avoid the issue of definition, and they report the status of the margin in terms of distance (in millimeters or fractions of millimeters) from ink to malignant cells.[102] The reality of margin assessment is that neither residual carcinoma nor subsequent local recurrence can be predicted with certainty based on margin assessment. Nevertheless, until further data are available, it is important to carefully assess margins because in some cases a clinical or gross examination alone is misleadingly negative (e.g., DCIS and ILC). Moreover, boosted radiation dosage may be incorporated in the plan in deference to positive margins. Margins are assessed most accurately on paraffin sections. Other methods exist, including intraoperative touch imprints,[106] but such methods have inherent limitations.

Allocation of Tissue for Ancillary Studies. As the average size of breast carcinoma at diagnosis has decreased, the demand for ancillary studies to supplement histopathologic prognostication has increased. This inverse relationship demands that the pathologist use sound clinical judgment in the allocation of fresh tissue. The prime goal is to identify the presence or absence of invasive carcinoma. No ancillary test can replace this critical prognostic factor. Although allocation of nonrepresentative tissue is indeed a pitfall, it is a much greater error in specimen management if the one diagnostic area of invasion is sent for an ancillary study. In this regrettable circumstance the tissue used for diagnosis does not contain the invasive component. How can such situations be avoided? First, small (<1 cm) carcinomas should not be sacrificed for ancillary studies (see Chap. 1). Hormone receptor studies may be performed on tissue sections from the paraffin block, with results that compare favorably with biochemical assays.[87] Similar techniques can be used for assessing level of proliferation. In practical terms, patients with invasive carcinomas less than 1 cm have good prognoses; additional studies are largely superfluous.[75] Larger lesions may be studied by ancillary methods because ample diagnostic tissue is available and the tissue studied is representative of the lesion. A touch imprint or frozen section helps to assure representation of the tumor itself and to assist in the accurate interpretation of results.

Although various publications have recommended one or another single parameter, we support the use only of those predictors of proven clinical utility. Others may be evaluated for research purposes, provided there is adequate tissue.

Clinical Management Based on Histopathology

A histopathologic diagnosis should indicate more than presence or absence of malignancy. The pathologist should address a number of questions. If a lesion is benign, is it indicative of increased risk? If a lesion is malignant, can it be managed conservatively? What is the likelihood of recurrence or death from a malignant process?

Patients at Increased Risk. Because epithelial proliferative lesions are not associated with any specific clinical or mammographic findings, their presence in a specimen cannot be predicted. The management of these risk-indicator lesions is different from the usual situation in which a particular diagnosis results in a specific therapy. Although long-term follow-up studies have assigned levels of risk, they do not lead to simple therapeutic decisions. Clinical management must consider the level of risk and the patient's level of anxiety, understanding and willingness to live with the probabilities of developing invasive carcinoma, and acceptance of long-term follow-up.

High-risk Lesions. The best characterized high-risk lesion, LCIS, indicates a risk of about nine to ten times that of the general population. Most advocate careful follow-up with close surveillance by mammography. In some patients, extirpation of breast tissue is appropriate. High-risk lesions such as LCIS are an important group to investigate in chemoprevention trials.[41]

Moderately Increased Risk Lesions. For women with atypical hyperplasia careful surveillance is required. Yearly mammograms and careful clinical examination twice a year are suggested.[107] The addition of a positive family breast cancer history increases the risk to that of LCIS.

Slightly Increased Risk Lesions. Those women with proliferative disease without atypia are at a slightly increased risk, no more than twice that of age-matched controls. Although of statistical significance, the medical management implications are unclear.[107] The current suggestion for management of women with only a slight increase in risk is yearly mammograms and self-examination. The level of risk that accompanies the ordinary patterns of hyperplasia should not elicit undue concern.[107]

Lesions Without Increased Risk. This group represents the majority of benign breast biopsies. Virtually all breast biopsies are characterized by some degree of fibrosis, small apocrine cysts, and lobule irregularity. Women with these changes can be reassured that their risk is no different from that of the general population.[2]

An important aspect of management of patients with histologic indicators of risk is the length of time for which this elevated risk persists. Clinical decisions should be based on knowledge of events in the ensuing 10 to 15 years and not beyond that time. This is the limit of likelihood that is derived from follow-up studies.[6] Especially for older women, the relative risk decreases after such a time interval.[6]

Patient management decisions in the setting of increased risk are difficult because no precise guidelines exist. The most important single factor is the individual woman's level of concern. If a high-risk lesion is detected it is not an emergent situation. Treatment decisions should be deliberative. For most women, mammographic surveillance is a widely accepted clinical alternative to extirpative surgery.

Management of Patients with Malignant Lesions. Clinical decisions regarding the treatment of malignant breast lesions must be based on stage of disease. For DCIS, considerations include size and type, patient preference for conservation, and sampling for detection. Small examples of mammographically detected, noncomedo DCIS have been treated by excision only without recurrence.[24, 25] Although total mastectomy is virtually curative for DCIS, it is clear that more conservative approaches, with or without radiotherapy, may suffice.[29] After diagnosis of DCIS, the presence of extensive microcalcifications within the residual breast tissue may weaken the power of mammographic follow-up, thus disallowing a conservative approach.

For invasive carcinomas therapeutic options should consider size and extent of the tumor and cosmetic result if conservation is desired. In some cases of large carcinomas or those with a diffuse growth pattern, mastectomy followed by reconstruction may be aesthetically most desirable.

For an excisional biopsy of carcinoma the following information should be supplied by the pathologist: (1) size, (2) type, (3) grade (with reference to grading system used), (4) status of margins, (5) peritumoral lymphovascular space involvement, (6) hormone receptor status, and (7) assessment of proliferative activity. This information, along with the lymph node status, allows stratification of patients into low-, intermediate-, and high-risk categories. Patients at low risk include those having pure special type carcinomas or low-grade or small (less than 1 cm) carcinomas of no special type (ductal).[74] Patients having large, high-grade carcinomas or those involving more than three lymph nodes are at high risk for recurrence, and they should be treated aggressively. Management of the intermediate-risk group of patients varies. For example, most patients having node-negative carcinomas greater than 2 cm receive some form of adjuvant therapy. Prognostic factors continue to be explored for stratification of this group of patients.

Acknowledgment

The authors are grateful to Dr. David L. Page for his helpful review of the manuscript.

PITFALLS FOR THE SURGEON

1. Excising a small, potentially malignant lesion in piecemeal fashion.
2. Submitting a biopsy that may be malignant in anything other than saline.
3. Failing to supply the pathologist with a clinical history.
4. Failing to orient the specimen for the pathologist.
5. Failing to corroborate with the mammographer when it is necessary to understand the relationship between a palpable finding and a mammographic finding that requires biopsy.
6. Not obtaining a specimen radiograph on a needle-localized excisional biopsy.
7. Failing to communicate to the pathologist the reason for the biopsy (mass, microcalcification) and what possibilities are anticipated on histologic examination.
8. Not obtaining a follow-up mammogram 2 to 3 months following a needle localization biopsy if the specimen radiograph was indeterminate and the tissue diagnosis was benign.
9. Failing to clarify features having an impact on specimen handling. For instance, margins are crucial if the patient is a candidate for conservation, but, if mastectomy has been planned for a diagnosis of carcinoma, margin assessment is a waste of resources.

PITFALLS FOR THE PATHOLOGIST

1. Misinterpreting DCIS that involves lobular units as LCIS. DCIS can sometimes be present within lobular units, mimicking the lobular distention of LCIS. In this setting, distinction is made on cytologic features; the cells of DCIS are larger and less uniform than LCIS.
2. Misinterpreting in situ disease (either DCIS or LCIS) involving sclerosing adenosis as invasive cancer. Lobular units involved by sclerosing adenosis may also be involved by the neoplastic cells of noninvasive carcinoma. The distortion of the sclerosed lobules may mimic invasion.
3. Misinterpreting DCIS associated with scarring as microinvasive carcinoma. Scarring can result in distortion, mimicking invasive carcinoma.
4. Misinterpreting radial scar for tubular carcinoma. A radial scar is a benign sclerotic lesion unassociated with previous trauma or surgery. An interlobular duct becomes scarred, and as it contracts it distorts surrounding interconnecting lobular units. The central portion of the scar often contains entrapped ductules, mimicking a tubular carcinoma.
5. Not recognizing a sparsely cellular ILC (see Fig. 5–15).
6. Misinterpreting a benign glandular inclusion (or nevus) in the capsule of a lymph node as a metastasis.
7. Misallocating tissue for ancillary studies. The greatest danger is in not reserving diagnostic tissue for the routine but essential microscopic diagnosis. An accurate histologic diagnosis takes precedence over any other study.
8. Misinterpreting retraction artifact around a tumor nest caused by tissue fixation as lymphatic vessel involvement by carcinoma. Lymphatic involvement should only be diagnosed when an endothelial-lined space is identified, preferably at the edge of the carcinoma.
9. Assuming that large examples of DCIS must have an invasive component. Although unusual, DCIS may attain palpable proportions. Thorough sampling is essential in these rare cases. The association of lymph nodal metastasis with DCIS is likely to have occurred in inadequately sampled large cases of DCIS.
10. Not identifying radiologically relevant calcifications in a needle localization specimen. Careful comparison of radiographed specimen slices with histopathologic findings is essential. Radiographing paraffin blocks and performing deeper sections may be necessary.

FURTHER READING

Page DL, Anderson TJ, Rogers LW. Epithelial hyperplasia and infiltrating carcinoma: major histological types. In: Page DL, Anderson TJ, eds. *Diagnostic Histopathology of the Breast.* Edinburgh: Churchill Livingstone; 1987: 120, 157.

Dupont WD, Page DL. Risk factors for breast cancer in women with proliferative breast disease. *N Engl J Med.* 1985;312:146.

Page DL, Dupont WD, Rogers LW, et al. Atypical hyperplastic lesions of the female breast: a long-term follow-up study. *Cancer.* 1985;55:2698.

Lagios MD, Margolin FR, Westdahl PR, et al. Mammographically detected duct carcinoma in situ: frequency of local recurrence following tylectomy and prognostic effect of nuclear grade on local recurrence. *Cancer.* 1989;63:618.

Page DL. Prognosis and breast cancer: recognition of lethal and favorable prognostic types. *Am J Surg Pathol.* 1991;15:334.

Elston CW, Ellis IO. Pathological prognostic factors in breast cancer. I. The value of histologic grade in breast cancer: experience from a large study with long-term follow-up. *Histopathology.* 1991;19:403.

Schnitt SJ, Abner A, Gelman R, et al. The relationship between microscopic margins of resection and the risk of local recurrence in patients treated with breast-conserving surgery and radiation therapy. *Cancer.* 1994;74:1746.

REFERENCES

1. Wellings SR, Jensen HM, Marcum RG. An atlas of subgross pathology of the human breast with special reference to possible precancerous lesions. *J Natl Cancer Inst.* 1975;55:231.
2. Dupont WD, Page DL. Risk factors for breast cancer in women with proliferative breast disease. *N Engl J Med.* 1985;312:146.
3. Page DL, Dupont WD, Rogers LW, et al. Atypical hyperplastic lesions of the female breast: a long-term follow-up study. *Cancer.* 1985;55:2698.
4. Hutter RVP, et al. Consensus meeting: is "fibrocystic disease" of the breast precancerous? *Arch Pathol Lab Med.* 1986;110:171.
5. Dupont WD, Page DL, Parl FF, et al. Long-term risk of breast cancer in women with fibroadenoma. *N Engl J Med.* 1994;331:10.
6. Dupont WD, Page DL. Relative risk of breast cancer varies with time since diagnosis of atypical hyperplasia. *Hum Pathol.* 1989;20:723.
7. Love SM, Gelman RS, Silen W. Fibrocystic "disease" of the breast: a non-disease. *N Engl J Med.* 1982;307:1010.
8. Haagensen DE, Jr. Is cystic disease related to breast cancer? *Am J Surg Pathol.* 1991;15:687.
9. London SJ, Connolly JL, Schnitt SJ, et al. A prospective study of benign breast disease and risk of breast cancer. *JAMA.* 1992;267:941.
10. Dupont WD, Parl FF, Hartmann WH, et al. Breast cancer risk associated with proliferative breast disease and atypical hyperplasia. *Cancer.* 1993;71:1258.
11. Page DL, Rogers LW. Combined histologic and cytologic criteria for the diagnosis of mammary atypical ductal hyperplasia. *Hum Pathol.* 1992;23:1095.
12. Page DL, Anderson TJ, Rogers LW. Epithelial hyperplasia. In: Page DL, Anderson TJ, eds. *Diagnostic Histopathology of the Breast.* Edinburgh: Churchill Livingstone; 1987: 120.
13. Kelsey JL, Horn-Ross PL. Breast cancer: magnitude of the problem and descriptive epidemiology. *Epidemiol Rev.* 1993;15:7.
14. Page DL. Cancer risk assessment in benign breast biopsies. *Hum Pathol.* 1986;17:871.
15. Page DL, Kidd TE, Dupont WD, et al. Lobular neoplasia of the breast: higher risk for subsequent invasive cancer predicted by more extensive disease. *Hum Pathol.* 1991;22:1232.
16. Rubin E, Alexander RW, Visscher DW, Urist MM, Maddox WA. Proliferative disease and atypia in biopsies performed for mammographically detected nonpalpable lesions. *Cancer.* 1988;61:2077.
17. Rosai J. Borderline lesions of the breast. *Am J Surg Pathol.* 1991;15:209.
18. Schnitt SJ, Connolly JL, Tavassoli FA, et al. Interobserver reproducibility in the diagnosis of ductal proliferative breast lesions using standardized criteria. *Am J Surg Pathol.* 1992;12:1133.
19. Haagensen CD. *Diseases of the Breast,* 3rd ed. Philadelphia: Saunders; 1986, 106.
20. Jensen RA, Page DL, Dupont WD, et al. Invasive breast cancer risk in women with sclerosing adenosis. *Cancer.* 1989;64:1977.
21. Page DL, Anderson TJ, Rogers LW. Infiltrating carcinoma: major histological types. In: Page DL, Anderson TJ, eds. *Diagnostic Histopathology of the Breast.* Edinburgh: Churchill Livingstone; 1987:157.
22. Lennington WJ, Jensen RA, Dalton LW, et al. Ductal carcinoma in situ of the breast: heterogeneity of individual lesions. *Cancer.* 1994;73:118.
23. Lagios MD, Margolin FR, Westdahl PR, et al. Mammographically detected duct carcinoma in situ: frequency of local recurrence following tylectomy and prognostic effect of nuclear grade on local recurrence. *Cancer.* 1989;63:618.
24. Schwartz GF, Finkel GC, Garcia JC, et al. Subclinical ductal carcinoma in situ of the breast: treatment by local excision and surveillance alone. *Cancer.* 1992;70:2468.
25. Page DL, Dupont WD, Rogers LW, et al. Intraductal carcinoma of the breast: follow-up after biopsy only. *Cancer.* 1982;49:751.
26. Betsill WL Jr, Rosen PP, Lieberman PH, et al. Intraductal carcinoma. Long-term follow-up after treatment by biopsy alone. *JAMA.* 1978;239:1863.
27. Ottesen GL, Graversen HP, Blichert-Toft M, et al. Ductal carcinoma in situ of the female breast: short term results of a prospective nationwide study. *Am J Surg Pathol.* 1992;16:1183.
28. Bellamy COC, McDonald C, Salter DM, et al. Noninvasive ductal carcinoma of the breast: the relevance of histologic categorization. *Hum Pathol.* 1993;24:16.
29. Solin LJ, Yeh I-T, Kurtz K, et al. Ductal carcinoma in situ (intraductal carcinoma) of the breast treated with breast-conserving surgery and definitive irradiation: correlation of pathologic parameters. *Cancer.* 1993;71:2532.
30. Holland R, Peterse J, Millis RR, et al. Ductal carcinoma in situ: a proposal for a new classification. *Sem Diag Pathol.* 1994;11:167.
31. Carter D, Orr SL, Merino MJ. Intracystic papillary carcinoma of the breast: after mastectomy, radiotherapy, or excisional biopsy alone. *Cancer.* 1983;52:14.
32. Foote F, Stewart F. Lobular carcinoma in situ: a rare form of mammary carcinoma. *Am J Pathol.* 1941;17:491.
33. Sonnenfeld MR, Frenna TH, Weidner N, et al. Lobular carcinoma in situ: mammographic-pathologic correlation of results of needle-directed biopsy. *Radiology.* 1991;181:363.
34. Pope T, Fechner R, Wilhelm M, et al. Lobular carcinoma in situ of the breast: mammographic features. *Radiology.* 1988;168:63.
35. Bartow SA, Pathak DR, Black WC, et al. Prevalence of benign atypical, and malignant breast lesions in populations at different risk for breast cancer. *Cancer.* 1987;60:2751.
36. Wheeler JE, Enterline HT, Roseman JM, et al. Lobular carcinoma in situ of the breast: long-term followup. *Cancer.* 1974;34:554.
37. Rosen PP, Lieberman PH, Braun DW Jr, et al. Lobular carcinoma in situ of the breast: detailed analysis of 99 patients with average follow-up of 24 years. *Am J Surg Pathol.* 1978;2:224.
38. Andersen JA. Lobular carcinoma in situ: a long-term follow-up in 52 cases. *Acta Pathol Microbiol Scand.* 1974;82:519.
39. Haagensen CD, Lane N, Lattes R, et al. Lobular neoplasia (so-called lobular carcinoma in situ) of the breast. *Cancer.* 1978;42:737.
40. Rosen PP, Braun DW Jr, Lyngholm B, et al. Lobular carcinoma in situ of the breast: preliminary results of treatment by ipsilateral mastectomy and contralateral breast biopsy. *Cancer.* 1981;47:813.
41. Morrow M. Pre-cancerous breast lesions: implications for breast cancer prevention trials. *Int J Radiat Oncol Biol Phys.* 1992;23:1071.
42. Dixon JM, Page DL, Anderson TJ, et al. Long term survivors after breast cancer. *Br J Surg.* 1985;72:445.
43. Fisher B, Redmond C, Fisher ER, et al. The contribution of recent NSABP clinical trials of primary breast cancer therapy to an understanding of tumor biology: an overview of findings. *Cancer.* 1980;46:1009.
44. Fu YS, Maksem JA, Hubay CA, et al. The relationship of breast cancer morphology and estrogen receptor protein status. In: Fenoglio CM, Wolff M, eds. *Progress in Surgical Pathology.* New York: Masson; 1981:65.
45. Wallgren A, Silfverward C, Eklund G. Prognostic factors in mammary carcinoma. *Acta Radiol.* 1976;5:1.

46. Page DL, Anderson TJ, Sakamoto G. Infiltrating carcinoma: major histological types. In: Page DL, Anderson TJ, eds. *Diagnostic Histopathology of the Breast.* New York: Churchill Livingstone; 1987:193.
47. Ellis IO, Galea M, Broughton N, et al. Pathologic prognostic factors in breast cancer. II. Histologic type. Relationship with survival in a large study with long term follow-up. *Histopathology.* 1992;20:479.
48. Anderson TJ, Lamb J, Donnan P, et al. Comparative pathology of breast cancer in a randomised trial of screening. *Br J Cancer.* 1991;64:108.
49. Cooper HS, Patchefsky AS, Krall RA. Tubular carcinoma of the breast. *Cancer.* 1978;42:2334.
50. McDivitt RW, Boyce W, Gersell D. Tubular carcinoma of the breast: clinical and pathological observations concerning 135 cases. *Am J Surg Pathol.* 1982;6:401.
51. Parl FF, Richardson LD. The histological and biological spectrum of tubular carcinoma of the breast. *Hum Pathol.* 1983;14:694.
52. Baker RR. Unusual lesions and their management. *Surg Clin N Am.* 1990;70:963.
53. Page DL, Dixon JM, Anderson TJ, et al. Invasive cribriform carcinoma of the breast. *Histopathology.* 1983;7:525.
54. Venable JG, Schwartz AM, Silverberg SG. Infiltrating cribriform carcinoma of the breast: a distinctive clinicopathologic entity. *Hum Pathol.* 1990;21:333.
55. Komari K, Sakamoto G, Sugano HH, et al. Mucinous carcinoma of the breast in Japan: a prognostic analysis based on morphologic features. *Cancer.* 1988;61:989.
56. Rasmussen BB, Rose C, Christensen IB. Prognostic factors in primary mucinous breast carcinoma. *Am J Clin Pathol.* 1987;87:155.
57. Clayton F. Pure mucinous carcinomas of the breast: morphologic features and prognostic correlates. *Hum Pathol.* 1986;17:34.
58. Donegan WL, Perez-Mesa CM. Lobular carcinoma—an indication for elective biopsy of the second breast. *Ann Surg.* 1972;176:178.
59. Fisher ER, Taylor M. Changing pattern of some pathologic parameters of mammary carcinoma. *Cancer.* 1973;32:1380.
60. Dixon JM, Anderson TJ, Page DL, et al. Infiltrating lobular carcinoma of the breast. *Histopathology.* 1982;6:149.
61. Haagensen CD. *Disease of the Breast.* 2nd ed. Eastbourne: Saunders; 1971.
62. Dixon JM, Anderson TJ, Page DL, et al. Infiltrating lobular carcinoma of the breast: an evaluation of the incidence and consequence of bilateral disease. *Br J Surg.* 1983;70:513.
63. Schnitt SJ, Connolly JL, Recht A, et al. Influence of infiltrating lobular histology on local tumor control in breast cancer patients treated with conservative surgery and radiotherapy. *Cancer.* 1989;64:448.
64. Silverstein MJ, Lewinsky BS, Waisman JR, et al. Infiltrating lobular carcinoma. Is it different from infiltrating duct carcinoma? *Cancer.* 1994;73:1673.
65. Rubens JR, Lewandrowski KB, Kopans DB, et al. Medullary carcinoma of the breast: overdiagnosis of a prognostically favorable neoplasm. *Arch Surg.* 1990;125:601.
66. Ridolfi RL, Rosen PP, Post A, et al. Medullary carcinoma of the breast . A clinical pathological study with 10 year follow-up. *Cancer.* 1977;40:1365.
67. Marcus JN, Watson P, Page DL, et al. Pathology and heredity of breast cancer in younger women. *Monogr Natl Cancer Inst.* 1994;16:23.
68. Berg JW, Hutter RVP. Breast cancer. *Cancer.* 1995;75:257.
69. Page DL. Prognosis and breast cancer: recognition of lethal and favorable prognostic types. *Am J Surg Pathol.* 1991;15:334.
70. McGuire WL. Breast cancer prognostic factors: evaluation guidelines (editorial). *J Natl Cancer Inst.* 1991;83:154.
71. Burke HB, Henson DE. Criteria for prognostic factors and for an enhanced prognostic system. *Cancer.* 1993;72:3131.
72. Carter CL, Allen C, Henson DE. Relation of tumor size, lymph node status, and survival in 24,740 breast cancer cases. *Cancer.* 1989;63:181.
73. Veronesi U, Marubini E, Del Vecchio M, et al. Local recurrences and distant metastases after conservative breast cancer treatments: partly independent events. *J Natl Cancer Inst.* 1995;87:19.
74. McGuire WL, Clark GM. Prognostic factors and treatment decisions in axillary-node negative breast cancer. *N Engl J Med.* 1992;326:1756.
75. Osborne CK. Prognostic factors for breast cancer: have they met their promise? *J Clin Oncol.* 1992;10:679.
76. Elston CW, Ellis IO. Pathological prognostic factors in breast cancer. I. The value of histologic grade in breast cancer: experience from a large study with long-term follow-up. *Histopathology.* 1991;19:403.
77. Fisher ER, Sass R, Fisher B, et al. Pathologic findings from the national surgical adjuvant project for breast cancer (protocol no 4). Discriminants for tenth year treatment failure. *Cancer.* 1984,53:712.
78. Contesso G, Mouriesse H, Friedman S, et al. The importance of histologic grade in long-term prognosis of breast cancer: a study of 1,010 patients, uniformly treated at the Institut Gustave-Roussy. *J Clin Oncol.* 1987,5:1378.
79. Henson DE, Ries L, Freedman LS, et al. Relationship among outcome, stage of disease, and histologic grade for 22,616 cases of breast cancer: the basis for a prognostic index. *Cancer.* 1991;68:2142.
80. Dalton LW, Page DL, Dupont WD. Histologic grading of breast carcinoma: a reproducibility study. *Cancer.* 1994;73:2765.
81. Frierson HF Jr, Wolber RA, Berean KW, et al. Interobserver reproducibility of the Nottingham modification of the Bloom and Richardson histologic grading scheme for infiltrating ductal carcinoma. *Am J Clin Pathol.* 1995;103:195.
82. Van Diest PJ, Baak JPA. The morphometric prognostic index is the strongest prognosticator in premenopausal lymph node-negative and lymph node-positive breast cancer patients. *Hum Pathol.* 1990;22:326.
83. Clayton F. Pathologic correlates of survival in 378 lymph node negative infiltrating ductal breast carcinomas: mitotic count is the best single predictor. *Cancer.* 1991,68:1309.
84. Sigurdsson H, Baldetorp B, Borg A, et al. Indicators of prognosis in node-negative breast cancer. *N Engl J Med.* 1990;322:1045.
85. Hedley DW, Clark GM, Cornelisse CJ, et al. Consensus review of the clinical utility of DNA cytometry in carcinoma of the breast. *Cytometry.* 1993;14:482.
86. Clark GM, McGuire WL. Steroid receptors and other prognostic factors in primary breast cancer. *Semin Oncol.* 1989;15:20.
87. Allred DC, Bustamante MA, Daniel CO, et al. Immunocytochemical analysis of estrogen receptors in human breast carcinomas. Evaluation of 130 cases and a review of the literature regarding concordance with the biochemical assay and clinical relevance. *Arch Surg.* 1990;125:107.
88. Allred DC. Should immunohistochemical examination replace biochemical hormone receptor assays in breast cancer? (editorial). *Am J Clin Pathol.* 1993;99:1.
89. Muss HB, Thor AD, Berry DA, et al. c-*erbB*-2 expression and response to adjuvant therapy in women with node-positive early breast cancer. *N Engl J Med.* 1994;330:1260.
90. Reynolds T. Breast cancer prognostic factors: the search goes on. *J Natl Cancer Inst.* 1994;86:480.
91. Silverstein MJ, Gierson ED, Waisman JR, et al. Axillary lymph node dissection for T1a breast carcinoma. Is it indicated? *Cancer.* 1994;73:664.
92. Borger J, Kemperman H, Hart A, et al. Risk factors in breast-conservation therapy. *J Clin Oncol.* 1994;12:653.
93. Schmidt-Ullrich RK, Wazer DE, DiPetrillo T, et al. Breast conservation therapy for early stage breast carcinoma with outstanding 10-year locoregional control rates: a case for aggressive therapy to the tumor-bearing quadrant. *Int J Radiat Oncol Biol Phys.* 1993;27:545.
94. Schnitt SJ, Abner A, Gelman R, et al. The relationship between microscopic margins of resection and the risk of local recurrence in patients treated with breast-conserving surgery and radiation therapy. *Cancer.* 1994;74:1746.
95. Schnitt SJ, Connolly JL, Harris JR, et al. Pathologic predictors of early local recurrence in stage I and II breast cancer treated by primary radiation therapy. *Cancer.* 1984;53:1049.
96. Egan RL, McSweeney MB. Multicentric breast carcinoma. *Recent Results Cancer Res.* 1984;90:28.
97. Rosen PP, Fracchia AA, Urban JA, et al. "Residual" mammary carcinoma following simulated partial mastectomy. *Cancer.* 1975;35:739.
98. Lagios MD, Westdahl PR, Margolin FR, et al. Ductal carcinoma in situ: relationship of extent of noninvasive disease to the frequency

of occult invasion, multicentricity, lymph node metastases and short-term treatment failures. *Cancer.* 1982;59:1309.
99. Patchefsky AS, Schwartz GF, Finkelstein SD, et al. Heterogeneity of intraductal carcinoma of the breast. *Cancer.* 1989;63:731.
100. Holland R, Hendricks JHCL, Verbeek ALM, et al. Extent, distribution, and mammographic/histologic correlations of breast ductal carcinoma in situ. *Lancet.* 1990;335:519.
101. Casey TT, Rodgers WH, Baxter JW, et al. Stratified approach to fine needle aspiration of the breast. *Am J Surg.* 1992;163:305.
102. Schnitt SJ, Connolly JL. Processing and evaluation of breast excision specimens: a clinically oriented approach. *Am J Clin Pathol.* 1992;98:125.
103. Fechner RE. Frozen section examination of breast biopsies: practice parameter. *Am J Clin Pathol.* 1995;103:6.
104. Graham RA, Homer MJ, Sigler CJ, et al. The efficacy of specimen radiography in evaluating the surgical margins of impalpable breast carcinoma. *AJR.* 1994;162:33.
105. Fisher ER, Sass R, Fisher B, et al. Pathologic findings from the National Surgical Adjuvant Breast Project (protocol 6). II. Relation of local breast recurrence to multicentricity. *Cancer.* 1986;57:1717.
106. Cox CE, Ku NN, Reintgen DS, et al. Touch preparation cytology of breast lumpectomy margins with histologic correlation. *Arch Surg.* 1991;126:490.
107. Page DL, Dupont WD. Management of the patient at high risk. In: Bland KI, Copeland EM III, eds. *The Breast: Comprehensive Management of Benign and Malignant Disease.* Philadelphia: Saunders; 1991:1046.

6

The Head and Neck

Leon Barnes and Jonas T. Johnson

Definition

For both surgeon and pathologist, the head and neck represent one of the most challenging areas of the entire human body. There are clear-cut reasons for this. First, biopsies from this region are, by necessity, often small, occasionally crushed, and, at times, difficult to orient for proper histologic processing, all of which may hamper pathologic interpretation. Second, some of the most complex tumors in the body are found in this region. Consider, for example, the numerous histologic subtypes of salivary gland and odontogenic tumors. Third, the anatomy is complicated. Unlike a resected portion of colon, in which the proximal and distal resection margins are easily determined, the head and neck region consists of a bewildering arrangement of cavities, sinuses, and spaces bound together by hollow muscular tubes. As a result, it is often difficult to determine what are true surgical margins and what are normal spaces in large specimens. One must truly think in three dimensions in order to evaluate head and neck tumors properly. Fourth, not all training programs in pathology offer a broad exposure to head and neck specimens and, accordingly, some pathologists feel insecure in their evaluation of tissue from this site. Finally, because human interchange is directed to and through this anatomic region, patient sensitivities to any surgical-cosmetic defects are often extreme.

For optimal patient care, it is essential that the pathologist and head-and-neck surgeon develop mutual respect and work together as a team. The key to the success of this team depends upon *communication* (see Chap. 1). This begins in the operating room, where the surgeon should provide, on the surgical pathology requisition form, a salient patient history, the source of the biopsy, and the clinical impression. Additional information—for example, as to whether or not the patient has received chemotherapy or irradiation or whether a given lesion has an appearance suspicious for verrucous carcinoma—can be of immense value to the pathologist.

Because of space constraints, it is impossible to discuss all surgical diseases of the head and neck. Instead we will focus on (1) margins of resection and the use of frozen sections in the head and neck, (2) common entities according to anatomic site of occurrence, and (3) neck dissections and the patient who presents with an unknown primary.

Margins of Resection

How widely should head and neck cancers be excised? The answer depends upon the anatomic site of origin and the histologic type and size of the tumor. For squamous cell carcinoma arising from a mucosal surface, a margin of 2 mm is sufficient in the larynx, while in the oral cavity and hypopharynx–cervical esophagus (where submucosal spread is common), margins of at least 5 and 10 mm, respectively, are desirable. In addition to mucosal margins, larger tumors may need consideration of soft tissue, osseous, cutaneous, and/or neural margins. This last consideration is particularly important in dealing with an adenoid cystic type carcinoma.

Supported in part by the Pathology Education and Research Foundation, Department of Pathology, University of Pittsburgh School of Medicine, and a grant from the Mary Hillman Jennings Foundation and the John R. McCune Foundation.

Traditionally, the pathologist evaluates margins of resection at the time of gross evaluation of the excised tumor; however, some surgeons prefer to remove the tumor and then separately sample designated margins. Either approach is acceptable. For larger, complex specimens, such as maxillectomies and cranial base resections, the surgeon may call the pathologist to the operating room to orient the specimen and point out margins of particular concern.

Because of the complex anatomy of the head and neck and the invasive potential of some tumors, it is sometimes necessary for the surgeon to remove a neoplasm in multiple parts rather than en bloc. In this instance, the surgeon assumes responsibility for identifying the margins of resection.

Frozen Sections

Frozen sections, or, as some prefer to call them, intraoperative consultations (since the tissue is not always frozen), are indispensable to the surgical oncologist. They offer a quick, usually definitive diagnosis that allows therapeutic decisions to be made while the patient is still in the operating room. In the head and neck region, they are used primarily to evaluate salivary gland tumors, lymph nodes, neck masses, disorders of the thyroid and parathyroid glands, and the adequacy of resection margins.

Although the procedure is 95 to 98% accurate, errors (false negative and false positive) do occur. Accordingly, as with any diagnostic procedure, there should be specific indications and contraindications for its use. Some of these are listed in Table 6–1.

Diagnostic errors are most often due to misinterpretation of the biopsy, inadequate sampling, technical problems, or lack of communication between the surgeon and pathologist. To minimize errors, we urge the pathologist to visit the operating room rather than communicate with the surgeon over an intercom or through a messenger. This allows the pathologist to acquire, first-hand, pertinent clinical history, to orient the specimen, and to visualize the pathology in vivo; furthermore, it affords direct review of the patient's clinical records and radiologic studies.

Table 6–1. Frozen Sections: Indications and Contraindications

Indications

1. To determine whether a tumor is benign or malignant. If malignant, more extensive surgery may be necessary.
2. To determine whether surgical margins are adequate.
3. To determine whether a biopsy is representative or diagnostic. Some biopsies may contain only necrotic debris and no viable tumor for evaluation.
4. To verify or confirm the identity of tissue removed. For example, in a parathyroidectomy, it may be difficult to distinguish a parathyroid gland from a lymph node clinically.
5. To hasten the identification of certain microorganisms, such as *Aspergillus*, rather than waiting days for the result of cultures.
6. To determine whether a lesion needs special handling, such as cultures for inflammatory processes or estrogen receptors for breast carcinomas.
7. To determine whether outpatients who travel long distances need to be hospitalized or can be allowed to return home.

Contraindications

1. When the results would not alter the operation.
2. If the tissue is heavily ossified or calcified.
3. If the biopsy is small and no additional tissue will be obtained for permanent histologic studies. Freezing and thawing of tissue results in artifacts that might interfere with subsequent histologic evaluation.
4. For certain lesions such as small cutaneous growths suspected of being malignant melanomas. Melanocytic lesions are difficult enough to diagnose with permanent sections, not to mention frozen sections.
5. To satisfy the surgeon's curiosity.
6. To tell the patient sooner about the diagnosis. Most patients are too obtunded from general anesthesia to comprehend the significance of a diagnosis anyway.

Premalignant Lesions

Premalignant lesions of the mucous membranes of the head and neck usually manifest as patches that are white (leukoplakia), red (erythroplasia, erythroplakia), or mixed white-red (speckled leukoplakia). Of the three, *erythroplasia* is the most ominous, since these lesions frequently show severe dysplasia, carcinoma in situ, or superficially invasive squamous cell carcinoma. Erythroplasias characteristically have poorly defined margins. They occur commonly in the oral cavity or oropharynx and infrequently in the larynx.

In contrast, *leukoplakias* exhibit a broad spectrum of histologic findings. Some show only surface keratinization without significant epithelial changes, while others demonstrate invasive, keratinizing, squamous-cell carcinoma. Leukoplakias occur on all mucous membranes and tend to have well-defined, easily visualized margins. *Speckled leukoplakias*, in turn, lie between leukoplakia and erythroplasia with regard to their clinical significance and histologic findings.

Treatment of these various lesions consists of identifying and eliminating the etiology (tobacco products, alcohol abuse, dental/denture problems), followed by incisional or excisional biopsy to assess the nature of the epithelial abnormality.

Oral Cavity

ANATOMY

The oral cavity extends from the skin/vermilion junction of the lips to the junction of the hard-soft palate above and the line of circumvallate papillae below. It is divided into seven major divisions: lips, anterior two thirds of the tongue (oral, mobile tongue), floor of mouth, buccal mucosa, upper and lower alveolar ridges, hard palate, and retromolar gingiva (retromolar trigone).[1]

BENIGN DISEASES

Common benign conditions of the oral cavity include cystic lesions of the jaws, mucoceles, ranulas, irritation fibromas, granular-cell tumors, and ameloblastomas.

Cysts and cystlike lesions of the jaws can be divided into two broad categories: (1) true cysts (those with an epithelial lining) versus pseudocysts (those without an epithelial lining) and (2) odontogenic versus nonodontogenic cysts.

The *odontogenic cysts* arise from or are associated with the tooth apparatus (Fig. 6–1). Since the subtypes share a similar histologic feature—namely, a squamous epithelial lining—accurate classification depends upon clinical-radiographic findings and the result of dental vitality testing. On roentgenographic exam, they appear as well-circumscribed, unilocular, sometimes multilocular, radiolucencies.

The *primordial cyst* (Fig. 6–1.1) is uncommon. It arises from the primitive tooth germ; as a result, normal tooth development fails to occur. The *eruption cyst* (Fig. 6–1.2) arises almost exclusively in children and represents an accumulation of fluid in soft tissue around an emerging tooth. The *radicular (periapical) cyst* is the most common odontogenic cyst (Fig. 6–1.3). It develops when a carious tooth is associated with inflammation and necrosis of the pulp. The inflammation spreads through the root of the tooth into the surrounding bone, where it eventually organizes and becomes a cyst. The tooth is characteristically nonvital (does not respond to electrical or thermal stimuli). If the tooth associated with a radicular cyst is extracted without the cyst, the cyst that remains is referred to as a *residual cyst* (Fig. 6–1.5). The *lateral periodontal cyst* is primarily a noninflammatory, developmental cyst lateral to the root of a vital tooth (Fig. 6–1.4). The *dentigerous cyst*, the second most frequent type of odontogenic cyst, is characteristically associated with the crown of an unerupted or developing tooth (Fig. 6–1.6).

Unless neglected, most odontogenic cysts are relatively harmless and are rarely the site of malignant change. The exception is the *odontogenic keratocyst*, especially the parakeratotic type. This cyst is locally aggressive, tends to recur, may be multiple, and is sometimes associated with the nevoid basal-cell carcinoma syndrome. It arises primarily in the posterior mandible and affects all age groups. It is also one of the few odontogenic cysts that can be diagnosed solely on its characteristic microscopic appearance, which consists of a thin squamous epithelial lining with nuclear palisading of the basal layer and an overlying corrugated surface of parakeratin.

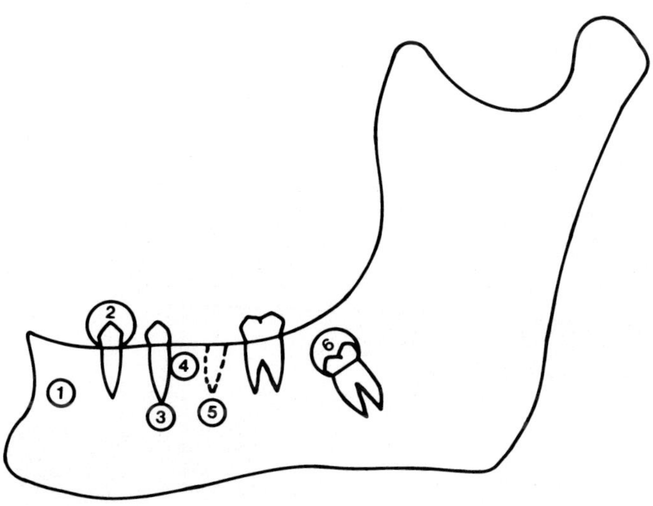

Figure 6–1. Location of odontogenic cysts. 1 = primordial cyst, 2 = eruption cyst, 3 = radicular cyst, 4 = lateral periodontal cyst, 5 = residual cyst, and 6 = dentigerous cyst.

Mucoceles arise from traumatic disruption of the ducts of minor salivary glands. As a result, mucus escapes into the soft tissue and elicits an inflammatory response. A mucocele typically presents as a solitary, 0.5-cm or less, blue, dome-shaped elevation on the lower lip and is especially common in "lip biters." *Ranulas* represent another type of mucus-retention phenomenon that present in the floor of the mouth on either side of the midline. They are larger than mucoceles and result from disruption of the excretory duct of the sublingual gland and, rarely, of the submandibular gland or as a result of blockage of the excretory duct with cystic accumulation of mucus distal to the obstruction. Infrequently, ranulas will herniate through the floor of the mouth into the neck, so-called plunging ranulas.

Irritation fibromas represent a localized fibrous tissue response to chronic trauma of the oral mucosa. They are usually seen on the lateral border of the tongue, the buccal mucosa, or the lower lip and rarely exceed 1 cm.

Granular-cell tumors are uncommon neoplasms of presumed neural origin that, in the past, have been inappropriately referred to as "granular-cell myoblastomas." They occur primarily on the tongue, usually the tip and lateral border, and rarely exceed 2 to 3 cm. Their smooth, firm, submucosal appearance contrasts with squamous-cell carcinoma of the tongue, which is usually ulcerated. They often induce pseudoepitheliomatous hyperplasia of the overlying squamous mucosa which in superficial biopsies can be mistaken by the pathologist for a squamous carcinoma. To avoid this mishap, any lesion suspected of being a granular cell tumor should be adequately biopsied.

The *ameloblastoma* is a histologically benign, sometimes locally aggressive odontogenic tumor that occurs primarily in the mandible (80 to 85% of all cases) and less commonly in the maxilla (15 to 20% of all cases). It is seen in all age groups, with a peak occurrence in adults averaging 35 to 45 years of age. On radiographic exam, it presents as a unilocular or multilocular radiolucency with well-defined, often sclerotic borders. The tumor is nonencapsulated and grows as large islands or anastomosing cords of cells, with prominent nuclear palisading of the peripheral cells. The centers of the tumor islands are composed of a loose stroma resembling stellate reticulum of the developing tooth. Six microscopic subtypes are recognized (follicular, plexiform, acanthomatous, basal cell, granular cell, and desmoplastic) but have no prognostic significance. Since curettage is associated with a 50 to 100% rate of recurrence, wide excision with a margin of 1 to 1.5 cm is advisable. Most ameloblastomas are radioresistant.

MALIGNANT DISEASES

Squamous-cell carcinoma is the most common malignant tumor of the oral cavity. The most frequent sites of origin are the lips, tongue, and floor of mouth.

Some 88 to 98% of all labial squamous-cell carcinomas occur on the lower lip, where they typically arise on the exposed vermilion border approximately halfway between the oral commissure and the midline. Most are well differentiated and, when small, are sometimes difficult to distinguish from actinic keratosis both clinically and microscopically. This is especially true when the lesions are accompanied by inflammatory changes. The majority of patients are men, usually between 50 and 80 years of age. Less than 10% of patients have cervical lymph node metastases at diagnosis. An elective neck dissection is therefore contraindicated. Local recurrence following initial excision varies from 5 to 20%. Distant metastases (i.e., below the clavicles) are exceptional. The average overall 5-year determinant survival is 82%.[2] (Determinant survival rate excludes those patients lost to follow-up or who die of other causes.) Poor prognostic features include (1) tumors larger than 2.0 cm, (2) occurrence on the upper lip or oral commissure, (3) perineural invasion, (4) greater than 6 mm depth of invasion, (5) mandibular involvement, and (6) cervical lymph node metastases, especially if there is extranodal spread.[2, 3]

The tongue is arbitrarily divided into an anterior two-thirds (oral or mobile tongue), which lies in the oral cavity, and a posterior one-third (base of tongue), which lies in the oropharynx. Some 70 to 75% of all lingual squamous-cell carcinomas arise on the anterior two-thirds and the remainder occur on the posterior one-third.

Approximately 75% of all carcinomas of the oral tongue present as painless ulcers on the lateral border. Tumors arising on the ventral or dorsal surface or tip are uncommon. Since the ulcerated area is often only the ''tip of the iceberg,'' the lesion must be palpated to assess its depth. At the time of diagnosis, 30% of patients will have clinically positive cervical lymph nodes and, if the tumor crosses the midline of the tongue, the incidence of contralateral or bilateral nodal metastases increases. The overall 5-year determinant survival for squamous-cell carcinoma of the oral tongue is 45 to 50%.[2]

The base of the tongue extends from the line of the circumvallate papillae to the undersurface of the tongue at the junction of the floor of the mouth. Since this area is not easily amenable to self-inspection, squamous-cell carcinomas in this site are typically quite advanced at presentation. Some 50 to 75% of patients will have cervical lymph node metastases at diagnosis, and 20 to 30% will either have or develop contralateral and/or bilateral nodal metastases during the course of their disease. The overall 5-year determinant survival rate is 25 to 30%.[2]

Squamous-cell carcinomas of the floor of the mouth typically arise laterally rather than in the midline. In 50 to 75% of cases, the tumor has extended beyond the floor of the mouth to involve the tongue, gingiva, anterior tonsillar pillar, or mandible. Some 30 to 60% of patients either have or will develop cervical lymph node metastases. Accurate assessment of the relationship of floor-of-mouth tumors to the mandible is crucial in determining optimal therapy. If the tumor is close to or involves the periosteum, a marginal mandibulectomy will generally provide a safe margin while maintaining the continuity of the mandible. If, on the other hand, the tumor invades the mandible, as 15 to 30% of floor-of-mouth tumors do, a segmental mandibulectomy is indicated. If the tumor invades the mandible, the tumor may propagate along the intraosseous inferior alveolar nerve and compromise an otherwise adequate margin of resection. Since intraoperative assessment of bone margins is difficult or impossible, the surgeon is wise to stage the degree of bone involvement with computed tomography (CT) or magnetic resonance imaging (MRI) and plan resection margins accordingly. The overall 5-year determinant survival rate for squamous-cell carcinoma of the floor of the mouth is 35 to 50%.[2]

Verrucous carcinoma is an exceedingly well-differentiated, nonmetastasizing, but locally aggressive variant of squamous-cell carcinoma which, on small biopsies, is often histologically indistinguishable from a squamous papilloma or nonspecific epithelial hyperplasia. As a result, close communication between the surgeon and pathologist is necessary to establish the correct diagnosis. The tumor is rarely seen in patients below the age of 50 years and, in the oral cavity, originates primarily from the lower alveolar ridge or buccal mucosa (Fig. 6–2). Risk factors include the use of tobacco (snuff and chewing tobacco), poor oral hygiene, and possibly the human papillomavirus.

Medina et al. have described variants of verrucous carcinoma that contain foci of conventional squamous-cell carcinoma, so-called hybrid tumors.[4] In their review of 104 verrucous carcinomas of the oral cavity, 19.2% were regarded as hybrid tumors. The incidence of local recurrence following treatment was higher in the hybrid group (30%) compared with that of pure verrucous carcinoma (18.2%). Their study underscores the importance of thorough microscopic sampling of verrucous carcinomas for foci of conventional squamous-cell carcinoma.

Oropharynx

ANATOMY

The oropharynx extends from the plane of the hard palate superiorly to the plane of the hyoid bone inferiorly

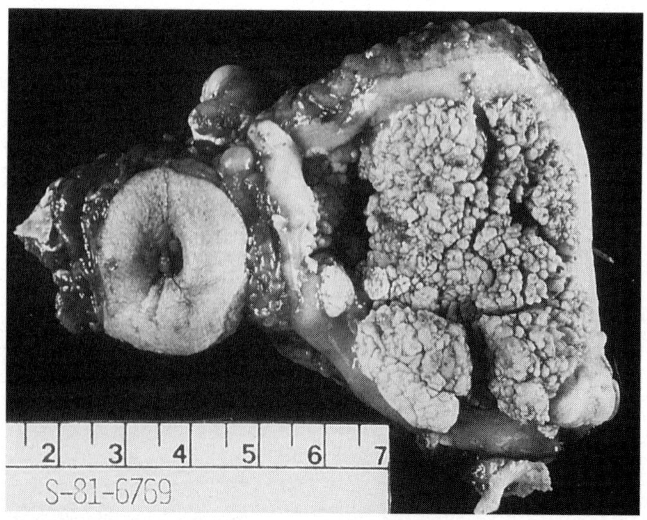

Figure 6–2. Large verrucous carcinoma of the buccal mucosa with involvement of overlying skin (note circular portion of skin on the left, with central ''dimple'').

and is continuous with the oral cavity through an opening termed the faucial isthmus. The junction of the hard and soft palates above, the line of the circumvallate papillae below, and the anterior tonsillar pillar laterally separate the oropharynx from the oral cavity. The oropharynx contains the soft palate, uvula, anterior and posterior tonsillar pillars, palatine tonsils, base of the tongue, vallecula, and posterior and lateral oropharyngeal walls.[1]

BENIGN DISEASES

At one time, tonsillectomy was the most common surgical procedure in the United States; however, subsequent studies of the patterns of upper respiratory tract diseases in infants and children have negated the need for routine *tonsillectomy*, since most youngsters have fewer upper respiratory infections as they get older. Presumably, this is due to maturation of their immune defenses.

However, tonsillectomy may be effective in reducing the incidence of tonsillitis in patients who are prone to recurring infection. One study suggests that children experiencing greater than 7 episodes per year, 4 episodes a year for 2 years, or 3 episodes a year for 3 years may benefit from tonsillectomy.[5]

Since tonsillectomy is not done during an episode of acute inflammation, pathologic evaluation of tonsils for recurrent tonsillitis generally shows only lymphoid hyperplasia with or without fibrosis or, at most, foci of superficial ulceration with residual acute inflammation of the surface or within the crypts. Granules of *Actinomyces* (sulfur granules) are commonly found in the tonsillar crypts and should not be confused with the disease actinomycosis, in which the organism invades the tissue and elicits an inflammatory response.

MALIGNANT DISEASES

Squamous-cell carcinoma and *malignant lymphoma* are the most common malignancies of the tonsils, accounting for 70 to 85% and 15% of all tonsillar malignancies, respectively. Because of their delicate lymphoid cellular composition, biopsies of the tonsils are more fragile and subject to crush artifact than tissue from most other sites in the head and neck. Some tonsillar carcinomas, especially those that arise from the base of the tonsillar crypts, are notorious for producing cystic cervical lymph node metastases that masquerade as a branchial cleft cyst or as a tumor of unknown origin, often without clinical abnormality on physical examination. As a result, diagnostic tonsillectomy is superior to biopsy for establishing the diagnosis.

A common misconception is that lymphomas do not ulcerate the tonsillar mucosa. Although lymphomas arise in the submucosa, they can involve the overlying mucosa and thereby result in ulceration. The most common problem for the pathologist dealing with small biopsies in regard to lymphoma is in its distinction from lymphoid hyperplasia, not from carcinoma.

Squamous-cell carcinoma of the tonsil occurs in patients over the age of 50 years and manifests as a ''sore throat'' or a neck mass. At the time of diagnosis, 50 to 75% will have clinically enlarged cervical lymph nodes. The overall 5-year determinant survival is about 40%.[2]

Nasopharynx

ANATOMY

The roof of the nasopharynx is the base of the skull, which slopes downward to become the posterior pharyngeal wall. The inferior limit is the plane of the hard palate. The anterior boundary is the choana, through which it is continuous with the nasal cavity. The lateral wall is composed of the torus tubarius, the eustachian tube orifice, and that portion of the mucosa of the fossa of Rosenmüller that extends to its apex and junction with the roof.[1]

BENIGN DISEASES

Symptomatic enlargement of the adenoids and angiofibromas are the most common benign conditions of the nasopharynx that require surgical intervention. *Enlarged adenoids* should be removed when they obstruct the nasopharyngeal orifice of the eustachian tube with repeated bouts of otitis media or when they occlude the nasal passages and cause labored breathing.

Angiofibroma, sometimes referred to as ''nasopharyngeal angiofibroma,'' arises from a fibrovascular nidus in the posterolateral wall of the nasal cavity but, following the lines of least resistance, secondarily involves the nasopharynx. It occurs almost exclusively in adolescent males, usually between the ages of 10 and 18 years, and manifests clinically as nasal obstruction, intermittent epistaxis, and facial deformity. Though histologically benign, this tumor can be locally destructive if neglected and may even extend intracranially in 5 to 20% of cases. If incompletely excised, it may recur. Histologically, the tumor is highly vascular and densely fibrous (Fig. 6–3). The blood vessels are usually but not invariably devoid of smooth muscle and therefore incapable of vasoconstriction. As a result, biopsies of angiofibromas may lead to profuse hemorrhage. Although

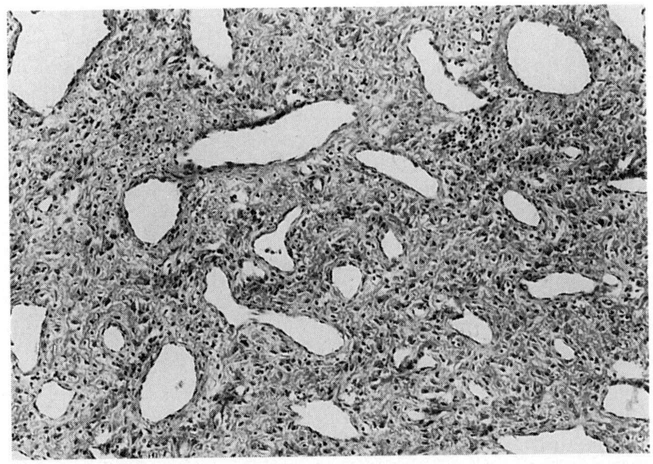

Figure 6–3. Angiofibroma. Note the fibrous stroma and the numerous blood vessels, which lack smooth muscle in their walls. Hematoxylin and eosin, ×100.

malignant change in angiofibromas has been recorded, in most cases this has followed unusually high doses of irradiation.

MALIGNANT DISEASES

Malignant lymphoma and nasopharyngeal carcinoma are the most common malignant tumors of the nasopharynx, and both are treated primarily by radiotherapy.

Nasopharyngeal carcinoma is one of the most common cancers in China and Southeast Asia but is relatively uncommon in the United States. The World Health Organization (WHO) divides nasopharyngeal carcinomas into three types: squamous-cell carcinoma (WHO I), nonkeratinizing carcinoma (WHO II), and undifferentiated carcinoma (WHO III). Prognosis depends partly on histologic type. Those carcinomas that show keratinization (squamous-cell carcinoma) tend to have a poorer prognosis than do those that lack keratinization (nonkeratinizing carcinoma and undifferentiated carcinoma). These latter types are also more responsive to irradiation therapy and are more closely associated with the Epstein-Barr virus than is squamous-cell carcinoma. According to Weiland, the 5-year survival rates for squamous-cell carcinoma, nonkeratinizing carcinoma, and undifferentiated carcinoma are 20, 35, and 60%, respectively.[6] Recently, some patients who have developed recurrent disease following initial radiotherapy have experienced long-term survival after surgical resection.[7]

Hypopharynx

ANATOMY

The hypopharynx extends from the plane of the hyoid bone superiorly to the lower border of the cricoid cartilage inferiorly. It consists of three regions: the pyriform sinuses, posterior pharyngeal wall, and postcricoid area. Although useful for descriptive purposes and classification, these divisions are continuous with one another and merge with the oropharynx, larynx, and cervical esophagus.[1]

BENIGN DISEASE

With the exception of sporadic occurrence of soft tissue tumors, such as lipomas or neurilemomas, benign neoplasms of the hypopharynx are infrequent.

MALIGNANT DISEASE

Squamous-cell carcinomas of the hypopharynx are about one-third as common as those of the larynx. Approximately 65 to 85% arise in the pyriform sinus, 10 to 20% on the posterior pharyngeal wall, and 5 to 15% in the postcricoid area.[2] Since the hypopharynx is not amenable to self-inspection, patients often present with advanced tumors. The most common symptoms are dysphagia, sore throat, otalgia, sensation of a foreign body in the throat, weight loss, and a neck mass.

Hypopharyngeal carcinomas are notorious for growing beneath intact mucosa and often extend well beyond their apparent clinical margins. Pyriform sinus tumors that extend to the apex of the sinus occasionally involve, either by direct extension or embolic spread, the ipsilateral lobe of the thyroid.

Some 65 to 75% of hypopharyngeal carcinomas are associated with cervical lymph node metastases. Other nodal groups can be metastatically involved as well: retropharyngeal nodes with posterior pharyngeal wall tumors and paratracheal nodes with postcricoid tumors. The 5-year determinant survival is 20 to 40%.[2]

Larynx

ANATOMY

The superolateral border of the larynx is delineated by the tip of the epiglottis and the aryepiglottic folds, while the inferior rim of the cricoid cartilage defines the lower extent. The larynx is divided into three regions: supraglottis, glottis, and subglottis.[1]

BENIGN DISEASE

Common benign conditions of the larynx are vocal cord nodules, squamous papillomas, and the "keratoses."

Vocal cord nodules (polyps, singer's nodules, screamer's nodules) are not true neoplasms but a stromal reaction to vocal abuse. They characteristically occur on the anterior half of the true vocal cord, may be single or multiple, may be unilateral or bilateral, and rarely exceed 1 cm. Simple excision together with vocal counseling is curative.

Squamous papillomas of the larynx are divided into nonkeratinized and keratinized types. Nonkeratinizing papillomas occur predominantly in children (juvenile papillomatosis), are often multiple, and are associated with the human papillomavirus types 6 and 11. Although they often recur following excision, they have little if any malignant potential (unless irradiated). Nonkeratinizing papillomas present as pink, often confluent growths. In contrast, keratinized papilloma occurs predominantly in adults and is usually a solitary white growth. They generally are not related to the human papillomavirus (HPV), but despite the fact that they show less tendency to recur, they may occasionally become malignant.

When the mucous membrane of the larynx is irritated, it may keratinize focally and form a white patch referred to clinically as "leukoplakia" or "keratosis." Some of these lesions are innocuous and will regress, while others are microscopically premalignant or malignant. For this reason, a surgeon may be asked to biopsy such a lesion.

MALIGNANT DISEASES

Squamous-cell carcinoma accounts for 95% of all malignant tumors of the larynx and, based on location, is divided into three major categories: glottic, supraglottic, and subglottic.

Glottic carcinomas arise from the true vocal cords or the anterior and posterior commissures. They represent 60 to 65% of all laryngeal carcinomas seen in the United

States.[2] They typically arise from the anterior half of the true vocal cord, manifest as hoarseness, and, collectively, are associated with an 80 to 85% 5-year survival.

Supraglottic carcinomas arise from the epiglottis, false vocal cords, ventricles, aryepiglottic folds, and/or arytenoids and represent 30 to 35% of all laryngeal carcinomas.[2] They tend to be bulky tumors and cause dysphagia, change in quality of the voice, otalgia, sensation of a foreign body in the throat, or a neck mass. Supraglottic carcinomas have cervical lymph node metastases in 40% of cases and carry a 5-year survival rate of 65 to 75%.

Subglottic carcinomas are the least common, representing no more than 5% of all laryngeal carcinomas.[2] The subglottis is defined as the region from 1 cm below the apex of the ventricles to the lower border of the cricoid cartilage. Subglottic carcinomas present with airway obstruction and often require tracheotomy. Although they have cervical lymph node metastases in only 15 to 20% of cases, the primary drainage is to the paratracheal lymph nodes and thyroid gland. Potential for successful treatment is negated if there are mediastinal metastases. The overall 5-year survival rate is 40%.

Unlike the above three categories, the term ''transglottic'' does not refer to an anatomic site within the larynx. Rather, it denotes any laryngeal tumor that crosses the ventricle in a vertical fashion to involve the supraglottis and glottis (and often the subglottis). Most transglottic carcinomas are probably primary glottic carcinomas with supraglottic extension. There are positive cervical lymph nodes in 45% of cases and these are associated with a 5-year survival of about 50%.

Nose and Paranasal Sinuses

ANATOMY

The nose and paired maxillary, ethmoid, frontal, and sphenoid sinuses form a functional unit referred to as the sinonasal tract. The nasal septum divides the nose internally into the right and left nasal cavities, each of which, in turn, communicates with the nasopharynx through openings called choanae. Each nasal cavity is subdivided into four areas: lateral wall, septum, floor, and roof.

The maxillary sinuses, the largest of the four sinuses, are usually symmetrical and located in the body of each maxilla. Each sinus is shaped like a pyramid, being based medially on the nasal cavity and projecting laterally to an apex in the zygoma. Each sinus has a roof, floor, and three walls—anterior, posterior, and medial. Ohngren's line, a theoretic plane extending from the medial canthus of the eye to the angle of the mandible, is sometimes used to divide the maxillary sinus into two divisions: anteroinferior (infrastructure) and superoposterior (suprastructure). Tumors that arise in the suprastructure have a poorer prognosis than those of the infrastructure.

BENIGN DISEASES

Sinonasal polyps (allergic polyps, inflammatory polyps, simple polyps) are nonneoplastic inflammatory swellings of the mucosa of the nose and paranasal sinuses. They may be unilateral or bilateral, single or multiple, and result in nasal obstruction, headaches, sneezing, and rhinorrhea. Etiologically, they may be related to allergies, vasomotor rhinitis, infections, and cystic fibrosis. Surgeons and pathologists should be aware that some sinonasal polyps may contain reactive histiocytes and fibroblasts that have been mistaken microscopically for rhabdomyosarcoma.

Inverted papillomas are histologically benign but locally aggressive head and neck tumors that, if neglected, may erode into the cranial cavity. They are more common in men by a ratio of 5:1, usually occur in patients between 40 and 70 years of age, and characteristically arise unilaterally in the nasal cavity in the region of the middle turbinate-ethmoid sinus. Microscopically, they are composed of hyperplastic ribbons of basement membrane–enclosed epithelium that grow into the underlying stroma (Fig. 6–4). The epithelium may be squamous, respiratory, or ''transitional.'' The treatment of choice for most inverted papillomas consists of a medial maxillectomy with meticulous removal of the mucosa from adjacent sinuses. If incompletely excised, they will recur. Because 5 to 15% of inverted papillomas are associated with squamous-cell carcinomas, thorough examination by the pathologist is essential.

MALIGNANT DISEASES

Numerous ''small round-cell tumors'' originate in the sinonasal tract. Such tumors are characterized by cells with prominent round nuclei and scant cytoplasm with or without mitoses and necrosis. This histologically similar but prognostically variable group of neoplasms includes *malignant lymphoma, extramedullary plasmacytoma, olfactory neuroblastoma, primitive neuroectodermal tumor, Ewing's sarcoma, embryonal rhabdomyosarcoma, malignant melanoma, anaplastic carcinoma,* and *invasive pituitary adenoma.* These tumors are often indistinguishable by routine hematoxylin and eosin microscopic evaluation and frequently require additional, time-consuming, specialized procedures, such as immunostaining and electron microscopy, for definitive diagnosis (see Chap. 2).

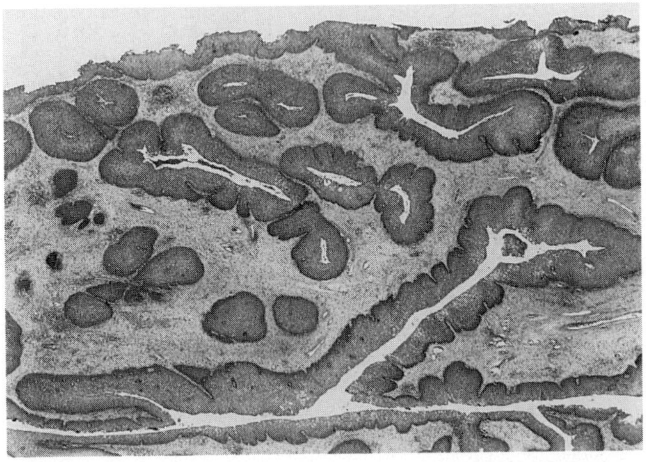

Figure 6–4. Inverted papilloma. Note the inverted growth of sharply demarcated islands of epithelium. Hematoxylin and eosin, ×100.

The *olfactory neuroblastoma* is the prototypical small round-cell tumor of the sinonasal tract. It occurs in all age groups (average 40 to 45 years) and typically arises as a polypoid intranasal mass attached high in the nasal cavity to the cribriform plate. Unilateral nasal obstruction and intermittent epistaxis with or without anosmia are the most common symptoms. The tumor may spread locally to involve the adjacent paranasal sinuses, orbit, or cranial cavity, or it may metastasize to cervical lymph nodes or to more distant sites. The overall 5-year survival is 50 to 60%.

Squamous-cell carcinoma involving the maxillary sinus is the most common sinonasal malignancy. It occurs more frequently in men (60 to 70% of cases) and affects individuals averaging 60 years of age. Signs and symptoms depend upon direction of tumor growth and are grouped accordingly: nasal, oral, ocular, facial, and neurologic. The 5-year survival ranges from 20 to 25%.

Ear—Temporal Bone

ANATOMY

The ear is divided into three compartments: external, middle, and inner. The external ear consists of the pinna, external auditory canal, and external surface of the tympanic membrane. The middle ear is composed of the tympanic cavity, eustachian tube, incus, stapes, malleus, tensor tympani and stapedius muscles, and the inner surface of the tympanic membrane. The inner ear contains the membranous and osseous labyrinths, which house the cochlear duct with its organ of hearing and the vestibular apparatus concerned with equilibrium.

BENIGN DISEASES

Otitis media is one of the most common pediatric diseases. It occurs in all age groups, with a peak incidence between 6 months and 3 years of age. It may be unilateral or bilateral and acute, subacute, or chronic, with or without an effusion. Most acute infections are associated with *Streptococcus pneumoniae* and *Haemophilus influenzae*. Occasionally otitis media, particularly the chronic form, may be associated with a polypoid accumulation of granulation tissue referred to as an *aural polyp*.

A *cholesteatoma* is also common and is a saclike accumulation of keratin within the middle ear or mastoid formed by aberrant keratinizing squamous epithelium. It is often accompanied by a malodorous discharge and hearing impairment and may lead to serious complications if neglected.

Paraganglioma (glomus tumor, chemodectoma) is the commonest tumor of the middle ear and the second most common tumor of the temporal bone, behind the *acoustic neuroma*. It arises from collections of paraganglion cells normally found in the adventitia of the jugular bulb, along the course of the nerve of Jacobson (branch of the glossopharyngeal nerve) or nerve of Arnold (branch of the vagus nerve). The term ''glomus jugulare'' is used when the tumor arises from the jugular bulb and the term ''glomus tympanicum'' is used when it arises from the middle ear. In practice, it may be impossible to determine the precise site of origin. In these instances, the all-inclusive term ''jugulotympanic paraganglioma'' is used. These tumors are three to six times more common in females, occur primarily in middle age, and present clinically with pulsatile tinnitus and conductive hearing loss. They are slow-growing neoplasms, but, if neglected, may extend intracranially. Since they are so vascular, jugulotympanic paragangliomas can often be diagnosed on angiograms. Surgical intervention requires caution (Fig. 6–5), and if biopsies prove necessary, they should be obtained intraoperatively (with frozen section evaluation).

Located within the dermis of the outer cartilaginous portion of the external auditory canal are a group of modified apocrine glands known as ceruminous glands. These glands can give rise to five distinct types of tumors: *ceruminous adenoma, ceruminous adenocarcinoma, pleomorphic adenoma, adenoid cystic carcinoma,* and *mucoepidermoid carcinoma.*

In the past, tumors of ceruminous glands have been referred to as ''ceruminomas'' without regard to histologic type or behavior. It is best to abandon this archaic term in favor of the above classification, which more accurately predicts behavior.

Tumors of the ceruminous glands are uncommon and, regardless of histologic type, present as polypoid or sessile masses with or without surface ulceration. Mechanical blockage of the external canal may lead to hearing loss, external otitis, or pruritus.

MALIGNANT DISEASES

Embryonal rhabdomyosarcoma and *squamous-cell carcinoma* are the most common malignant tumors of the middle ear. Rhabdomyosarcoma occurs primarily in children under 5 years of age and presents as a polypoid lesion that is often mistaken, both clinically and pathologically, for an aural polyp. Close attention to cytologic details, augmented with immunostains for muscle markers (myoglobin, desmin) allow distinction. Because of close proxim-

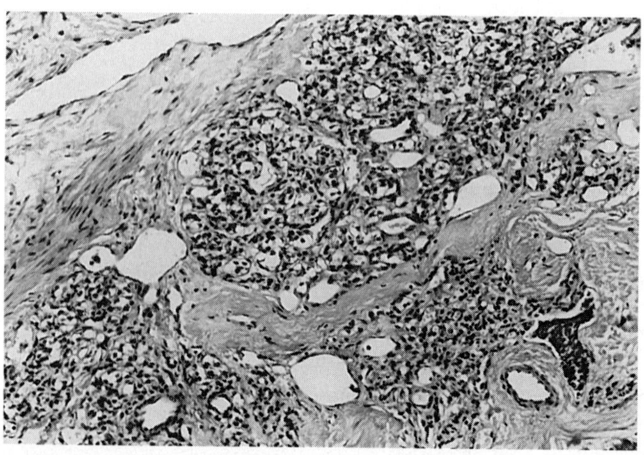

Figure 6–5. Jugulotympanic paraganglioma. The tumor cells grow in small clusters (referred to as *Zellballen*), which are sometimes difficult to appreciate in small, crushed biopsies. Note the prominent vascularity. Hematoxylin and eosin, ×200.

ity to the central nervous system, tumor seeding of the meninges with neurologic signs and symptoms is not uncommon. The overall 3-year relapse-free survival rate for rhabdomyosarcoma of the middle ear–mastoid is 45%.

Squamous-cell carcinoma of the middle ear–mastoid is symptomatically similar to cholesteatoma, often accounting for delay in diagnosis. Any biopsies from this area that show dysplasia should be regarded as suspicious for carcinoma, since cholesteatomas rarely if ever show this feature. A combination of surgery and radiation generally offers the best chance of cure. About 15% of patients will have cervical lymph node metastases and 10% will develop systemic metastases. The overall 5-year survival is about 25 to 30%.[2]

Salivary Glands

ANATOMY

The major salivary glands are paired and symmetrical. The parotid gland, the largest salivary gland, lies in front of the ear and extends from the zygomatic arch superiorly to just below the angle of the mandible inferiorly. Although a single anatomic unit, it is customarily divided into two lobes separated by the facial nerve and its branches. The larger superficial or lateral lobe composes 70 to 80% of the gland and lies lateral to the facial nerve, whereas the smaller deep or medial lobe lies medial to the nerve. The main excretory duct of the parotid gland, Stensen's duct, empties into the oral cavity through a small papilla on the buccal mucosa opposite the second upper molar tooth. In contrast to the other salivary glands, the parotid contains a large number of intraglandular lymph nodes that may (1) show nonspecific hyperplasia and clinically masquerade as a tumor, (2) give rise to primary lymphomas, or (3) harbor metastases from tumors arising in other sites.

The submandibular gland lies in the posterior floor of the mouth between the tongue, mandible, and hyoid bone. Its excretory duct, Wharton's duct, opens into the floor of the mouth, near the lingual frenulum.

The sublingual gland, the smallest of the three major glands, rests upon the mylohyoid muscle near the mandibular symphysis just beneath the mucosa of the floor of the mouth. The gland has several minor salivary ducts—ducts of Rivinus—some of which empty separately into the oral cavity while others join to form the major excretory duct, Bartholin's duct, which opens either into or adjacent to Wharton's duct in the region of the lingual frenulum.

BENIGN AND MALIGNANT DISEASES

The most common presentation of a salivary gland tumor is an asymptomatic mass located under normal-appearing soft tissue. These neoplasms may be clinically indistinguishable from chronic inflammatory diseases. In one series, over 85% of patients who were operated upon for removal of a submandibular mass were found to have chronic inflammatory disease with sialoadenitis and sialolithiasis.[8] In contrast, over 75% of patients who present with a discreet mass in the parotid gland will have a neoplasm. In general, 15 to 25% of all parotid, 40 to 60% of all submandibular, and 80 to 90% of all sublingual gland neoplasms are malignant.[9]

Patients with *chronic sialoadenitis* with stone formation often present with a history of recurring infection and swelling with eating. Radiographic confirmation of calculus improves diagnostic accuracy; however, 20% of submandibular and 80% of parotid calculi do not contain calcium and are therefore radiolucent.

The nature of salivary gland masses can often be confirmed with fine needle aspiration biopsy (FNAB) (see Chap. 3). The prudent physician, however, is aware of the potential for sampling errors. If the clinical situation strongly suggests a neoplasm, appropriate diagnostic steps should be made to confirm this possibility regardless of FNAB results.

Imaging with CT and MRI is used to determine three-dimensional relationships of malignant salivary gland tumors. By contrast, modern imaging is rarely needed to evaluate benign neoplasms or inflammatory disease. Signs of malignancy include motor nerve paralysis, cervical adenopathy, and fixation to skin and other structures. The presence of pain and rapid growth, while sometimes worrisome, often fails to distinguish inflammatory disease from malignancy.

The heterogeneity of tumor types encountered in the salivary glands is a challenge even to experienced pathologists (Table 6–2). For this reason, many head and neck surgeons caution against the use of frozen section in therapeutic decision making when managing salivary gland malignancy. This strategy applies especially to those situations in which the integrity of the facial nerve is at stake or when a potentially disfiguring resection is being considered. In our medical center, radical excision of salivary tumors is never performed based on an FNAB or frozen section diagnosis. Instead, the pathologist bases diagnoses on permanent histologic sections. If indicated, the patient is then

Table 6–2. Abridged Classification of Salivary Gland Tumors

Benign	**Malignant**
Pleomorphic adenoma	*Low Grade*
Basal cell adenoma	Mucoepidermoid carcinoma
Warthin's tumor	Acinic-cell carcinoma
Oncocytoma	Adenoid cystic carcinoma
Myoepithelioma	Basal-cell adenocarcinoma
Sebaceous adenoma	Epithelial-myoepithelial carcinoma
Canalicular adenoma	Myoepithelial carcinoma
Papillary cystadenoma	Polymorphous low-grade adenocarcinoma
	Carcinoma ex pleomorphic adenoma (some)
	Papillary cystadenocarcinoma
	High Grade
	Mucoepidermoid carcinoma
	Carcinoma ex pleomorphic adenoma (some)
	Salivary duct carcinoma
	Undifferentiated carcinoma
	Squamous-cell carcinoma

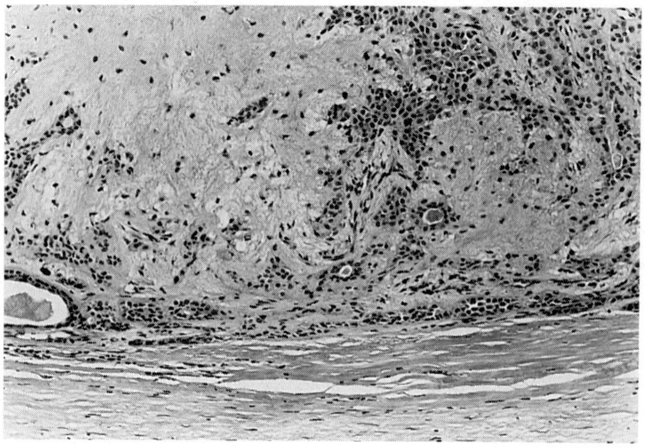

Figure 6–6. Pleomorphic adenoma composed of epithelial cells lying in a myxochondroid stroma. Note the fibrous tumor capsule at the bottom. Hematoxylin and eosin, ×200.

taken back to the operating room for a definitive procedure following thorough evaluation and informed consent.

Ideally, benign salivary gland neoplasms are removed en bloc by doing a superficial (lateral) parotid lobectomy with facial nerve dissection or submandibular gland excision. Simple enucleation was abandoned due to the high rate of recurrence following removal of pleomorphic adenoma by this method (Fig. 6–6). Excision of a cuff of extraglandular tissue is unnecessary when dealing with benign neoplasms. This is in contrast to most malignant salivary gland tumors, which are best treated with wide local excision to include a cuff of uninvolved soft tissue. If, however, the patient presents with normal facial motion and it is possible to dissect the tumor off the nerve, most head and neck oncologists believe that the continuity of the facial nerve should be maintained. The indication for neck dissection is controversial unless palpable adenopathy exists; in this case, neck dissection should be accomplished. Postoperative irradiation therapy is advocated with high-grade salivary gland neoplasms.

The Neck and Neck Dissections

NECK

Branchial cleft cyst is one of the most common benign conditions of the neck. It arises from remnants of the second branchial apparatus entrapped in a cervical lymph node and characteristically presents along the anterior border of the upper one-third of the sternocleidomastoid muscle in patients between 20 and 40 years of age. Occasionally it is associated with a sinus tract or fistula.

Such cysts produce cosmetic deformities and are often the sites of recurrent inflammation. Carcinomas arising in branchial cleft cysts, however, are extremely rare and most alleged cases, on long-term follow-up, turn out to be examples of cystic cervical lymph node metastases from a clinically occult squamous cell carcinoma, most often from the tonsil.

NECK DISSECTION

It has been almost a century since the technique for and principles of neck dissection were introduced in the United States. Neck dissection is an effective means to control early metastatic disease and is now embraced as an ideal method to stage squamous-cell carcinoma that originates on the mucosal surfaces of the upper aerodigestive tract. Neck dissection can be classified as either therapeutic or elective (Table 6–3).

Therapeutic neck dissection is performed for patients who present with cervical metastases. The presence of metastatic disease need not be confirmed preoperatively if histologic evidence of squamous-cell carcinoma has been obtained from a primary site that drains to the involved cervical lymph nodes.

Elective neck dissection is the removal of cervical lymph nodes in patients with no clinical evidence of metastasis but significant risk for occult cervical metastasis based upon the size and site of the primary malignant tumor.

The *classic radical neck dissection* encompasses an en bloc resection of the soft tissues between the clavicle inferiorly, the mandible superiorly, the trapezius posteriorly, and the visceral compartment anteriorly; it includes the internal jugular vein, sternocleidomastoid muscle, and spinal accessory nerve. The deep cervical fascia forms the deep boundary of resection whereas the platysma serves as a superficial boundary. The brachial plexus, phrenic nerve, vagus nerve, hypoglossal nerve, and carotid artery system are identified and preserved.

The morbidity associated with routine resection of the spinal accessory nerve has prompted surgeons to experiment with dissection and preservation of the spinal accessory nerve in selected patients. Experience indicates that selected patients with cervical metastases are effectively treated with *modified neck dissections* with preservation of the spinal accessory nerve. Other modifications include preservation of the internal jugular vein with or without the sternocleidomastoid muscle. The efficacy of such functional operations is not entirely proven in the presence of metastatic cervical adenopathy. Accordingly, most head and neck surgeons recommend routine use of postoperative irradiation therapy in patients with metastatic adenopathy following modified procedures.

Conventional wisdom holds that the initial node involvement with metastatic squamous-cell carcinoma can be pre-

Table 6–3. Classification of Neck Dissections

1. Radical neck dissection
2. Modified radical neck dissection
3. Selective neck dissection
   A. Supraomohyoid neck dissection (levels I, II, III)
   B. Posterolateral neck dissection (levels II, III, IV, V) and removal of suboccipital and retroauricular nodes
   C. Lateral neck dissection (levels II, III, IV)
   D. Anterior compartment neck dissection (level VI)
4. Extended radical neck dissection

Source: Modified from Robbins KT, ed. *Pocket Guide to Neck Dissection, Classification and TNM Staging of Head and Neck Cancer.* Alexandria, VA: American Academy of Otolaryngology and Head and Neck Surgery Foundation, Inc.; 1991:13, with permission.

dicted based on the site of the primary lesion. While nomenclature has varied over the years, a widely used method is to label the *levels* of the neck I to VI (Fig. 6–7). Selective removal of lymph nodes from certain levels based upon the likelihood of metastatic disease is termed *selective neck dissection*. Important structures such as the sternocleidomastoid muscle, internal jugular vein, and spinal accessory nerve are selectively preserved. In reality, this approach is a biopsy or staging procedure. Patients who are subsequently found to have occult metastases are referred for adjuvant irradiation therapy.

Since selective neck dissections lack anatomic landmarks and consist of a mass of lymph nodes embedded in soft tissue, meaningful pathologic evaluation requires orientation by the surgeon. Indeed, orientation of any neck dissection, whether radical, modified, or selective, is helpful and well advised. For instance, the in situ boundary between levels II and III is the hyoid bone, while the boundary between levels III and IV is the cricothyroid membrane. These boundaries can be identified in the tissue specimen by placement of one or more long sutures.

In their assessment of neck dissections, pathologists should indicate the number of positive lymph nodes, their location (level), size range, and extranodal spread of tumor. Johnson et al. found extranodal spread to be an important

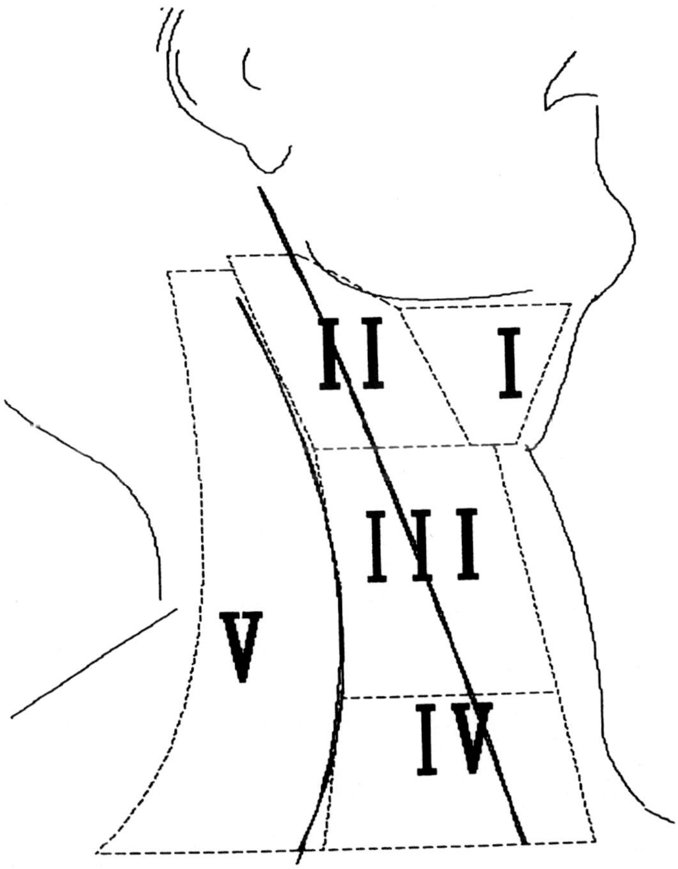

Figure 6–7. Diagram showing the various levels of the neck. Level I contains the submental and submandibular nodes, level II the upper jugular nodes, level III the midjugular nodes, level IV the lower jugular nodes, and level V the posterior cervical nodes. Level VI, not depicted, contains the anterior neck nodes.

prognostic indicator associated with a reduced disease-free interval that warrants the use of postoperative irradiation.[10] The presence of vascular and perineural invasion should also be described, since these findings may have an impact on prognosis.

Unknown Primary

With careful evaluation, a primary tumor will be uncovered in over 95% of patients who present with metastases in cervical lymph nodes. Prognosis in the remaining 5% of patients depends upon many factors, including the histologic type and degree of differentiation of the tumor, number and location of the positive cervical lymph nodes, presence or absence of extranodal spread (fixed nodes), and, possibly, whether or not the primary tumor is subsequently found.

The prototypic patient with an unknown primary in the head and neck is a male about 60 years of age who presents with a solitary upper or midjugular lymph node (stage N1), with or without fixation, that harbors a squamous-cell carcinoma. Patients with multiple positive cervical nodes (stages N2 to N3) are less common, while those with isolated supraclavicular nodes generally have an adenocarcinoma metastatic from a primary focus below the clavicles.

A thorough physical and panendoscopic examination, the latter preferably under anesthesia, is essential. The patient's symptoms may also point to the primary (e.g., decreased hearing—nasopharynx (eustachian tube); hoarseness—larynx; dysphagia and otalgia—pharynx). The exact location of the positive lymph node in the neck and knowledge of lymphatic drainage patterns from mucosal sites in the head and neck may also suggest a likely origin.

Unless a surgeon is prepared to treat the neck definitively at the time of biopsy, the temptation to excise the positive lymph node before thorough evaluation should be resisted. To do so may cause fibrosis that complicates future neck dissection or may produce local or distant dissemination of tumor. Fine needle aspiration biopsy is an alternative to excisional biopsy, since it avoids these complications (see Chap. 3).

Any mucosal irregularity should be biopsied and submitted for histologic evaluation. Random sampling, or "blind biopsies" of sites that are difficult to inspect, is favored by many surgeons. These include the nasopharynx, base of tongue, and pyriform sinus. Since some tonsillar carcinomas are exceedingly small, a diagnostic tonsillectomy ipsilateral to the adenopathy (rather than random biopsy) may be more effective. The pathologist must examine the entire tonsil, since some of these tumors are easily missed on gross inspection alone.

If a primary site cannot be found after thorough evaluation, the patient should still undergo curative treatment, since the prognosis is not as dismal as once thought. At our medical center, most patients with an unknown primary are treated with modified neck dissection with removal of the sternocleidomastoid muscle and preservation of the spinal accessory nerve and internal jugular vein assuming that the latter structures are not involved by tumor. External beam irradiation is given postoperatively in a port extending from the nasopharynx to the clavicle.

In an evaluation of 113 patients with cervical metastases from squamous carcinoma and no known primary, Maulard et al. found the overall 3- and 5-year actuarial survival to be 51 and 38%, respectively.[11] In this same study, the 5-year survival was 62, 40, and 19%, respectively, for N1, N2, and N3 stage lymph nodes.

The incidence of subsequent location of the primary tumor during or following treatment ranges from 4 to 30%.[11–13] The impact of primary site identification upon prognosis is controversial. Coker et al. reported a 5-year survival of 60% if the primary tumor remained occult versus 30% if it were identified.[12] In contrast, Barrie et al. observed no significant difference in survival whether or not the tumor was found (31 and 32% 5-year determinant survival, respectively).[14]

Acknowledgments

The authors extend their sincere thanks and appreciation to Donna Bowen for secretarial assistance and to Linda Shab and Jeffrey D. Levis for medical illustrations.

PITFALLS FOR THE SURGEON

1. Failure to provide pertinent clinical information to the pathologist for evaluation of tissue specimens.
2. Failure to orient large, complex specimens and to delineate levels of selective neck dissections for the pathologist.
3. Enucleating parotid tumors for fear of damaging the facial nerve rather than performing a superficial (lateral) parotid lobectomy.
4. Excising neck masses before proper clinical evaluation.

PITFALLS FOR THE PATHOLOGIST

1. Inability to visualize the three-dimensional anatomy of tumors for selection and evaluation of appropriate resection margins.
2. Evaluating cystic and fibroosseous lesions of the jaws without reviewing or having knowledge of radiographic and clinical findings.
3. Mistaking benign mucosal biopsies for malignancy on the basis of oblique or tangential orientation of the biopsies within the paraffin blocks.
4. Mistaking radiation-induced changes for malignancy.

FURTHER READING

Barnes L, ed. *Surgical Pathology of the Head and Neck.* New York: Dekker; 1985.

Barnes L, Peel RL, eds. *Head and Neck Pathology: A Text/Atlas of Differential Diagnosis.* New York: Igaku-Shoin; 1990.

Bluestone CD, Stool SE, eds. *Pediatric Otolaryngology*, 2nd ed. Philadelphia: Saunders; 1990.

Ellis GL, Auclair PL, Gnepp DR, eds. *Surgical Pathology of the Salivary Glands.* Philadelphia: Saunders; 1991.

Myers EN, Suen JY, eds. *Cancer of the Head and Neck*, 2nd ed. New York: Churchill-Livingstone; 1989.

Regezi JA, Sciubba JJ, eds. *Oral Pathology: Clinical-Pathologic Correlations.* Philadelphia: Saunders; 1989.

REFERENCES

1. Beahrs OH, Henson DE, Hutter RVP. *American Joint Committee on Cancer: Manual for Staging of Cancer*, 4th ed. Philadelphia: Saunders; 1992.
2. Barnes L, Johnson JT. Pathological and clinical considerations in the evaluation of major head and neck specimens resected for cancer. Part I. In: Sommers SC, Rosen PP, Fechner RE, eds. *Pathology Annual.* Vol 21. Norwalk, CT: Appleton-Century-Crofts; 1986:173.
3. Frierson HF Jr, Cooper PH. Prognostic factors in squamous cell carcinoma of the lower lip. *Hum Pathol.* 1986;17:346.
4. Medina JE, Dichtel W, Luna MA. Verrucous-squamous carcinoma of the oral cavity: A clinicopathologic study of 104 cases. *Arch Otolaryngol.* 1984;110:437.
5. Paradise JL. Tonsillectomy and adenoidectomy. In: Bluestone CD, Stool SE, eds. *Pediatric Otolaryngology*, 2nd ed. Philadelphia: Saunders; 1990:915.
6. Weiland LH. Nasopharyngeal carcinoma. In: Barnes L, ed. *Surgical Pathology of the Head and Neck.* New York: Dekker; 1985:453.
7. Fee WE Jr, Roberson JB, Goffinet DR. Long-term survival after surgical resection for recurrent nasopharyngeal cancer after radiotherapy failure. *Arch Otolaryngol Head Neck Surg.* 1991; 117:1233.
8. Gallia LJ, Johnson JT. The incidence of neoplastic versus inflammatory disease in major salivary gland masses diagnosed by surgery. *Laryngoscope.* 1981;91:512.
9. Barnes L, Johnson JT. Pathologic and clinical considerations in the evaluation of major head and neck specimens resected for cancer. Part II. In: Sommers SC, Rosen PP, Fechner RE, eds. *Pathology Annual.* Vol 21. Norwalk, CT: Appleton-Century-Crofts; 1986:83.
10. Johnson JT, Myers EN, Bedetti CD, et al. Cervical lymph node metastases: Incidence and implications of extracapsular spread. *Arch Otolaryngol.* 1985;111:534.
11. Maulard C, Housset M, Brunel P, et al. Postoperative radiation

therapy for cervical lymph node metastases from an occult squamous cell carcinoma. *Laryngoscope*. 1992;102:884.
12. Coker DD, Casterline PF, Chambers RG, et al. Metastases to lymph nodes of the head and neck from an unknown primary. *Am J Surg*. 1977;134:517.
13. Bataini JP, Rodriquez J, Jaulerry C, et al. Treatment of metastatic neck nodes secondary to an occult epidermoid carcinoma of the head and neck. *Laryngoscope*. 1987;97:1080.
14. Barrie JR, Knapper WH, Strong EW. Cervical nodal metastases of unknown origin. *Am J Surg*. 1970;120:466.

7

The Eye and Ocular Adnexa

James A. Garrity and R. Jean Campbell

Definition

The orbit, globe, and ocular adnexa, because of their location, mark a surgical crossroads between multiple specialties. These specialties include otorhinolaryngology, plastic surgery, and, occasionally, neurosurgery. The eye and the attached extraocular muscles, however, most often fall within the exclusive domain of the ophthalmic surgeon. The same may be stated in regard to pathologic examination of tissue from these areas, which is done largely by pathologists specialized in ophthalmic pathology.

The goal of this chapter is to introduce the reader to somc of thc more common disease processes occurring within and around the globe, orbit, and ocular adnexa and to suggest approaches to the practical management of these problems.

Because the biopsy specimen from these areas may be limited in amount, the surgeon is encouraged to communicate with the pathologist *before* the operation. When this communication occurs, the tissue can be handled in the most appropriate manner with regard to frozen section, appropriate fixative solution, and histopathologic studies. Such preoperative planning maximizes the information obtained from a small specimen.

This chapter is divided into separate anatomic and functional units, beginning with the eyelids and proceeding posteriorly to consider the conjunctiva, globe, orbit, and finally the optic nerve. The symptoms, signs, and management are discussed in relation to each anatomic site, and the pathologic features of the more important lesions are discussed in the order below.

Eyelids: Hemangioma, chalazion, sebaceous gland carcinoma, basal-cell carcinoma, squamous-cell carcinoma, pigmented lesions, and benign neoplasms (papilloma, xanthelasma, cutaneous horn)
Conjunctiva: Papilloma, carcinoma, nevus, primary acquired melanosis (PAM)
Globe: Trauma, retinoblastoma, melanoma, metastasis
Orbit: Metastasis, hemangioma, pleomorphic adenoma and adenoid cystic carcinoma of the lacrimal gland, rhabdomyosarcoma, inflammatory and lymphocytic infiltrates
Optic nerve: Glioma, meningioma

Eyelids

Regardless of the pathologic process, many of the symptoms and signs of eyelid involvement are the same. Symptoms relating to a mass may produce pain, swelling, and even blurred vision if the upper eyelid is involved. Recurrent irritation and bleeding are features of some eyelid neoplasms. Some malignancies may be entirely asymptomatic and are detected coincidentally on routine clinical examination.

Mattering about the eyelids is a nonspecific sign. It occurs most often with a conjunctivitis but is also produced by lesions of the eyelid. Such lesions include a chalazion or even a malignant lesion (such as sebaceous gland carcinoma). The presence of ancillary signs, such as conjunctival retraction and scarring, is helpful in this situation; if these signs are present, a biopsy is mandated.

Management of eyelid lesions may be considered on the basis of age. In the pediatric population, most lesions are benign. A capillary hemangioma in a child, which characteristically enlarges and becomes dusky when the child cries, probably typifies most such lesions. The majority of capillary hemangiomas are best managed by observation only; with time, sclerosis will occur with resolution. Hemangiomas that are large, cause amblyopia, or fail to resolve may be managed with local steroid injection or sometimes with laser therapy.

Chalazion may occur in both the adult and pediatric populations. This entity is a granulomatous reaction to a dysfunctional sebaceous gland (Fig. 7–1). Lesions that are not responsive to local measures require incision and curettage. In a young child, a general anesthetic is required. Large chalazia often have an accompanying pyogenic granuloma of the adjacent conjunctiva, which may create clinical diagnostic confusion. Effective treatment of the chalazion will result in resolution of the conjunctival pyogenic granuloma.

Material obtained from curettage shows a granulomatous reaction to empty fat spaces (Fig. 7–1). These fat spaces are the characteristic microscopic finding for these lesions.

Management of chalazion in the adult does not differ from that in the child. However, in adult patients, the examiner should be extremely cautious in approaching persistent or recurrent chalazia, particularly those that occur at the same location; such features are a warning that a carcinoma of the sebaceous gland may be present. Any lesion that involves the margin of the eyelid or the immediately adjacent area requires careful examination for eyelash loss, which is a finding specifically suggestive of a malignant process. Sebaceous gland carcinoma is well known to masquerade as a recurrent chalazion or as a persistent unilateral blepharoconjunctivitis (Fig. 7–2). Such lesions require a full-thickness wedge biopsy of the eyelid and, if positive, excision until intraoperative tumor-free margins are obtained (Fig. 7–3).

Sebaceous gland carcinoma constitutes only 1 to 2% of all malignant neoplasms of the eyelid, but the eyelid is the most common site for this tumor.[1] Its early recognition is important because it is highly invasive and may lead to early lymph node involvement. The microscopic finding of pagetoid change within the epithelium is the telltale signal for an underlying sebaceous gland carcinoma (Fig. 7–4). On occasion, the overlying epithelium may show in situ squamous-cell carcinoma.

Basal-cell carcinoma is, of course, the most common malignant lesion of the eyelid and is most often found in the lower eyelid.[2–4] As mentioned, loss of eyelashes is an important sign, suggests malignancy, and mandates biopsy (Fig. 7–5). A raised, pearly appearance with telangiectatic vessels is typical. Surgical excision with attention to tumor-free margins is of the utmost importance. When removing the lesion as a whole, indicate to the pathologist, preferably with a marker pen or a peripheral suture, the orientation of the margins—such as superior, inferior, nasal, and temporal. When this marking is done, tumor involvement of a margin can be accurately reported with regard to site, and the surgeon may judiciously proceed with further surgery. Another option is to send a separate margin from the edges of excision after the main mass has been excised. If many

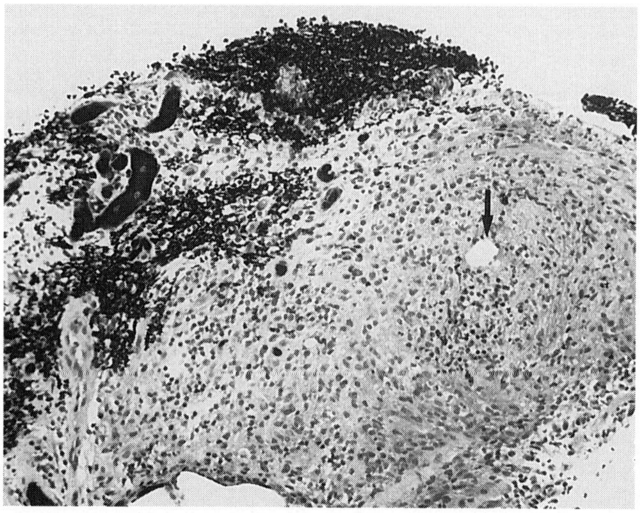

Figure 7–1. Chalazion; granulomatous reaction with empty fat spaces *(arrow)*. Hematoxylin and eosin, ×160.

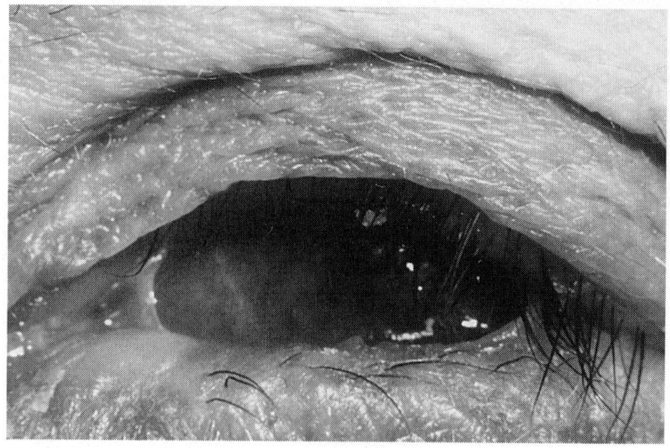

Figure 7–2. Sebaceous gland carcinoma of upper and lower eyelids in an 82-year-old woman. Note loss of upper and lower eyelashes with symblepharon.

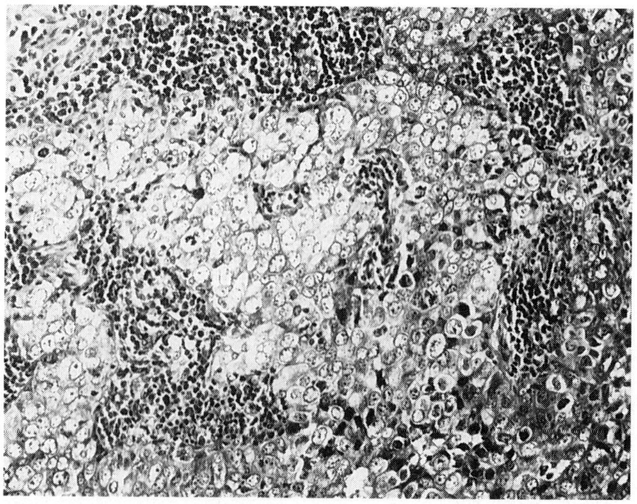

Figure 7–3. Poorly differentiated sebaceous gland carcinoma. The tumor is composed of poorly differentiated, pale, foamy cells resembling normal sebaceous epithelium. Overlying adjacent epithelium shows changes seen in Figure 7–4. Hematoxylin and eosin, ×160.

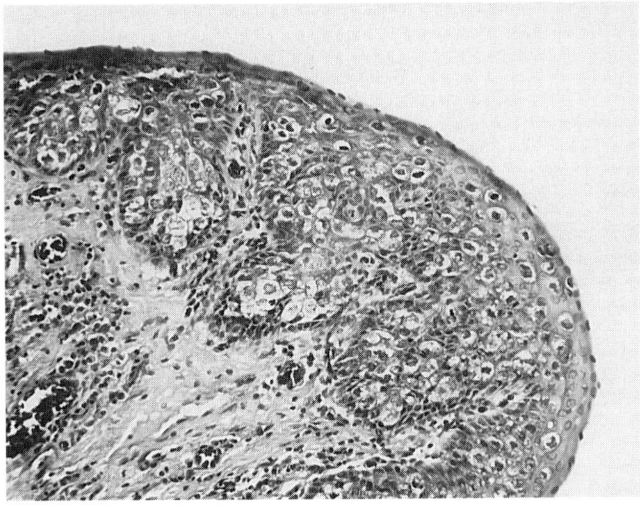

Figure 7–4. Pagetoid cells in epithelium of eyelid associated with underlying sebaceous carcinoma. Hematoxylin and eosin, ×160.

''margins'' are submitted at the same time, it is important to make sure that each specimen is correctly labeled to avoid confusion in the pathology laboratory and in the operating room. Histologically, the lesion may be of the nodular, basosquamous, or adenoid cystic type, or it may be of the morphea form. The latter type is particularly aggressive because of its ill-defined margins (Fig. 7–6). This form has the highest recurrence rate of all histologic types (see Chap. 4).

Squamous-cell carcinoma constitutes approximately 5% of all malignant tumors of the eyelid.[2–4] Like basal-cell carcinoma, it is found most frequently on the lower eyelid, but it is more frequent on the upper eyelid than basal-cell carcinoma. Elderly, fair-skinned persons are typically affected. The lesion can arise de novo, in actinic keratosis, in previously irradiated skin, or in patients with xeroderma pigmentosa. Clinically, the lesion may appear as an elevated, indurated plaque or a nodule that is subject to ulceration. Wide local excision, with monitoring of the margins by frozen sections, is usually curative. Metastases are unusual, in contrast to the behavior of squamous-cell carcinoma at other sites.

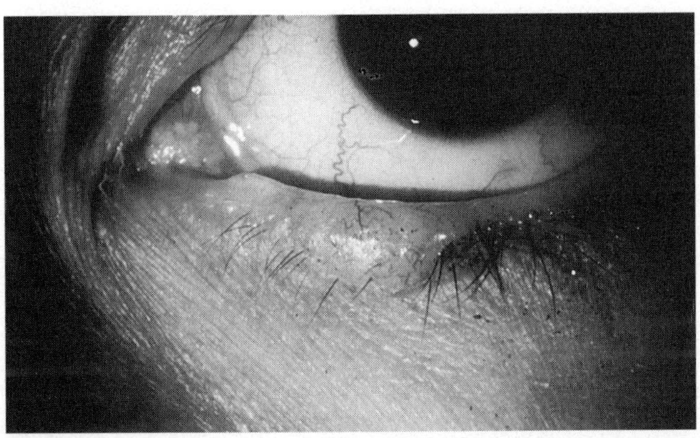

Figure 7–5. Basal-cell carcinoma of medial lower lid in a 37-year-old woman. Note pearly appearance with telangiectasia and loss of eyelashes.

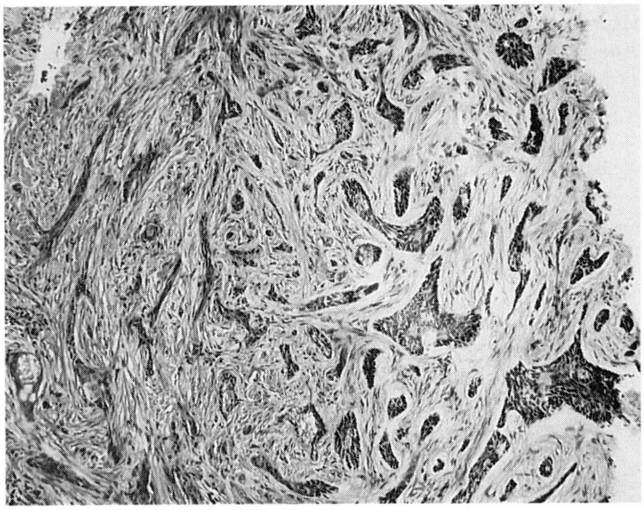

Figure 7–6. Basal-cell carcinoma of medial lower eyelid in a 67-year-old man. This morpheaform variant shows constricted nests of proliferating basal cells in desmoplastic background. Hematoxylin and eosin, ×160.

Pigmented lesions around the eyelid may be benign or malignant. A benign lesion is typified by the nevus, which can be located on the surface of the eyelid or on the eyelid margin. A history of growth associated with the hormonal influences of puberty or pregnancy is common. Of the three histologic types—junctional, intradermal, and compound—only the junctional type presents as a flat lesion. Whereas an elevated nevus on the surface of the eyelid is amenable to excision, a lesion of the eyelid margin is shaved flush with the surrounding surface whenever possible in order to avoid notches in the margin of the eyelid.

Malignant melanoma constitutes only 1% of eyelid malignancies. Nevertheless, because melanoma is the cause of most deaths from cutaneous malignancies in general, it should be suspected and excised early.

There are four types of malignant melanoma: lentigo maligna, superficial spreading melanoma, nodular melanoma, and acral lentiginous melanoma. The most frequent type is the superficial spreading variety. Initially, growth occurs in a horizontal plane; only later does it proceed in a vertical plane. Prognosis correlates with the depth of tumor invasion (Clark classification) and with measured maximal thickness of the tumor (Breslow classification).[5]

Among the most common lesions of the eyelid are squamous papilloma and xanthelasma. The former is usually pedunculated, is often friable, and frequently occurs at the eyelid margin among the eyelashes. Excision or cautery is usually effective. Xanthelasma is yellowish-tan and usually flat. The patient may or may not have elevated serum lipid values. Removal is usually for cosmesis. Necrobiotic xanthogranuloma has the same coloration but tends to be elevated and is more firm or indurated. This lesion, which in itself is benign, can be associated with paraproteinemia, sometimes reflecting underlying multiple myeloma.[6]

Other benign lesions include seborrheic keratosis, keratoacanthoma, and cutaneous horn. A word of caution is required for the cutaneous horn. This should never be shaved but rather excised, because the raised epithelial base from which it arises may harbor a malignancy. The superficial horny projection typically consists of microscopically benign keratin layers regardless of whether the base is actinic keratosis or basal-cell or squamous-cell carcinoma.

Disease entities that may become malignant include actinic keratosis, radiation dermatitis, xeroderma pigmentosa, and Bowen's disease. Bowen's disease manifests as an erythematous, scaly, keratotic plaque with sharply defined edges that may have elevated margins. It consists of intraepithelial squamous-cell carcinoma and occurs predominantly in fair-skinned, middle-aged men. Associated malignancy of the gastrointestinal tract has been reported with Bowen's disease of the lid and skin.

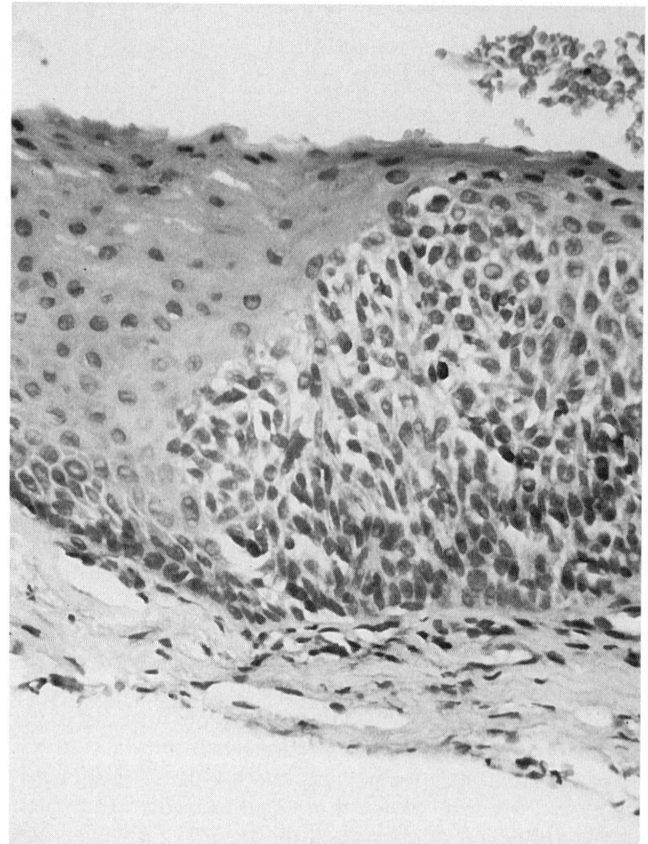

Figure 7–8. In situ squamous-cell carcinoma of conjunctiva. Note sharp line of demarcation between normal and malignant epithelium. Hematoxylin and eosin, ×250.

Conjunctiva

The conjunctiva is a mucous membrane that lines the inner aspect of the eyelids (palpebral conjunctiva) and the exposed surface of the globe (bulbar conjunctiva). Some of its important functions include the secretion of mucus, protection against infection, and maintenance of a smooth, gliding surface between the globe and the eyelids. Most of the epithelium is of the stratified columnar type except at the limbus and the palpebral margins, where it is of the stratified squamous type. The goblet cells are most numerous in the inferior fornix, and it is this site that is amenable to biopsy for aid in the diagnosis of systemic disease. Such diseases include sarcoidosis, cystinosis, and cerebrosidase deficiency. Local diseases include lymphoma and amyloidosis. The biopsy material may be obtained with use of a topical or local anesthetic. The specimen should be placed on a flat mount such as a piece of sponge or a piece of paper (cut from the wrapping of surgical gloves, Fig. 7–7) that has previously been moistened in the fixative of choice.[7] The specimen should *never* be placed on a dry mount because the specimen first adheres and dries on contact and then stretches as the mount saturates with fluid. Stretching causes distortion of the tissue, with severe artifactual obscuration in microscopic appearance.

Neoplasms may occur anywhere on the bulbar or palpebral conjunctiva; however, the limbus (corneoscleral junction) is the most common site for pinguecula, pterygia, and malignant epithelial lesions.

Conjunctival intraepithelial neoplasia (CIN) (Fig. 7–8) may be gelatinous or leukoplakic in appearance.[8] It may be sessile or polypoid. The latter, if occurring as a single lesion in an adult, must be distinguished from a benign papilloma of viral origin (Fig. 7–9). In children, papillomas tend to be multiple. If CIN with pagetoid features is de-

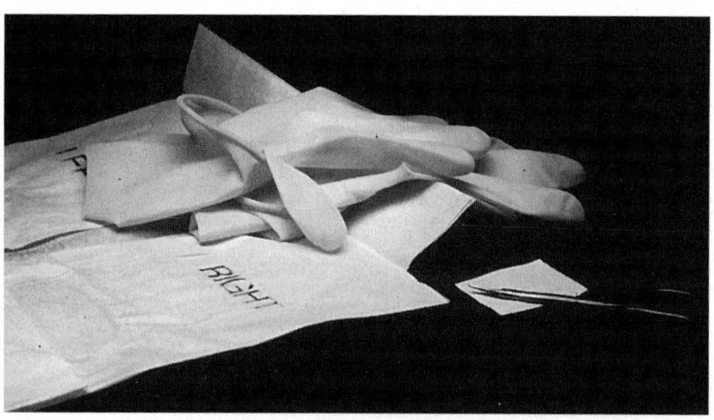

Figure 7–7. Piece of paper cut from glove wrapping serves as a flat mount for a conjunctival biopsy specimen. Paper must be moistened in fixative before tissue is applied to surface.

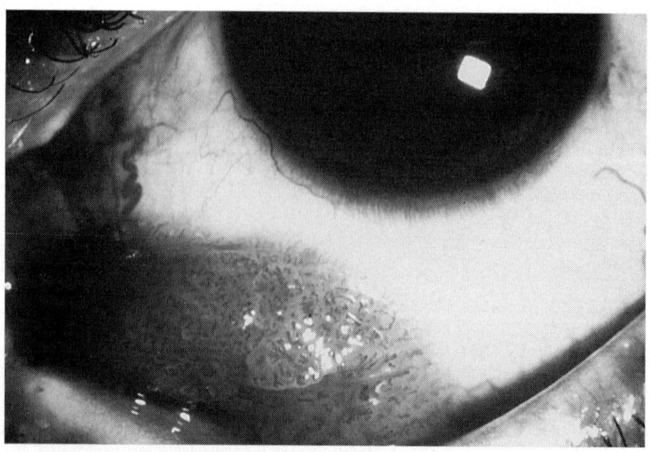

Figure 7–9. Single benign conjunctival polyp in an adult.

tected in the palpebral conjunctiva (Fig. 7–4), an adjacent sebaceous-cell carcinoma should be suspected and examination and a wedge biopsy of the eyelid should be performed. Management of CIN or in situ squamous-cell carcinoma includes excision and cryotherapy of the bed. If the lesion involves the corneal epithelium, it is critical that Bowman's layer be left intact, because this layer is an important barrier to neoplasia and inflammation; if breached, the possibility of neoplastic invasion or infection into the underlying stroma arises.

Nevi are common in the conjunctiva. Increase in pigmentation is associated with hormonal changes, such as occur with pregnancy or the onset of adolescence; sudden changes in coloration during this period may cause the patient to seek professional advice. The growth of epithelial inclusion cysts with goblet secretion may lead to the expansion of a nevus and bring the patient in for professional advice. The vast majority of these lesions are benign and are either compound or subepithelial nevi (Fig. 7–10).[9]

Primary acquired melanosis (PAM) is a condition that occurs in the middle years of life; it may wax and wane. For any associated nodular lesion that develops, biopsy must be done, because melanoma may develop in PAM after many years. If an initial biopsy of a pigmented area shows the features of cellular nesting within the epithelium *without* atypical features, then the clinical course will be benign. If, however, the cellular appearances are atypical, recurrence with malignant change is a strong possibility.[10] As a general rule, pigmented lesions, whatever their site, should be examined by permanent sections and not by frozen section. Pigment obscures cellular detail and bleaching cannot be performed on frozen tissue.

Globe

Ocular trauma with disruption of structure and loss of function is the most common indication for enucleation. This is performed to eliminate pain or reduce the risk of sympathetic ophthalmia. Trauma to the face frequently includes the eye. The nature of the injury may be blunt, perforating, or penetrating. A perforating injury of the globe is defined as one with both an entry and an exit wound. A penetrating global injury has only an entrance wound.[11]

In the examination of such a globe, either during operation or subsequently during pathologic examination,[12–14] the sclera beneath the extraocular muscles must be carefully inspected to assess the full posterior extent of the scleral wound. At times it is difficult to identify the exact nature of dark tissue that protrudes through a scleral wound. The pathologist may be asked to examine this prolapsed tissue with intraoperative frozen section. If retina is identified, the surgeon is justified in proceeding with a primary enucleation. The possibility of an intraocular foreign body should not be overlooked. A foreign body that contains copper is renowned for causing suppurative endophthalmitis.

Retinoblastoma is the most common primary malignant tumor of childhood. It usually presents with leukocoria or strabismus. Persons who have the hereditary form of the disease may have bilateral tumors. Those with sporadic disease tend to have unilateral tumors. Children with the hereditary form are at risk for the development of a second primary tumor. Commonly, this second primary tumor is an osteosarcoma. The sarcomatous change may occur at a remote site or in the field of radiation. Members of the same family who do not have a retinoblastoma are also at risk for the development of an osteosarcoma.[15]

Malignant melanoma of the uvea is the most common primary malignant tumor of the eye in the adult; the most common site is the posterior choroid. Usually it appears as an elevated lesion of variable pigmentation. Current treatment includes enucleation, with or without preoperative irradiation, or brachytherapy alone. Tumors less than 5 mm at base and less than 3 mm in height are usually observed.[16–18] Should metastatic disease occur, the liver is the most frequently affected site.

For evaluation of a patient for the possibility of melanoma metastases, specialties other than ophthalmology, in particular hematology-oncology, should be recruited into the effort. A diagnostic liver biopsy will show histologic

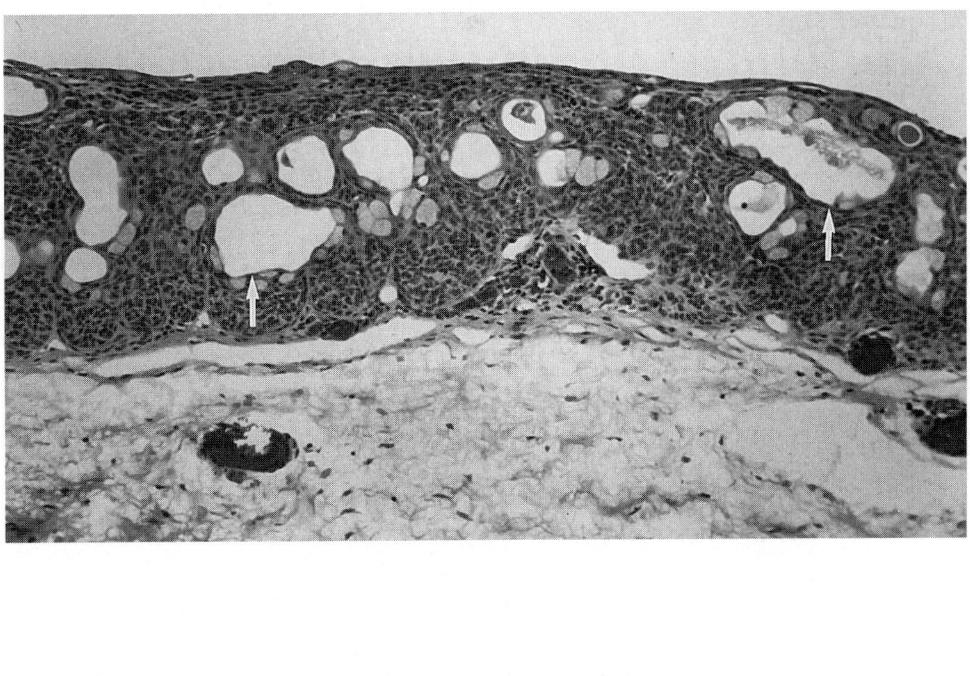

Figure 7–10. Conjunctival nevus in a 10-year-old boy. Nests of benign nevus cells occupy subepithelial tissues together with epithelial inclusion cysts *(arrows)*, the growth of which had caused enlargement of the lesion. Hematoxylin and eosin, ×160.

findings that are commonly of a mixed cellular pattern of spindle and epithelioid cells. The microscopic slides from previous operations should always be reviewed.

The most common malignant uveal tumor is in fact a metastasis, usually to the posterior choroid but on rare occasions to the iris or ciliary body. The most common primary sources for such metastases are breast, lung, and colon. Once uveal metastases are present, the median life expectancy is approximately 1 year. The notable exception to such behavior is metastatic carcinoid; patients with metastasis of these low-grade endocrine tumors have been known to survive for up to 8 years.[19] If the patient has symptoms, the metastases, whatever the source, are best treated with radiation.

Orbit

It is in the orbit where the specialties of ophthalmology, neurosurgery, otorhinolaryngology, and plastic surgery overlap considerably. Biopsy specimens from this area may, at times, be difficult to obtain and are small. In these situations, preoperative communication between the surgeon and pathologist is essential. Some of the more common orbital tumors and inflammations likely to be encountered are briefly reviewed.

Primary orbital tumors can be considered on the basis of age. In the pediatric population, the most frequent orbital tumor is cystic, typically a dermoid or epidermoid cyst.[20] The most frequent malignant tumor is a rhabdomyosarcoma; histopathologically, the picture ranges from a spindle-cell variant with few mitotic figures to a small round-cell anaplastic variety. In most instances, the diagnosis is confirmed by immunohistochemistry. When the differential diagnosis is as limited as it is in pediatric orbital tumors, sometimes even a very small tissue sampling, such as aspiration cytology biopsy, allows the pathologist to establish a definitive diagnosis.

In the adult, the most frequent benign tumor is the cavernous hemangioma. The most frequent malignant tumor is non-Hodgkin's lymphoma.[21] In anticipation of this possibility, it is of the utmost importance to freeze part of the tissue that is obtained at operation for immunohistochemistry and other molecular studies. The biopsy specimen should be of sufficient size to allow both this and enough tissue in formalin for good-quality conventional slides. Surface antigens may be destroyed by formalin fixation, and thus the type of lymphocytic infiltrate, either benign or malignant, cannot be determined with accuracy. Freezing all the tissue is unsatisfactory because the cellular and nuclear detail of the cells is distorted by the freezing process. Most orbital lymphomatous infiltrates are low-grade tumors of the B phenotype, often localized to this area, in keeping with tumor of mucosa-associated lymphoid tissue (see Chap. 17).

Primary tumors of the lacrimal gland are more frequent in the adult population and closely resemble minor salivary gland tumors. The pleomorphic adenoma (benign mixed tumor) is the most common benign epithelial tumor in this region. Among epithelial malignancies, adenoid cystic carcinoma is the most frequent; however, lymphomatous involvement of the lacrimal gland is even more frequent.

Secondary tumors are those that invade the orbit from adjacent anatomic structures, such as the sinuses, the eyelids, or the globe itself. The most frequent type of secondary tumor is the squamous-cell carcinoma that arises in a nasal sinus.[21] It is essential that the uninvolved eye be examined by an ophthalmologist before radical surgery is performed. This examination is needed because the prognosis in such a patient may be poor, and if the sight in the eye of the non–tumor-involved orbit is significantly decreased, it is highly undesirable to render the patient blind in the final days of life.

Metastatic tumors are most commonly from the breast and lung, but a wide variety of sources are possible. The patient may present with orbital findings, most notably when the primary lesion is in the kidney or the lung. In general, with the notable exception of metastatic carcinoid, the prognosis is poor. Tissue from fine-needle biopsy of such lesions often requires immunohistochemical study to define the tumor type. Such study can be performed on paraffin sections from the cytology cell block.

In regard to the various orbital inflammations (such as orbital myositis or inflammatory dacryoadenitis), any or all of the structures in the orbit (extraocular muscles, perioptic meninges, lacrimal gland, or other soft tissues) may be involved. The presentation usually includes pain, swelling, proptosis, and loss of function. The response to systemic steroids may be dramatic.[2, 21, 22]

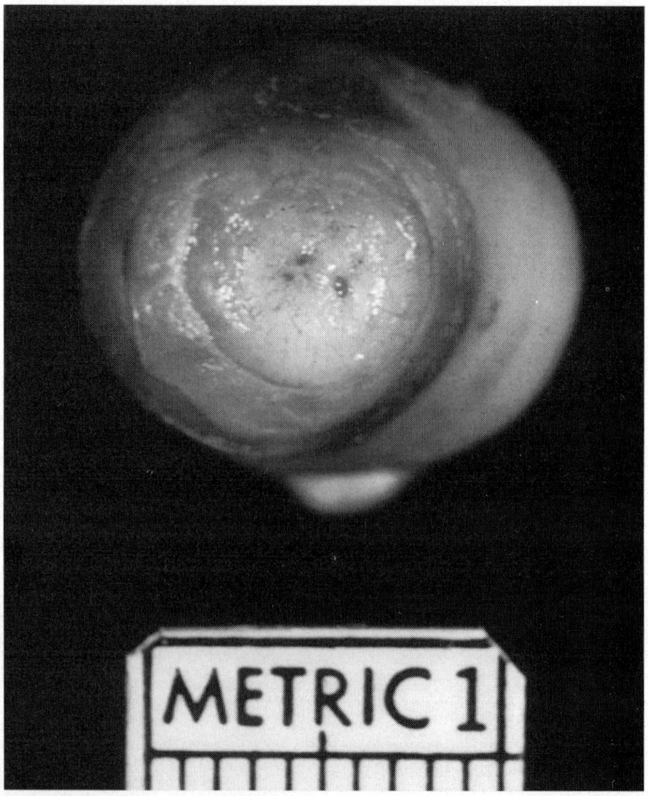

Figure 7–11. Optic nerve glioma in a 9-year-old boy. Gross section of optic nerve shows increased size and reactive thickening of surrounding layer of meninges.

The inflammatory infiltrate usually consists of an admixture of acute and chronic inflammatory cells. The proportion of each varies from case to case, but eosinophils are usually a prominent feature. On occasion, inflammation is angiocentric and angiodestructive. The presence of granulomatous inflammation with vasculitis suggests Wegener's granulomatosis.[23] It is important to refer the patient to an internist for the appropriate evaluation, which will include estimation of serum levels of cytoplasmic antineutrophil cytoplasmic antibody (c-ANCA) and perinuclear antineutrophil cytoplasmic antibody (p-ANCA).[24] The therapeutic response to corticosteroids is usually not as dramatic as in an idiopathic inflammatory process, and antimetabolites may ultimately be needed for control.

Infiltrates within the orbit that are predominantly lymphocytic must be considered to be malignant until proved otherwise by immunohistochemical studies on tissue that has been snap-frozen at the time of biopsy. A polyclonal reaction pattern supports the diagnosis of a benign reactive proliferation.

Optic Nerve

Juvenile pilocytic astrocytoma can arise in the substance of the optic nerve. Some regard this as a hamartoma, others as a low-grade astrocytoma. Whatever its exact nature, it grows slowly and is commonly associated with a reactive proliferation of the leptomeninges. It remains confined to the nerve by the dura. Most patients are managed by observation alone. Excision of the optic nerve distal to the chiasm is an option for patients who already have visual loss or who suffer extreme proptosis with pain. Radiotherapy and chemotherapy have been used for symptomatic tumors of the chiasm and hypothalamus.

In children, astrocytoma must be distinguished from a primary meningioma of the optic nerve sheath. This latter process is capable of highly aggressive growth and may invade the eye itself as well as the optic nerve. Most meningiomas of the optic nerve sheath are of the meningotheliomatous growth pattern. When biopsy of the optic nerve sheath reveals spindle-shaped cells, this finding signifies reactive hyperplasia of the meninges that accompanies an underlying glioma rather than a fibrous meningioma (Fig. 7–11). The typical patient with an optic nerve sheath meningioma is a middle-aged woman. Management is generally conservative, although, in selected cases, surgical excision of the tumor and the optic nerve or external beam radiation therapy is indicated. Many meningiomas have surface receptors for estrogens or progesterone; thus, hormonal manipulation for the control of tumor growth is a potential future therapy.

PITFALLS FOR THE SURGEON

1. Inadequate preoperative planning with the pathologist. Discussion should include differential diagnosis; this allows proper handling of tissue, proper utilization of fresh tissue, and selection of proper fixative.
2. A biopsy specimen from an area that is not representative of the pathologic process or one without enough tissue to allow definitive studies.
3. Failure to orient the excised specimen adequately or failure to send a separate margin for determination of tumor-free margins.
4. Failure to suspect eyelid malignancy in cases of persisting chalazion or a lesion associated with loss of eyelashes.
5. Failure to inform the patient after delayed pathologic results are obtained.

PITFALLS FOR THE PATHOLOGIST

1. Failure to discuss questions or problems concerning a case with the surgeon.
2. Failure to identify surgical margins of biopsy specimens and anatomic landmarks of enucleation specimens.
3. Failure to allocate frozen tissue for biopsy specimens suspicious for lymphoma.
4. Freezing of the whole biopsy specimen (this should never be done).
5. Need for multiple-step sections in suspected cases of sebaceous carcinoma.
6. Necessity to identify by history and examination intraocular lens prosthesis. Eye must be sectioned coronally.
7. Frozen section of deeply pigmented lesions (this should be avoided).

FURTHER READING

Havener VR. Basic principles for the submission and management of ophthalmic specimens for histopathology. *Vet Clin North Am Small Anim Pract*. 1980;10:497.

Margo CE, Grossniklaus HE. *Ocular Histopathology: A Guide to Differential Diagnosis*. Philadelphia: Saunders; 1991.

Torczynski E. Preparation of ocular specimens for histopathologic examination. *Ophthalmology*. 1981;88:1367.

REFERENCES

1. Wolfe JT III, Yeatts RP, Wick MR, et al. Sebaceous carcinoma of the eyelid: Errors in clinical and pathologic diagnosis. *Am J Surg Pathol*. 1984;8:597.
2. Spencer WH, ed. *Ophthalmic Pathology: An Atlas and Textbook*, 3rd ed. Philadelphia: Saunders; 1985.
3. Boniuk M, Zimmerman LE. Eyelid tumors with reference to lesions confused with squamous cell carcinoma: II. Inverted follicular keratosis. *Arch Ophthalmol*. 1963;69:698.
4. Boniuk M, Zimmerman LE. Eyelid tumors with reference to lesions confused with squamous cell carcinoma: III. Keratoacanthoma. *Arch Ophthalmol*. 1967;77:29.
5. Breslow A. Thickness, cross-sectional areas and depth of invasion in the prognosis of cutaneous melanoma. *Ann Surg*. 1970;172:902.
6. Bullock JD, Bartley GB, Campbell RJ, et al. Necrobiotic xanthogranuloma with paraproteinemia: Case report and a pathogenetic theory. *Ophthalmology*. 1986;93:1233.
7. Erie JC, Collyer SK, Campbell RJ. Dehydrated cucumber slice as a mount for conjunctival biopsy specimens. *Am J Ophthalmol*. 1985;99:539.
8. Erie JC, Campbell RJ, Liesegang TJ. Conjunctival and corneal intraepithelial and invasive neoplasia. *Ophthalmology*. 1986;93:176.
9. Folberg R, Jakobiec FA, Bernardino VB, Iwamoto T. Benign conjunctival melanocytic lesions: Clinicopathologic features. *Ophthalmology*. 1989;96:436.
10. Folberg R, McLean IW, Zimmerman LE. Primary acquired melanosis of the conjunctiva. *Hum Pathol*. 1985;16:129.
11. Morris DA. Ocular trauma. In: Garner A, Klintworth GK, eds. *Pathobiology of Ocular Disease*, 2nd ed. New York: Dekker; 1994:387.
12. Campbell RJ. Examination of eyes and their adnexae. In: Ludwig J, ed. *Current Methods of Autopsy Practice*, 2nd ed. Philadelphia: Saunders; 1979:120.
13. Campbell RJ. Ophthalmic pathology for the general pathologist. In: Weinstein RS, Graham AR, eds. *Advances in Pathology and Laboratory Medicine*. Vol 6. Chicago: Mosby-Year Book; 1993:547.
14. Jakobiec FA, Zimmerman LE. Symposium on ophthalmic surgical pathology: Part I. Introduction. *Hum Pathol*. 1982;13:98.
15. Abramson DH, Ellsworth RM, Kitchin FD, Tung G. Second nonocular tumors in retinoblastoma survivors: Are they radiation-induced? *Ophthalmology*. 1984;91:1351.
16. Folberg R, Verdick R, Weingeist TA, Montague PR. The gross examination of eyes removed for choroidal and ciliary body melanomas. *Ophthalmology*. 1986;93:1643.
17. Prophet E. Technique for processing eye specimens. *Histo-Logic* 1976;6:75.
18. Tasman W, Jaeger EA, eds. *Duane's Clinical Ophthalmology*. Vols I–V. Philadelphia: Lippincott; 1993.
19. Balestrazzi E, di Tondo U, delle Noci N, Blasi MA. Metastasis of bronchial carcinoid tumour to choroid. *Ophthalmologica*. 1989;198:104.
20. Kodsi SR, Shetlar DJ, Campbell RJ, et al. A review of 340 orbital tumors in children during a 60-year period. *Am J Ophthalmol*. 1994;117:177.
21. Henderson JW. *Orbital Tumors*, 3rd ed. New York: Raven Press; 1994.
22. Kennerdell JS, Dresner SC. The nonspecific orbital inflammatory syndromes. *Surv Ophthalmol*. 1984;29:93.
23. Bullen CL, Liesegang TJ, McDonald TJ, DeRemee RA. Ocular complications of Wegener's granulomatosis. *Ophthalmology*. 1983;90:279.
24. Jennette JC, Wilkman AS, Falk RJ. Anti-neutrophil cytoplasmic autoantibody-associated glomerulonephritis and vasculitis. *Am J Pathol*. 1989;135:921.

8

The Nervous System

M. Beatriz S. Lopes, Bernd W. Scheithauer, and David G. Piepgras

Considerations of the nervous system are not the exclusive province of the neurosurgeon. Peripheral nerves and their disorders extend to every organ system and tissue. Indeed, skeletal muscle and nerve biopsies are most often performed by plastic or general surgeons. Even the *central* nervous system, with its surrounding structures giving rise to various soft tissue and osseous lesions, may be encountered by specialists in head-and-neck, orthopedic, plastic, or dermatologic surgery. Malformations and disease processes of this system sometimes lead to encounters that are unexpected and unintentional!

Perhaps more so than in other organ systems, diagnosis in neuropathology requires integration of four parameters: (1) morphologic examination of the lesion, (2) topographic analysis of the lesion, (3) correlation of histology with neuroimaging, and (4) evaluation of these findings in light of clinical data. Regardless of diagnostic considerations or biopsy site (brain, spinal cord, nerve, or muscle), integration of morphologic and clinical data is essential.

The purpose of this chapter is threefold: to describe the most common diseases affecting the nervous and neuromuscular systems, to discuss diagnostic pitfalls and their therapeutic implications, and to make recommendations for obtaining and handling surgical specimens.

Central Nervous System

ANATOMIC DESCRIPTION

The central nervous system (CNS) is protected by the skull and vertebral column and by the multilayered meninges. The latter are of mesenchymal derivation and consist of three layers: (1) the dura, the most superficial layer formed of dense collagenous tissue; (2) the arachnoid, a thin membrane composed largely of meningothelial cells, which serves to contain and direct the flow of cerebrospinal fluid (CSF); and (3) the pia, a delicate layer closely applied to the brain and spinal cord. Accordingly, the meninges delimit three potential spaces between the skull and brain: the epidural, subdural, and subarachnoidal. Within the skull, the dura adheres to the inner table of the calvaria. Its folds form basic anatomic landmarks that separate the compartments of the CNS. These include the falx, a midline fold separating the left and right cerebral hemispheres, and the tentorium, which separates the middle from the posterior fossa. Additionally, the dural layers envelope the major venous sinuses, including the superior and inferior sagittal, the transverse and sigmoid sinuses, and in the parasellar region the cavernous sinus. The intracranial contents thus lie within two compartments, the supra- and the infratentorial spaces. Supratentorial structures include the cerebral hemispheres and the deep gray nuclei (the basal ganglia, thalamus, and hypothalamus). The cerebellum and the brainstem are infratentorial in location.

In the spinal canal the meninges also form three anatomic compartments: the extradural space (between the dura and the spine, there being no adhesion to the bone), the intradural-extramedullary space (within the dura but outside the substance of the spinal cord), and the intramedullary region (consisting of the spinal cord proper). Several anatomic sites surrounding the CNS represent important surgical and pathologic landmarks in that lesions arise specific to these locations, and their involvement engenders specific differential diagnoses. These sites include the sellar and suprasellar regions, the cavernous sinus, the cerebellopontine angle, the pineal region, and the base of the skull.

MALFORMATIONS AND RESTS

Spina Bifida and Related Spinal Lesions

Defects of neural tube closure are among the most frequent congenital anomalies of the CNS.[1] Architecturally varied, these malformations involve the spine or calvaria or both and are often associated with developmental abnormalities of overlying bony structures and soft tissues. Those involving the spinal cord tend to be situated in the posterior midline. Less frequently occurring neural tube closure defects include cranial dysraphisms such as anencephaly and encephaloceles.

Spinal dysraphisms include a spectrum of defects of the vertebral column and spinal cord. The spectrum ranges from spina bifida occulta, an asymptomatic, innocuous defect of spinal lamina, to extensive rachischisis, a devastating process characterized by wide exposure, deformity, and dysplasia of neural tissue. Spinal dysraphisms primarily affect the lumbar region and decrease in incidence both rostrally and caudally. Two major forms represent a source of surgical material. Meningomyeloceles are a defect in or absence of the posterior vertebral arches accompanied by the formation of a connective tissue sac, often very delicate, which contains the dorsally displaced spinal cord and nerve roots (Fig. 8–1). In severe deformities, the neural structures are unprotected by overlying muscle, subcutaneous tissue, or even skin, a precarious situation rendering these vital tissues susceptible to direct trauma and infection. In these cases, immediate surgery is indicated to mobilize adjacent tissues to protect the neural elements. Meningomyeloceles are often associated with malformation of the hindbrain and cerebellum (Chiari malformation), with obstruction of the cerebrospinal fluid (CSF) pathways, especially of the aqueduct of Sylvius, leading to hydrocephalus. A milder degree of dysraphism, without involvement of neural structures, is the meningocele. Here, the malformative dural sac extends through a defect in the spinal canal, but there is no extension of the spinal cord or other neural elements into the cyst. Meningoceles represent only the minority (10 to 20%) of spinal dysraphic lesions[2] and are often asymptomatic.

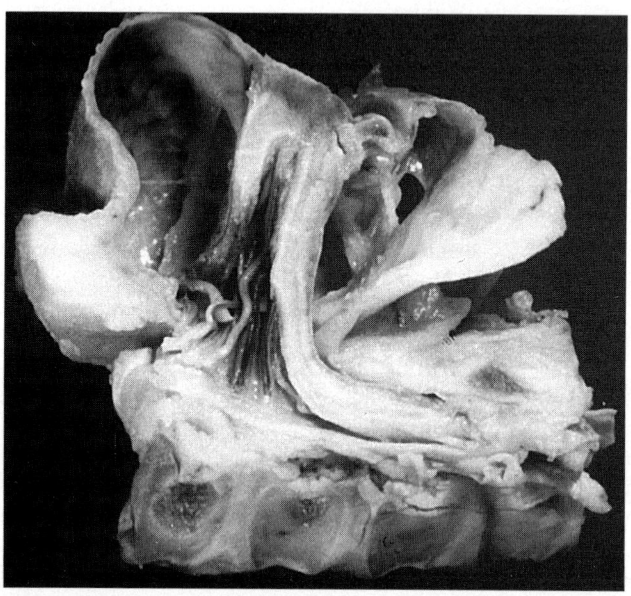

Figure 8–1. Meningomyelocele. Note upward displacement of the spinal cord and nerve roots as well as their attachment to the meningocele sac. Spinal column lies below. Provided by Dr. H. N. Harrison, Redding, California.

Encephaloceles

The encephalocele is the cranial counterpart of meningomyelocele, consisting of herniated but otherwise well-formed cerebral tissue associated with a defect of overlying cranial bone. Such lesions are far less common than spinal dysraphisms.[2] Most occur in the occipital region and are found typically in the midline.[3] In the frontal area, encephaloceles involve the frontoethmoidal junction, with cerebral tissue protruding into the nose, the ethmoid sinus, or the orbit, a situation predisposing to CSF leakage and meningitis, either spontaneously or following a misguided surgical procedure. In all such cases careful neuroimaging assessment of brain and bony structures is first required to define the skull defect because the previously described serious sequelae may follow simple nasal excision.

An important mimicker of frontal encephalocele is the "nasal glioma," a neuroglial heterotopia involving the skin or nasal mucosa or both; some extend inferiorly to form an intranasal polyp. Microscopically these vary from disorganized, largely glial lesions intimately admixed with fibrous tissue to relatively well-organized tissues resembling cerebral cortex, in some cases accompanied by poorly formed leptomeninges.

Arachnoid Cysts

Arachnoid cysts comprise about 1% of all intracranial, space-occupying lesions.[4] They are benign and extraparenchymal in location and arise within the arachnoid membrane. Microscopically, they are lined by a delicate layer of collagen and arachnoidal cells and are filled with a fluid resembling CSF. Arachnoidal cysts occur in both children and adults, with male predominance at all ages.[2] Although they occur at all levels of the neuraxis, approximately half arise in the temporal region and involve the sylvian fissure. Favored sites in the posterior fossa include the cerebellopontine angle and the cerebellar vermis.[5] Spinal examples are uncommon.

Congenital or primary arachnoidal cysts are believed to be developmental in origin, the result of splitting of the arachnoid membrane with secondary accumulation of CSF.[2] The reason for their enlargement is unclear. Proposed mechanisms invoke osmotic pressure or the mechanical "valve effect" of intracystic CSF upon a defect in the wall. In some instances, a communication with the subarachnoid space is found.[6] Acquired or secondary arachnoidal cysts may develop after trauma or infection. As spectacular as intact cysts may be by virtue of their size and compressive effects (Fig. 8–2), they are often asymptomatic, incidental findings. In cases with symptoms due to mass effect, surgical correction is indicated. Interestingly, excision of a portion of the cyst wall and communication

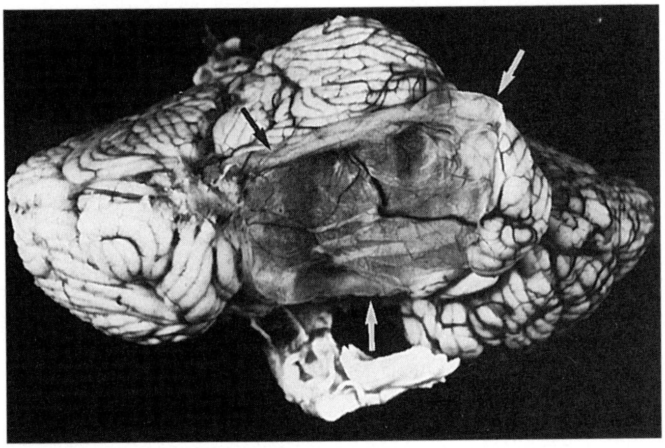

Figure 8–2. Arachnoid cyst of midline cerebellum *(arrows)*. Note the thin-walled nature of the cyst and its displacement of cerebellar parenchyma.

of the cyst with the CSF cisterns is not always effective. A shunting procedure of the cyst is also an option.

PRIMARY CENTRAL NERVOUS SYSTEM TUMORS

Intraoperative Diagnosis

Optimal surgical management of CNS tumors requires intraoperative pathology consultation to facilitate decision making. In most instances, this process includes microscopic confirmation of the presence of a neoplasm, determining whether it is primary or secondary, benign or malignant, and, if primary, of a morphologic type that may lend itself to complete excision. Improved sensitivity of neuroimaging, coupled with the increased use of stereotactic biopsy, has expanded the pathologist's role to include assessment of whether the biopsy findings are consistent with the imaging abnormality. The diminutive nature of many biopsy specimens, particularly those obtained by needle and fine forceps, emphasizes the importance of combining the cytologic smear method with conventional frozen section interpretation.

Both the pathologist and the neurosurgeon must understand that the process of intraoperative diagnosis is only the first step in specimen assessment and that it has limitations. A final diagnosis, one correlating cytologic and histologic features, tumor growth pattern relative to underlying parenchyma, and clinical data with imaging characteristics, awaits review of permanent sections.

An intraoperative diagnosis is jeopardized when a smear or frozen section is interpreted without consideration of clinical information and neuroimaging data. The development of a differential diagnosis depends upon factors such as patient age, clinical presentation, duration of symptoms, and gross operative findings. Patient age and tumor location, in particular, become major factors in elaborating a differential diagnosis for CNS tumors (Table 8–1). Clear communication and a collegial relationship between pathologist and neurosurgeon greatly facilitate the diagnostic effort and reduce the likelihood of ''beginner's errors.''

Although frozen sections provide a good working if not always precise diagnosis, several centers have recommended the cytologic smear technique for intraoperative evaluation of CNS biopsy findings.[7–11] The smear method also provides useful information regarding the cellular composition of either reactive or neoplastic processes. In our collective experience, smear interpretations concur with final diagnoses made on permanent sections in 90 to 95% of cases, a range comparable to that achieved by the frozen section approach.[9] The great advantage of the smear method resides in its suitability for the study of minute fragments of tissue, allowing retention of a good portion, if not the majority of the specimen for optimal processing. Indeed, considering the weight of a stereotactic biopsy specimen and the cost of the surgical procedure, the tissue obtained is arguably the most costly material on earth! Imprint preparations, although produced less often than smears, are better suited for the examination of specimens firm or fibrous in nature, e.g., metastatic carcinomas in dural tissue.[11] Scraping the surfaces of such tissue to make smears often ruptures the cells and introduces crush artifact in the tissue block.

Approach to the Specimen

As previously stated, intraoperative tissue review should be regarded as a preliminary step, one providing information useful in operative decision making. Care must be taken to conserve tissue needed for permanent sections and, in some cases, for special procedures. Indiscriminate freezing of entire specimens should be avoided. Cauterized tissue and samples from suction bottles are usually inadequate because such specimens show distortion and obscuration of cellular and architectural features.

In the case of brain tumors, in particular, material should be set aside for routine histology, special histochemical stains, and for immunostaining. Because of the tissue-sparing nature of smear or imprint preparations, even small specimens may suffice for special analyses such as ultrastructural study. The latter requires only a 1- to 2-mm fragment and, in difficult cases, may be pivotal for diagnosis. In cases suspicious for hematopoietic disorders, fresh tissue should be submitted for flow cytometric studies and for the assessment of tumor clonality (see Chapter 17). Chromosomal abnormalities in brain tumors, some of diagnostic importance, can be identified using viable, fresh tissue submitted for cytogenetic analysis. Immediate freezing of specimens (with liquid nitrogen or similar methods) preserves their potential for molecular diagnosis. In cases of a possible infectious nature, specimens should be obtained for microbial culture. To avoid contamination of such specimens in the frozen section laboratory, they should be submitted to the microbiology laboratory directly from the operating room.

Topographic Classification

Topographic and histologic features are relevant not only to the diagnosis of CNS neoplasms but also play a role in determining prognosis and treatment. As previously mentioned, location within the CNS is a major factor in narrowing down the differential diagnosis of tumors occurring

Table 8–1. Topographic Distribution of Tumors of the Central Nervous System by Patient Age

Location	Children/Adolescents	Adults
Supratentorium		
Cerebral hemispheres	Astrocytoma Anaplastic astrocytoma Pleomorphic xanthoastrocytoma Pilocytic astrocytoma Ependymoma Oligodendroglioma Ganglioglioma Desmoplastic infantile ganglioglioma, astrocytoma PNET	Astrocytoma Anaplastic astrocytoma Glioblastoma multiforme Metastatic carcinoma Oligodendroglioma Ependymoma PNET Meningioma
Corpus callosum	Astrocytoma Anaplastic astrocytoma Oligodendroglioma	Astrocytoma Anaplastic astrocytoma Glioblastoma multiforme
Lateral ventricle	Ependymoma Choroid plexus papilloma (> carcinoma) Central neurocytoma Subependymal giant-cell astrocytoma	Ependymoma Subependymoma Choroid plexus papilloma Central neurocytoma Meningioma
Third ventricle	Ependymoma Choroid plexus papilloma (> carcinoma)	Colloid cyst Ependymoma
Region of third ventricle	Pilocytic astrocytoma Oligodendroglioma Ependymoma	Astrocytoma, anaplastic astrocytoma, glioblastoma Oligodendroglioma Ependymoma
Optic nerve and chiasm	Pilocytic astrocytoma	Meningioma Pilocytic astrocytoma
Pineal region	Germ-cell tumors Pineoblastoma	Germ-cell tumors Pineocytoma Pineoblastoma
Pituitary-sellar region	Craniopharyngioma Germ-cell tumor	Pituitary adenoma Meningioma Germ-cell tumor Metastasis Chordoma/chondrosarcoma
Infratentorium		
Cerebellum	Medulloblastoma Pilocytic astrocytoma Dermoid cyst	Hemangioblastoma Metastatic carcinoma Astrocytoma (diffuse or pilocytic) Medulloblastoma
Fourth ventricle	Ependymoma Choroid plexus papilloma (> carcinoma)	Ependymoma Choroid plexus papilloma Subependymoma
Cerebellopontine angle	Ependymoma Choroid plexus papilloma	Schwannoma Meningioma Epidermoid cyst Choroid plexus papilloma Glomus jugulare tumor
Brainstem	Astrocytoma (diffuse or pilocytic) Anaplastic astrocytoma Glioblastoma multiforme	Astrocytoma Anaplastic astrocytoma Glioblastoma multiforme
Spinal region	Ependymoma Astrocytoma (pilocytic or diffuse) Meningioma	Ependymoma Astrocytoma (pilocytic or diffuse) Hemangioblastoma Meningioma Schwannoma Neurofibroma Paraganglioma

Modified from Scheithauer BW, Central nervous system and pituitary. *In* Silva EG, Kramer BB, eds. *Intraoperative Pathologic Diagnosis*, Baltimore: Williams & Wilkins; 1987.

in both adult and pediatric populations. Approximately 70% of the tumors appearing in childhood arise in the infratentorial compartment whereas the great majority of tumors in adults are supratentorial. A topographic distribution of tumors in relation to patient age is provided in Table 8–1.

Histologic Classification of Brain Tumors

Tumors of the CNS account for a small but significant portion of all human tumors. Their spectrum, as evidenced by the new World Health Organization (WHO) Classification (Table 8–2), is very broad.[12, 64] In children, the CNS is the second most common site of primary tumors. The distribution and categories of neoplasms that arise in the CNS of children and adults reflect their distinctive histogenesis. The presumed lack of a normal reserve or progenitor cell population in the adult brain stands in contrast to the presence of several such cell populations in the immature nervous system. These cells are thought to be vulnerable to neoplastic transformation,[13] which is reflected in differences in the location, incidence, and types of malignant tumors encountered in adults and children. In children, cerebellar medulloblastoma is the most common malignant tumor whereas in adults it is glioblastoma multiforme (astrocytoma grade IV). Radiologic and operative data as well as such factors as patient age and tumor site serve to quickly narrow down the differential. Diagnoses should not be rendered without clinical data.

In the following discussion, salient clinical features of the most common CNS tumors will be reviewed. Table 8–2 provides a concise summary of common lesions. For a more detailed description of CNS tumors, the reader is referred to major neuropathology texts.[12, 14–16]

Neuroepithelial Tumors with Glial Differentiation

Regardless of patient age, gliomas are the most common CNS tumors. Collectively, they represent nearly 50% of tumors in both the adult and pediatric population. Gliomas are classified according to predominant cell type, a feature presumably reflecting their histogenesis. Gliomas are classified as astrocytomas of varying type, oligodendrogliomas, ependymomas, and mixed gliomas, most of which are oligoastrocytomas (Table 8–2).

Astrocytic Tumors

Astrocytomas are proliferations of neoplastic astrocytes. Such tumors vary greatly, both in morphology and biologic behavior. Astrocytomas are divided into two major groups according to their tendency to infiltrate surrounding brain parenchyma: diffusely infiltrating astrocytomas versus circumscribed astrocytomas. The latter category includes several variants, all of which are more favorable than diffusely infiltrative astrocytomas with their tendency to become increasingly malignant with time.

Diffusely Infiltrating Astrocytomas with Unfavorable Prognosis. This grouping of glioma comprises nearly 75% of all astrocytic neoplasms[14] and forms a spectrum of lesions that vary in differentiation and degree of malig-

Table 8–2. Tumors of Neuroepithelial Tissue WHO Classification (1993)

Astrocytic Tumors
Astrocytoma: variants: fibrillary, protoplasmic, gemistocytic
Anaplastic (malignant) astrocytoma
Glioblastomas: variants: giant-cell glioblastoma, gliosarcoma
Pilocytic astrocytoma
Pleomorphic xanthoastrocytoma
Subependymal giant-cell astrocytoma (usually in association with tuberous sclerosis)

Oligodendroglial Tumors
Oligodendroglioma
Anaplastic (malignant) oligodendroglioma

Ependymal Tumors
Ependymoma: variants: cellular, papillary, clear-cell
Anaplastic (malignant) ependymoma
Myxopapillary ependymoma
Subependymoma

Mixed Gliomas
Oligoastrocytoma
Anaplastic (malignant) oligoastrocytoma
Others

Choroid Plexus Tumors
Choroid plexus papilloma
Choroid plexus carcinoma

Neuroepithelial Tumors of Uncertain Origin
Astroblastoma
Polar spongioblastoma
Gliomatosis cerebri

Neuronal and Mixed Neuronal-Glial Tumors
Gangliocytoma
Dysplastic gangliocytoma of cerebellum (Lhermitte-Duclos)
Desmoplastic infantile ganglioglioma
Dysembryoplastic neuroepithelial tumor
Ganglioglioma
Anaplastic (malignant) ganglioglioma
Central neurocytoma
Paraganglioma of the filum terminale
Olfactory neuroblastoma (esthesioneuroblastoma): variant: olfactory neuroepithelioma

Pineal Parenchymal Tumors
Pineocytoma
Pineoblastoma
Mixed pineoblastoma/pineocytoma

Embryonal Tumors
Medulloepithelioma
Neuroblastoma: variant: ganglioneuroblastoma
Ependymoblastoma
Retinoblastoma
Primitive neuroectodermal tumors (PNETs)
- Medulloblastoma: variants: desmoplastic medulloblastoma, medullomyoblastoma, melanotic medulloblastoma
- Cerebral or spinal PNETs

From Kleihues P, Burger PC, Scheithauer BW. *Histological Typing of Tumours of the Central Nervous System,* 2nd ed. New York: Springer-Verlag; 1993.

nancy. Even the relatively low-grade forms are prognostically unfavorable, the 10-year survival being 20%. According to the 1993 WHO classification,[12, 64] these lesions include the *astrocytoma* (grade II astrocytoma), *anaplastic astrocytoma* (grade III astrocytoma), and *glioblastoma multiforme* (grade IV astrocytoma). A comparative summary of the criteria used for grading astrocytic tumors is presented in Table 8–3. Diffusely infiltrating astrocytomas are characterized by remarkable intratumoral heterogeneity, both morphologic and genetic.[17, 18] This is particularly the case as they undergo progressive anaplastic transformation. The frequency of this shift to higher grade is the basis for a poor prognosis with this grouping of astrocytic neoplasms.

The astrocytomas are relatively well-differentiated, diffusely infiltrative neoplasms that most often occur in young to middle-age adults. Although such tumors may arise anywhere along the neuraxis, their site of predilection is related to patient age; in adults, they more commonly affect the cerebral hemispheres, whereas in children most arise in the brainstem. Radiographically, grossly, and microscopically, such low-grade astrocytomas have ill-defined margins and show diffuse infiltration of brain parenchyma (Fig. 8–3*A*). Their microscopic appearance varies, most tumors being either fibrillary or gemistocytic in type (Fig. 8–3*B* and *C*). Cytologic smears permit a ready diagnosis (Fig. 8–3*D*). Surgical treatment consists of incomplete resection; as a result, astrocytomas show a high rate of recurrence. Anaplastic transformation occurs in up to 50% of recurrent cases,[19] but is seen less often in pediatric patients.[20] The long-term mortality rate is high.

Anaplastic astrocytoma, the intermediate member of the spectrum of diffusely infiltrative astrocytic neoplasms, exhibits more malignant features than does the well-differentiated astrocytoma. Nonetheless, its microscopic appearance falls far short of that of glioblastoma multiforme. As in the case of astrocytoma, anaplastic astrocytomas arise most frequently in the cerebral hemispheres, but on average in patients 10 years older. The majority of anaplastic astrocytomas arise by anaplastic transformation from astrocytoma;[14] however, some anaplastic tumors apparently do arise de novo. Microscopically, anaplastic astrocytomas exhibit greater cellularity than do astrocytomas and show more in the way of nuclear pleomorphism, hyperchromasia, and mitotic activity. In the present WHO grading scheme, mitotic activity distinguishes these tumors.[12] High cellularity and an attendant increase in vascularity correlate particularly well with MRI findings of signal heterogeneity or focal contrast enhancement.

Glioblastoma multiforme is the most malignant form of diffuse astrocytic tumor and shows frankly anaplastic morphology. It represents 15 to 20% of all intracranial tumors, about 50% of gliomas in adults. Glioblastomas arise later in life than do astrocytomas or anaplastic astrocytomas, with peak incidence in thc 5th and 6th decades.[15] A significant proportion represents anaplastic progression of preexisting astrocytoma or anaplastic astrocytoma,[14, 19, 21] but glioblastomas can arise de novo. As in lower-grade variants of diffuse astrocytic tumors, glioblastomas arise primarily in the cerebral hemispheres of adults, whereas in the pediatric age group the brainstem is most often affected.[22] In contrast-enhanced CT or MRI scans, these tumors often appear as "ring lesions" with central areas of necrosis surrounded by enhanced zones of viable tumor (Fig. 8–4*A*). The differential diagnosis of this imaging abnormality includes metastatic carcinoma, abscess, and lymphoma. Whereas many glioblastomas are grossly invasive tumors with ill-defined margins, others appear more circumscribed, their necrotic center being surrounded by viable, highly cellular, and vascular tumor.

Microscopically, glioblastoma shows a remarkable morphologic spectrum, hence the designation "multiforme." Most distinct are the cytologic appearances. Whereas many tumors consist of obvious spindle-shaped fibrillary astrocytes, others show gemistocytic, small-cell, giant-cell, or epithelioid features. However, diagnosis of glioblastoma is not based so much on the appearance of the cellularity but on other features. Common features include those previously described under anaplastic astrocytoma, e.g., hypercellularity, nuclear pleomorphism, and mitotic activity, with the addition of endothelial proliferation and/or necrosis

Table 8–3. Grading Systems for Diffusely Infiltrating Astrocytomas (Comparison of the WHO, St. Anne/Mayo, and the Rubinstein Systems)*

Classification	Grade 2 or Astrocytoma	Grade 3 or Anaplastic Astrocytoma	Grade 4 or Glioblastoma Multiforme
WHO[64]	Nuclear atypia No mitoses No endothelial proliferation No necrosis	Nuclear atypia Mitoses No endothelial proliferation No necrosis	Nuclear atypia Mitoses Endothelial proliferation and/or necrosis
St. Anne/Mayo[65] (This method is based upon the presence or absence of 4 criteria, including nuclear atypia, mitoses, endothelial proliferation, and necrosis)	1 criterion	2 criteria	3 or 4 criteria
Rubinstein[14]	Low cellularity Nuclear atypia Scant mitoses No endothelial proliferation No necrosis	Increased cellularity Nuclear atypia Mitoses Endothelial proliferation No necrosis	Hypercellularity Nuclear atypia Mitoses Endothelial proliferation and necrosis

*Three-tier grading schemes based upon subjective criteria also include those of Ringertz[66] and of Burger et al.[15]
The Kernohan scheme is a four-tier method, which, unlike all of the above, includes pilocytic tumors among those graded.

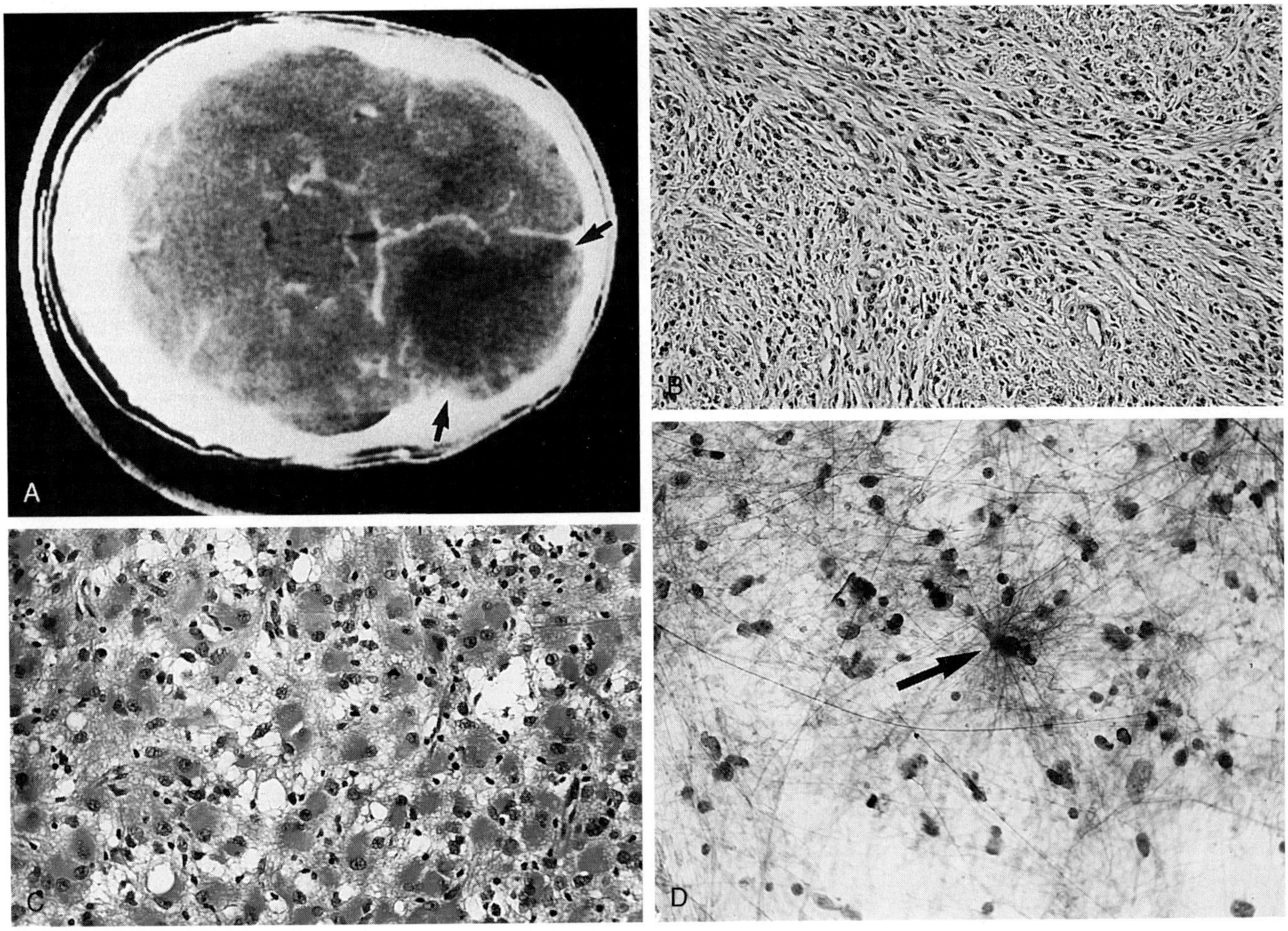

Figure 8–3. Diffusely infiltrative low-grade glioma (fibrillary astrocytoma). *A,* Contrast-enhanced CT scan. Such infiltrative gliomas *(arrows)* exhibit relatively low to moderate cellularity and are unassociated with a significant increase in vascularity; they lack contrast enhancement. *B,* Microscopic features of grade 2 fibrillary astrocytoma: note spindling cellular pattern. *C,* Microscopic features of grade 2 gemistocytic astrocytoma: note large, round, granular cells. *D,* This smear preparation from grade 2 astrocytoma of fibrillary type demonstrates scattered neoplastic cells with nuclear pleomorphism and variable hyperchromasia. Note their apparent lack of cytoplasm, a feature typical of isolated infiltrating cells. At the center is a stellate reactive astrocyte *(arrow)* with its symmetrically radiating processes. Sharply delineated, long processes crossing the field represent residual axons within the parenchyma. Hemalum-phloxine stain.

(Fig. 8–4*B*). Glioblastomas spread within the nervous system, a factor contributing to its poor prognosis. Common routes of spread include the white matter tracts (particularly the corpus callosum with resultant bilateral involvement of the cerebral hemispheres), the ventricular system, and craniospinal leptomeninges. Glioblastomas are the most aggressive of all the gliomas. Median survival is less than 12 months. Younger patients often experience somewhat longer survivals.[23] Surgical management consists of first providing sufficient tissue for definitive diagnosis and then resecting as much tumor as possible without causing unacceptable neurologic morbidity.

Relatively Circumscribed Astrocytomas with Favorable Prognosis. This second grouping of astrocytomas includes tumors that, in terms of their radiographic and gross appearances, are relatively circumscribed neoplasms when compared with the diffuse astrocytomas previously discussed. This category includes pilocytic astrocytoma, pleomorphic xanthoastrocytoma, and subependymal giant cell astrocytoma. Collectively, these tumors all exhibit distinctive clinicopathologic features, tend to be slow growing, and have a much more favorable prognosis. This is due not only to their relative circumscription but to the fact that they occur in younger patients and show less tendency to undergo anaplastic transformation. With surgical resection the majority of patients do well.

Pilocytic astrocytomas typically occur in children and young adults and are commonly situated in the cerebellum[24] and in the midline structures of the supratentorial region, including the third ventricle, hypothalamus, and optic tracts. Relatively few arise in the cerebral hemispheres (Fig. 8–5*A*).[25] Fully two thirds of spinal cord astrocytomas are of pilocytic type.[26] Typical examples are cystic with a solid component that takes the form of a mural nodule. Histologically, pilocytic astrocytomas are characterized by a biphasic architectural pattern. One element consists of elongated, bipolar cells arranged in compact fascicles and associated with Rosenthal fiber formation. The other element is loosely textured, microcystic tissue formed from stellate, less-elongated cells accompanied by granular or

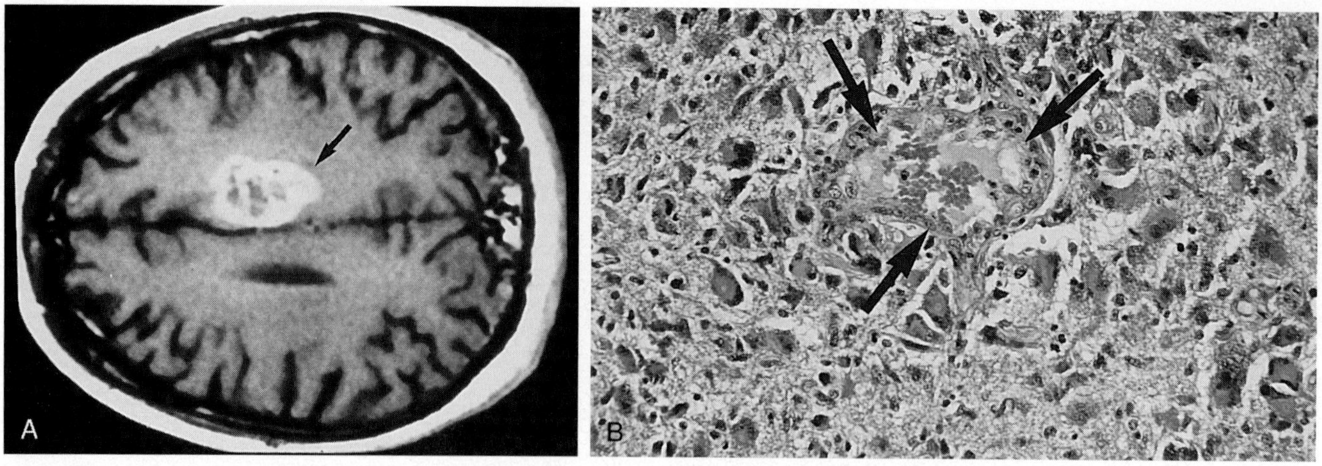

Figure 8–4. Diffusely infiltrative high-grade astrocytoma. *A,* This grade 4 lesion (glioblastoma multiforme) shows ring enhancement corresponding to a highly cellular and vascular element, central hypodensity which equates with necrosis, and a surrounding hypodense zone of parenchymal infiltration by isolated tumor cells, as well as of edema *(arrow)*. *B,* Microscopic appearance of grade 4 astrocytoma (glioblastoma multiforme). Key features distinguishing this common tumor from the closely related grade 3 (anaplastic) astrocytoma are endothelial proliferation *(arrows)* and necrosis.

hyalin bodies (Fig. 8–5*B*). Anaplastic transformation of pilocytic astrocytoma is a rare event occurring in less than 1% of cases.[27]

Pleomorphic xanthoastrocytomas (PXAs) are superficially situated tumors affecting the cerebral hemispheres, particularly the temporal lobe. Most are diagnosed in children and young adults with a long history of seizures.[28] On imaging they appear as superficially situated, often cystic, contrast-enhancing masses. The tumors frequently show involvement of the leptomeninges and associated cyst formation. The histologic hallmark of pleomorphic xanthoastrocytoma is its cellular pleomorphism, featuring spindle to polygonal to giant astrocytes, some of which are lipid vacuolated and exhibit bizarre, often multiple hyperchromatic nuclei (Fig. 8–6). Cytoplasmic nuclear pseudoinclusions are commonly seen as are eosinophilic granular bodies. A characteristic feature of PXA is the presence of a dense intercellular reticulin network delineating either individual cells or clusters or fascicles of cells (Fig. 8–6). This delicate, distinctive stroma is not uniformly distributed but is most conspicuous in areas of leptomeningeal involvement and about the often prominent vasculature. Microfoci of chronic inflammation are also common. In general, PXAs are associated with a relatively favorable prognosis. Many patients survive long term after resection alone. Anaplastic transformation occurs in approximately 10% of cases. There are currently no histopathologic criteria for recognition of risk for such malignant change. In the WHO

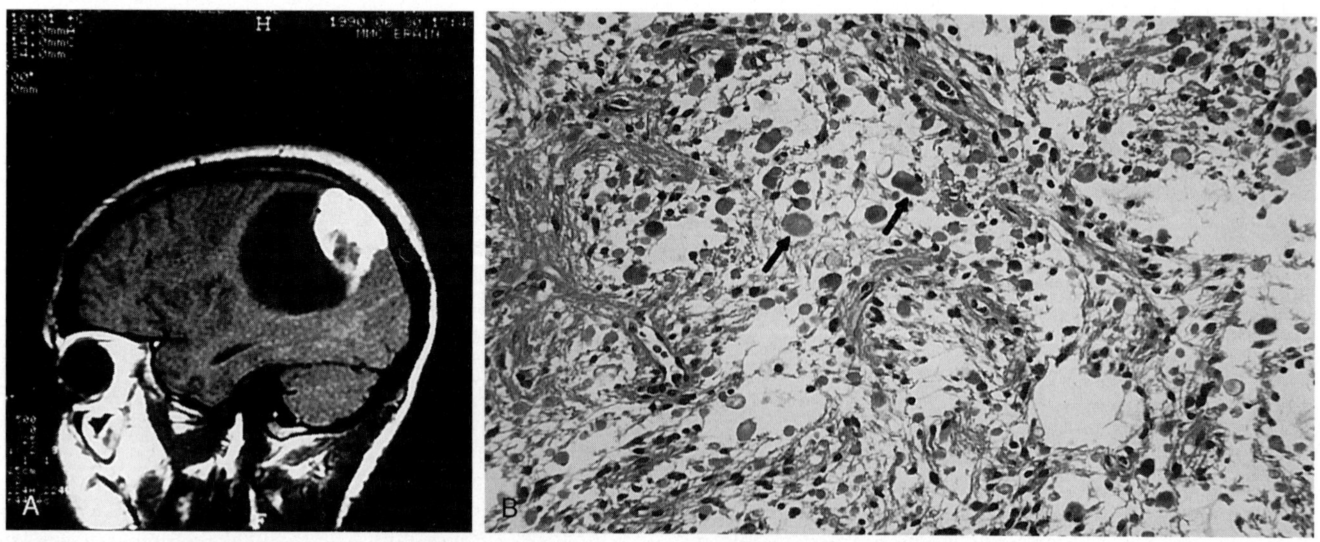

Figure 8–5. Circumscribed, favorable astrocytoma, pilocytic type. *A,* MRI with contrast. This classic supratentorial example consists of a mural nodule of solid tumor within a cyst. Contrast enhancement is typical of pilocytic astrocytomas and, in contrast to diffuse astrocytic tumors, is not indicative of high-grade malignancy. *B,* Microscopic features of pilocytic astrocytoma. This, the most common of astrocytomas with favorable prognosis, shows considerable histologic variation, ranging from bipolar spindle cells *(left)* to less fibrillary cells engaged in microcyst formation. The latter pattern predominates in this example and is associated with granular body formation *(arrows)*.

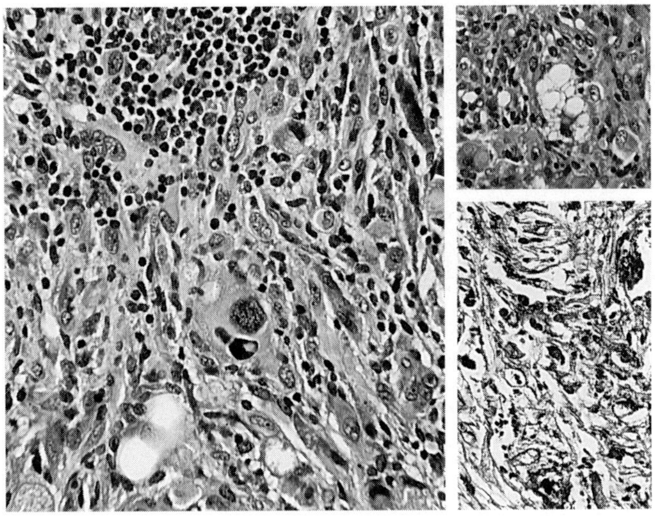

Figure 8–6. Microscopic features of pleomorphic xanthoastrocytoma include cellular pleomorphism, varying numbers of giant cells, some of which may be lipidized *(inset, upper right),* paucity or absence of mitoses, foci of chronic inflammation *(upper left),* and an intercellular pattern of reticulin deposition *(inset, lower right)* The latter is most apparent in the leptomeningeal component. Despite these appearances this tumor is relatively favorable.

classification, PXAs are considered grade II tumors, only a minority of which become grade III.[12]

Subependymal giant cell astrocytomas typically arise in the 1st or 2nd decade of life, usually in patients with tuberous sclerosis.[14, 29] Imaging shows them to be contrast enhancing and often calcified (Fig. 8–7*A*). Grossly, subependymal giant cell astrocytomas are remarkably circumscribed, nodular tumors arising anteriorly in the wall of the lateral ventricles at the level of the basal ganglia. Obstructive hydrocephalus is common. The tumors are morphologically diverse and consist in varying proportions of spindle, polygonal, and characteristic ganglionlike cells in a fibrillar matrix (Fig. 8–7*B*). Calcifications are commonly seen. Despite the occasional finding of atypia, mitoses, and even necrosis, subependymal giant cell astrocytomas are associated with a uniformly favorable prognosis.[29] Surgical resection is indicated only when the tumor becomes symptomatic, usually with obstruction of CSF flow. In such cases, partial resection may be sufficient. Radical resection at the expense of neurologic impairment is rarely justified.

Oligodendrogliomas

Estimates put the frequency of oligodendrogliomas at approximately 5 to 15% of intracranial gliomas.[30] Although the majority occurs in adults, with a peak incidence in the 4th and 5th decades, oligodendrogliomas comprise about 5% of gliomas in childhood and adolescence.[30, 31] Clinically, most oligodendrogliomas progress very slowly and are often associated with a long history of seizures.[31] They occur at any level of the neuraxis, most frequently the cerebral hemispheres, particularly the frontotemporal region.[32] Contiguous lobes are commonly involved.[31] Tumors with bilateral components represent approximately 20% of cases.[30] With neuroimaging studies or gross pathologic examination, oligodendrogliomas can be seen to involve not only white matter but also the overlying cortex with obliteration of the gray-white junction (Fig. 8–8*A*); calcifications are evident in up to 70% of cases.[33] Cystic changes are uncommon but may be seen in large tumors. Oligodendrogliomas are relatively vascular tumors, and spontaneous hemorrhage may occasionally be seen.

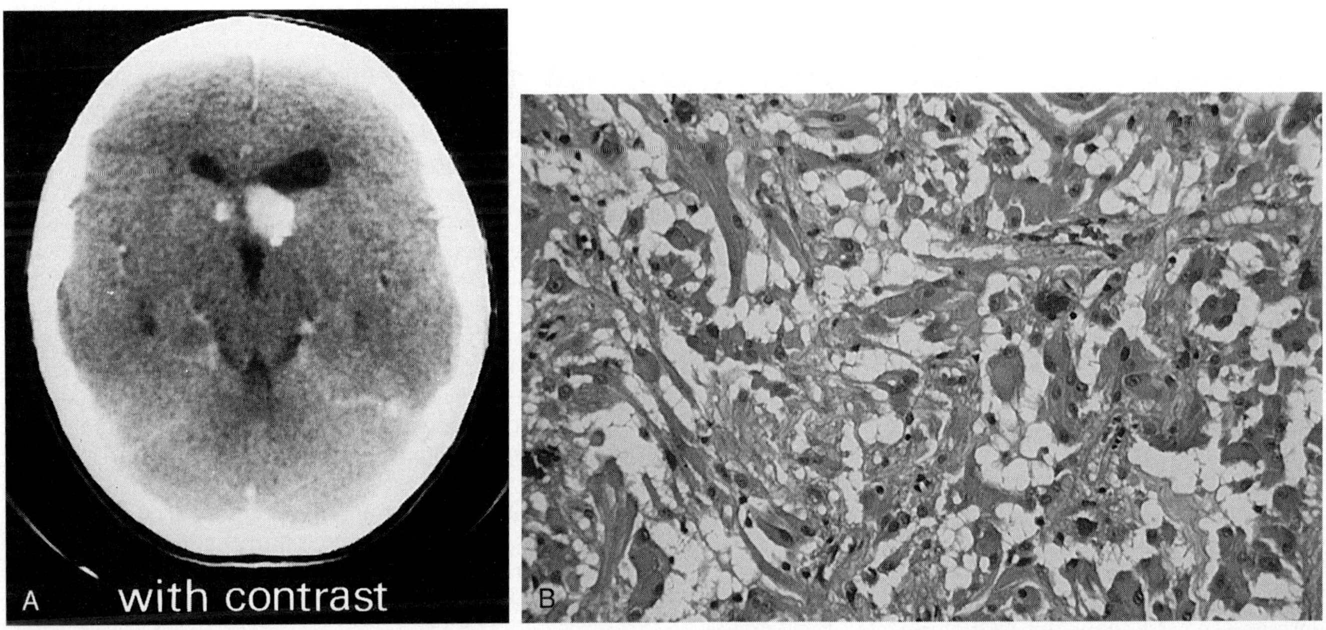

Figure 8–7. Subependymal giant cell astrocytoma. *A,* Head CT with contrast. Such tumors are typically tuberous sclerosis associated, appear as contrast-enhancing masses overlying the head of the caudate nucleus, and obstruct the foramen of Monro. *B,* Microscopic study reveals spindle and epithelioid cells with a perivascular orientation. Such tumors are biologically benign, even when showing mitotic figures or foci of necrosis.

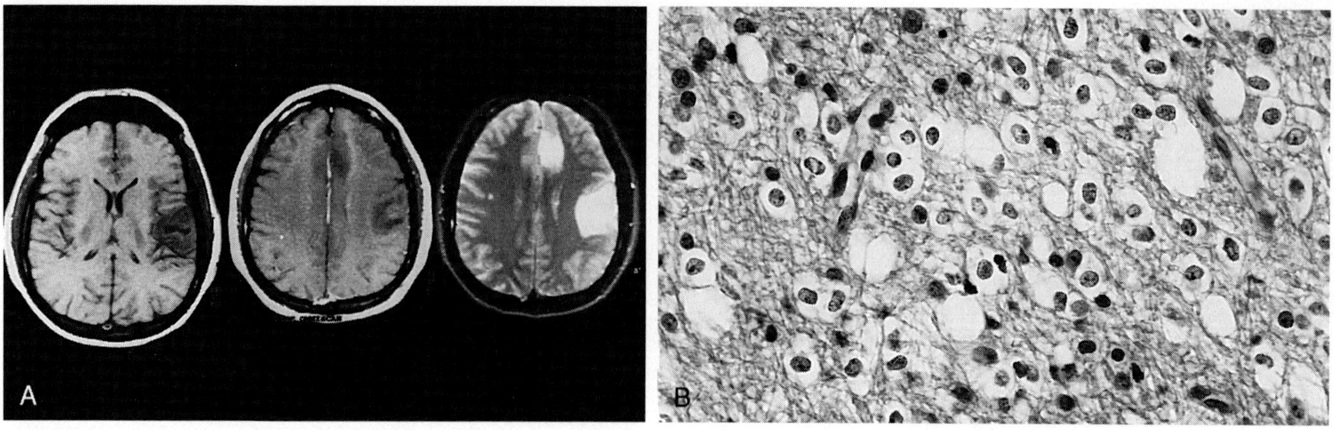

Figure 8–8. Oligodendroglioma. *A,* This MRI sequence (T1, T1 with contrast, and T2 studies) shows the tumor to be relatively demarcated and to involve both the white matter and overlying cerebral cortex. Secondary cortical involvement is typical of oligodendrogliomas. *B,* Microscopy reveals residual axons readily visible as processes enmeshing tumor cells with their typical conspicuous perinuclear clearing. The latter is a diagnostically helpful artifact, one resulting from delayed fixation. Perinuclear clearing is not evident in frozen sections or in promptly fixed specimens.

As with other gliomas, oligodendrogliomas exhibit a spectrum of histologic differentiation, one without prognostic implication. Common to all are cellular uniformity, round nuclei, scant processes, ''geometric'' acutely branching capillaries, and scattered microcalcifications. A helpful diagnostic feature, present only in permanent sections, is clear perinuclear halo formation (Fig. 8–8*B*). Other tumors feature a rim of cytoplasm and small fibrillary processes (gliofibrillary oligodendrocytes) or an eccentric plump cell body (minigemistocytes). Such cellular variations are of no prognostic significance.[34] Although the great majority of oligodendrogliomas are well differentiated and slow growing, a minority behaves more aggressively.[35] The latter represents anaplastic oligodendrogliomas; their incidence corresponds to 3.5% of new malignant gliomas in one series.[35] Pleomorphism and brisk mitotic activity are often seen in anaplastic variants, as are proliferative vascular changes such as thickening of vessel walls or conspicuous endothelial proliferation. Similar to diffuse astrocytic tumors, anaplastic oligodendrogliomas can represent either anaplastic transformation of preexisting low-grade tumors or can arise de novo. Microscopically and in neuroimaging studies, anaplastic oligodendrogliomas frequently demonstrate areas of necrosis.[33] Such tumors, when showing other features of anaplasia, are still oligodendrogliomas, albeit of high grade. They must not be confused with glioblastoma, in that the latter are by definition grade IV astrocytomas. Particularly in well-defined, low-grade oligodendrogliomas located in polar regions of the cerebral hemispheres, the goal of surgical treatment is gross total excision, provided this can be accomplished without producing major neurologic deficit.

Ependymomas

Ependymomas represent approximately 5% of intracranial gliomas.[14] Children and adolescents are affected more often than are adults. Pediatric ependymomas usually arise in the fourth ventricle whereas those of adults are located primarily in the spinal cord. Ependymomas are reported to represent as many as 60% of spinal cord gliomas.[36] Multiple spinal cord ependymomas typically arise in the setting of neurofibromatosis 2 (NF-2). Circumscription and contrast enhancement is common to all (Fig. 8–9*A*). Unlike other gliomas and regardless of location, ependymomas are grossly and microscopically well-demarcated tumors with ''pushing borders'' (Fig. 8–9*B*). Tumors with intraventricular components may spread through the ventricular system via foramina, such as the foramen of Luschka in the lateral recess of the fourth ventricle. This notwithstanding, only a small minority seed the subarachnoid space.

A characteristic histologic feature of ependymomas is radial orientation of the processes of tumor cells around blood vessels, resulting in pseudorosette formation (Fig. 8–9*C*). True ependymal rosettes and epithelial-lined tubules, although pathognomonic of ependymal neoplasia, are less commonly seen (Fig. 8–9*D*). Ependymomas are among the most cellular of gliomas. Most are composed of compact sheets of uniform cells and, at least focally, a variably fibrillar matrix. The cells possess round-to-oval nuclei and small-to-moderate quantities of cytoplasm and are arranged in an epithelial-like manner or lie within a process-rich, clearly glial background. The WHO classification recognizes three histologic forms of ependymoma: cellular, papillary, and clear-cell. These tumor variants have essentially the same clinical behavior, but their recognition as ependymomas is important to avoid confusion with anaplastic gliomas, choroid plexus tumors, and oligodendrogliomas, respectively. Occasional mitotic figures, atypical nuclei, and foci of necrosis may be present in ependymomas without indicating anaplastic change. Intraoperatively, a plane of demarcation between tumor and brain or spinal cord can usually be established. Gross total excision is the goal. In the fourth ventricle, attachment to or infiltration of the ventricular floor precludes total resection.

Anaplastic Ependymoma

Anaplastic transformation of ependymomas can occur at any site but is relatively infrequent in the spinal cord.[14] A

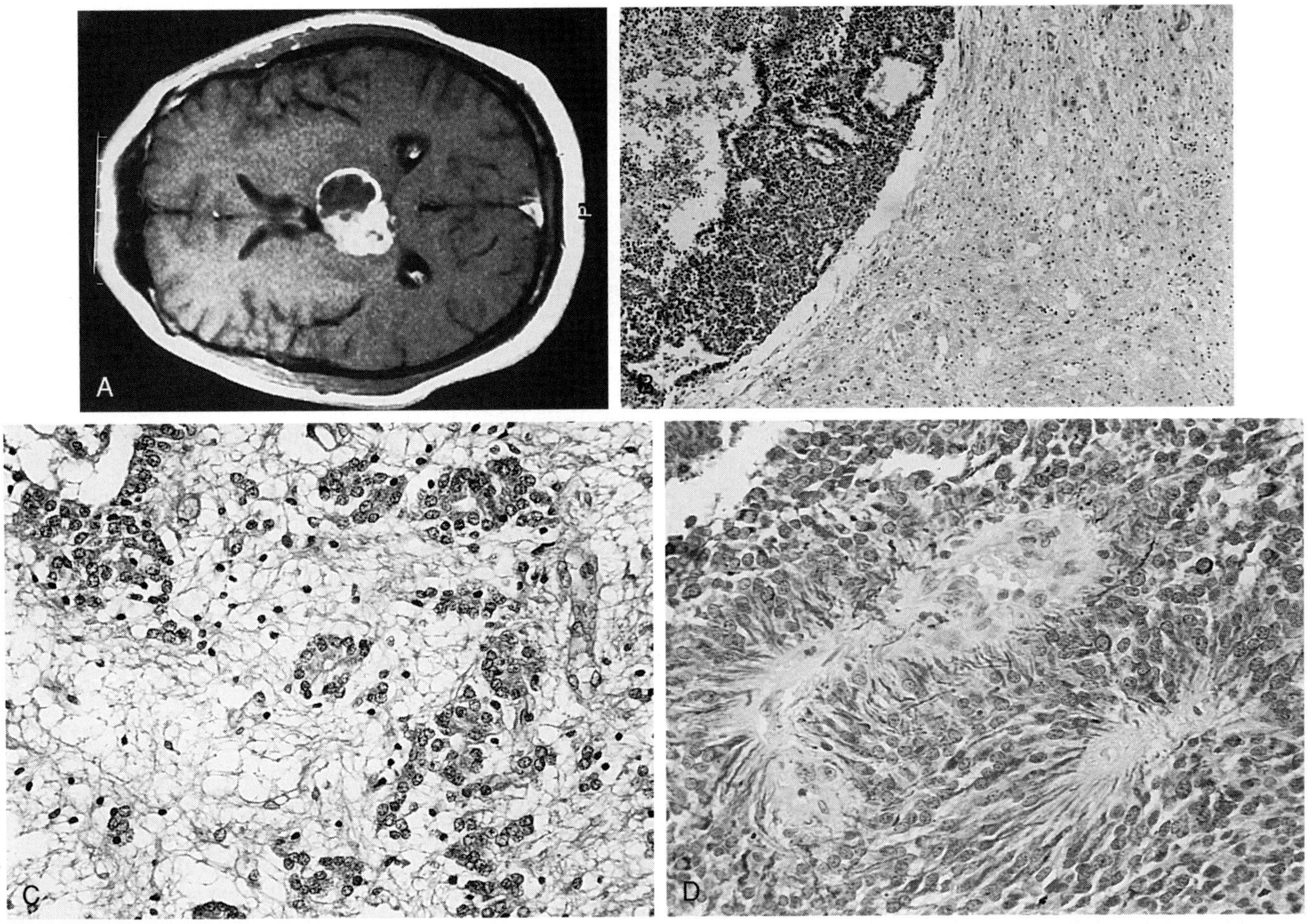

Figure 8–9. Ependymoma. *A,* Head CT shows relatively demarcated, noninfiltrative form of glioma typically situated adjacent to the ependyma and contrast enhancing. As in the case of pilocytic astrocytoma, contrast enhancement is a typical feature and is not indicative of high-grade malignancy. Cyst formation is common. *B,* This low-power view of a hematoxylin and eosin (H&E) stained section illustrates the high cellularity and sharp demarcation that such tumors show relative to surrounding brain parenchyma. A characteristic histologic feature is the formation of perivascular pseudorosettes *(C)* and true rosettes with lumens *(D)*. The latter are uncommonly seen. *C,* GFAP immunostain; *D,* H&E stain.

clinically reliable grading scheme for ependymomas has not yet been devised. Histologic criteria alone have limited significance;[37, 38] however, histologic grade in conjunction with such factors as patient age and DNA ploidy analysis permits distinction of low- from high-grade tumors.[39] Anaplastic ependymomas have increased cellularity, brisk mitotic rate, and endothelial proliferation. Unlike the diffuse gliomas such as astrocytoma and oligodendroglioma, neither nuclear atypia nor necrosis reliably serves to distinguish ordinary from anaplastic ependymoma. Despite the dense cellularity that characterizes anaplastic tumors, recognizable features of ependymoma, particularly pseudorosette formation, generally persist.

Myxopapillary Ependymomas

The myxopapillary ependymoma is a morphologically distinct variant of ependymoma that, with few exceptions, is restricted to the cauda equina.[40] Most occur in adults during the 3rd or 4th decades. Presenting symptoms include pain, asymmetric sensorimotor deficits, and sphincter dysfunction (''cauda equina syndrome''). Grossly, the tumors appear either as delicately encapsulated discrete, sausage-shaped masses arising from the filum terminale or as disrupted tumors associated with local tumor seeding. Secondary spinal nerve root involvement is common. Extradural lesions arising in either the post- or presacral regions are far less common and presumably arise from ependymal rests. Myxopapillary ependymomas show varying proportions of elongated, fibrillary, glial-appearing cells together with epithelial-like cells arranged around perivascular accumulations of mucin. These tumors should be removed intact; their rupture or piecemeal extraction forfeits the chance of a surgical cure. Recurrence and extensive CSF seeding are more likely for tumors locally disseminated or subtotally resected. Long-term survival is nonetheless the rule. Postoperative radiotherapy is indicated for lesions that cannot be totally removed intact. The differential diagnosis of this tumor includes paraganglioma and schwannoma.

Subependymoma

Asymptomatic subependymomas are well-circumscribed tumors that arise in the walls of the fourth ventricle.[41] In contrast, symptomatic tumors, which are very uncommon, may involve any level of the ventricular system, including the septum pellucidum, foramen of Monro, and on rare occasions the center of the spinal cord. Symptoms are generally related to hydrocephalus, the result of obstruction of CSF flow, or to intratumoral hemorrhage. Subependymomas consist of cells exhibiting ependymal and astrocytic differentiation. Tumor cells are typically arranged in clusters surrounded by skeins of long, fibrillary tumor cell processes. Although the histogenesis of subependymomas remains unclear, the same distinct cellular pattern is seen in some ependymomas, suggesting a close relationship between these two tumors. Clinical behavior is even more favorable than that of pure ependymomas; even subtotal removal results in long-term improvement. Tumor location and successful resection appear to be the most important prognostic factors.[42]

Embryonal Tumors (Medulloblastoma)

As the most common malignant CNS tumors of childhood, medulloblastomas comprise approximately one quarter of all intracranial tumors in the pediatric age group.[43] Their peak incidence is at the end of the 1st decade. Medulloblastoma is the prototype of primitive neuroepithelial neoplasms.[14] The new WHO classification (Table 8–2) applies the generic designation of ''primitive neuroectodermal tumor'' (PNET) to small-cell embryonal tumors that appear to be composed of primitive neuroepithelial progenitor cells expressing divergent glioneuronal differentiation. Morphologically, they appear similar throughout the CNS. Currently, the designation PNET is limited to medulloblastoma and similar neoplasms arising at other sites within the CNS. Medulloblastomas are by far the most common form of PNET and of embryonal tumors in general.[44]

Most medulloblastomas arise in the roof of the fourth ventricle and commonly fill the fourth ventricle, producing symptoms of increased intracranial pressure. Less often, particularly in adults, they are situated laterally in the cerebellar hemisphere (Fig. 8–10*A* and *B*). In diagnostic imaging studies they appear as solid contrast-enhancing tumors. The desmoplastic variant, a tumor found more commonly in adults, frequently involves the cerebellar hemispheres. Grossly, ordinary medulloblastomas are soft and clearly demarcated from surrounding brain. Necrosis may be multifocal or confluent, but massive necrosis is uncommon. Seeding by CSF may be apparent either early or late in the disease course (Fig. 8–10*C*). Medulloblastomas are markedly cellular neoplasms typically composed of small cells with scant cytoplasm, variably hyperchromatic nuclei, and ill-defined cell borders (Fig. 8–10*D*). Although poorly differentiated by routine light microscopy, a significant proportion of medulloblastomas show neuroblastic differentiation in the form of neuroblastic rosettes (Fig. 8–10*E*); immunostaining for neuronal markers, particularly synaptophysin, can be demonstrated in 95% of cases.[44, 45]

Several variants of medulloblastoma have been identified, the most frequent being the desmoplastic form (10 to 12%).[46] This behaves clinically similarly to the usual type but is distinctive in microscopic appearance with a biphasic architecture featuring pale nodules or follicles of differentiating tumor cells, lying within a reticulin-rich desmoplastic stroma composed of small primitive neuroepithelial cells. Other rare variants of medulloblastoma included in the WHO classification are (1) anaplastic or large-cell medulloblastoma,[47] a particularly aggressive lesion; (2) medullomyoblastoma, which shows striated muscle cell differentiation; and (3) melanotic medulloblastoma (Table 8–2). The relationship of these latter variants to the more conventional medulloblastoma is unclear.

Top surgical priorities are removal or debulking of tumor and clearing obstruction of CSF pathways, particularly at the fourth ventricle. Even when total removal is achieved adjuvant postoperative therapy is indicated—craniospinal irradiation or chemotherapy or both.

Meningothelial Tumors

Meningiomas are dural tumors derived from arachnoidal cells.[14, 48] They account for about 15% of intracranial tumors[14] and about 25% of intraspinal tumors.[36] Most meningiomas become clinically apparent in midlife but occasional cases are seen in childhood. In adults there is a marked female predominance (3:1); in childhood and in the elderly no sex predilection is apparent.[14] Meningiomas are multiple in nearly 8% of cases and large numbers of lesions are associated with NF-2.[14, 49]

Meningiomas may arise at any level of the neuraxis, but there are sites of predilection. In neuroimaging studies strong contrast enhancement is the rule; in addition, the periphery of the lesion may exhibit a ''dural tail'' (Fig. 8–11*A*). Supratentorially, they most frequently arise along the falx (Fig. 8–11*B*), over the cerebral convexity, on the tuberculum sellae, in the parasellar region, in the olfactory grooves, and along the sphenoidal ridge. Pineal region examples are infrequent. Also uncommon are intraventricular meningiomas, tumors thought to arise from arachnoidal cells within choroid plexus stroma. The posterior fossa, the cerebello-pontine angle or, more anteriorly, the petroclival junction are commonly affected sites. Spinal canal meningiomas most often affect the thoracic and cervical regions, not the lumbar level. Most meningiomas are globular, well-demarcated, dural-based masses without a discernible capsule. Limited peritumoral spread or dural hypervascularity is the basis of the dural tail sign (Fig. 8–11*C*), which is often detected with contrast-enhanced CT or MRI scans. An exception to the globular morphology is the meningioma ''en plaque,'' a carpetlike tumor growth that typically affects the skull base, particularly over the sphenoid ridge and clivus. Meningiomas are typically slow-growing lesions. Many displace brain while invading dura and bone. Tumors abutting or invading bone may produce hyperostosis, a distinctive radiographic abnormality.

Histologically, meningiomas are divided into four general categories (Table 8–4) that roughly reflect aggressiveness and malignant potential: meningioma, atypical meningioma, papillary meningioma, and anaplastic (malignant) meningioma. A bewildering complexity of variant patterns overlaps these categories; these patterns are itemized in the new WHO classification.[12, 50, 64] The range is broad and includes epithelial, mesenchymal, and mixed phenotypes (Fig. 8–11*D* and *E*). The most common examples of each are meningothelial (syncytial), fibrous, and transitional meningiomas. Microcystic, secretory, and chordoid tumors are

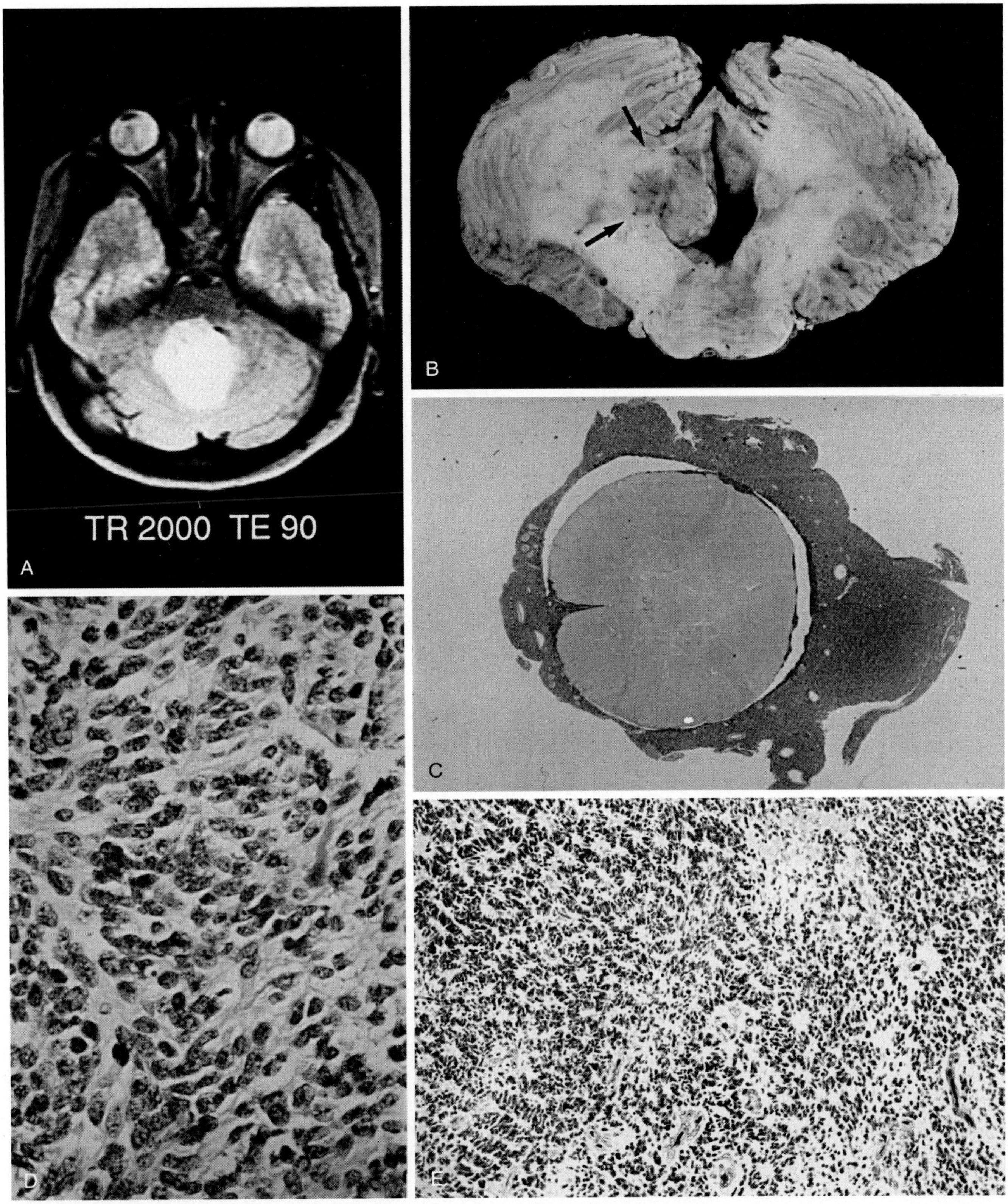

Figure 8–10. Medulloblastoma. *A,* MRI with contrast. This form of primitive neuroectodermal tumor arises within the cerebellum, more often in the vermis than the hemispheres. Many extend into the fourth ventricle. Medulloblastomas are typically solid, relatively demarcated, and contrast enhancing on CT and MRI scans. *B,* This horizontal section of the cerebellum shows the tumor *(arrows)* to arise within the vermis and to compromise the fourth ventricle. Cerebrospinal seeding has led to the formation of a cerebellopontine angle mass and widespread leptomeningeal involvement. *C,* This transverse whole-mount section of the spinal cord shows extensive leptomeningeal dissemination as well as tumoral encasement of the otherwise unremarkable cord. *D,* This pediatric tumor of the cerebellum is a distinctive form of PNET, one often associated with loss of chromosome 17p and a relatively good response to therapy. The majority are composed of hyperchromatic, carrot-shaped cells *(D).* Homer-Wright rosettes are commonly seen and are indicative of neuroblastic differentiation *(E).*

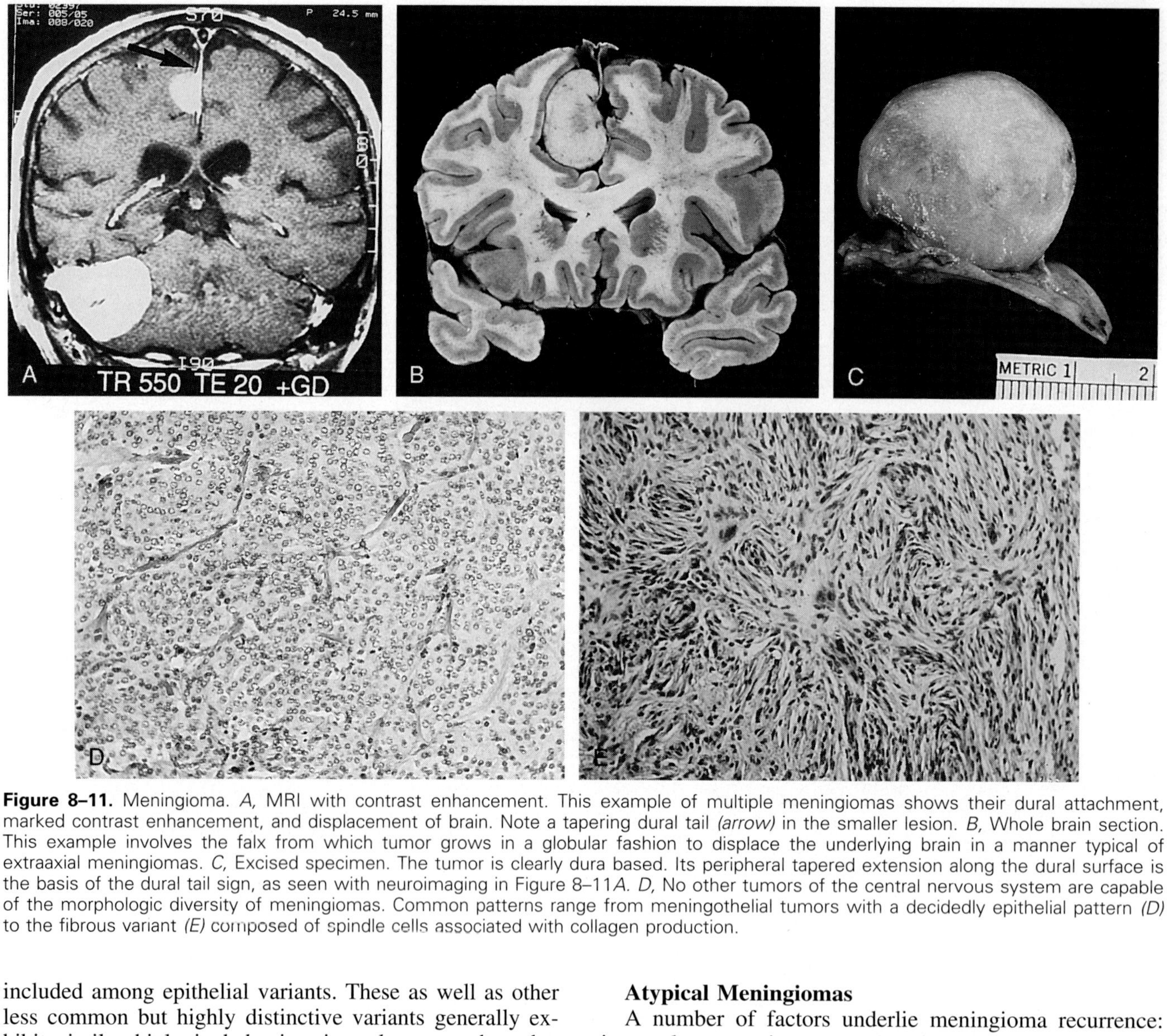

Figure 8–11. Meningioma. *A,* MRI with contrast enhancement. This example of multiple meningiomas shows their dural attachment, marked contrast enhancement, and displacement of brain. Note a tapering dural tail *(arrow)* in the smaller lesion. *B,* Whole brain section. This example involves the falx from which tumor grows in a globular fashion to displace the underlying brain in a manner typical of extraaxial meningiomas. *C,* Excised specimen. The tumor is clearly dura based. Its peripheral tapered extension along the dural surface is the basis of the dural tail sign, as seen with neuroimaging in Figure 8–11*A*. *D,* No other tumors of the central nervous system are capable of the morphologic diversity of meningiomas. Common patterns range from meningothelial tumors with a decidedly epithelial pattern *(D)* to the fibrous variant *(E)* composed of spindle cells associated with collagen production.

included among epithelial variants. These as well as other less common but highly distinctive variants generally exhibit similar biologic behavior, i.e., slow growth and a tendency toward local recurrence after excision. Some variants are associated with peculiar systemic disease manifestations; examples include Castleman's disease in the chordoid variant, polyclonal gammopathy and iron-refractory anemia with lymphoplasmacytic tumors, extreme peritumoral edema with microcystic tumors, measurable carcinoembryonic antigen (CEA) production by secretory meningiomas, and inordinately aggressive behavior by the clear-cell and papillary variants.[50–53]

Among "garden variety" meningiomas are the meningotheliomatous and transitional tumors; these display the most typical microscopic meningothelial features, including lobules of cells with poorly defined cell borders (meningothelial tumors) and fascicles or whorls of plump to elongated cells in a variably collagen-rich stroma, often with abundant psammoma bodies (transitional tumors). The designation "psammomatous meningioma" is applied to these tumors when such calcific bodies are a conspicuous feature. Fibrous meningiomas are marked by cellular spindling and collagen deposition.

Atypical Meningiomas

A number of factors underlie meningioma recurrence: incomplete resection, tumor location, the presence of peritumoral satellite nodules, histologic features of atypia, and the presence of bone, soft tissue, or brain invasion. Although all meningiomas have the potential for recurrence, microscopic atypia increases the likelihood. The morphologic features of atypical meningiomas are not sufficient for definite diagnosis of malignancy but include hypercellularity, nuclear pleomorphism with nucleolar prominence, increased mitotic activity, sheetlike growth pattern, and necrosis often associated with palisading of tumor cells. These features are encountered more often in meningothelial or transitional tumors and less so in fibrous or other more specialized variant patterns. Features of atypia are not uniformly distributed throughout a given tumor, a factor mandating thorough tissue sampling and microscopic examination by the pathologist.

Papillary Meningiomas

The papillary meningioma, a rare variant occurring in young patients, is particularly aggressive, regarded by some to be malignant.[52, 53] It is characterized by the formation of

Table 8–4. Tumors of the Meninges WHO Classification (1993)

Tumors of Meningothelial Cells

Meningioma (histologic types)
- Meningothelial (syncytial)
- Transitional/mixed
- Fibrous (fibroblastic)
- Psammomatous
- Angiomatous
- Microcystic
- Secretory
- Clear-cell
- Chordoid
- Lymphoplasmacyte-rich
- Metaplastic variants (xanthomatous, myxoid, osseous, cartilaginous)

Atypical meningioma
Papillary meningioma
Anaplastic (malignant) meningioma
- Variants of histologic types of meningioma
- Papillary

Mesenchymal, Nonmeningothelial Tumors

Benign Neoplasms

Osteocartilaginous tumors
Lipoma
Fibrous histiocytoma
Others

Malignant Neoplasms

Hemangiopericytoma
Chondrosarcoma
Malignant fibrous histiocytoma
Rhabdomyosarcoma
Meningeal sarcomatosis

Primary Melanocytic Lesions

Diffuse melanosis
Melanocytoma
Malignant melanoma: variant: malignant melanomatosis

Tumors of Uncertain Histogenesis

Hemangioblastoma

From Kleihues P, Burger PC, Scheithauer BW. *Histological Typing of Tumours of the Central Nervous System,* 2nd ed. New York: Springer-Verlag; 1993.

pseudopapillae, not due to necrosis but to loss of cellular cohesion. Specimens removed by ultrasonic aspiration or excised with electrocautery are obscured by artifacts that interfere with histologic assessment. Specimens should be submitted before subjecting the tumor to such methods.

Anaplastic (Malignant) Meningiomas

Anaplastic meningiomas display obviously malignant histologic features. Although there is no sharp distinction between highly atypical and anaplastic meningiomas, the latter often show marked nuclear and cellular pleomorphism, a high mitotic index, and extensive geographic, palisading necrosis. Frank brain invasion, which may or may not be apparent to the surgeon, is indicative of malignancy, regardless of the presence of histologic anaplasia. Thus, when the size of the specimen permits, careful microscopic assessment of its periphery for the tumor-brain interface is mandatory. This is particularly critical for cases in which irregular tumor border and peritumoral edema are evident in preoperative neuroimaging studies.

It is not uncommon to encounter meningiomas as incidental findings with head CT and MRI scans or at postmortem examination of the elderly. When symptomatic, usually due to mass effect, resection of the tumor with involved dura is the treatment of choice. It is of note that, in the parasagittal and parasellar regions, meningiomas may extend into the venous (superior sagittal and cavernous) sinuses, thus precluding their total removal. Likewise, plaque-shaped tumors on the skull base tend to be unresectable and are prone to recurrence. In such cases, depending upon clinical factors such as patient age and neurologic status, postoperative radiation therapy may be indicated.

Pitfalls in the Diagnosis of CNS Tumors

In most cases, accurate diagnosis of an intracranial neoplasm is straightforward based on combined clinical and pathologic features. However, ''look-alikes'' do occur. These include not only primary and secondary tumors of the nervous system, but a variety of non-neoplastic conditions that simulate neoplasia.

Normal Anatomy Versus Glioma

Oligodendrocytes are normally encountered in considerable number within fiber tracts of the white matter. Their linear orientation and frequent perivascular concentration, as well as their tendency to aggregate about cortical neurons, should not be interpreted as evidence of infiltrative glioma. Cortical neurons are occasionally surrounded by as many as eight normal oligodendrocytes, a finding that mimics ''satellitosis.'' The proper diagnosis depends upon careful correlation of clinical and imaging data, as well as requiring nuclear atypia for cases of glioma.

The finding of ganglion cells, particularly in a small biopsy, prompts consideration of a ganglion cell neoplasm such as ganglioglioma. Ganglion cells are often focally aggregated in spinal cord segments, in the hippocampus, and in the cerebellum (dentate nucleus and roof nuclei) and are found normally individually scattered within temporal lobe white matter. In and of themselves, or when overrun by glioma, such cells should not be overinterpreted as neoplastic because the prognosis of ganglioglioma is far more favorable than that of infiltrative gliomas.

Particularly with small biopsy intraoperative frozen section or smear preparations, cerebellum may show sheetlike arrays of granular neurons that at first glance mimic medulloblastoma. Their uniform distribution, round rather than oval- or carrot-shaped nuclei, distinct solitary nucleoli, lack of mitotic activity, and association with Purkinje cells permit recognition as normal tissue.

Gliosis Versus Glioma

Astrocytic cells respond nonspecifically to pathologic processes with hypertrophy and, to a lesser extent, with proliferation—a process termed gliosis. It may be acute, as in infarction, subacute, as in abscess or demyelination, or chronic, as in arteriovenous malformation, craniopharyngioma, or hemangioblastoma. Subacute gliosis is characterized by enlargement of astrocytic cell bodies with accentuation of their symmetrically radiating processes (Fig. 8–12*A*). Such cells are uniformly distributed and best defined by immunostains for glial fibrillary acid protein (GFAP). In comparison with acute or subacute gliosis, gemistocytic astrocytomas, the tumors with which they are most readily confused, are more cellular, less organized proliferations that show distinct nuclear atypia and occasional mitotic figures. Mitoses are very infrequent in gliosis. In contrast to astrocytomas, reactive astrocytes do not form secondary structures such as subpial, subependymal, perivascular, or perineuronal aggregations of neoplastic cells. Similarly, they are not associated with neovascularity or endothelial proliferation. When gliosis is chronic, the cells become more fibrillar and may be mistaken for those of fibrillary astrocytoma. Long-standing gliosis may also be accompanied by Rosenthal fiber formation, a finding that prompts consideration of pilocytic astrocytoma (Fig. 8–12*B*). Nuclear changes in long-standing gliosis, particularly in the setting of prior irradiation, include variation in nuclear shape and staining density (Fig. 8–12*C*). Such ''degenerative atypia'' has no associated mitotic activity. A similar process also occurs in the ventricular regions, involving proliferation of subependymal glial and ependymal cells in response to acute or chronic irritation. In chronic ependymal reaction, rosettes or even ependymal canals may form immediately beneath intact, otherwise normal ependyma.

Infarct Versus Glioma

In subacute and organizing phases of infarction, reactive cellularity may be dense and easily mistaken for glioma. Both the neuroimaging appearance of infarcts, affecting known vascular distributions, and clinical data indicating an abrupt or stepwise evolution are helpful in distinguishing them from gliomas. The latter respect no vascular boundaries and are associated with progressive, often steadily accelerating signs and symptoms. Whereas in their acute phases infarcts are not contrast enhancing, they soon become so. The capillaries within and surrounding an infarct are often markedly proliferative (Fig. 8–13) but lack the endothelial proliferation and glomeruloid architecture that characterize the vasculature of high-grade gliomas. Like demyelinating disease (see next section), well-developed infarcts are characterized by an influx of both lipid-rich histiocytes (''gitter'' cells) and neutrophils, followed in turn by small numbers of lymphocytes and by prominent reactive astrocytes exhibiting a prominent stellate array of tapering processes.

Glioma Versus Demyelinating Disease

Central inflammatory diseases can mimic CNS tumors in both clinical presentation and neuroimaging. This problem

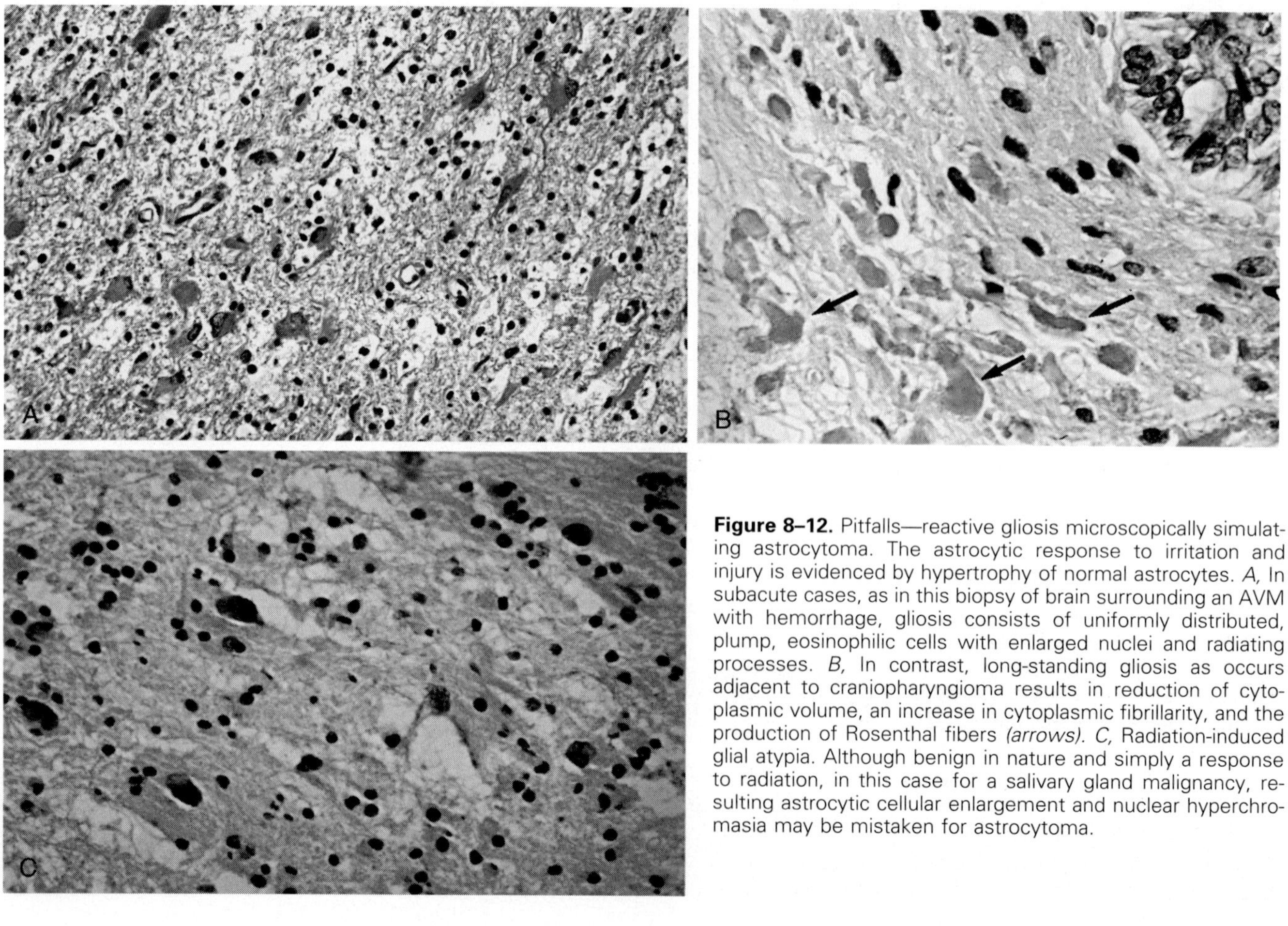

Figure 8–12. Pitfalls—reactive gliosis microscopically simulating astrocytoma. The astrocytic response to irritation and injury is evidenced by hypertrophy of normal astrocytes. *A,* In subacute cases, as in this biopsy of brain surrounding an AVM with hemorrhage, gliosis consists of uniformly distributed, plump, eosinophilic cells with enlarged nuclei and radiating processes. *B,* In contrast, long-standing gliosis as occurs adjacent to craniopharyngioma results in reduction of cytoplasmic volume, an increase in cytoplasmic fibrillarity, and the production of Rosenthal fibers *(arrows)*. *C,* Radiation-induced glial atypia. Although benign in nature and simply a response to radiation, in this case for a salivary gland malignancy, resulting astrocytic cellular enlargement and nuclear hyperchromasia may be mistaken for astrocytoma.

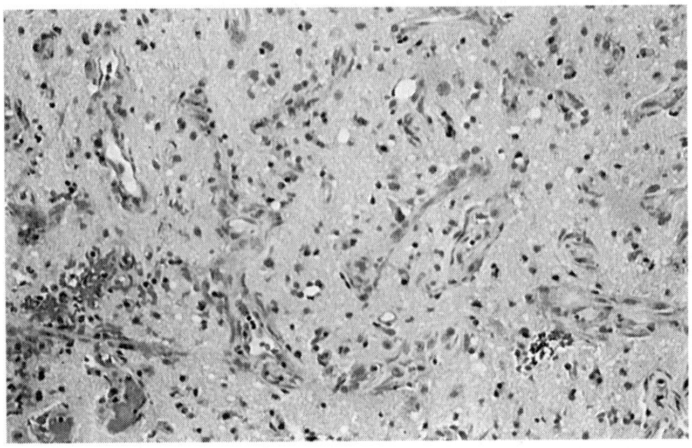

Figure 8–13. Pitfalls—infarct. Note the presence of capillary proliferation, an early event, and dense accumulation of histiocytes, a feature of well-established lesions. Infarcts are distinguished from glioma by their high content of histiocytes and lack of nuclear atypia.

frequently arises in the setting of demyelinating disease. In some patients, one predominant lesion, rather than multiple lesions (multiple sclerosis), is manifested, the others being small or undetectable. In such patients the clinical and imaging features are those of a space-occupying process with mass effects[54]—the picture of glioma. Such cases present a challenge to the pathologist in that such a misdiagnosis of tumor may lead to a neurologically devastating resection.

Histologically, demyelinating disease features moderately cellular lesions composed of conspicuous, plump astrocytes accompanied by a diffuse and perivascular infiltrate of foamy macrophages with perivascular concentrations of lymphocytes and occasional plasma cells. Although the reactive astrocytes appear increased in number, instead they represent hypertrophic resident astrocytes. Their uniform distribution and stellate configuration generally permit ready distinction from neoplastic astrocytes; however, those in chronic plaques may show nuclear variation and hyperchromasia. The degree of inflammation reflects the ''activity'' of the process. Necrosis may be seen in large or rapidly evolving lesions.

Key to diagnosis of demyelinating lesions is the recognition of macrophages, not mistaking them for neoplastic oligodendrocytes or astrocytes. The distinction is made readily with smear preparations, which show vacuolization of macrophage cytoplasm and the stellate configuration of reactive astrocytes. Special histochemical and immunohistochemical stains also facilitate the diagnosis of demyelinating disease. Stains for myelin (Luxol-fast blue) and for axons (Bodian or Bielschowsky) demonstrate virtual loss of myelin with preservation of axonal processes, respectively. Immunostains for macrophages and lymphocytes confirm their presence, in favor of demyelinating disease.[55] Immunostain for GFAP serves to highlight the stellate configuration and the uniform distribution of reactive astrocytes.

Progressive Multifocal Leukoencephalopathy Versus Glioma

Caused by an oncogenic papovavirus, progressive multifocal leukoencephalopathy (PML) is the only viral infection to be regularly mistaken for glioma. It occurs almost exclusively in immunocompromised patients and is a multifocal process that on CT or MRI scans has a typical appearance. Although the essential lesion is demyelination, the accompanying astrocytosis is markedly atypical featuring large, hyperchromatic, and often bizarre nuclei and mitotic figures, some abnormal. However, other characteristics of glioma, e.g., secondary structure formation, vascular proliferation, and necrosis, are lacking. Helpful diagnostic features of PML include a background of numerous histiocytes (uncommon in gliomas) and oligodendroglial cells with nuclei replaced by a wine-red inclusion. In contrast to other demyelinating diseases, lymphocytic infiltrates are not a feature of PML. Electron microscopy and virus-specific immunohistochemical stains are diagnostic.

Primary Versus Tumor-Induced Syrinx

Slowly growing spinal cord neoplasms may be associated with the formation of a syrinx, an intramedullary cystic space filled with fluid. Such spaces form within cord parenchyma and do not represent dilations of the central canal. Tumors showing a tendency toward syrinx induction include astrocytomas, particularly pilocytic types, ependymoma, and capillary hemangioblastoma. Such a syrinx is often larger than the tumor responsible for its development. Preoperative imaging, particularly contrasted MRI of the spinal cord, is critical for detecting and locating the causative lesion and in directing an appropriate surgical approach. Syrinx formation can also be idiopathic or caused by non-neoplastic processes, such as trauma. The syrinx fluid associated with tumors is typically dark and heavily protein-rich, whereas that of non-neoplastic syringes is highly variable in character. Cytologic examination of the fluid is useless. The major pitfall involving biopsy of the wall of a syrinx, regardless of cause, is misdiagnosis as astrocytoma. Such samples consist of variably compact gliotic tissue containing reactive astrocytes, some with degenerative nuclear atypia. Such tissue is generally hypocellular, but long-standing syrinx tissue may be sufficiently cellular with Rosenthal fiber formation as to simulate astrocytomas, particularly in small biopsies. Occasional samples also show scattered histiocytes or hemosiderin deposits. The lesion termed ''central canal syrinx,'' associated with an abnormality at the craniocervical junction such as the Chiari malformation, is more appropriately designated hydromyelia. Its fluid content is in reality CSF, in contrast to that of a neoplasm-associated syrinx. Ascending and descending intramedullary extensions of posttraumatic syrinx are often hydromyelic as well.

Abscess Versus Glioblastoma

Particularly in fragmented biopsy specimens, well-developed abscesses can resemble glioblastoma microscopically. In the absence of frank pus, the operative appearance may also be that of a necrotic tumor (Fig. 8–14*A*). Abscesses vary in their cellular composition over time in accordance with a consistent progression: there is an early predominance of neutrophils, subsequent acquisition of lymphocytes, plasma cells, and histiocytes, and the presence of

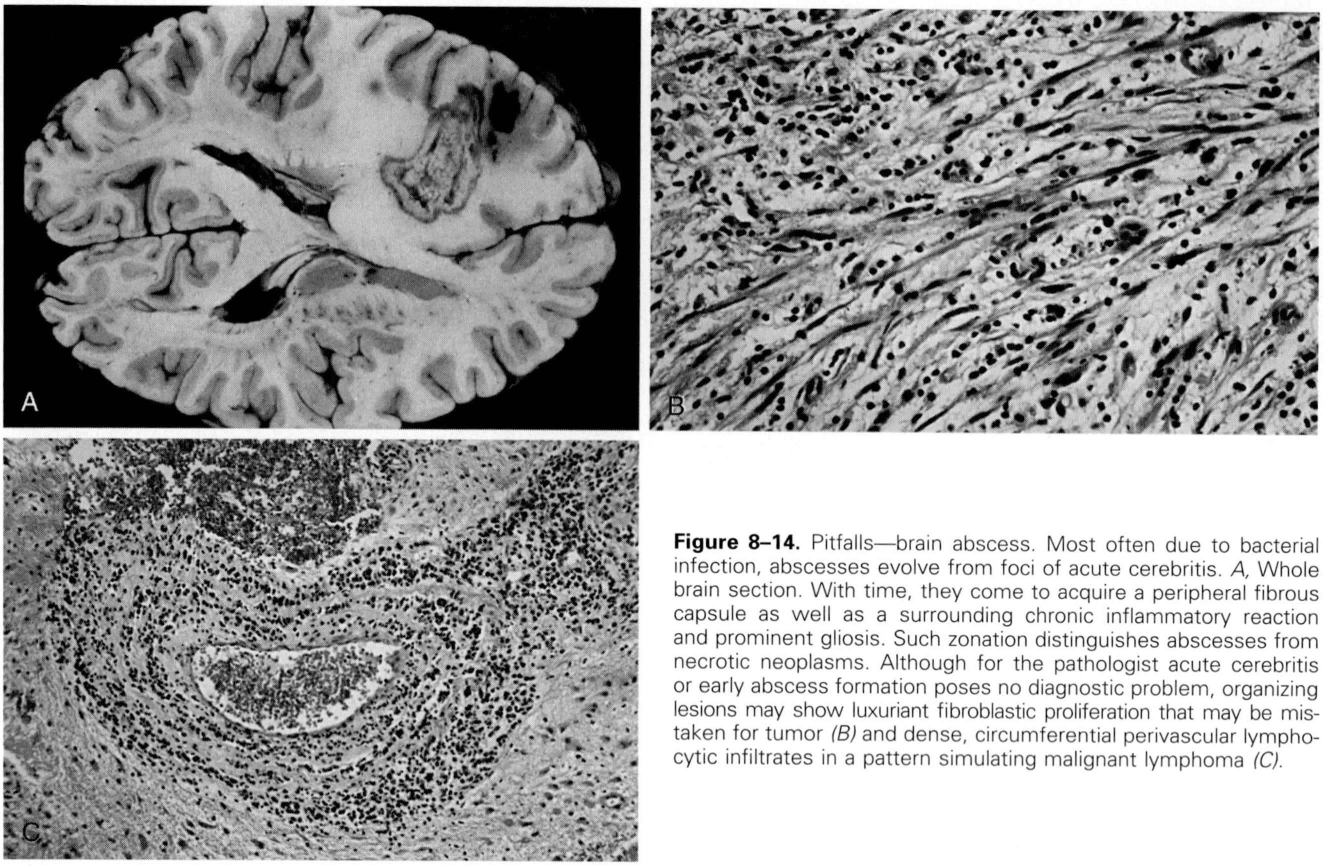

Figure 8–14. Pitfalls—brain abscess. Most often due to bacterial infection, abscesses evolve from foci of acute cerebritis. *A,* Whole brain section. With time, they come to acquire a peripheral fibrous capsule as well as a surrounding chronic inflammatory reaction and prominent gliosis. Such zonation distinguishes abscesses from necrotic neoplasms. Although for the pathologist acute cerebritis or early abscess formation poses no diagnostic problem, organizing lesions may show luxuriant fibroblastic proliferation that may be mistaken for tumor *(B)* and dense, circumferential perivascular lymphocytic infiltrates in a pattern simulating malignant lymphoma *(C).*

surrounding reactive astrocytes. The latter are most noticeable at the periphery of the lesion where other cellular elements are less prominent. Abscesses are laminar in architecture and consist, from center to periphery, of necrosis, leukocytic exudate, capillary proliferation with histiocytic reaction, and gliosis. Selective sampling of an organizing abscess with fibrous capsule formation and chronic inflammation may result in misdiagnosis (Fig. 8–14*B* and *C*).

Only rarely do glioblastomas contain large numbers of neutrophils. Furthermore, their vascular reaction is more frequently characterized by endothelial proliferation with glomeruloid structures. Lastly, glioblastomas are composed of large numbers of cytologically atypical astrocytes. The latter, unlike the reactive astrocytes of gliosis accompanying abscess, penetrate surrounding brain parenchyma, showing a tendency to infiltrate fiber tracks as well as nearby gray matter and to form their own intrinsic structure.

Metastatic Neoplasia Versus Glioma

Metastatic neoplasms can involve the brain or meninges. In the latter situation they resemble meningiomas (Fig. 8–15*A*). In either location they are characterized by circumscription (Fig. 8–15*B* and *C*) and may be multifocal. In most instances the diagnosis is straightforward, with known prior extracranial malignancy. Metastatic carcinomas and melanomas far outnumber sarcomas. Any of these may mimic glioblastoma. Pathologic features of metastases that aid in their recognition include abrupt tumor margins, relative lack of microvascular proliferation, and absence of elongated cells with multipolar processes.

Metastatic melanomas are frequently accompanied by hemorrhage and, at low magnification, tend to form pseudopapillae surrounded by zones of necrosis. In the absence of either obvious or stainable melanin, the identification of melanomas requires performance of immunostains. Melanomas are S-100 protein and HMB-45 immunoreactive and, in contrast to gliomas, are GFAP negative. Metastatic carcinomas often show sheetlike growth or vague glandular patterns where neoplastic cells show nuclear molding. The intercellular cohesion so typical of carcinoma cells is most readily appreciated with smear preparations. Special stains for epithelial markers are important in the identification of carcinoma, but caution is recommended in the choice of immunostains for cytokeratin. High molecular weight cytokeratin antibodies frequently show cross-reactivity with GFAP, strongly staining neoplastic as well as reactive astrocytes. This is not a problem with antibodies for low molecular weight cytokeratin.

Ependymomas, like metastases, are characterized by remarkable circumscription. Low-grade ependymomas sometimes show focal epithelial membrane antigen (EMA) immunoreactivity, a feature characteristic of carcinoma cells, but they are nonreactive for low molecular weight cytokeratin. Metastatic adenocarcinomas, particularly papillary forms, can mimic papillary ependymoma and choroid

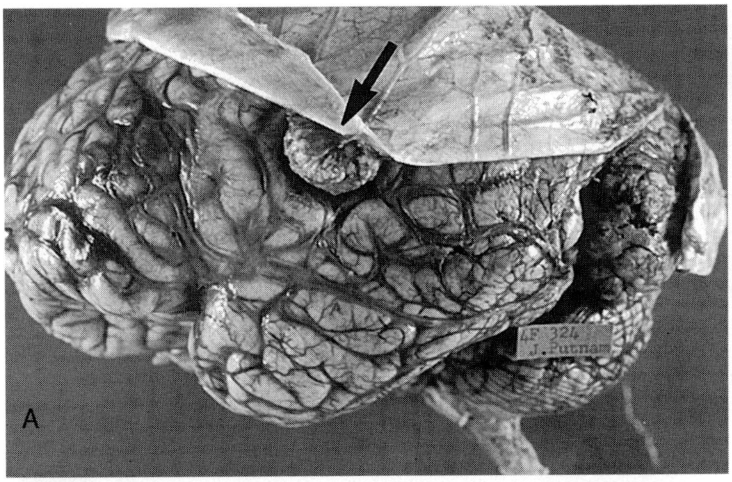

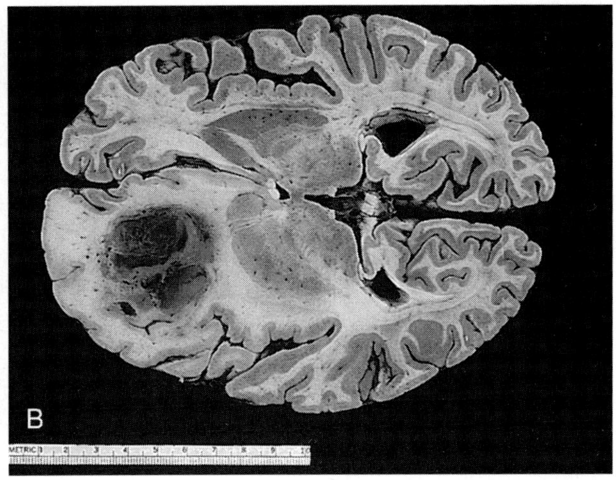

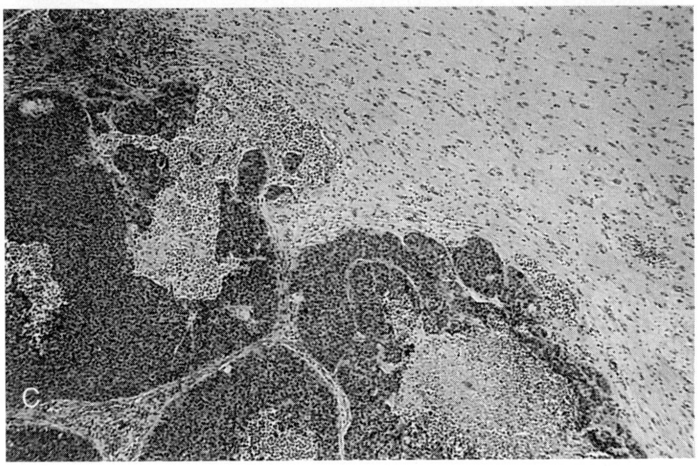

Figure 8–15. *A,* Metastatic carcinoma of the dura. Such tumors may be globular or diffuse in their pattern of growth. Globular lesions such as this breast carcinoma *(arrow)* displace underlying brain and may mimic meningioma. *B,* Metastatic carcinoma in brain. Parenchymal metastases are characterized by circumscription and accompanying edema. Multiplicity is common. When the deposits are small, they tend to center upon the junction of gray and white matter. This example of metastatic oat-cell carcinoma of lung in a 62-year-old man involves a frontal lobe, is well demarcated, associated with edema, and produces considerable mass effect. *C,* Microscopic features of metastatic carcinoma. Unlike the vast majority of gliomas, metastatic carcinomas typically form sharply demarcated deposits, ones often associated with necrosis. The surrounding brain shows edema and gliosis.

plexus carcinoma; in contrast to metastatic carcinoma, both occur in young children. In addition, choroid plexus carcinomas, unlike metastatic carcinomas, lack EMA and CEA reactivity. Instead, they exhibit vimentin, low molecular weight cytokeratin, S-100 protein, and on occasion GFAP staining. Immunoreactivity for GFAP is seen more regularly in papillary ependymoma.

The distinction of medulloblastoma from metastatic small-cell carcinoma is only rarely a problem. Only in the adult setting does this differential arise. Small-cell carcinomas typically show extensive necrosis, lack the desmoplasia so frequently seen in medulloblastomas in adults, show less tendency for rosette formation, and have a much higher mitotic index. The Azzopardi phenomenon, i.e., impregnation of vessel walls by nucleic acids, is a common feature of small-cell carcinoma, but is only rarely encountered in medulloblastoma.

Meningioma: "The Great Masquerader"

Of all tumors affecting the nervous system, no others exhibit such a broad range of morphology as do meningiomas (Fig. 8–11*D* and *E*). As previously mentioned, most are solitary, globular, dura-based masses (Fig. 8–11*B* and *C*), but a minority grow in a diffuse manner, are entirely intraparenchymal or intraventricular, or are even extradural in location. Therefore, the pathologist must be familiar, not only with the many histologic patterns of this common neoplasm, but also with the differential diagnosis of tumors in such locations. Although communication with the surgeon, attention to radiographic studies, and extensive tissue sampling will nearly always lead to correct diagnosis, special methods such as immunostaining or electron microscopy are useful in any equivocal cases.

BRAIN BIOPSY IN SITUATIONS OTHER THAN NEOPLASMS

Patients with non-neoplastic disease may require brain biopsy. Conditions that warrant such a diagnostic strategy include dementia or focal, multifocal, or diffuse encephalopathy in an effort to diagnose such disorders as neurodegenerative diseases, metabolic and storage diseases, and vasculitis. Specific identification of an infectious process, be it protozoal, fungal, bacterial, or viral, may also necessitate brain biopsy. An optimal diagnostic evaluation requires special attention to specimen handling. Coming into the operating room, the pathologist should become oriented to the anatomic relationships of the biopsy specimen. When possible, the biopsy should derive from an area of CT or MRI abnormality, preferably a neurologically ''silent'' location such as the anterior frontal or temporal lobes or from the cerebellum. The surgeon should be encouraged to obtain more than a minute fragment, e.g., a full-thickness biopsy of leptomeninges with surface vasculature, attached cortex, and underlying white matter. A separate piece of overlying dura should also be obtained. Specimen cautery induces major artifacts and should be avoided.

Although the need to provide a preliminary diagnosis is understandable, particularly in cases of suspected infection, vasculitis, or neoplasm, frozen sections should be kept at a minimum to conserve precious tissue. Instead, smear preparations are preferable for preliminary diagnosis to confirm that the specimen is representative. In addition to allocating some tissue for conventional permanent sections, tiny portions of both cortex and white matter should be fixed for potential electron microscopy. Lastly, a portion of each should be frozen and stored at −70°C for special studies, e.g., polymerase chain reaction (PCR) analysis for suspected viral infection. If infection is suspected, microbiologic specimens should be submitted directly to the microbiology facility from the operating room rather than via the pathology laboratory to avoid contamination. Processes affecting the basal leptomeninges and cranial nerves should be biopsied in those areas most affected, where samples are most likely to be diagnostic.[56]

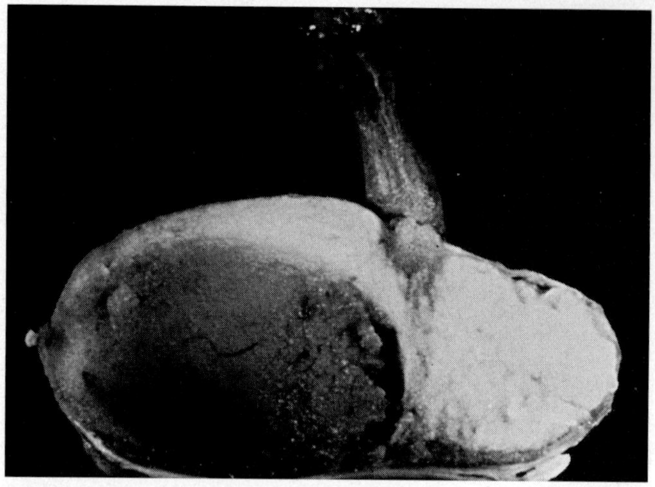

Figure 8–16. Pituitary adenoma in sagittal section. This microadenoma, defined as a tumor 1 cm or less in size, displaces surrounding anterior lobe tissue and abuts the dural capsule of the gland. Microscopic invasion of adjacent dura is seen in the majority of cases wherein dura is sampled. The pituitary stalk *(upper)* and posterior lobe *(right)* are unremarkable. Provided by Dr. Kalman Kovacs, Toronto, Ontario, Canada.

Pituitary Gland

Although not arising in what is strictly a part of the nervous system, pituitary tumors affect neighboring intracranial structures, e.g., the suprasellar space, third ventricle, and cavernous sinuses. This gland and its diseases are thus treated by the neurosurgeon. Because transsphenoidal approach is most commonly employed for sellar tumors, both otolaryngologist and neurosurgeon are frequently involved in such cases.

Pituitary adenomas comprise more than 75% of surgical specimens from the sellar region. Correlation of clinical and biochemical data is of particular diagnostic importance because of the broad spectrum of endocrinologic manifestations produced by pituitary adenomas. Clinically, adenomas may appear as "functioning" tumors, i.e., associated with a clinical syndrome resulting from tumoral hormone production (hyperprolactinemia, acromegaly/gigantism, Cushing's disease), or as nonfunctioning tumors. In the latter situation, patients present with symptoms resulting from compression of adjacent neural structures, usually visual field defects related to optic chiasm compression or signs of hypopituitarism. Diabetes insipidus is rarely seen. Adenomas are somewhat arbitrarily divided into microadenomas, defined as tumors up to 1 cm in size (Fig. 8–16), and macroadenomas, large tumors prone to suprasellar extension. Approximately 40% of adenomas invade surrounding dura or bone. Meaningful classification of pituitary adenomas requires not only conventional paraffin sections, but special methods, particularly immunostaining and sometimes electron microscopy.[15, 16] These methods identify tumoral production of certain hormones, an issue of particular importance in the distinction of prolactinomas from pituitary stalk section effect, and specifically identify adenoma subtypes in cases not associated with serum hormone elevations. The issue of tissue conservation again becomes significant. Suction removal of these soft tumors should be avoided until tissue free of microscopic artifact has been obtained and set aside for pathologic studies.

Intraoperative diagnosis of pituitary lesions may be problematic when specimens are small. This is particularly the case in adenomas of Cushing's disease and in prolactinomas occurring in reproductive-age females. In such instances, indiscriminate frozen section is to be avoided. Instead, smears or touch preparations are preferable; they permit the identification of adenomas, minimize tissue utilization, and represent a useful permanent record of the pathology. In smear preparations the cytologic features of the cells, particularly uniformity and prominence of nucleoli, serve to distinguish adenomas from the cellular heterogeneity that characterizes normal adenohypophyseal cells. Reticulin stains greatly aid in the distinction of normal from adenomatous tissue. Mechanical artifacts may induce changes easily mistaken for metastatic carcinoma.

Peripheral Nervous System

Cranial and spinal nerve roots supply the functionally defined voluntary (sensorimotor) and autonomic systems with nerves that ramify in every organ and tissue. Whether intracranial or distal within extremities, these nerves are prone to similar diseases, both neoplastic and non-neoplastic.

NERVE SHEATH TUMORS

This category includes tumors derived from supportive or stromal cells of peripheral nerves including Schwann cells and perineurial cells as well as fibroblasts. Although traumatic neuromas produce painful masses, these are not neoplasms but reparative proliferations of intertwined nerve processes and nerve sheath elements. Variants include am-

Table 8–5. Tumors of Cranial and Spinal Nerves WHO Classification (1993)

Schwannoma (neurilemoma, neurinoma) variants: cellular, plexiform, melanotic
Neurofibroma: variants: circumscribed, plexiform
Malignant peripheral nerve sheath tumor (MPNST) (neurogenic sarcoma, anaplastic neurofibroma, malignant schwannoma): variants: epithelioid MPNST with divergent mesenchymal and/or epithelial differentiation; melanotic

From Kleihues P, Burger PC, Scheithauer BW. *Histological Typing of Tumours of the Central Nervous System,* 2nd ed. New York: Springer-Verlag; 1993.

putation neuroma and Morton's (intermetatarsal) neuroma. The majority of nerve sheath neoplasms are schwannomas (neurilemomas) and neurofibromas (Table 8–5).[64] Schwannomas consist exclusively of Schwann cells. In contrast, neurofibromas consist of Schwann cells together with perineurial cells, fibroblasts, and transitional cells. As a result, some authors consider neurofibromas to be hamartomas rather than neoplasms. Both lesions exhibit distinctive anatomic and histologic features. Schwannomas tend to be solitary and arise more frequently from cranial and spinal nerve roots than from peripheral nerves. Grossly, their pattern of growth is as a solid encapsulated mass, one eccentric to the parent nerve, which remains intact alongside the tumor. Degenerative changes including lipid accumulation and cystic change are common (Fig. 8–17*A*), and "degenerative nuclear atypia" should not be misinterpreted as evidence of malignancy (Fig. 8–17*B*). Neurofibromas, by contrast, are commonly multiple and usually involve major peripheral nerves or their branches. The majority of cutaneous nerve sheath tumors are neurofibromas. Unlike

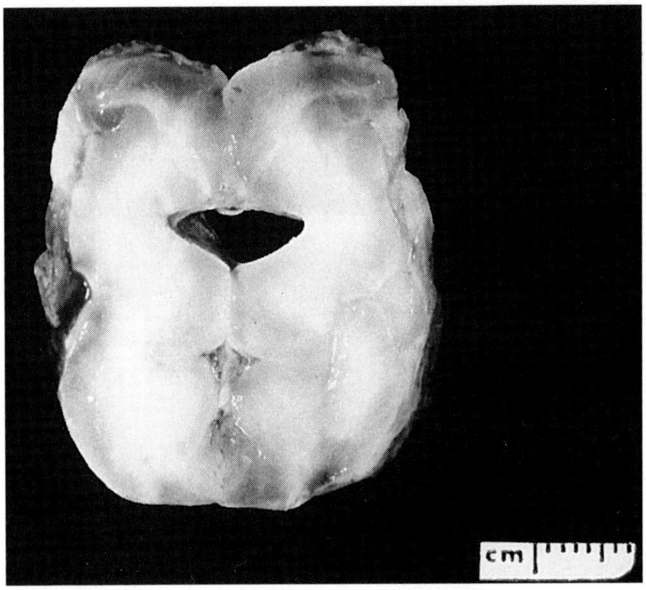

Figure 8–18. Neurofibroma. Unlike schwannomas, neurofibromas grow and spread within the substance of the nerve, have a somewhat translucent appearance, lack yellow coloration attributable to lipid accumulation, and show little or no tendency to cystic change.

schwannomas, neurofibromas symmetrically enlarge the parent nerve in a fusiform fashion; they grow within the nerve substance and lack their own capsule (Fig. 8–18).

Schwannomas and neurofibromas occur either sporadically or in the setting of neurofibromatosis (NF). Multiple neurofibromas arise in NF-1 (von Recklinghausen's disease or peripheral neurofibromatosis), whereas multiple schwannomas are associated with NF-2 (central neurofibromatosis) or with a little known condition termed

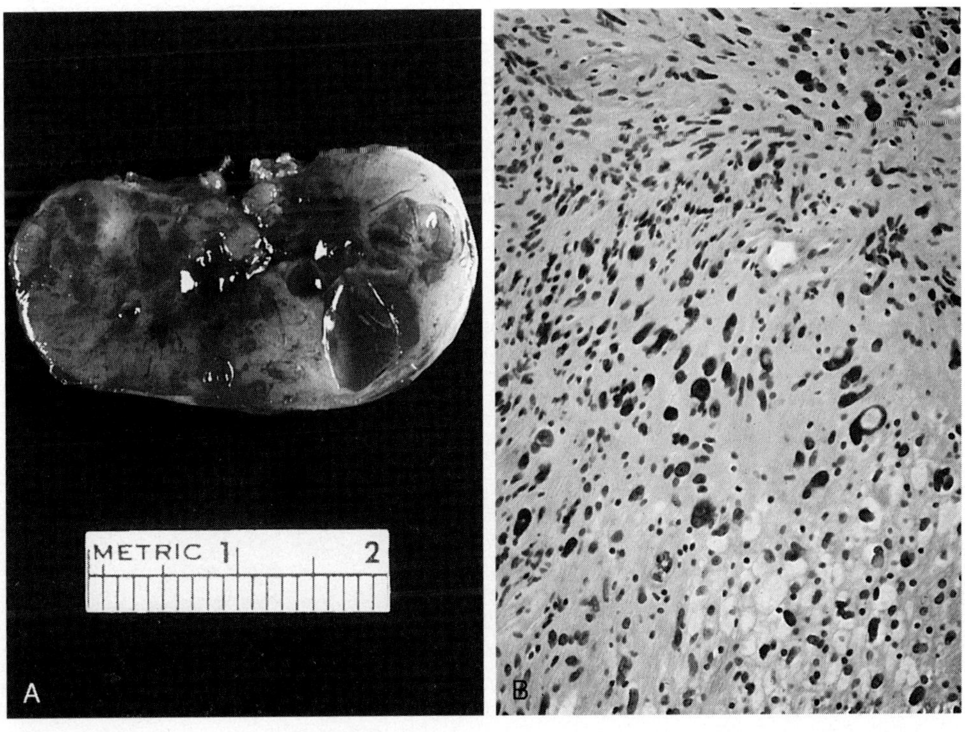

Figure 8–17. Schwannoma. *A,* Gross appearance. Typical of this tumor is its eccentric manner of growth relative to the parent nerve (not shown), patchy yellow discoloration, and tendency to undergo cystic degeneration. *B,* Microscopic features of "ancient schwannoma." Despite their benign nature, schwannomas of long standing may show a degree of degenerative nuclear atypia readily mistaken for malignancy. Unlike sarcomas of peripheral nerves, such tumors typically lack mitotic activity.

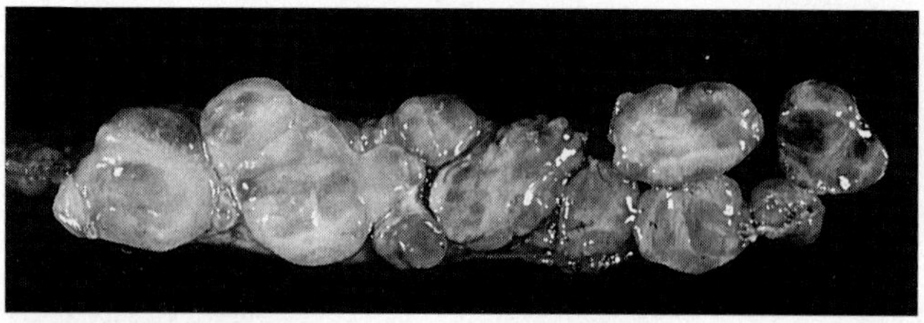

Figure 8–19. Plexiform neurofibroma. Such tumors involve multiple nerve fascicles, are typically mucoid in texture, and often defy gross total removal. Their finding is virtually pathognomonic of von Recklinghausen's disease (NF-1). Careful tissue sampling is of importance in that 5% of such tumors undergo sarcomatous transformation.

schwannomatosis. Neurofibromas are the principal lesions of NF-1, being far more common than schwannomas. Plexiform neurofibromas are diagnostic of NF-1 (Fig. 8–19), whereas bilateral acoustic schwannomas are pathognomonic of NF-2. Important surgical considerations surround the resection of nerve sheath tumors. Short of diffuse cutaneous tumors, the removal of neurofibroma necessarily involves resection of the parent nerve with resultant loss of its function. By contrast, with careful dissection, schwannomas can be removed without sacrifice of the parent nerve, preserving its function. The same is true of ''cellular schwannomas,'' benign tumors that, owing to their cellularity, are often mistaken for malignant peripheral nerve sheath tumors. Unlike neurofibromas, schwannomas almost never become malignant (see Chapter 18).

Malignant peripheral nerve sheath tumors (MPNSTs) are often large, partially necrotic tumors that spread within the parent nerve. Anaplastic transformation of schwannomas is an extremely rare event and most MPNSTs are derived from neurofibromas.[57] Their overall incidence in the general population is very low (approximately 0.001%), but is much higher among patients with NF-1 (4.6%).[57] In this setting a high incidence of MPNST is observed in children and young adults.[57–59] Radiation-induced MPNSTs have been reported to occur in patients both with and without NF-1[57, 58]; the latency period is generally about 1 decade.

Because MPNSTs often arise in neurofibromas (Fig. 8–20*A* and *B*), sampling is of importance, particularly in large tumors. The transition may be gradual or abrupt and focal or multifocal. A single biopsy of a transformed neurofibroma may not be representative and may miss the sarcomatous element. The majority of MPNSTs are high-grade tumors featuring necrosis or hemorrhage. Their microscopic appearance varies considerably, ranging from conventional spindle-cell lesions (Fig. 8–20*B*) to epithelioid variants that mimic carcinoma. Rare MPNSTs show differentiation toward skeletal muscle (''Triton tumors''), bone, cartilage, or even bonafide epithelium—mucin-producing, squamous, or neuroendocrine. Such variants are more often observed in NF-1, but also occur in sporadic tumors.[60]

The treatment of MPNST is primarily surgical, the goal being complete tumor resection with confirmed adequate margins. Sacrificing the parent nerve is implicit. In the extremities this approach is often feasible and preferable to amputation. In addition to peritumoral soft tissue margins, proximal and distal nerve margins must also be examined because MPNST may extend considerable distances within the parent nerve. For centrally situated lesions, such as in the brachial or lumbosacral plexus regions, resection with wide margins is rarely possible and tumor recurrence is the rule. If in these cases the diagnosis can be established through needle or incisional biopsy, preoperative chemotherapy and radiation therapy followed by debulking surgery has been advocated (see Chapter 18).

The prognosis of MPNST relates not only to resectability but also to tumor size, location, and to association with NF-1; more centrally situated tumors, those greater than 5 cm in greatest dimension, and those occurring in the setting of NF-1 have a particularly poor prognosis.[57] Tumors associated with NF-1 are more often centrally located, large, high grade, and prone to early recurrence and to metastasis. Histologic grade is not a powerful prognostic indicator.

PERIPHERAL NERVE BIOPSIES FOR NON-NEOPLASTIC DISORDERS

Peripheral nerve biopsy is indicated for the evaluation of a number of peripheral neuropathies, particularly to assess fiber and interstitial pathology. Diseases that may underlie such neuropathies include amyloidosis, vasculitis

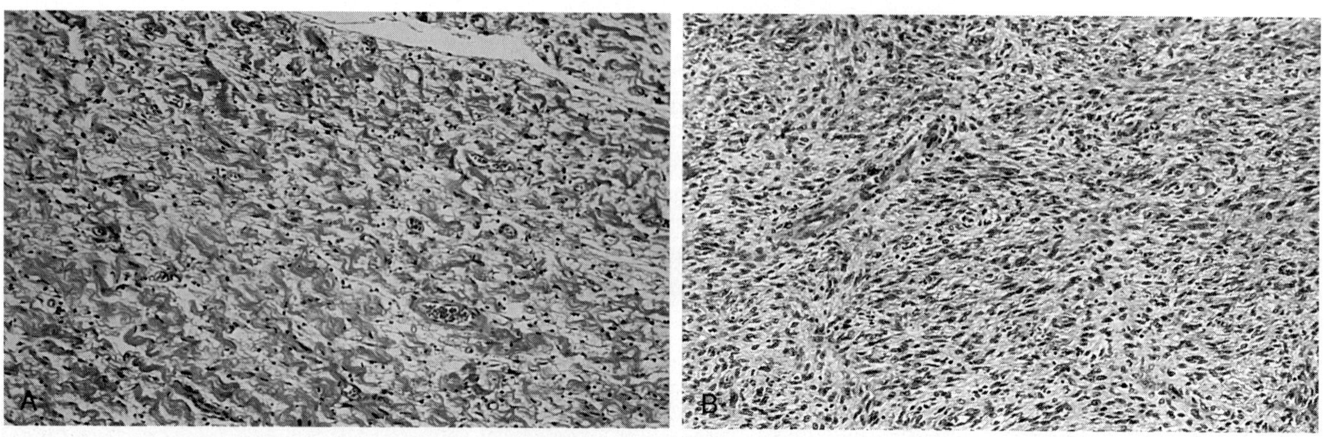

Figure 8–20. Microscopic features of neurofibroma *(A)* in which has arisen a high-grade MPNST *(B)*. Fully half of MPNSTs arise in transition from a preexisting neurofibroma, thus underscoring the necessity of a generous biopsy to avoid sampling error and underdiagnosis.

(systemic and localized), sarcoidosis, and inherited conditions such as metachromatic leukodystrophy. The sural nerve is ideal because of its accessibility, predictable location, absence of extensive branching, the limited neurologic deficit resulting from biopsy, and the extensive information available standardizing its normal morphology (e.g., fiber type, numbers, size, and distribution). The specimen should be long enough to provide adequate tissue; this includes material for histopathologic studies (2.5 to 3 cm), resin embedding and teased fiber preparations (2.5 to 3 cm), and possibly frozen tissue as well. Particular care should be taken to avoid grasping or stretching the nerve. Artifacts produced during nerve removal are common and can impair pathologic interpretation. For a detailed description of the biopsy technique the reader is referred to an authoritative text.[61] The protocol used in the Peripheral Nerve Center at the Mayo Clinic is designed to prevent retraction of nerve fibers; once exposed and before transection, the sural nerve is gently tied at the proximal end and a hooked end of a 10-mg weight (a bent insulin needle can also be used) is inserted into the nerve approximately 2.5 to 3 cm distally. The first segment is immediately suspended in 2% buffered (pH 7.4) paraformaldehyde at 10°C. The next 2.5 to 3 cm segment is removed in a similar manner and is immersed in 2.5% buffered glutaraldehyde. If possible, a third segment should be removed and immediately frozen in cooled isopentane suspended in liquid nitrogen. The presence of a pathology technician experienced in collecting nerve biopsies in the operating room is required to implement this procedure.

Skeletal Muscle

Interpretation of muscle biopsy results relies upon close collaboration among the neurologist, surgeon, and pathologist. Muscle biopsies are performed primarily for two purposes: (1) the investigation of a suspected primary neuromuscular disease and (2) the diagnosis of systemic disease with associated neuromuscular abnormalities, such as vasculitis and sarcoidosis. Whereas systemic diseases can be diagnosed by standard histopathologic techniques, the detailed studies of muscle fibers essential for diagnosis of primary neuromuscular diseases can be performed only on frozen sections with special enzymatic and histochemical stains. In exceptional cases such studies can be complemented by electron microscopy, which serves to identify specific structural abnormalities, e.g., mitochondrial myopathies. Alternatively, the performance of biochemical assays may be required in the setting of metabolic disease. In summary, muscle biopsy samples cannot be handled as standard surgical pathology specimens with routine formalin fixation and paraffin embedding.

The preferred site for muscle biopsy is determined by the clinical features of the disease. The most useful information is derived from a muscle that is clinically affected to only a moderate degree. A severely involved muscle, one with advanced fiber loss and fat substitution, or one only minimally involved should be avoided. The same is true of muscles previously subjected to electromyographic needle placement because these may exhibit focal necrosis and inflammatory infiltrates—misleading features that interfere with interpretation. In general, biopsy of a single muscle is adequate for diagnosis. The frequently selected muscles are the biceps or deltoid in the upper extremities and the quadriceps or gastrocnemius in the lower extremities. Depending upon the specific clinical presentation, other muscles may be selected. In certain situations, the site chosen permits inclusion of other structures in the same procedure; for example, in cases requiring both muscle and nerve biopsy, the sural nerve can be taken in conjunction with the gastrocnemius muscle. Muscle specimens can be obtained either by open excision or by needle biopsy. Although open muscle biopsies provide larger, more readily oriented specimens with minimal tissue distortion, in some instances needle biopsies may be preferable, e.g., in children or in patients requiring sequential biopsies over the course of disease. The major disadvantage of needle biopsies is small specimen size, a factor that may preclude a complete analysis. In muscle biopsy, careful and gentle handling of the tissue is critical to prevent artifact. To minimize the deterioration of enzyme activity, muscle samples must be processed almost instantaneously. A technician or the pathologist should be present in the operating room. The specimen for histochemical study should be promptly frozen in isopentane cooled in liquid nitrogen and the specimen for electron microscopy fixed without delay. A discussion of muscle pathology is beyond the scope of this chapter. The reader is referred to authoritative texts.[62,63]

PITFALLS FOR THE SURGEON

1. Proceeding to cranial or intracranial procedures without first integrating clinical and radiologic data.
2. Attempting transnasal excision of a lesion of the upper nose without first excluding encephalocele, with its characteristic bony defects, by radiologic studies.
3. Inadequately sampling a brain tumor by not including the tumor's periphery or interface with brain, as well as its central or contrast-enhancing elements.
4. Unnecessarily producing severe neurologic impairment with extensive resection of a prognostically favorable variant of astrocytoma.

Continued

5. Mistaking brain abscess for glioblastoma on the basis of observed central necrosis.
6. Inadequately sampling brain for non-neoplastic disease: biopsying an area not affected, taking too small or too superficial a biopsy, failing to sample dura and leptomeninges, or by not sending sterilely procured tissue directly to the microbiology laboratory.
7. Removing a pituitary tumor entirely by suction without excising a portion intact and unaffected by artifact for pathologic examination.
8. Obtaining only a small biopsy from a large tumor of peripheral nerve sheath. Because there is often great variation in composition, malignant elements can readily be missed.
9. Introducing artifact into biopsied peripheral nerve by compressing or stretching the sample.
10. Proceeding with biopsy of nerve or skeletal muscle (for non-neoplastic disorders) without first coordinating with the pathologist to facilitate rapid and correct allocation of the sample for special study needs.
11. Selecting the wrong muscle to biopsy, one either uninvolved by disease or in too advanced a stage of degeneration for specific diagnosis.

PITFALLS FOR THE PATHOLOGIST

1. Attempting to diagnose CNS tumors without consideration of clinical and radiologic (neuro-imaging) data.
2. Failing to retain enough biopsied CNS tissue, apart from that used for intraoperative frozen section or preferably smear preparation interpretation, to assure good permanent sections for definitive diagnosis.
3. Misdiagnosing glial tumors as malignant based simply upon cellular pleomorphism. Several prognostically favorable tumors show such features, including pilocytic astrocytoma, pleomorphic xanthoastrocytoma, and subependymal giant-cell astrocytoma.
4. Failing to thoroughly sample CNS gliomas; such tumors often show wide variation in histologic anaplasia.
5. Mistaking normal CNS tissue for neoplasm, particularly with intraoperative frozen sections. Oligodendrocytes in normal white matter pathways can simulate oligodendrogliomas; the apparent increase in glial cells in the white matter of seizure specimens or about vascular malformations may simulate glioma; normal neurons in temporal lobe white matter or in spinal cord biopsies may simulate ganglion-cell lesions; cerebellar neurons can mimic medulloblastoma.
6. Misdiagnosing non-neoplastic processes as brain tumors: reactive gliosis, infarct, demyelinating disease, or PML as glioma; abscess as glioblastoma; gliosis in the wall of a benign spinal cord syrinx as tumor-associated syrinx.
7. Mistaking metastatic neoplasms, carcinoma more often than lymphoma or sarcoma, as primary brain tumors or meningiomas.
8. Failing to conserve adequate brain tissue, apart from that used for frozen sections or preferably smear preparations, biopsied for non-neoplastic disease to permit definitive diagnosis. Optimal tissue free of operative or freezing artifact is always needed for conventional permanent sections. Depending upon clinical-operative findings, tissue allocations may also include tissue for microbial culture, glutaraldehyde-fixed tissue for electron microscopy, and even sterile fresh tissue for tissue culture assays.
9. Failing to classify selected pituitary adenomas, according to hormone production, by means of immunostaining or to set aside a minute fragment for electron microscopy.
10. Basing a diagnosis of malignancy in schwannoma upon cellularity and occasional mitotic figures; this is a frequent finding without implication for aggressive behavior. Cellular schwannoma is a well-characterized benign tumor that recurs infrequently and does not metastasize.

11. Inadequately sampling a large neurofibroma, particularly a plexiform lesion; malignant transformation can be a localized phenomenon.
12. Failing to properly allocate tissue from muscle or nerve biopsies to allow appropriate special study methods.

FURTHER READING

Russell DS, Rubinstein LJ. *Pathology of Tumours of Nervous System.* 5th ed. Baltimore: Williams & Wilkins; 1989.

Burger PC, Scheithauer BW, Vogel FS. *Surgical Pathology of the Nervous System and Its Coverings.* 3rd ed. New York: Churchill Livingstone; 1991.

Kleihues P, Burger PC, Scheithauer BW. *Histologic Typing of Tumours of the Central Nervous System.* 2nd ed. New York: Springer Verlag; 1993.

Burger PC, Scheithauer BW. Tumors of the central nervous system. In: *Atlas of Tumor Pathology.* 3rd ser. Fascicle 10. Washington, DC: Armed Forces Institute of Pathology; 1994.

Engel AG. The muscle biopsy. In: Engel AG, Franzini-Armstrong C, eds. *Myology.* Vol. 1, 2nd ed. New York: McGraw-Hill; 1994:822–831.

Dyck PJ, Giannini C, Lars A. Pathologic alterations of the nerve. In: Dyck PJ, Thomas PK, eds. *Peripheral Neuropathy.* Philadelphia: Saunders; 1993:514–596.

REFERENCES

1. Copp AJ. Neural tube defects. *Trends Neurosci.* 1993;16:381–383.
2. Friede RL. *Developmental Neuropathology.* 2nd ed. Berlin: Springer-Verlag; 1989.
3. Caviness VS, Evrard P. Occipital encephalocele: a pathologic and anatomic analysis. *Acta Neuropathol.* 1975;32:245–255.
4. Naidich TP, McLone DG, Radkowski MA. Intracranial arachnoid cysts. *Pediatr Neurosci.* 1985;2:112–122.
5. Rengachary SS, Watanabe I, Brackett CE. Pathogenesis of intracranial arachnoid cyst. *Surg Neurol.* 1987;9:139–144.
6. von Wild K. Arachnoid cysts of the middle cranial fossa. *Neurochirurgia.* 1992;5:177–182.
7. Adams JH, Graham DI, Doyle D. *Brain Biopsy: The Smear Technique for Neurosurgical Biopsies.* Philadelphia: Lippincott; 1981.
8. Burger PC. Use of cytological preparations in the frozen section diagnosis of central nervous system neoplasia. *Am J Surg Pathol.* 1985;5:344–354.
9. Daumas-Duport C, Scheithauer BW, Kelly PJ. A histologic and cytologic method for the spatial definition of gliomas. *Mayo Clin Proc.* 1987;62.435–449.
10. Chandrasoma PT, Apuzzo MLJ. *Stereotactic Brain Biopsy.* New York: Igaku-Shoin; 1989.
11. Martinez AJ, Pollack I, Hall WA, Lunsford LD. Touch preparations in the rapid intraoperative diagnosis of central nervous system lesions. A comparison with frozen sections and paraffin-embedded sections. *Mod Pathol.* 1988;1:378–384.
12. Kleihues P, Burger PC, Scheithauer BW. *Histological Typing of Tumours of the Central Nervous System.* 2nd ed. Berlin: Springer-Verlag; 1993.
13. Kleihues P, Aguzzi A, Wiestler OD. Cellular and molecular aspects of neurocarcinogenesis. *Toxicol Pathol.* 1990;18:193–203.
14. Russell DS, Rubinstein LJ. *Pathology of Tumours of the Nervous System.* 5th ed. London: Edward Arnold; 1989.
15. Burger PC, Scheithauer BW, Vogel FS. *Surgical Pathology of the Nervous System and its Coverings.* 3rd ed. New York: Churchill Livingstone; 1991.
16. Burger PC, Scheithauer BW. Tumors of the central nervous system. In: *Atlas of Tumor Pathology.* 3rd Ser. Fascicle 10. Washington, DC: Armed Forces Institute of Pathology; 1994.
17. Bigner DD, Bigner SH, Pontn J, et al. Heterogeneity of genotypic and phenotypic characteristics of fifteen permanent cell lines derived from human gliomas. *J Neuropathol Exp Neurol.* 1981;40:201–229.
18. Jenkins RB, Kimmel DW, Moertel CA, et al. A cytogenetic study of 53 human gliomas. *Cancer Genet Cytogenet.* 1898;39:253–279.
19. Laws ER Jr, Taylor WF, Clifton MB, Okazaki H. Neurosurgical management of low-grade astrocytoma of the cerebral hemispheres. *J Neurosurg.* 1984;61:665–673.
20. Jay V, Parkinson D, Becker L, Chan FW. Cell kinetic analysis in pediatric brain and spinal tumors: a study of 117 cases with Ki-67 quantitation and flow cytometry. *Pediatr Pathol.* 1994;14:253–276.
21. Dropcho EJ, Wisoff JH, Walker RW, Allen JC. Supratentorial malignant gliomas in childhood: a review of fifty cases. *Ann Neurol.* 1987;22:355–364.
22. Georges PM, Noterman J, Flament-Durand J. Glioblastoma in childhood. *J Neuro-Oncol.* 1983;1:275–278.
23. Chandler KL, Prados MD, Malec M, Wilson CB. Long-term survival in patients with glioblastoma multiforme. *Neurosurgery* 1993;32:716–720.
24. Hayostek CJ, Shaw EG, Scheithauer B, et al. Astrocytomas of the cerebellum. A comparative clinicopathologic study of pilocytic and diffuse astrocytomas. *Cancer.* 1993;72:856–869.
25. Forsyth PA, Shaw EG, Scheithauer BW, et al. Supratentorial pilocytic astrocytomas. A clinicopathologic, prognostic and flow cytometric study of 51 patients. *Cancer.* 1993;72:1335–1342.
26. Minehan K, Scheithauer B, Shaw E, Onofrio B. Astrocytic tumors of the spinal cord (abstract). *J Neuropathol Exp Neurol.* 1993;52:289.
27. Tomlinson FH, Scheithauer BW, Hayostek CJ, et al. The significance of atypia and histologic malignancy in pilocytic astrocytoma of the cerebellum: a clinicopathologic and flow cytometric study. *J Child Neurol.* 1994;9:301–310.
28. Kepes JJ. Pleomorphic xanthoastrocytoma: the birth of a diagnosis and a concept. *Brain Pathol.* 1993;3:269–274.
29. Shepherd CW, Scheithauer BW, Gomez MR, et al. Subependymal giant cell astrocytoma: a clinical, pathological, and flow cytometric study. *Neurosurgery.* 1991;28:864–868.
30. Mørk SJ, Lindegaad K-F, Halvorsen TB, et al. Oligodendroglioma: incidence and biological behavior in a defined population. *J Neurosurg.* 1985;63:881–889.
31. Shaw EG, Scheithauer BW, O'Fallon JR, et al. Oligodendrogliomas: the Mayo Clinic experience. *J Neurosurg.* 1992;76:428–434.
32. Fortuna A, Celli P, Palma L. Oligodendrogliomas of the spinal cord. *Acta Neurochir.* 1980;52:305–329.
33. Huk WJ, Gademann G, Friedmann G. *Magnetic Resonance Imaging of the Central Nervous System Diseases.* Berlin: Springer-Verlag; 1990.
34. Kros JM, Van Eden CG, Stefanko SZ, et al. Prognostic implications of glial fibrillary acidic protein containing cell types in oligodendrogliomas. *Cancer.* 1990;66:1204–1212.
35. Cairncross JG, Macdonald DR, Ramsay DA. Aggressive oligodendroglioma: a chemosensitive tumor. *Neurosurgery.* 1992;31:78–82.
36. Slooff JL, Kernohan JW, MacCarty CS. *Primary Intramedullary Tumors of the Spinal Cord and Filum Terminale.* Philadelphia: Saunders; 1964.
37. Ross GW, Rubinstein LJ. Lack of histopathological correlation of malignant ependymomas with postoperative survival. *J Neurosurg.* 1989;70:31–36.
38. Schiffer D, Chi A, Giordana MT, et al. Histologic prognostic factors in ependymoma. *Child's Nervous System.* 1991;7:177–182.
39. Keating G, Scheithauer BW, Groover RV, et al. Pediatric ependymoma: the relation of histologic and flow cytometric parameters to prognosis. *Mod Pathol.* 1993;6(1):120A.
40. Sonneland PRL, Scheithauer BW, Onofrio BM. Myxopapillary ependymoma: clinicopathologic study and immunocytochemical study of 77 cases. *Cancer.* 1985;56:883–893.

41. Scheithauer BW. Symptomatic subependymoma: report of 21 cases with review of the literature. *J Neurosurg.* 1978;49:689–696.
42. Lombardi D, Scheithauer BW, Meyer FB, et al. Symptomatic subependymoma: a clinicopathological and flow cytometric study. *J Neurosurg.* 1991;75:583–588.
43. Zulch KJ. *Brain Tumors. Their Biology and Pathology.* 3rd ed. Berlin: Springer-Verlag; 1986.
44. Tomlinson FH, Scheithauer BW, Meyer FB, et al. Medulloblastoma. I. Clinical, diagnostic, and therapeutic overview. *J Child Neurol.* 1992;7:142–155.
45. Kleihues P, Aguzzi A, Shibata T, Wiestler OD. Immunohistochemical assessment of differentiation and DNA replication in human brain tumors. In: Fields WS, ed. *Primary Brain Tumors. A Review of Histologic Classification.* New York: Springer-Verlag; 1989:123–132.
46. Katsetos CD, Herman MM, Frankfurter A, et al. Cerebellar desmoplastic medulloblastomas. A further immunohistochemical characterization of the reticulin-free pale islands. *Arch Pathol Lab Med.* 1989;113:1019–1029.
47. Giangaspero F, Rigobello L, Badiali M, et al. Large-cell medulloblastomas. A distinct variant with highly aggressive behavior. *Am J Surg Pathol.* 1992;16:687–693.
48. Kepes JJ. *Meningiomas. Biology, Pathology, and Differential Diagnosis.* New York: Masson; 1982.
49. Nakasu S, Hirano A, Shimura T, Llena JF. Incidental meningiomas in autopsy study. *Surg Neurol.* 1987;27:319–322.
50. Scheithauer BW. Tumors of the meninges: proposed modifications of the World Health Organization classification. *Acta Neuropathol.* 1990;80:343–354.
51. Zorludemir S, Scheithauer BW, Hirose T, et al. Clear cell meningioma: a clinicopathologic study of a potentially aggressive variant of meningioma. *Am J Surg Pathol.* 1995;19(5):493–505.
52. Ludwin SK, Rubinstein LJ, Russell DS. Papillary meningioma: a malignant variant of meningioma. *Cancer.* 1975;36:1363–1373.
53. Pasquier B, Gasnier F, Pasquier B, et al. Papillary meningioma. Clinicopathologic study of 7 cases and review of the literature. *Cancer.* 1986;58(2):299–305.
54. Giang DW, Posuri KR, Eskin TA, et al. Multiple sclerosis masquerading as a mass lesion. *Neuroradiology.* 1992;34:150–154.
55. Zagzag D, Miller DC, Kleinman GM, et al. Demyelinating disease versus tumor in surgical neuropathology. *Am J Surg Pathol.* 1993;17:537–545.
56. Cheng TM, O'Neill BP, Scheithauer BW, Piepgras DG. Chronic meningitis and the role of meningeal or cortical biopsy. *Neurosurgery.* 1994;34(4):590–596.
57. Ducatman BS, Scheithauer BW, Piepgras DG, et al. Malignant peripheral nerve sheath tumors. A clinicopathological study of 120 cases. *Cancer.* 1986;57:2006–2021.
58. Wanebo JE, Malik JM, VandenBerg SR, et al. Malignant peripheral nerve sheath tumors. A clinicopathologic study of 28 cases. *Cancer.* 1993;71:1247–1253.
59. Matsui I, Tanimura M, Kobayashi N, et al. Neurofibromatosis type 1 and childhood cancer. *Cancer.* 1993;72:2746–2754.
60. Ducatman BS, Scheithauer BW. Malignant peripheral nerve sheath tumors with divergent differentiation. *Cancer.* 1984;54:1049–1057.
61. Dyck PJ, Giannini C, Lars A. Pathologic alterations of the nerve. In: Dyck PJ, Thomas PK, eds. *Peripheral Neuropathy.* Philadelphia: Saunders; 1993:514–596.
62. Cumming WJK, Fulthorpe JJ, Hudgson P, Mahon M. *Color Atlas of Muscle Pathology.* London: Mosby-Wolfe; 1994.
63. Engel AG. The muscle biopsy. In: Engel AG, Franzini-Armstrong C, eds. *Myology.* Vol 1. 2nd ed. New York: McGraw-Hill; 1994:822–831.
64. Kleihues P, Burger PC, Scheithauer BW. *Histological Typing of Tumours of the Central Nervous System,* 2nd ed. New York: Springer-Verlag; 1993.
65. Daumas-Duport C, Scheithauer B, O'Fallon J, Kelly P. Grading of astrocytomas: A simple and reproducible grading method. *Cancer* 1988;62:2152–2165.
66. Ringertz N. Grading of gliomas. *Acta Pathol Microbiol Scand.* 1950;27:51–64.

9

Endocrine Pathology

Martha A. Zeiger and Ralph H. Hruban

Definition

Communication between surgeon and pathologist is essential for the proper management of patients with endocrine neoplasms. The questions posed to the pathologist include the following: (1) Does the cytology or pathology specimen show endocrine tissue? (2) If so, does the tissue represent hyperplasia, adenoma, or carcinoma? and (3) In the case of a metastatic endocrine tumor with an unknown primary, can the primary endocrine tumor be identified by clinical, biochemical, microscopic, or immunocytochemical methods? These decisions arise at various points during patient care, particularly after fine needle aspiration biopsy (FNAB); intraoperatively, at the time of frozen section; and during final pathologic evaluation of permanent sections. Each crucial surgical decision depends upon the accurate interchange of information between the pathologist and the surgeon.

This chapter addresses the cytologic, frozen section, and final pathologic analyses of thyroid, parathyroid, and adrenal neoplasms. Our intent is to strengthen the surgeon's insight into pathology in order to facilitate surgical decision making.

Thyroid Pathology

THYROID NODULE

Three issues are addressed during the evaluation of a patient with a thyroid nodule. First, what is the likelihood that the nodule is malignant? Second, if it is malignant, what is its microscopic type? Third, does the patient have evidence of metastatic spread? Fortunately, only about 5 to 10% of thyroid nodules are malignant, and the majority of these are localized to the thyroid gland.[1]

Clinical history is crucial in the patient with a thyroid nodule and should be directed at determining risk factors for thyroid malignancy. For example, a history of radiation therapy to the neck for tonsillar or thymic enlargement or for acne should be elicited. Similarly, patients with a family history of multiple endocrine neoplasia (MEN) type IIa or IIb (Table 9–1), or a family history of medullary carcinoma of the thyroid (MCT) are at increased risk for developing MCT. Finally, the clinician must suspect a thyroid malignancy in patients with hoarseness, respiratory stridor, dyspnea, or a rapidly growing thyroid mass. Such relevant clinical findings should be shared with the pathologist.

FINE NEEDLE ASPIRATION BIOPSY

Although thyroid nodules are evaluated by other techniques, including ultrasound, thyroid scan, and thyroid

Table 9–1. Multiple Endocrine Neoplasia Syndromes

Type I	Pituitary adenoma Hyperparathyroidism Pancreatic islet cell tumors
Type IIA	Hyperparathyroidism Medullary carcinoma of the thyroid Pheochromocytoma
Type IIB	Hyperparathyroidism Medullary carcinoma of the thyroid Pheochromocytoma Mucosal neuromas and ganglioneuromas Marfanoid habitus

function tests, fine needle aspiration (FNA) biopsy has emerged as the favored primary diagnostic modality for thyroid nodules.[2–5] Surgeons rely on this method for convenient preoperative screening of patients with suspect clinical findings. All cellular aspiration material should be evaluated by a cytopathologist, whether the lesion is cystic or solid. The technique for FNA of the thyroid is addressed in more detail in Chapter 3.

The results of FNA are divided into four categories: (1) *benign or negative,* including colloid, cyst, or thyroiditis; (2) *suspect or indeterminate,* including Hürthle cell, follicular neoplasm, or findings suggestive of malignancy; (3) *malignant or positive,* including papillary, medullary, or anaplastic thyroid cancer, metastatic carcinoma, or lymphoma; and, finally, (4) *unsatisfactory* for cytopathologic evaluation.[4] Patients with benign or negative cytology and a benign clinical picture do not need surgery and may be followed with serial physical examinations. Malignant or suspicious FNA cytology results require that the patient undergo definitive surgery. One caveat, however, is that patients with cytology suspicious for lymphoma or anaplastic thyroid cancer need an incisional thyroid biopsy for diagnosis. When either lymphoma or anaplastic carcinoma is confirmed, the patients receive chemotherapy or radiation therapy, respectively. Similarly, if the FNA shows metastatic carcinoma, treatment of the primary tumor must be addressed. If the FNA is unsatisfactory, a second aspiration should be obtained for more definitive cytopathology. Cystic lesions can yield false-negative results on FNA, and recurrent cyst fluid accumulation may indicate need for thyroid resection. De los Santos and colleagues reported on 221 patients with FNA of the thyroid nodule, and the only false-negative FNA cytology occurred in a single case with a cystic lesion.[6]

A collective review of more than 18,000 FNA specimens showed an average rate of 69% benign aspiration results, 3.5% malignant, 10% suspect, and 17% nondiagnostic.[4] The false-negative rate was 1 to 11%; the false-positive

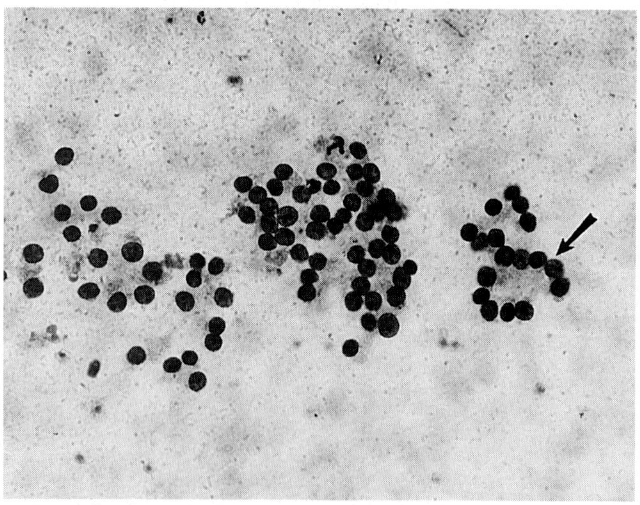

Figure 9–1. Cytology of a follicular neoplasm of the thyroid. As is typical for follicular neoplasms, the cells in this follicular adenoma form a small follicle *(arrow).* The nuclei do not overlap and contain uniform chromatin. Distinction from well-differentiated follicular carcinoma is not possible on the basis of such preparations.

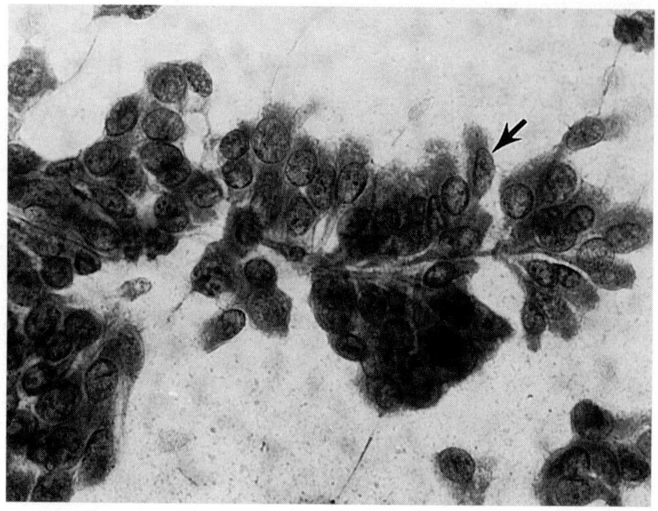

Figure 9–2. Cytology of a papillary carcinoma of the thyroid. Note the papillary architecture of the tissue fragment, the overlapping nuclei, and the nuclear grooves *(arrow)* in this Papanicolaou-stained preparation.

rate, 1 to 8%. Of those patients who required operations (i.e., those with either malignant or suspect cytopathology), 32% later proved to have a thyroid malignancy. Of greater concern, however, is the possibility of missing a thyroid malignancy because of a false-negative FNA. However, in a study by Grant et al. of 439 patients with benign cytopathology, only 0.7% developed thyroid cancer after an average follow-up of 6.1 years.[7]

The evaluation of FNAs of the thyroid should include both cytologic slides (smears) and histologic preparations (cell block sections). The diagnostic accuracy of FNA is excellent for papillary, anaplastic, and medullary carcinomas (Figs. 9–1 and 9–2). However, because the diagnosis of follicular carcinoma is based on noncytologic criteria (capsular invasion and vascular invasion), FNAs of follicular lesions are inconsistent predictors of malignancy (Figs. 9–1, 9–3 to 9–5).

Papillary carcinomas of the thyroid have distinct cyto-

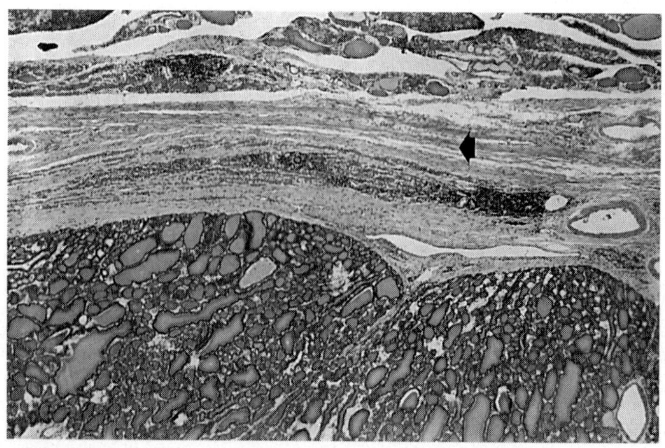

Figure 9–3. Follicular adenoma of the thyroid. This adenoma *(bottom)* is entirely separated from adjacent normal thyroid *(top)* by a complete capsule *(arrow).*

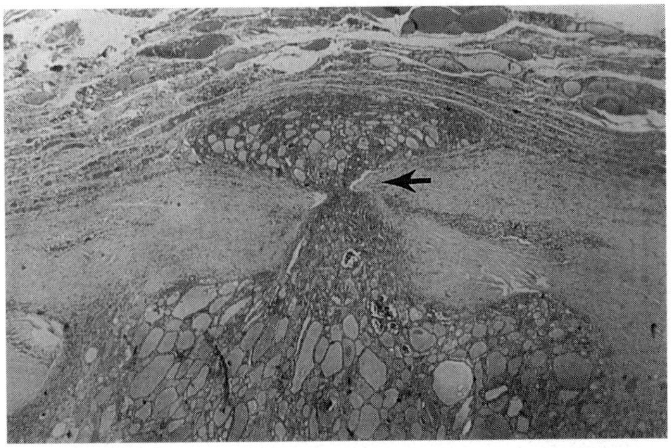

Figure 9–4. Transcapsular penetration *(arrow)* in a follicular carcinoma of the thyroid. The presence of transcapsular penetration in a follicular neoplasm is diagnostic of a carcinoma.

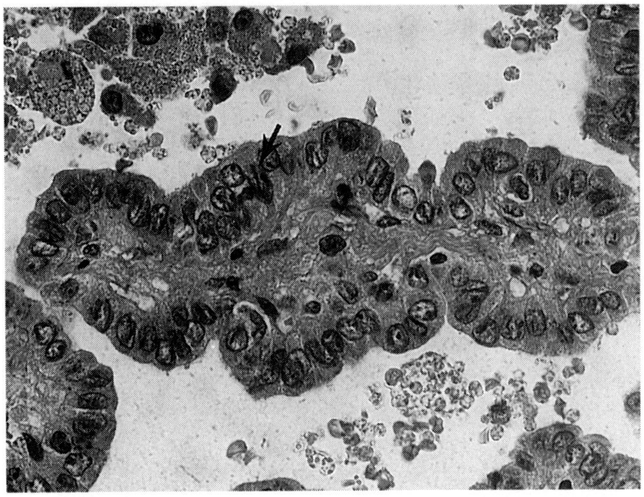

Figure 9–6. Papillary carcinoma of the thyroid. Note the overlapping optically clear nuclei with nuclear grooves *(arrow)* as well as the tumor papillary architecture.

logic features that are easily recognized on FNA (Figs. 9–2, 9–6, and 9–7). These include papillary fronds, psammoma bodies, and characteristic nuclear features. The nuclei of papillary carcinomas are clear, with finely dispersed chromatin; they tend to overlap and often contain nuclear grooves or intranuclear cytoplasmic inclusions. In contrast, the cytologic features of *medullary carcinoma* are variable. Aspirates from medullary carcinomas often show single cells or small groups of spindle-shaped cells. The nuclei may be uniform or show marked pleomorphism. Clumps of extracellular amyloid, when present, support the diagnosis of medullary carcinoma (Fig. 9–8). Because of its variable appearance on FNA, immunohistochemical staining for calcitonin is often necessary to establish the diagnosis of a medullary carcinoma (Figs. 9–8 to 9–11).

Interpretation of *follicular neoplasms* by FNA is more problematic, and the surgeon must accept the inherent limitations of cytologic evaluation of these neoplasms. Because the diagnosis of follicular carcinoma rests on transcapsular and vascular invasion, FNA biopsy from the center of a follicular neoplasm is not sensitive for diagnosing follicular carcinoma; however, useful information can be gleaned. Follicular carcinomas often have a solid, microfollicular, or trabecular growth pattern and, if seen on FNA, these architectural patterns should raise concerns. Only occasionally do higher-grade follicular carcinomas manifest cytologic atypia and abundant mitotic figures. By contrast, FNA of a ''goiter'' or a colloid nodule usually yields well-formed macrofollicles; therefore, aspirates showing macrofollicles are more likely to be benign. Despite these generalities, FNA evaluation of follicular lesions rarely distinguishes between a benign and a malignant neoplasm; surgery is usually required for definitive diagnosis (see Figs. 9–1 and 9–3 to 9–5).[8]

Just as FNA of a thyroid nodule is useful *within the confines of its limitations,* so too is the *intraoperative frozen section.* If the surgeon recognizes the limitations of utilizing a frozen section diagnosis, it can be a useful

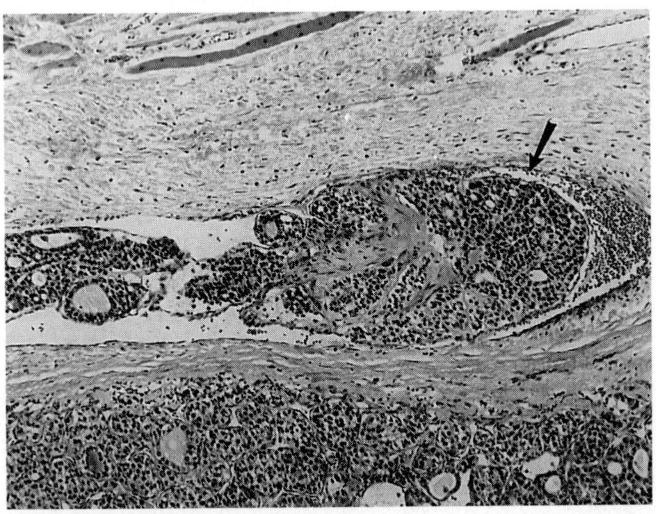

Figure 9–5. Vascular invasion *(arrow)* in a follicular carcinoma of the thyroid. The presence of vascular invasion in a follicular neoplasm is diagnostic of a carcinoma.

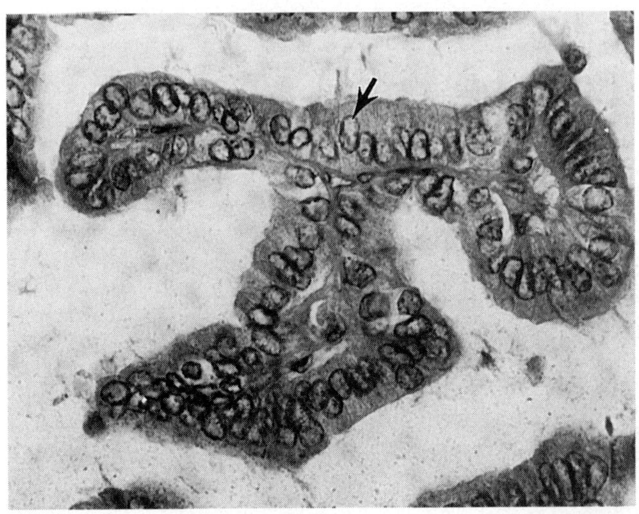

Figure 9–7. Papillary carcinoma of the thyroid. Nuclear clearing *(arrow)* is prominent in this case.

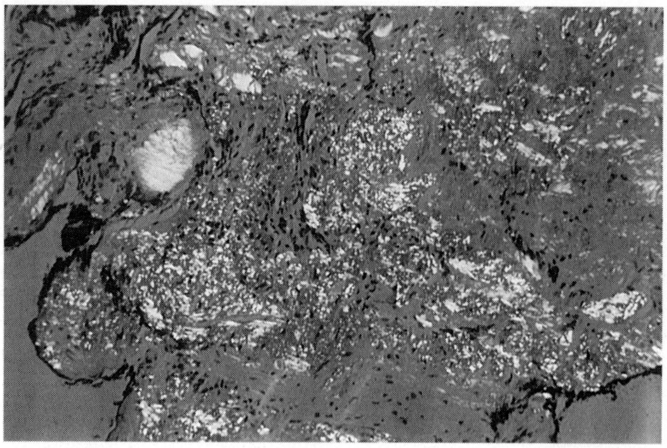

Figure 9–8. Amyloid in a medullary carcinoma of the thyroid. This section has been stained with the Congo Red stain and then polarized. Note the characteristic apple-green birefringence of amyloid, appearing white in this photomicrograph.

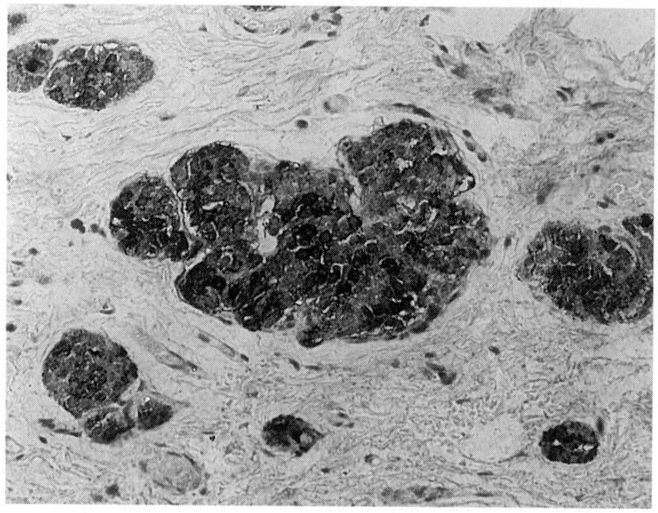

Figure 9–10. Immunohistochemical stain for calcitonin in a primary medullary carcinoma. Note the intense cytoplasmic staining, indicating the expression of calcitonin by the neoplastic cells.

technique. There are *two main limitations* of frozen section diagnosis: first, *distinguishing a follicular adenoma from a follicular carcinoma* (see Figs. 9–3 to 9–5) and, second, *distinguishing a follicular neoplasm from the follicular variant of papillary carcinoma* (Fig. 9–12). Follicular carcinomas are distinguished from follicular adenomas by the presence of transcapsular penetration and vascular invasion. A *follicular carcinoma* cannot be ruled out until the entire capsule is examined microscopically. Because it is neither practical nor reliable to examine an entire lesion microscopically at the time of frozen section, the probability of a false-negative frozen section interpretation cannot be eliminated. Even after careful intraoperative microscopic examination, *microscopic foci of transcapsular or vascular invasion will sometimes be identified in permanent sections.* Surgeons must be aware of these limitations while planning the postoperative management of patients.

Similarly, the follicular variant of papillary carcinoma can be difficult to recognize on frozen sections (see Fig. 9–12).[9] This neoplasm has a predominantly follicular architecture and can closely mimic follicular carcinomas in frozen section; however, cellular features disclose its true nature: optically clear nuclei with intranuclear inclusions and nuclear grooves. Unfortunately, these nuclear features are largely dependent on artifacts of fixation and are not present in frozen sections. Although the follicular variant of papillary carcinoma is difficult to diagnose on frozen section, this mistake can be avoided if the results of the frozen section and the FNA are integrated. *A lesion with follicular architecture on frozen section and papillary nuclei on FNA is most likely a follicular variant of papillary carcinoma* (compare Figs. 9–2 with 9–12).

In summary, based upon FNA biopsy, the patient should undergo surgery if the cytology is positive or suspicious for ''follicular neoplasm'' or papillary or medullary carcinoma. In a series of 641 patients reported by Grant et al., all FNA biopsies interpreted as diagnostic for malignancy

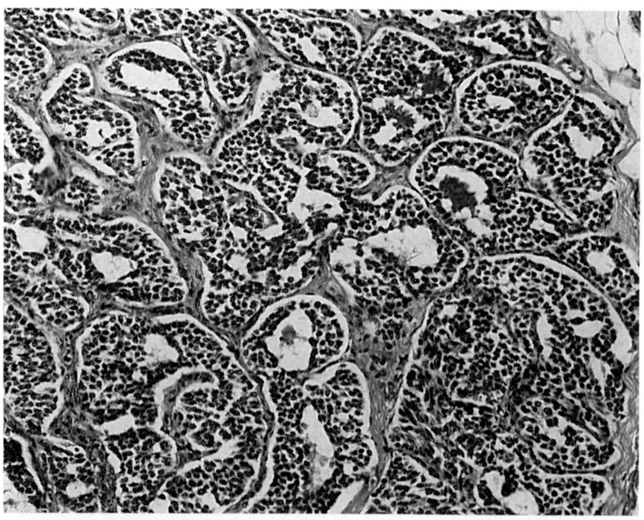

Figure 9–9. Medullary carcinoma of the thyroid. The neoplastic cells form prominent nests in this case. Most of the cells are rather uniform, but focal spindling is present.

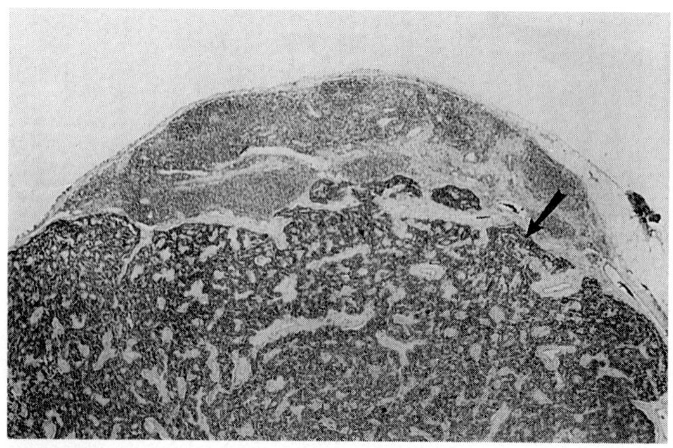

Figure 9–11. Immunohistochemical stain for calcitonin in a metastatic medullary carcinoma. Notice how intensely the metastasis stains *(bottom half, arrow)* compared with the absence of staining in the residual nonneoplastic lymphoid tissue *(top third).*

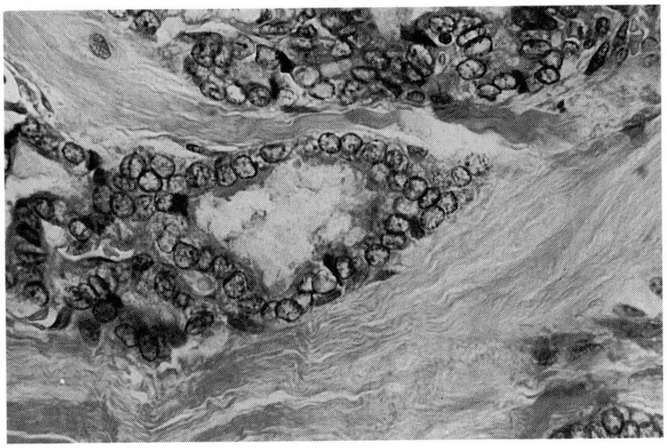

Figure 9–12. Follicular variant of papillary carcinoma of the thyroid. Note how the nuclear features in this carcinoma are similar to those seen in the papillary carcinoma illustrated in Figure 9–7.

proved to be malignant thyroid tumors, whereas 23% of patients with suspicious FNA and less than 1% of patients with benign FNA were found to harbor malignancy. Three percent of patients with an unsatisfactory FNA proved to actually have a malignancy.[7]

Although TNM staging for thyroid carcinomas exists, most authors use histology, patient age, sex, size of the lesion, extent of tumor invasion, and lymph node involvement as determinants for the surgical procedure—unilateral lobectomy or near-total, subtotal, or total thyroidectomy. Medullary carcinoma of thyroid requires, at a minimum, total thyroidectomy and central compartmental lymph node dissection.[10] Bilateral or ipsilateral modified radical neck dissection should also be considered in a patient with clinically positive lymph nodes.[11, 12] Follicular and papillary carcinomas require unilateral lobectomy, unilateral lobectomy on the side of the lesion and a contralateral near-total lobectomy, or a total thyroidectomy. The procedure used depends on (1) the surgeon's treatment bias regarding unilateral versus bilateral thyroid lobectomy for well-differentiated thyroid cancer, (2) the age and sex of the patient, (3) tumor type and size, and (4) among follicular cancers, the extent of capsular invasion.[13–23] A problem arises when frozen sections reveal a well-encapsulated follicular neoplasm but permanent sections show a follicular carcinoma. Controversy exists over the indication for completion thyroidectomy in these patients.[13, 14, 19, 21–23] Optimum treatment for thyroid carcinoma (unilateral lobectomy versus total thyroidectomy) is unresolved and should prompt further reading.[16–23]

Parathyroid Pathology

Patients undergo surgery for primary, secondary, or tertiary hyperparathyroidism and, rarely, for parathyroid carcinoma. Patients with primary hyperparathyroidism have elevated parathyroid hormone (PTH) levels in the face of hypercalcemia. Approximately 80% of patients with primary hyperparathyroidism harbor a parathyroid adenoma, 20% have parathyroid hyperplasia, and less than 1% have a parathyroid carcinoma.[10] Only a very small percentage of patients have multiple parathyroid adenomas.[24] Hyperparathyroidism in patients with chronic renal failure is usually due to secondary hyperparathyroidism, whereas patients with functioning kidney transplants and hyperparathyroidism usually have so-called tertiary hyperparathyroidism.[10] This represents parathyroid hyperfunction originally induced by renal failure that has subsequently become autonomous. Patients who have marked hypercalcemia, palpable neck mass, symptoms secondary to hypercalcemia, and no evidence of metastatic disease should be suspected of having parathyroid carcinoma.

Intraoperative interchange between surgeon and pathologist is essential for distinguishing between parathyroid adenoma and parathyroid hyperplasia. Ideally, the surgeon should identify all four glands and the adenoma or adenomas should be removed or, in the case of hyperplasia, all but the equivalent of a normal-sized parathyroid gland (approximately 30 to 40 mg) should be removed. This remnant may be left in situ on a well-vascularized pedicle or transplanted to the sternocleidomastoid or brachioradialis muscle.[25, 26] The pathologist's intraoperative responsibility is to determine whether or not the biopsied tissue is parathyroid tissue. It is the *role of the surgeon to determine whether the patient has evidence of hyperplasia, with all four glands appearing abnormally enlarged, or whether the patient harbors one or more adenomas.* The surgeon also plays a central role in the diagnosis of parathyroid carcinoma by reporting the invasive nature of a lesion to the pathologist. If such is the case, the patient requires removal of all tumor-bearing tissue, including lymph nodes.[27–30]

Generally, the sequence of the operation for hyperparathyroidism is as follows. Unless a parathyroid adenoma has been localized preoperatively, one side of the neck is first explored. If an adenoma is located on that side, it is removed and sent to pathology for frozen section confirmation. The second parathyroid gland on that side is then located. If the second gland appears normal, a small biopsy is obtained to confirm that it is parathyroid. The opposite side of the neck is then explored for evidence of a second adenoma. The two remaining parathyroids are visualized to confirm that they are of normal size, but they are not biopsied. If more than one of the glands appears abnormally large, the surgeon must suspect parathyroid hyperplasia. In this case, all but 30 to 40 mg of parathyroid tissue from one gland is removed. The decision to leave parathyroid tissue within the neck and mark it with a hemoclip or to transplant the tissue into the forearm depends upon whether or not the patient has MEN or is undergoing a repeated operation (see Table 9–1).[25, 26] In general, if the patient has a history of MEN or if the procedure is being repeated for hyperplasia, the parathyroid remnant should be transplanted to the forearm for easier patient management and follow-up.[25, 26]

Parathyroid adenomas are clonal neoplasms that result in single gland enlargement.[31] For the pathologist, the distinction between adenoma and hyperplasia is frequently very difficult to make. Ideally, adenomas are well encapsulated and are composed of chief or oxyphil cells arranged in sheets or nests, devoid of fat (Figs. 9–13 and 9–14).

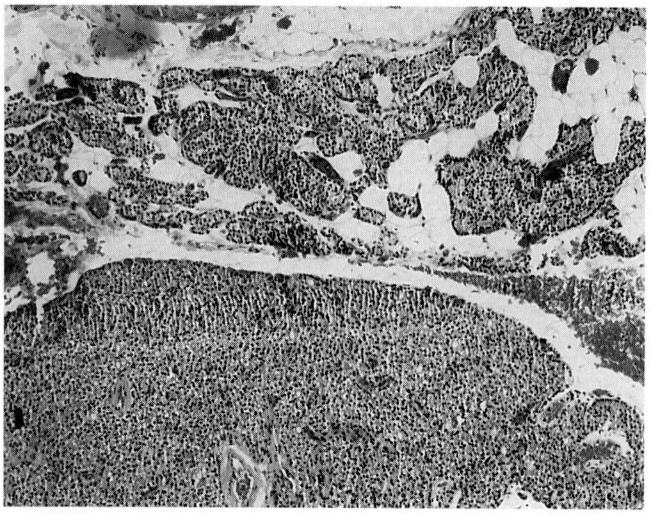

Figure 9–13. Parathyroid adenoma. The absence of fat in the adenoma *(bottom half)* separates it from the residual normal parathyroid *(top half).*

They range from 300 mg to several grams. Another helpful clue for diagnosis of adenoma is the presence of a thin rim of residual normal, fatty parathyroid tissue. Unfortunately, this feature can seldom be identified.

In contrast, parathyroid hyperplasia shows enlargement of all four glands. Hyperplastic glands usually lack the capsules of adenomas and typically retain more fat than do adenomas. Nonetheless, it is often extremely difficult to distinguish parathyroid hyperplasia from parathyroid adenoma purely by microscopic criteria. It is therefore very helpful for the surgeon to sample one normal-appearing gland in addition to any apparent adenomas.[32–36]

Parathyroid carcinomas can also be difficult to distinguish from adenomas on microscopic grounds alone, but clinical and pathologic clues can help distinguish these two entities. Parathyroid carcinomas are aggressive neoplasms that infiltrate adjacent connective tissues and other structures. It is therefore important that the surgeon tell the pathologist if a parathyroid neoplasm is adherent to adjacent structures. Microscopically, parathyroid carcinomas are recognized by their trabecular (ribbonlike) architecture, with fibrous bands, vascular invasion, and mitotic figures.

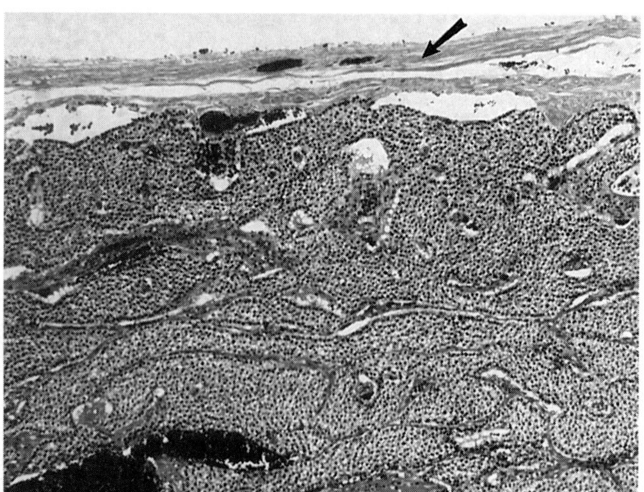

Figure 9–14. Parathyroid adenoma. This adenoma is well encapsulated *(arrow).*

Adrenal Pathology

The indications for adrenalectomy include benign nonfunctioning adrenal tumors (''incidentalomas'') greater than 4 cm; primary bilateral adrenocortical hyperplasia; functioning adrenal tumors, such as pheochromocytomas; aldosteronomas; adrenal tumors causing Cushing's syndrome; and, finally, adrenocortical carcinomas and malignant pheochromocytomas.

The advent of high-resolution radiologic imaging has vastly increased detection of clinically unsuspected adrenal tumors, or so-called incidentalomas. If serum and urinary corticosteroids/catecholamine levels are normal and the tumor is less than 4 to 5 cm in size, the patient may safely be followed by serial computed tomography (CT) scans. If one suspects metastatic disease based upon the patient's history, one may then obtain a CT-guided needle aspiration for confirmation. Any tumor that is larger than 4 to 5 cm or is hormone-secreting warrants surgical excision.

ADRENAL ADENOMA VERSUS HYPERPLASIA VERSUS CARCINOMA

Difficulty in distinguishing hyperplasia from adenoma, and adenoma from carcinoma, is a common problem in endocrine surgery. The adrenal gland is no exception. The differential diagnosis of primary hyperaldosteronism and primary hypercortisolism (Cushing's syndrome) is particularly common. The distinction between aldosterone-producing adenoma and hyperaldosteronism due to bilateral adrenocortical hyperplasia can be particularly difficult, since a nonfunctioning adenoma may accompany bilateral hyperplasia.[37–39] And unless the patient presents with a large invasive adrenal tumor or with metastatic disease, establishing the diagnosis of aldosterone-producing adrenal carcinoma may also be extremely difficult.

In general, elevated serum aldosterone levels with low serum renin levels and hypokalemia will help to confirm the diagnosis of primary hyperaldosteronism. The differentiation between adenoma (''aldosteronoma'') and bilateral adrenocortical hyperplasia is best made by postural response studies.[38] A CT scan will identify an adenoma, and surgery should be directed at the side with the adenoma if confirmed by postural studies. Other localization studies include ^{131}I-6 β-iodomethylnorcholesterol (NP-59) scan or adrenal vein venous sampling for serum aldosterone.[39]

Differential diagnostic evaluation for primary hypercortisolism is similar to that for primary hyperaldosteronism.[37] The differential diagnosis for *primary adrenal* causes of Cushing's syndrome includes glucocorticoid-producing adrenal adenoma and bilateral adrenocortical hyperplasia. If biochemical studies show elevated 24-hour urinary free cortisol levels, low plasma ACTH, and failure to suppress cortisol levels with high-dose dexamethasone, a CT scan is used to differentiate between an adenoma and primary bilateral adrenocortical hyperplasia.[37] Once again, however, a nonfunctioning adenoma may exist in the presence of bilateral hyperplasia.[37] The iodocholesterol scan may also help by showing either unilateral (adenoma) or bilateral uptake (adrenocortical hyperplasia).[37] After the diagnosis has been made and the appropriate surgery accomplished (unilateral versus bilateral adrenalectomy), microscopic confirmation is the pathologist's responsibility.

Primary adrenal neoplasms originate in cortex (adenoma, carcinoma) or in medulla (pheochromocytoma, neuroblastoma). Adrenal cortical adenomas may be either functional or nonfunctional clinically. They are usually solitary and encapsulated and they tend to compress surrounding adrenal tissue, with resulting atrophy. By contrast, hyperplastic adrenal cortical nodules are poorly defined, unencapsulated, and often multiple. The majority of adenomas are yellow and weigh less than 100 g. They are composed of either clear lipid-containing cells (Cushing's syndrome, hyperaldosteronism) or eosinophilic cells (feminizing or virilizing syndromes). Even though they are benign, adenomas may exhibit bizarre-appearing cells microscopically, with large pleomorphic nuclei. Unfortunately, no single feature can be used to separate adrenal adenomas from adrenocortical carcinomas. Cumulative experience associates the following features with malignancy: weight greater than 100 g, mitotic counts greater than 60 per 50 high-power fields, bizarre mitoses, and vascular invasion.[40–43] Multiple-parameter scoring systems are therefore useful for predicting outcome.

MALIGNANT VERSUS BENIGN PHEOCHROMOCYTOMA

Pheochromocytomas are adrenal medullary neoplasms that are capable of synthesizing and secreting catecholamines. These mediators are responsible for the patient's presenting symptoms: hypertension, palpitations, sweating, headaches, and paroxysmal attacks. Extraadrenal pheochromocytomas, or paragangliomas, are found anywhere from the base of the skull to the lower genitourinary tract, including the aortic bifurcation (organ of Zuckerkandl), bladder, mediastinum, and heart as well as carotid and glomus jugular bodies. Pheochromocytomas follow the "10% rule": 10% are familial, 10% malignant, 10% extra-adrenal, 10% multifocal, and 10% arise in children.[44]

The preoperative evaluation of the patient includes either 24-hour levels of urinary norepinephrine, epinephrine, dopamine, total metanephrines, and vanillylmandelic acid or the clonidine suppression test. This is followed by localization studies, including CT or magnetic resonance imaging (MRI) scans, or preferably, a ^{131}I-metaiodobenzylguanidine (^{131}I-MIBG) scan.[45] Preoperatively, the patient should be managed pharmacologically with both alpha- and beta-adrenergic receptor blockade.

Pheochromocytoma can be multifocal. Therefore, unless the pheochromocytoma is metastatic or is locally invasive, differentiating between malignant and benign conditions is a challenge. Final pathologic differentiation is often determined by the patient's postoperative course. Intraoperatively, therefore, the surgeon should remove all grossly evident disease and avoid tumor spillage.[45]

Pathologically, pheochromocytomas are rare neoplasms of the adrenal medulla related embryologically to paragangliomas. Grossly, pheochromocytomas are well-circumscribed, large (3 to 5 cm), and gray to dark red on fresh-cut section. Pheochromocytomas can show a variety of microscopic growth patterns, including trabecular, nesting, and diffuse patterns. As is the case with adrenal cortical neoplasms, it can be difficult to diagnose malignancy in a pheochromocytoma. Features favoring malignancy include large size (greater than 700 g), extraadrenal location, extensive necrosis, numerous mitoses (greater than 1 per 10 high-power fields), and vascular invasion.

Immunohistochemical Stains for Endocrine Tumors

On occasion, a patient will present to the surgeon with a metastatic endocrine tumor of unknown primary or with a tumor suspected to be a metastasis from a known-site-of-origin endocrine tumor (Fig. 9–15). Identification of the lesion's origin can often be achieved by immunocytochemical staining.

The development of monoclonal and polyclonal antibodies for immunohistochemical staining has had a major impact on the practice of endocrine pathology (see Chap. 2). The three main uses for immunohistochemistry in endocrine pathology are (1) to demonstrate neuroendocrine differentiation in a poorly differentiated neoplasm that is otherwise hard to classify, (2) to determine the specific tissue type of origin of a neuroendocrine tumor, and (3) to provide prognostic information.

Three immunohistochemical stains are commonly employed: chromogranins, synaptophysin, and neuron-specific enolase (NSE). The *chromogranins* are a family of acidic polypeptides that probably function as carrier proteins in

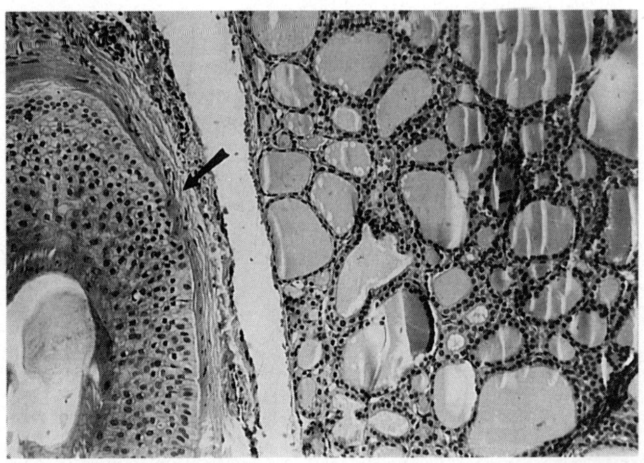

Figure 9–15. Metastatic follicular carcinoma of the thyroid. This follicular carcinoma metastasized to the scalp. A hair follicle is present on the left *(arrow)* and the follicular cancer is on the right. Even in this metastasis, the microscopic characteristics of the follicles are not overtly malignant.

neurosecretory granules. For this reason, they are very sensitive markers for neuroendocrine differentiation[46–47] and are expressed in a diversity of neoplasms, including islet cell tumors, pheochromocytomas, pituitary adenomas, parathyroid adenomas, and carcinoid tumors. Similarly, the expression of *synaptophysin,* an acidic transmembrane glycoprotein, is also a relatively sensitive and specific marker of neuroendocrine differentiation.[48] Neuron-specific enolase is an enzyme expressed in a variety of endocrine neoplasms, but, unfortunately, most commercially available antibodies to NSE lack the sensitivity necessary for them to be useful.[48] Furthermore, despite its name, expression of this enzyme is not entirely specific to neuroendocrine differentiation.

A wide variety of immunohistochemical stains is currently available for demonstration of the cell of origin (direction of differentiation) of a neuroendocrine neoplasm. Whereas a detailed discussion of all of these is beyond the scope of this chapter, several of the thyroid markers deserve note. *Thyroglobulin* is expressed by normal follicular cells of the thyroid and by most neoplasms derived from follicular cells.[8] Although not all follicular carcinomas express this marker, its presence in a metastatic carcinoma strongly suggests origin from follicular cells of the thyroid.[8,49] Similarly, the expression of *calcitonin* can demonstrate C-cell origin of a neoplasm[50,51] (see Figs. 9–10 and 9–11). Not only does calcitonin expression demonstrate a medullary carcinoma but the intensity of the staining can help to predict its behavior[52]: heavy staining correlates with an indolent course.[51,52]

In summary, immunohistochemical staining is an integral part of the endocrine pathologist's armamentarium. In addition to the uses described, the method is used to confirm neuroendocrine differentiation of a metastatic neuroendocrine carcinoma as well as to provide prognostic information for patients with these tumors.

PITFALLS FOR THE SURGEON

1. Expecting the pathologist to distinguish benign versus malignant follicular neoplasm of the thyroid by either FNA or intraoperative frozen sections.
2. Assuming that a thyroid neoplasm with follicular appearance at intraoperative frozen section is follicular and not papillary carcinoma, as anticipated by FNA, since papillary thyroid carcinomas often have a considerable or even predominant follicular architecture.
3. Insisting that the pathologist distinguish between parathyroid adenoma and hyperplasia on the basis of sampling only one enlarged gland. This decision should be made by the surgeon, based upon identification and biopsy of more than one gland.
4. Failing to resect a pheochromocytoma in its entirety based upon intraoperative surgical and pathologic findings suggesting that it is benign. Such tumors are occasionally capable of malignant (metastatic) behavior.

PITFALLS FOR THE PATHOLOGIST

1. Relying on cytologic atypia rather than capsular or vascular invasion as a criterion to distinguish benign from malignant follicular thyroid tumors.
2. Relying on papillary versus follicular organization of a thyroid carcinoma to classify it rather than on the cytologic features that characterize papillary carcinoma.
3. Using cellular pleomorphism as a criterion for diagnosing endocrine tumors as malignant when this is often not helpful (e.g., thyroid adenomas, adrenal cortical adenomas, pheochromocytomas).

FURTHER READING

Gharib H, Goellner J. Fine-needle aspiration biopsy of the thyroid: an appraisal. *Ann Intern Med.* 1993;118:282–289.

LiVolsi VA. *Surgical Pathology of the Thyroid.* Philadelphia: Saunders; 1990.

Lowhagen T, Willems J, Lundell G, et al. Aspiration biopsy cytology in diagnosis of thyroid cancer. *World J Surg.* 1981;5:61.

Mazzaferri E. Management of a solitary thyroid nodule. *N Engl J Med.* 1993;328:553–559.

Mendelsohn G, Wells SA, Baylin SB. Relationship of tissue carcinoembryonic antigen and calcitonin to tumor virulence in medullary thyroid carcinoma: An immunohistochemical study in early, localized and virulent disseminated stages of disease. *Cancer.* 1984;54:657.

Tielens ET, Sherman SI, Hruban RH, et al. Follicular variant of papillary thyroid carcinoma: A clinicopathologic study. *Cancer.* 1994;73:424.

Uribe M, Grimes M, Fenoglio-Preiser C, et al. Medullary carcinoma of the thyroid gland: Clinical, pathological and immunohistochemical features with review of the literature. *Am J Surg Pathol.* 1985;9:577.

Wang C. The anatomic basis of parathyroid surgery. *Ann Surg.* 1976;183:271–275.

Weiss L, Medeiros L, Vickery A. Pathologic features of prognostic significance in adrenocortical carcinoma. *Am J Surg Pathol.* 1989;13:202.

REFERENCES

1. Udelsman R. Thyroid cancer. In: Cameron JL, ed. *Current Surgical Therapy*. Philadelphia: Decker; 1992:568.
2. Lowhagen T, Willems J, Lundell G, et al. Aspiration biopsy cytology in diagnosis of thyroid cancer. *World J Surg*. 1981;5:61.
3. Lowhagen T, Granberg P, Lundell G, et al. Aspiration biopsy cytology (ABC) in nodules of the thyroid gland suspected to be malignant. *Surg Clin North Am*. 1979;59:3.
4. Gharib H, Goellner J. Fine-needle aspiration biopsy of the thyroid: An appraisal. *Ann Inter Med*. 1993;118:282.
5. Mazzaferri E. Management of a solitary thyroid nodule. *N Engl J Med*. 1993;328:553.
6. de los Santos E, Keyhani-Rofagha S, Cunningham J, et al. The dilemma of malignant lesions. *Arch Intern Med*. 1990;150:1422.
7. Grant C, Hay I, Gough I, et al. Long-term follow-up of patients with benign thyroid fine-needle aspiration cytologic diagnoses. *Surgery*. 1989;106:980.
8. LiVolsi VA. *Surgical Pathology of the Thyroid*. Philadelphia: Saunders; 1990.
9. Tielens ET, Sherman SI, Hruban RH, et al. Follicular variant of papillary thyroid carcinoma: A clinicopathologic study. *Cancer*. 1994;73:424.
10. Edis A, Grant C, Egdahl R. *Manual of Endocrine Surgery*, 2nd ed. New York: Springer-Verlag; 1975:238.
11. Ellenhorn J, Shah J, Brennan M. Impact of therapeutic regional lymph node dissection for medullary carcinoma of the thyroid gland. *Surgery*. 1993;114:1078.
12. Buhr H, Kallinowski F, Raue F, et al. Microsurgical neck dissection for occultly metastasizing medullary thyroid carcinoma. *Cancer*. 1993;72:3685.
13. van Heerden J, Hay I, Goellner J, et al. Follicular thyroid carcinoma with capsular invasion alone: A nonthreatening malignancy. *Surgery*. 1992;112:1130.
14. Shaha A, Jaffe B. Completion thyroidectomy: A critical appraisal. *Surgery*. 1992;112:1148.
15. McConahey W, Hay I, Woolner L, et al. Papillary thyroid cancer treated at the Mayo Clinic, 1946 through 1970: Initial manifestations, pathologic findings, therapy, and outcome. *Mayo Clin Proc*. 1986;61:978.
16. DeGroot L, Kaplan E, McCormick M, et al. Natural history, treatment, and course of papillary thyroid carcinoma. *J Clin Endocrinol Metab*. 1990;71:414.
17. Mazzaferri E. Papillary thyroid carcinoma: Factors influencing prognosis and current therapy. *Semin Oncol*. 1987;14:315.
18. Hay I, Grant C, van Heerden J, et al. Papillary thyroid microcarcinoma: A study of 535 cases observed in a 50-year period. *Surgery*. 1992;112:1139.
19. Cady B, Rossi R. An expanded view of risk-group definition in differentiated thyroid carcinoma. *Surgery*. 1988;104:947.
20. Allo M, Christianson W, Koivunen D. Not all "occult" papillary carcinomas are "minimal." *Surgery*. 1988;104:971.
21. Clark O, Levin K, Zeng Q, et al. Thyroid cancer: The case for total thyroidectomy. *Eur J Cancer Clin Oncol*. 1988;24:305.
22. Van De Velde C, Hamming J, Goslings B, et al. Report of the consensus development conference on the management of differentiated thyroid cancer in the Netherlands. *Eur J Cancer Clin Oncol*. 1988;24:287.
23. Baldet L, Manderscheid J, Glinoer D, et al. The management of differentiated thyroid cancer in Europe in 1988: Results of an international survey. *Acta Endocrinol*. 1989;120:547.
24. Tezelman S, Shen W, Shaver JK, et al. Double parathyroid adenomas: Clinical and biochemical characteristics before and after parathyroidectomy. *Ann Surg*. 1993;218:300.
25. Fraker D, Travis W, Merendino J, et al. Locally recurrent parathyroid neoplasms as a cause for recurrent and persistent primary hyperparathyroidism. *Ann Surg*. 1991;213:58.
26. Carty S, Norton J. Management of patients with persistent or recurrent primary hyperparathyroidism. *World J Surg*. 1991;15:716.
27. Wang C, Gaz R. Natural history of parathyroid carcinoma. *Am J Surg*. 1985;149:522.
28. Streeten E, Weinstein L, Norton J, et al. Studies in a kindred with parathyroid carcinoma. *J Clin Endocrinol Metab*. 1992;75:362.
29. Vetto J, Brennan M, Woodruf J, et al. Parathyroid carcinoma: Diagnosis and clinical history. *Surgery*. 1993;114:882.
30. Fyfe S, Hoover L, Zuckerbraun L, et al. Parathyroid carcinoma: Clinical presentation and treatment. *Am J Otolaryngol*. 1990;11:268.
31. Arnold A, Staunton CE, Kim HG, et al. Monoclonality and abnormal parathyroid hormone genes in parathyroid adenomas. *N Engl J Med*. 1989;318:658.
32. Wang C. The anatomic basis of parathyroid surgery. *Ann Surg*. 1976;183:271.
33. Gilmour J. The embryology of the parathyroid glands, the thymus and certain associated remnants. *J Pathol Bacteriol*. 1937;45:507.
34. Grimelius L, Akerstrom G, Johansson H, et al. Anatomy and histopathology of human parathyroid glands. *Pathol Annu*. 1981;16:1.
35. Akerstrom G, Malmaeus J, Bergstrom S. Surgical anatomy of human parathyroid glands. *Surgery*. 1984;95:14.
36. Alveryd A. Parathyroid glands in thyroid surgery. *Acta Chir Scand (Suppl)*. 1968;389:9.
37. Zeiger M, Nieman L, Cutler G, et al. Primary bilateral adrenocortical causes of Cushing's syndrome. *Surgery*. 1991;110:1106.
38. Herf S, Teates D, Tegtmeyer C. Identification and differentiation of surgically correctable hypertension due to primary aldosteronism. *Am J Med*. 1979;67:397.
39. Noth R, Biglieri E. Primary hyperaldosteronism. *Med Clin North Am*. 1988;72:1117.
40. Hough A, Hollifield J, Page D, et al. Prognostic factors in adrenal cortical tumors: A mathematical analysis of clinical and morphologic data. *Am J Clin Pathol*. 1979;72:390.
41. van Slooten H, Schaberg A, Smeenk D, et al. Morphologic characteristics of benign and malignant adrenocortical lesions. *Cancer*. 1985;55:766.
42. Weiss L, Medeiros L, Vickery A. Pathologic features of prognostic significance in adrenocortical carcinoma. *Am J Surg Pathol*. 1989;13:202.
43. Weiss L. Comparative histology of 43 metastasizing and non-metastasizing adrenocortical tumors. *Am J Surg Pathol*. 1984;8:163.
44. Shapiro B, Gross M. Pheochromocytoma. *Crit Care Clin*. 1991;7:1.
45. Ito Y, Fujimoto Y, Obara T, et al. Clinical significance of associated nodular lesions of the adrenal in patients with aldosteronoma. *World J Surg*. 1990;14:330.
46. Weiler R, Fischer-Colbrie R, Schmid KW, et al. Immunological studies on the occurrence and properties of chromogranin A and B and secretogranin in endocrine tumors. *Am J Surg Pathol*. 1988;12:877.
47. Schimd KW, Fischer-Colbrie R, Hagn C, et al. Chromogranin A and B and secretogranin II in medullary carcinomas of the thyroid. *Am J Surg Pathol*. 1987;11:551.
48. Elias JM. *Immunohistopathology: A Practical Approach to Diagnosis*. Chicago: ASCP Press; 1990.
49. Harach HR, Franssila KO. Thyroglobulin immunostaining in follicular thyroid carcinoma. *Histopathology*. 1988;13:43.
50. Uribe M, Grimes M, Fenoglio-Preiser C, et al. Medullary carcinoma of the thyroid gland: Clinical, pathological and immunohistochemical features with review of the literature. *Am J Surg Pathol*. 1985;9:577.
51. Mendelsohn G, Wells SA, Baylin SB. Relationship of tissue carcinoembryonic antigen and calcitonin to tumor virulence in medullary thyroid carcinoma: An immunohistochemical study in early, localized and virulent disseminated stages of disease. *Cancer*. 1984;54:657.
52. Mendelsohn G, Saad MF, Ordonez NG. The prognostic value of calcitonin immunostaining in medullary carcinoma of the thyroid. *J Clin Endocrinol Metab*. 1984;59:850.

10

The Mediastinum

Nancy Lee Harris and Earle W. Wilkins, Jr.

Definition

WHAT IS THE MEDIASTINUM?

The word "mediastinum" means "median septum." In current medical usage, it is defined as the anatomic compartment bounded superiorly by the plane of the thoracic inlet (outlined by the manubrium and first ribs), inferiorly by the diaphragm, and laterally by the mediastinal parietal pleura of the left and right thoracic cavities. It thus contains all the thoracic viscera except the lungs. Its three major components—the airways, the esophagus, and the heart and great vessels—are included by custom in descriptions of the systems to which they belong. This chapter addresses the common pathologic conditions of the other tissues of the mediastinum: the thymus, lymph nodes, nerves, and connective tissues. The discussion is restricted to disorders that cause mass lesions requiring histopathologic diagnosis.

Its location in the midline of the chest renders access to the mediastinum difficult, and the associated presence of large vessels and airways makes exploration hazardous. In addition, the tissues of the mediastinum, like the retroperitoneum, have a propensity for fibrosis in response to diverse pathologic processes. This combination of factors often leads to difficulty in histopathologic interpretation of biopsy specimens from the mediastinum, since they are likely to be small, fibrotic, and crushed. Mass lesions of the mediastinum are often lymphoid and may be either neoplastic or infectious, requiring special techniques such as microbial cultures, immunophenotyping, or electron microscopy for diagnosis. The role of the surgeon in diseases of the mediastinum ranges from providing diagnostic tissue so that other physicians can proceed with definitive treatment (as, for example, in lymphoma) to providing definitive surgical treatment (as in thymoma and mediastinal cysts). Both the surgeon and the pathologist must have a clear idea of the preoperative differential diagnosis and the goals of the operative procedure so that the specimen may be handled appropriately.

Anatomy of the Mediastinum

Knowledge of the anatomy of the mediastinum is useful in the diagnosis of mediastinal masses. The incidence of primary tumors and cysts, nonneoplastic conditions, and metastatic tumors differs in relation to the anatomic compartments of the mediastinum.

The mediastinum is divided into three compartments: anterosuperior, middle (also called the visceral compartment), and posterovertebral (a new term replacing "posterior" to emphasize the paravertebral location of most posterior mediastinal tumors) (Fig. 10–1). These are not exact anatomic divisions but rather regional designations that facilitate radiographic and surgical descriptive localization of tumors. The normal constituents of the various mediastinal compartments determine the types of pathologic conditions that arise in each (Table 10–1).[1] By far the most common tumors found in the mediastinum are metastatic carcinomas, usually of pulmonary origin. These are found in the anterosuperior and middle mediastinum, which contains the majority of mediastinal lymph nodes.

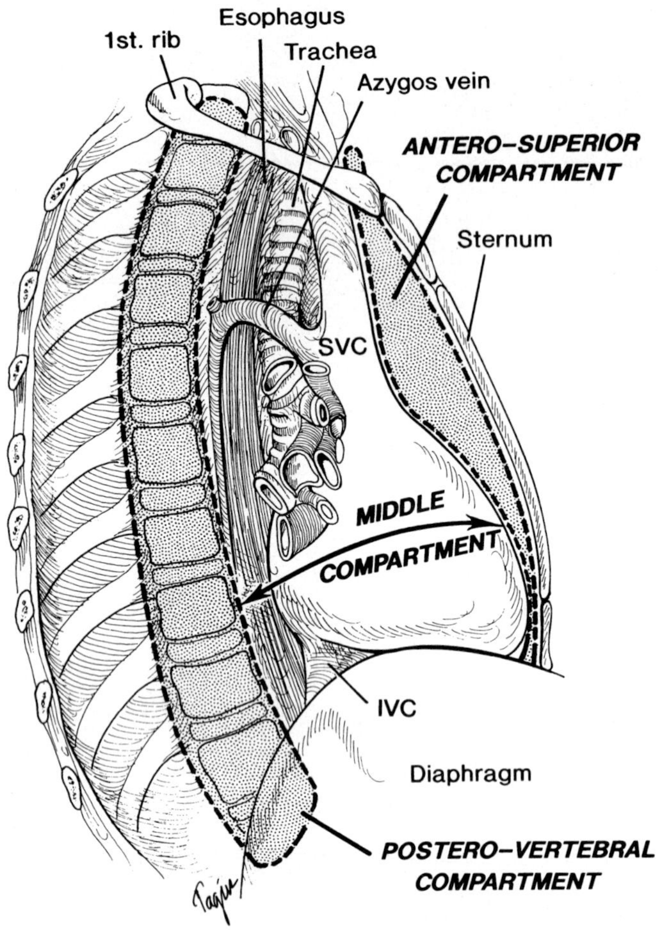

Figure 10–1. Diagram of mediastinal compartments: anterosuperior, middle (visceral), and posterovertebral. SVC = superior vena cava; IVC = inferior vena cava.

Frequency of Primary Mediastinal Tumors and Cysts

The anterosuperior mediastinum is the site of the majority of primary mediastinal tumors, accounting for over half of all tumors (Table 10–1). The posterior mediastinum is next, comprising just over one-quarter, and the middle is the least frequent site. The incidence of the various tumor types varies in different age groups (Table 10–2). In adults, thymoma, lymphoma (usually Hodgkin's disease or large-cell lymphoma), and neurogenic tumors (usually neurilemoma or neurofibroma) are the most common (15 to 20% each), followed by germ-cell tumors (10%). Mesenchymal tumors, carcinomas of unknown origin, and other rare conditions make up the rest. In children, neurogenic tumors (usually ganglioneuroma or neuroblastoma) are most common (35%), followed by lymphoma, usually lymphoblastic (25%), and germ-cell tumors, usually mature teratoma (10%). Mesenchymal tumors, often vascular, and other rare tumors account for the remainder. Cysts (pericardial, bronchogenic, or enteric) account for about 20% of primary mediastinal masses in adults and children.[1]

Diagnostic Procedures

PREOPERATIVE EVALUATION

Two basic tenets govern the diagnosis of mediastinal disease. First, evaluation begins with a careful history and detailed physical examination. Second, radiographic studies provide morphologic but not histologic analysis of mediastinal abnormalities.

The detection of mediastinal pathology often begins with the standard chest radiograph, including posterior-anterior (PA) and lateral views. The right and left anterior oblique views may be added to project abnormalities away from the normal cardiovascular structures of the thorax. No mediastinal tumor should be approached without computed tomography (CT). It provides cross-sectional imaging, which helps to delineate superimposed structures, as well as high-contrast resolution, which assists in defining the size, shape, and density of a mass lesion and the nature of adjacent structures. In the middle (visceral) compartment of the mediastinum, the simultaneous use of contrast medium distinguishes vascular structures from solid tumors.

Other Studies

Magnetic resonance imaging (MRI) is especially useful in defining vascular structures and in assessing vertebral involvement. It does not permit visualization of calcification. Angiography is the ultimate technique for topographic mapping of vascular structures. The practical value of radionuclide imaging is limited to ^{99m}Tc pertechnetate or ^{131}I study of substernal or ectopic thyroid. Detection of tumor markers in serum may suggest a diagnosis, particularly alpha-fetoprotein (AFP) for germ-cell tumor, beta–human chorionic gonadotropin (beta-hCG) for choriocarcinoma, and catecholamines for pheochromocytoma.

BIOPSY TECHNIQUES

Surgical access for biopsy of tumors in the various mediastinal compartments is governed by the complex visceral anatomy of the thorax. There are four biopsy techniques: percutaneous needle biopsy, mediastinoscopy, anterior mediastinotomy (Chamberlain procedure), and video-assisted thoracoscopy (VAT) (Table 10–3). In general, the anterior mediastinum is approached by mediastinotomy or thoracoscopy, the middle mediastinum by mediastinoscopy or mediastinotomy, and the posterior mediastinum by thoracoscopy.

Percutaneous Needle Biopsy. This is usually performed by the aspiration technique, which minimizes the possibility of pneumothorax should the pleura or lung be transgressed during the approach.[2] Interpretation of the specimen requires an expert cytopathologist. Lymphomas are particularly difficult to diagnose by this technique. Implantation of malignant tumors by fine needle aspiration biopsy (FNAB) is apparently rare. Its greatest applicability is proving that a lesion is cystic. In the case of a pericardial cyst, it may also achieve definitive therapy (see Chap. 3).

Mediastinoscopy. Cervical mediastinoscopy is most useful for evaluating lymph nodes in the middle mediastinum along the trachea and proximal bronchi. Its greatest role is

Table 10–1. Mediastinal Compartments, Contents, and Pathologic Conditions

Compartment	Definition	Contents	Pathology	Percent[a]
Anterosuperior	Anterior and superior to pericardial sac	Trachea Esophagus Great vessels Thymus Lymph nodes Nerves (vagus, phrenic) Fat Connective tissue	*Primary Tumors/Cysts* Thymoma (30%)[a] Lymphoma (25%) Germ-cell tumors (20%) Cysts (5%) Thymic or bronchogenic Mesenchymal (4%) Carcinoid (thymic) Primary carcinoma *Other Conditions* Metastatic carcinoma Castleman's disease Sarcoidosis Histoplasmosis	56%
Middle	Visceral compartment, between anterior and posterior compartments	Heart Great vessels Phrenic nerves Carina and bronchi Lymph nodes Connective tissue	*Primary Tumors/Cysts* Cysts (60%) Pericardial Bronchogenic Lymphoma (20%) Mesenchymal (10%) Paraganglioma *Other Conditions* (As for anterosuperior)	19%
Posterovertebral	Posterior to pericardial sac	Esophagus Descending aorta Azygos vein Thoracic duct Nerves (vagus, sympathetic, intercostal) Lymph nodes Fat Connective tissue	*Primary Tumors/Cysts* Neurogenic (50%) Cysts (30%) Bronchogenic Enteric Mesenchymal (10%) *Other Conditions* Meningioma Extramedullary hematopoiesis	25%

[a]Frequency of primary tumors and cysts in Duke University Medical Center series of 441 cases, from Davis and Sabiston.[1]

in staging lung carcinomas, but it may also be helpful in diagnosing mediastinal lymphomas and granulomatous diseases.[3, 4] The location of the incisions for mediastinoscopy and mediastinotomy are shown in Figure 10–2. Three principal areas are not accessible to evaluation by the mediastinoscope: prevascular nodes in the anterior mediastinum, subaortic (aortic window) nodes, and posterior subcarinal nodes.[3, 4] The location of the accessible as well as the inaccessible nodes is illustrated in Figure 10–3. A primary mediastinal mass visualized by mediastinoscopy should be aspirated prior to biopsying to make sure that it is not a vascular structure (see "Pitfalls for the Surgeon").

Table 10–2. Summary of Primary Mediastinal Tumors and Cysts

Tumor	Adults (%)	Children (%)
Neurogenic tumors	21	35
Thymoma	19	
Lymphoma	13	25
Germ-cell tumor	10	10
Cysts	18	16
Mesenchymal tumors	6	10
Endocrine tumors	6	
Carcinomas of unknown primary	5	2
Other	2	2

Mediastinotomy. The biopsy approach by anterior parasternal mediastinotomy, known as the Chamberlain procedure,[5] is most useful for biopsy of anterior mediastinal tumors. It provides access to the anterior mediastinum, including the paratracheal and azygos nodes on the right and the cardiopulmonary window and subaortic nodes on the left (Figs. 10–4 and 10–5).[6] The left paratracheal and posterior subcarinal nodes are not accessible by this technique.

Thoracoscopy. The ultimate role of thoracoscopy, using the VAT surgical methodology, in the resection of mediastinal tumors has not been determined. However, through properly positioned ports, almost any mediastinal tumor is accessible for biopsy. Sugarbaker points out that the technique can be used both for obtaining adequate biopsy specimens and for the resection of benign lesions such as thymic, pericardial, and bronchogenic cysts.[7]

Table 10–3. Types of Biopsy Procedures and Their Utility

Biopsy Type	Accessible Areas	Major Utility
Needle aspiration biopsy	Anterior and middle mediastinum	Cysts (diagnosis and treatment)
Mediastinoscopy	Middle mediastinum	Staging lung cancer Lymphoma (diagnosis)
Mediastinotomy	Anterior and middle mediastinum	Anterior mediastinal tumors (diagnosis)
Thoracoscopy	Anterior and posterior mediastinum	Tumor diagnosis Resection of benign cysts and certain tumors

WHEN SHOULD A BIOPSY BE DONE?

The advisabilityof biopsying anterosuperior mediastinal tumors, particularly suspected thymomas, is debated because of the hypothetical risk of disrupting the tumor capsule and increasing the likelihood of subsequent implantation and relapse. Since the report of Dahlgren and Nordenstrom using the double-needle technique, it is accepted that tumor implantation does not result from FNAB[2]; however, concern about the open biopsy technique persists. We were unable to find documentation of this complication in the literature. Nonetheless, Shields recommends that "biopsy of suspected thymoma preoperatively, unless the lesion is clearly nonresectable, is unnecessary and may even be contraindicated, because the capsule of the tumor of necessity must be violated by any invasive technique."[8]

Since lymphomas and germ-cell tumors may resemble thymoma clinically and radiologically and since appropriate management differs, biopsy may be desirable prior to definitive surgery. Furthermore, since a histologic classification of thymoma predictive for both the likelihood of invasion and prognosis is now available,[9, 10] biopsy of thymomas is indicated for predicting the likelihood of resectability and determining the need for adjuvant therapy such as radiation. Finally, as noted by Davis and Sabiston, "poorly differentiated malignant tumors of the anterosuperior mediastinum, particularly thymomas, lymphomas, germ cell tumors, and primary carcinomas, can have remarkably similar . . . morphologic appearances. Diagnoses based on examination of frozen sections are therefore frequently incorrect, and, similarly, therapeutic decisions based on frozen section examination may be in error."[1] For this reason, if the selection of operative procedure (biopsy only versus definitive resection) depends upon a precise histopathologic diagnosis, preoperative biopsy is required.

The following practical approach is suggested:

1. In a patient with myasthenia gravis and an anterosuperior mediastinal mass, the diagnosis of thymoma is so likely that biopsy is unnecessary if the tumor appears resectable by noninvasive studies.
2. In the absence of myasthenia gravis, if the tumor is well circumscribed on CT scan and there is no enlargement of lymph nodes or evidence of invasion of adjacent structures, the tumor is likely to be either a stage I or II thymoma or a seminoma, both of which require resection; in this situation biopsy may not be necessary. Furthermore, this is the one situation in which the thymoma may be encapsulated, so that disruption of the capsule by biopsy might be an issue. Rare cases of primary mediastinal large B-cell lymphoma may be confined to the thymus, and resection of these is unnecessary; this may be an acceptably small risk, since it is rare and since no harm (except an unnecessary thoracotomy) will result (see Case 1–2, Chap. 1).
3. If lymph nodes are enlarged, if there is evidence of invasion of adjacent structures, or if there is evidence of the superior vena cava (SVC) syndrome, there is a significant possibility that the tumor is lymphoma or nonseminomatous germ-cell tumor. In this case, an attempt should be made to obtain diagnostic tissue by biopsy before carrying out a definitive surgical procedure. In a tumor of this type, capsular invasion has by definition already occurred; therefore iatrogenic capsular disruption is not a concern.

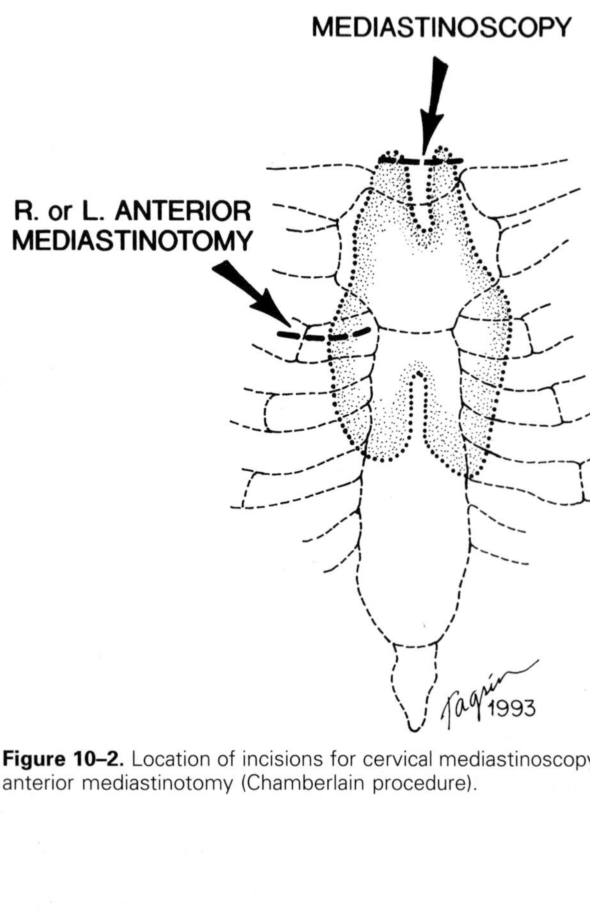

Figure 10–2. Location of incisions for cervical mediastinoscopy and anterior mediastinotomy (Chamberlain procedure).

WHAT TYPE OF BIOPSY SHOULD BE DONE?

In the differential diagnosis of primary anterosuperior mediastinal tumors, FNAB has limited utility. The epithe-

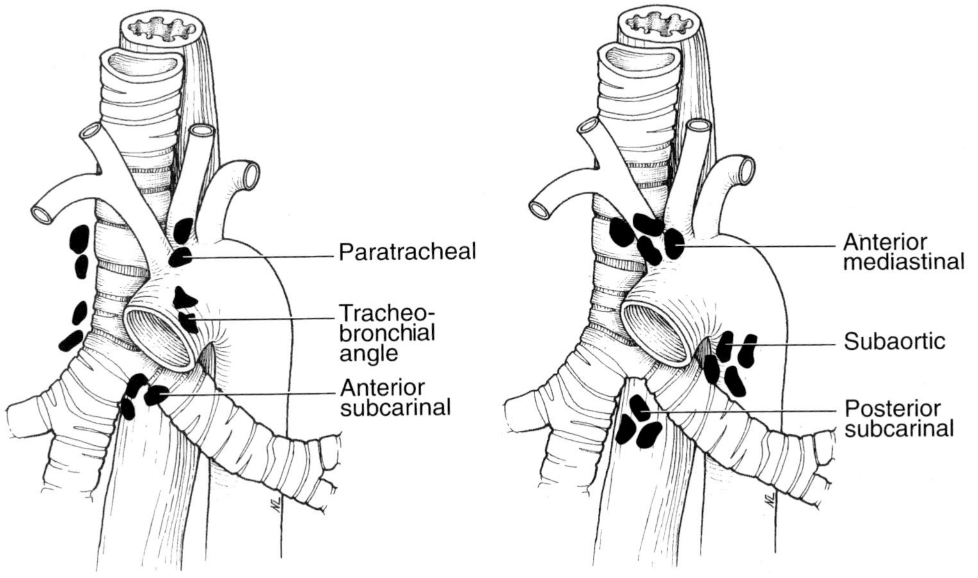

Figure 10–3. Location of mediastinal lymph nodes, illustrating on the left those accessible for biopsy by cervical mediastinoscopy and on the right those inaccessible by this technique. (Reprinted with permission from Ginsberg RJ, Rice TW, Goldberg M, et al. Extended cervical mediastinoscopy. *J Thorac Cardiovasc Surg.* 1987;94:673–678.)

lial cells of thymoma or of germ-cell tumor and the large cells of lymphoma all resemble one another cytologically. The lymphocytes of a cortical thymoma may resemble those of a lymphoblastic lymphoma or the background lymphocytes of Hodgkin's disease. Similar problems will be encountered with cutting needle biopsies. Special immunohistologic techniques can be performed on these types of specimens, but they are often suboptimal and inconclusive on small specimens, only delaying the definitive diagnosis. For the diagnosis of these tumors, a piece of tissue at least 1 to 2 cm in diameter is usually required to demonstrate the typical cytologic and architectural features that distinguish one tumor from another. Unless there is a compelling clinical reason to avoid anesthesia, it may be more efficient and cost-effective to proceed directly to an open biopsy procedure. Because of their location, anterosuperior mediastinal tumors are usually readily accessible via either cervical mediastinoscopy or mediastinotomy, and satisfactory tissue can usually be obtained by either method.

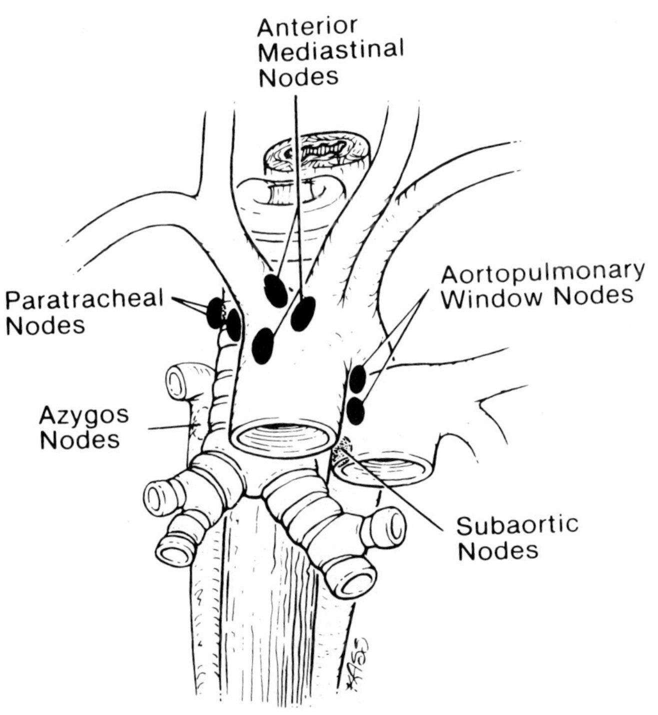

Figure 10–4. Locations of mediastinal lymph nodes accessible by anterior mediastinotomy. The left paratracheal nodes are inaccessible by mediastinotomy, and the posterior subcarinal nodes are not accessible by either cervical mediastinoscopy or mediastinotomy. (Reprinted with permission from LoCicero J III. Mediastinotomy. In: Shields TW, ed. *Mediastinal Surgery.* Philadelphia: Lea & Febiger; 1991: chap 12.)

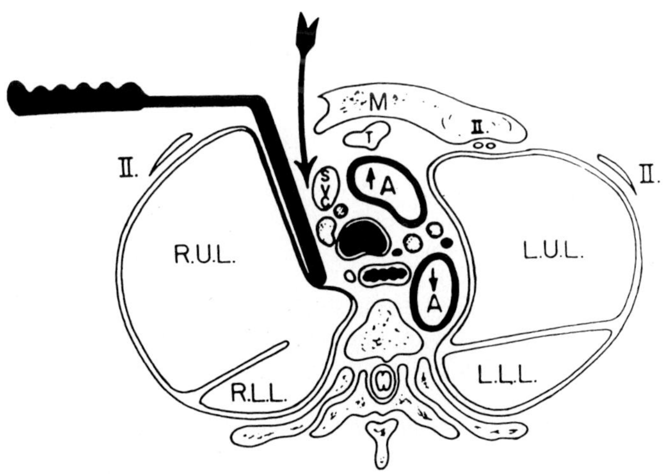

Figure 10–5. A cross-sectional view (similar to a CT section) showing access to the middle mediastinum using a right second costal cartilage mediastinotomy. RUL = right upper lobe of lung; RLL = right lower lobe; LUL = left upper lobe; LLL = left lower lobe; A = aorta; M = manubrium sternum; II = second rib; T = thymus. (Reprinted with permission from the Society of Thoracic Surgeons. McNeill TM, Chamberlain JM. Diagnostic anterior mediastinotomy. *Ann Thorac Surg.* 1966;2:532–539.)

HANDLING OF THE BIOPSY SPECIMEN AND THE ROLE OF INTRAOPERATIVE FROZEN SECTION

Biopsy specimens from mediastinal masses should always be sent fresh (the entire specimen) to the pathologist for intraoperative determination of specimen adequacy and for preparation of tissue for special diagnostic techniques. There is no role for intraoperative diagnosis followed by immediate resection of anterosuperior mediastinal masses except possibly for confirmation of strongly suspected clinical diagnoses in the limited situations previously described. In contrast, the nature of cystic lesions, neurogenic tumors, and metastatic carcinoma can often be established with reasonable certainty on intraoperative frozen section. Frozen sections can also be used selectively to evaluate the status of margins during definitive resection of a tumor; the surgeon must guide the pathologist to areas of particular suspicion, since complete intraoperative evaluation of all margins is impractical.

Histopathologic and Clinical Features of Primary Mediastinal Diseases

NEOPLASMS

Thymoma

Clinical Features. Patients with thymoma are virtually always adults, with a wide age range (20 to 80 years); the peak is in the third through the fifth decades (Table 10–4). Between 10 and 80% of patients in various series have myasthenia gravis (MG); the incidence of MG is greater in older patients and in selected series from major neurologic hospitals, but in unselected series it is, overall, about 40%.[11–14] Other associated conditions such as pure red-cell aplasia and hypogammaglobulinemia are much less common. Thymoma may be discovered incidentally on chest x-ray, but most non-MG patients have symptoms related to a superior mediastinal mass, such as cough and dyspnea. Superior vena caval syndrome occurs in 1 to 2% and is an ominous prognostic sign, indicating advanced local invasion.

On radiologic studies, thymomas are solid or partially cystic masses, usually well circumscribed, in the anterosuperior mediastinum. Lymph node enlargement is so uncommon that its presence alone speaks strongly against the diagnosis of thymoma.

Thymomas usually behave as either benign or low-grade malignant tumors with a propensity for local invasion and recurrence and a minuscule rate of true metastasis. The vast majority of metastases are intrathoracic in the form of pleural seeding; hematogenous metastases to lung and bone are much less common.

Gross Appearance. Thymomas, even when invasive, generally appear as more or less well-circumscribed masses, often with a bosselated or lobulated surface. They may occur anywhere within the thymus but are most commonly found at the base, or isthmus, where the right and left lobes join. The consistency ranges from fleshy to firm, and there are often areas of cystic degeneration (Fig. 10–6).

Histopathology. Thymoma is a tumor of thymic epithelial cells and is thus the only true thymic neoplasm.[12, 15] Carcinoid tumors, germ-cell tumors, and lymphomas may all arise in the thymus, but these are tumors of cells that can be found elsewhere in the body and are thus not uniquely thymic neoplasms.

Thymomas closely resemble the normal thymus. All thymomas contain neoplastic thymic epithelial cells, and most contain non-neoplastic lymphocytes of the types normally found in the thymus. While some classifications subdivide them according to the relative proportions of lymphocytes and epithelial cells, these tumors can more usefully be classified according to the morphology of the epithelial cells (Fig. 10–6). The Müller-Hermelink classification has five categories of thymoma and has predictive value both for invasiveness and risk of relapse and death (Table 10–5).[10, 11, 15, 16]

Medullary thymomas are composed of bland oval or spindle cells resembling those of the thymic medulla, with few lymphocytes. They are usually encapsulated (85%) and, even when invasive, do not recur or metastasize.

Mixed thymomas have areas of medullary thymoma admixed with areas of organoid thymoma (see subsequent discussion); these tumors too are usually encapsulated and do not recur even when invasive.

Organoid thymomas contain areas resembling both normal thymic cortex and medulla, usually have a lobular architecture, and very closely resemble the normal thymus. They are invasive about 40% of the time and carry a small but definite risk of late relapse when invasive.

Cortical thymomas have large, pale epithelial cells identical to those of the normal thymic cortex, with preservation of a lobular architecture, but the epithelial cells are more numerous and the lymphocytes less densely packed than in either normal cortex or organoid thymomas. Cortical thymomas carry a risk of invasiveness and relapse similar to that of organoid thymoma in some series and considerably higher in other series.

Well-differentiated thymic carcinoma is composed predominantly of epithelial cells that resemble those of cortical thymoma but with a moderate degree of cytologic atypia and occasional mitotic figures. Their architecture is less regularly lobular, with areas of dense fibrosis. They are almost always invasive. They carry a significant risk of early relapse, even with minimal invasion. This type accounted for all the relapses and deaths from thymoma occurring within 10 years in a large series of cases from Massachusetts General Hospital.[10]

Unlike the tumors that resemble normal thymic epithelium and are considered thymomas, there are rare, poorly differentiated carcinomas that resemble carcinomas of other sites and appear to have arisen in the thymus. Several morphologic types have been described; the two most common are squamous cell and lymphoepitheliomalike carcinomas, but small-cell, spindle-cell, and basaloid types have also been described. These have a much poorer prognosis than thymoma.[17, 18]

Staging. Thymomas are staged according to the extent of invasion, most often according to the system of Masaoka (Table 10–6).[19] Even using the Müller-Hermelink histologic classification, stage is still a powerful factor in predicting

Table 10–4. Clinical Features of Common Pathologic Conditions of the Mediastinum

Tumor	Age[a] and Sex	Common Symptoms	Special Tests	Primary Location	LN[b]
Anterosuperior					
Thymoma	3–5; M=F	Myasthenia (10–50%), cough, dyspnea, SVC	Anti-ACHE or striated muscle antibody	Thymus	No
Lymphomas					
Hodgkin's disease	2–3; M<F	Fever, pruritus, alcohol-induced pain		Thymus and/or nodes	Yes
Large-cell lymphoma	2–4; M<F	Cough, dyspnea, SVC		Thymus +/− nodes	Yes
Lymphoblastic lymphoma	2–3; M>>F	Fever, cough, dyspnea, SVC	WBC (leukemia); bone marrow asp	Thymus +/− nodes	Yes
Germ-Cell Tumors					
Teratoma	2–3; M=F	Cough, dyspnea		Thymus	No
Seminoma	2–5; M only	Cough, dyspnea, SVC (10–20%)		Thymus +/− nodes	Rare
Nonseminomatous	3–4; M>>>>F	Cough, dyspnea, SVC (20%)	AFP, HCG	Thymus, lung, distant mets	Often
Other Conditions					
Metastatic carcinoma	5–8; M=F	Related to primary tumor		Lymph nodes	Yes
Sarcoidosis	3–4; M=F	Cough	Low CD4 Angiotensin-converting enzyme	Lymph nodes (usually hilar), lungs	Yes
Infectious granuloma	Any age	Cough, fever	Skin tests	Lymph nodes, lungs	Yes
Castleman's disease	2–4	None	None	Lymph node	Yes
Middle					
Bronchogenic cyst	Any age M=F	None; infants: cough, dyspnea	None	Postcarinal	No
Pericardial cyst	Adult M=F	None	None	Pericardiophrenic angle	No
Paraganglioma	Adult	MEN	^{131}I-MIBG scan[c]	Periarterial	No
Pheochromocytoma	M=F	Pheochromocytoma syndrome	VMA[d]	Paraspinal	No
Other Conditions (see "Anterosuperior")					
Posterovertebral					
Neurogenic Tumors					
Neurilemoma	3–5; M=F	None; rare cord compression with dumbbell tumor (60%)	None	Paraspinal; intraspinal component in 10% (dumbbell)	No
Neurofibroma	3–5; M=F	Neurofibromatosis	None	Like neurilemoma	No
Ganglioneuroma	Children	Diarrhea (VIP)	None	Paraspinal	No
Ganglioneuroblastoma	Children	Diarrhea (VIP)	None	Paraspinal	No
Neuroblastoma	Children (<4 yr)	Cough, dysphagia, diarrhea (VIP)	None	Paraspinal; distant mets	Often
Enteric cyst	Children > adults; M=F	Dysphagia	None	Paraesophageal	No

[a]Peak decades of incidence.
[b]Lymph nodes involved.
[c]^{131}I-metaiodobenzylguanidine.
[d]Vanillylmandelic acid.
Abbreviations: HCG = human chorionic gonadotropin, AFP = alpha-fetoprotein, SVC = superior vena cava syndrome, MEN = multiple endocrine neoplasia, VIP = vasoactive intestinal peptide, ACHE = acetylcholinesterase, mets = metastases.

outcome.[10, 13, 14, 20] Staging is a cooperative endeavor requiring both surgeon and pathologist. The surgeon must carefully examine the thorax at the time of thymectomy to determine whether the tumor has invaded adjacent structures and to look for pleural "drop" metastases. If the tumor is invasive but resectable, areas of involved pericardium or lung should also be removed.

Small fragments of pericardium, lung, or nerve may not be as readily identifiable in a resection specimen as they are in situ. The specimen should be oriented and marked

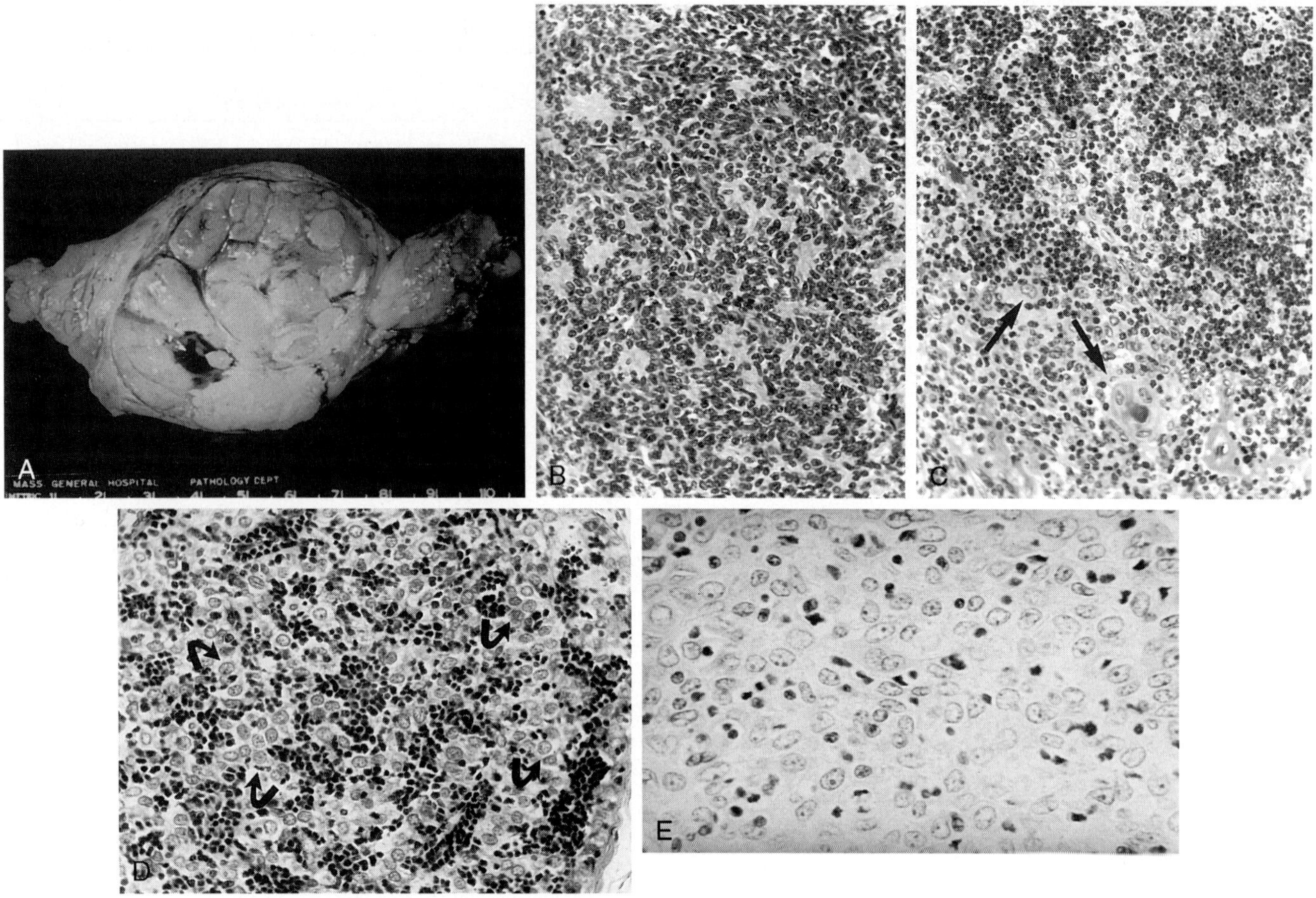

Figure 10–6. Thymoma. *A,* Gross photograph, showing large, encapsulated tumor. *B–E,* Microscopic sections illustrating histologic subtypes of thymoma according to the Müller-Hermelink classification. *B,* Medullary thymoma, with small oval- to spindle-shaped cells. *C,* Organoid thymoma, with zones featuring numerous lymphocytes and other areas of epithelial cells *(arrows),* closely resembling normal thymus. *D,* Cortical thymoma, with large, pale epithelial cells *(arrows)* and many lymphocytes. *E,* Well-differentiated thymic carcinoma; the epithelial cells are smaller than those of cortical thymoma, with nuclear irregularity, moderate mitotic activity, and relatively few lymphocytes. This tumor may be confused with (large-cell) lymphoma in small biopsy specimens or on intraoperative frozen section.

with sutures or other means to indicate to the pathologist the location and identity of any important adherent structures. The specimen should be delivered promptly to the pathologist so that proper fixation can be achieved. Particularly if a preoperative histologic diagnosis of thymoma has not been made, tissue should be prepared for immunohistologic and electron microscopic study, in anticipation that other tumors will enter into the differential diagnosis (see Chap. 2 and Case 1–3 in Chap. 1).

Treatment and Outcome. Treatment depends on stage and histologic subtype, but complete thymectomy, with removal of all anterior mediastinal fat, is the primary mo-

Table 10–5. Thymoma: Correlation of Histologic Type with Stage: Analysis of 122 Cases at Massachusetts General Hospital

Histologic Type	No. of Cases (%)	Stage I (%)	Stage II (%)	Stage III (%)	Stage IV (%)
Medullary	8 (7)	5 (62)	3 (38)	0	0
Mixed	34 (28)	22 (65)	12 (35)	0	0
Organoid	20 (16)	11 (55)	7 (35)	2 (10)	0
Cortical	22 (18)	10 (45)	8 (36)	4 (18)	0
Well-differentiated thymic (carcinoma)	32 (26)	0	6 (19)	21 (66)	5 (16)
High-grade carcinoma	2 (2)	0	0	2 (100)	0
Unclassifiable	4 (3)	2 (50)	1 (25)	1 (25)	0
Total	122	50 (41)	37 (30)	30 (25)	5 (4)

Source: From Quintanilla-Martinez L, Wilkins EJ, Ferry J, Harris N: Thymoma: Morphologic subclassifications correlates with invasiveness and immunohistologic features: A study of 122 cases. *Hum Pathol* 1993;24:958–969, with permission.

Table 10–6. Masaoka Staging of Thymoma[a]

Stage I	Macroscopically completely encapsulated, with no microscopic extracapsular extension
Stage II	Microscopic invasion through the capsule (IIA) Macroscopic invasion of mediastinal fat or mediastinal pleura (IIB)
Stage III	Invasion into adjacent structures (pericardium, visceral pleura, lung, vena cava)
Stage IV	A. Pleural or pericardial dissemination B. Lymphatic or hematogenous metastasis

[a]No staging system for thymoma has yet been recommended by the American Joint Committee on Cancer.

dality.[13, 14, 20] Encapsulated (stage I) thymomas require no additional therapy after thymectomy, regardless of histologic type. Minimally invasive (stage II) thymomas of medullary and mixed types are usually cured by resection alone. However, even completely resected stage II thymomas of organoid, cortical, or well-differentiated thymic carcinoma type have potential for recurrence, and stage III thymomas, particularly the well-differentiated thymic carcinoma type, have a relatively high recurrence rate.[10] Radiation therapy has been shown to decrease the risk of recurrence of stage II thymomas and is used in virtually all stage III thymomas and in unresectable cases.[21] Because of the poor prognosis of well-differentiated thymic carcinomas, the efficacy of more intensive postoperative adjunctive therapy, including chemotherapy, needs further evaluation.

Lymphomas: Hodgkin's Disease, Large-Cell and Lymphoblastic Types

Lymphomas derive from cells of the immune system. Although they most commonly arise in lymphoid tissues, they can occur virtually anywhere in the body in extranodal sites. In the mediastinum, lymphomas most often involve anterosuperior mediastinal lymph nodes and/or thymus, but they can also involve the peribronchial lymph nodes of the middle mediastinum. Three major types of lymphoma arise in the mediastinum: Hodgkin's disease, large-cell lymphoma, and lymphoblastic lymphoma. Occasionally, patients with low-grade lymphomas may present with mediastinal lymphadenopathy, but in this situation disease is present in other sites as well, and the diagnosis can be made without invading the mediastinum.

Different types of lymphoma call for different types of therapy. The surgeon's role in the care of the patient with mediastinal lymphoma is to provide sufficient tissue to the pathologist in a condition that will permit optimal fixation and special diagnostic studies, and, of course, to avoid unnecessary radical surgery on the basis of a misdiagnosis (clinical or frozen section) of thymoma or germ-cell tumor (see Case 1–3, Chap. 1). If the type of mediastinal tumor is uncertain by clinical and radiologic criteria and by intraoperative frozen section, definitive surgery should be deferred until permanent histologic sections are available for accurate diagnosis.

Hodgkin's Disease

Clinical Features. Hodgkin's disease (HD) can occur at any age, but the peak incidence is in the second through fourth decades. It is rare in very young children (Table 10–4).[22] Patients with mediastinal HD are usually adolescents or young adults with the nodular sclerosis subtype (see below), who present with symptoms related to local nodal enlargement, such as cough or dyspnea. Surprisingly, SVC syndrome is relatively uncommon, even in the presence of massive mediastinal disease. However, airway compromise can be a significant problem in patients with large masses.

The majority of patients with mediastinal HD also have disease outside the mediastinum—usually cervical or occasionally axillary lymphadenopathy. In radiologic studies the tumor may appear as either a solitary mass, usually in the thymus, as multiple enlarged separate lymph nodes, or both.[22] In contrast to thymoma, lymph node enlargement is usually present. When the thymus is involved epithelial proliferation and cystic change can occur, mimicking thymoma.

Gross Appearance. At operation, the tumor is virtually always invasive and involves multiple lymph nodes. As in thymoma, the presence of sclerosis in HD makes the involved nodes firm, and they are often densely adherent to one another and to pericardium or pleura. The dense sclerosis may complicate biopsy. Unfortunately, superficial specimens are often nondiagnostic (see Chap. 17).

Histopathology. A detailed description of the pathology and subclassification of HD is found in Chapter 17. Mediastinal tumors are usually of the nodular sclerosis (NS) type, in which fibrous bands enclose cellular nodules of lymphocytes, histiocytes, eosinophils, plasma cells, and lacunar variants of Reed-Sternberg cells.[23] The diagnosis requires identification of diagnostic Reed-Sternberg cells in the appropriate cellular background. Because of the lymphocytic background and the lobular architecture as well as the presence of proliferating thymic epithelium in some cases, HD may be difficult to distinguish from thymoma in small biopsy specimens and particularly on frozen section. In some cases, broad sheets of lacunar cells may be present—so-called syncytial variant or lymphocyte-depleted NS—causing difficulty in distinction from large-cell lymphoma or germ-cell tumors. Finally, because of the prominent inflammatory components, which may be granulomatous, distinction from sarcoidosis and infectious processes may be difficult in small specimens (see "Pitfalls for the Pathologist").

Staging. Details of staging and treatment are covered in Chapter 17. Patients who present with mediastinal HD in the absence of cervical or axillary nodal involvement are rarely found to have disease below the diaphragm and are often treated with radiation therapy, without staging laparotomy. Patients with mediastinal masses more than one-third of the thoracic width do poorly with radiation therapy alone because of the large volume of lung and heart that would have to be included within the radiation port. For this reason, chemotherapy is used, sometimes for subsequent radiation. Most other patients will undergo staging laparotomy to determine extent of disease. Localized disease is managed with radiation therapy alone, while disseminated disease requires chemotherapy.

Outcome. The majority of patients with Hodgkin's disease are cured, and survival depends almost entirely on the stage of the disease at the time of the diagnosis.[22]

Diffuse Large B-Cell Lymphoma

Clinical Features. Patients with primary large B-cell lymphoma of the mediastinum are most commonly young adults in their third and fourth decades; females predominate (Table 10–4).[24–30] They are virtually always symptomatic because of a rapidly enlarging anterosuperior mediastinal mass, with cough, dyspnea, and often SVC syndrome (30%). Radiologic studies show a solid mass in the region of the thymus, usually with enlarged nodes and evidence of invasion of adjacent structures. In contrast to HD, extramediastinal nodal involvement is rare at presentation.

Gross Appearance. The tumors are similar in appearance to HD; they may either be firm, because of sclerosis, or soft and fleshy. Most involve the thymus but also show widespread local invasion at the time of diagnosis; a few cases have been completely confined to the thymus, suggesting that they may indeed originate there (Fig. 10–7).[25, 27]

Histopathology. The tumors have a diffuse growth pattern and show variable amounts of fine or dense sclerosis, which does not form nodules, as in HD, but rather divides the tumor cells into small nests, mimicking carcinoma. The tumor cells are similar in size to those of well-differentiated thymic carcinoma or seminoma and, like these tumors, have abundant pale or clear cytoplasm. The nuclei vary from oval to irregular or "cleaved," with one or more prominent nucleoli; there is often a rather brisk mitotic rate (Fig. 10–7). Areas of normal thymus may be found in large biopsy specimens or in resected tumors. Immunophenotyping studies have shown that the majority of primary mediastinal large-cell lymphomas are of B-cell origin.[27, 29, 30]

This tumor has often been misdiagnosed in the past as thymoma, germ-cell tumor, or HD and has been defined as a distinct entity in only the last decade. Because of its resemblance to other common mediastinal tumors, it cannot be reliably diagnosed on frozen section. In fact, immunohistologic studies are often necessary to confirm the diagnosis on permanent sections. Electron microscopy may be useful in some cases.

Staging. Since all patients are treated with chemotherapy, staging laparotomy is not performed. The staging system used is the same as that for large-cell lymphoma at other sites (see Chap. 17).

Treatment and Outcome. Treatment is always with combination chemotherapy, using regimens effective against large-cell lymphomas arising in other sites, with or without radiation therapy. The prognosis is not as favorable as that of HD, but it is not significantly worse than that for large-cell lymphoma in general; 5-year median survivals are 40 to 60% in most series.[26] Relapses tend to be extranodal, involving sites such as the liver, gastrointestinal (GI) tract, kidney, ovary, and central nervous system (CNS).

Lymphoblastic Lymphoma

Clinical Features. Lymphoblastic lymphoma (LBL) is most common in children and young adults, with a sharp peak in the second and third decades and a striking male predominance (Table 10–4).[31, 32] However, the tumor can occur in older adults as well. Patients usually present with symptoms of an anterior mediastinal mass: cough, dyspnea,

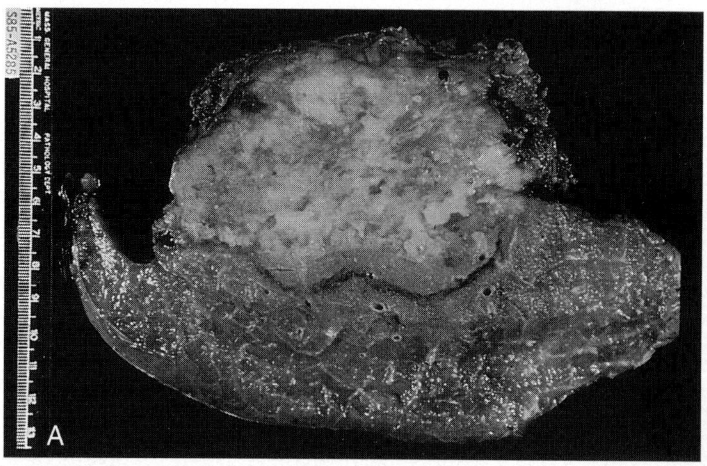

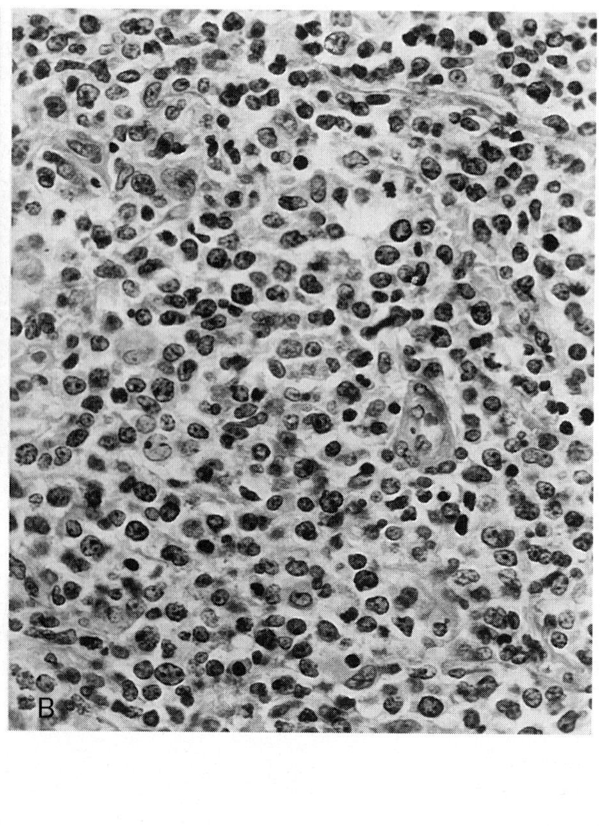

Figure 10–7. Primary mediastinal large B-cell lymphoma. *A,* Gross photograph, showing a large tumor invading the lung. *B,* Photomicrograph showing large lymphoid cells with fine, compartmentalizing sclerosis mimicking a nonlymphoid tumor, such as seminoma or well-differentiated thymic carcinoma (see Chap. 1, Case 1–3).

and often SVC syndrome. In contrast to HD and mediastinal large-cell lymphoma, LBL is usually a systemic disease, with involvement of the thymus and mediastinal nodes and other supradiaphragmatic nodes; malignant pleural effusions and bone marrow involvement, as well as CNS involvement, are common. Mediastinal LBL is one end of a spectrum of lymphoblastic neoplasia, with T-cell acute lymphoblastic leukemia at the other end. The distinction is distributional. The presence of bone marrow involvement arbitrarily decides terminology: if the marrow is negative, it is lymphoma; if the marrow is positive, it is leukemia.

Gross Appearance. The involved thymus and lymph nodes are generally soft and fleshy, resembling other small round-cell tumors and lacking the fibrotic quality of HD and large-cell lymphoma. The infiltrate often extends diffusely into perithymic and perinodal fat, which gives the fat an indurated quality.

Histopathology. The neoplastic lymphoblasts are smaller than those of large-cell lymphoma or thymoma and only slightly larger than normal lymphocytes. They have dispersed, primitive-appearing chromatin, scant cytoplasm, inconspicuous nucleoli, and a high mitotic rate.[31] Most cases have the immunophenotype of immature T cells, often similar to those normally found in the thymus, but rare cases are composed of immature B-cells. On a small biopsy specimen, it may be difficult to distinguish lymphoblasts from the immature lymphoid cells found in normal thymic cortex or the cortical areas of lymphocyte-rich thymomas. The differential diagnosis may also include other small round-cell tumors of childhood, such as neuroblastoma, as well as small-cell carcinoma, granulocytic sarcoma, and large-cell lymphoma.

Special Pathologic Studies. Immunophenotyping studies on fresh frozen tissue or cell suspensions are usually needed for the diagnosis and subclassification of lymphoblastic lymphoma/leukemia. Electron microscopy can be useful in distinguishing LBL from other small round-cell tumors.

Staging. Since all patients receive chemotherapy, staging laparotomy is not performed. Because of the high frequency of bone marrow and CNS involvement, bone marrow biopsy and aspirate and cerebrospinal fluid (CSF) examination are always done. In children, it may be convenient to have these procedures performed under the anesthesia used for the diagnostic biopsy.

Treatment and Outcome. Treatment is with aggressive combination chemotherapy, usually with CNS prophylaxis; children have a relatively high likelihood of cure, but the prognosis in adults is less favorable.[32]

Germ-Cell Tumors

Clinical Features. Mediastinal germ-cell tumors occur in the same age group as testicular germ-cell tumors (predominantly males in the third and fourth decades) (Table 10–4), and may be any of the same histologic types: teratoma, seminoma (dysgerminoma), embryonal carcinoma, yolk sac (endodermal sinus) tumor, and choriocarcinoma, or a mixture of these. Children are most likely to have mature teratomas. Patients are always symptomatic from a large anterosuperior mediastinal mass and may have SVC syndrome (20%). The majority of nonseminomatous types have elevation of serum HCG or AFP, and these tests should be done on all males of this age group with an anterosuperior mediastinal mass.

Gross Appearance. Mature teratomas are often cystic (dermoid cyst) and may contain hair, sebaceous material, and teeth, like gonadal germ-cell tumors. The gross features of the other germ-cell tumors are not distinctively different from those of other malignant tumors: they are lobulated, often invasive solid masses that may have areas of necrosis (Fig. 10–8*A*). Choriocarcinoma is typically hemorrhagic.

Histopathology. The histopathology of mediastinal germ-cell tumors is identical to that of gonadal tumors.[33] Teratomas contain all germ-cell layers, with mature or immature endodermal, mesodermal, and ectodermal derivatives, including skin and skin appendages, hair, teeth, muscle, cartilage, fibrous tissue, and nerves as well as parenchymal, glandular, and endocrine tissue. Malignant teratomas contain immature embryonic tissues. Seminomas are composed of uniform round cells with abundant clear cytoplasm, which is usually glycogen-rich; their size is similar to that of the cells of thymoma and large-cell lymphoma, and they may be arranged in nests with numerous stromal lymphocytes, giving rise to a differential diagnosis that includes thymoma and lymphoma (Fig. 10–8*B*). A prominent granulomatous reaction is sometimes seen, which, on small biopsy specimens, may raise the question of sarcoidosis or infectious processes. Embryonal carcinoma is characterized by large cells with pleomorphic, atypical nuclei and abundant basophilic cytoplasm, which form papillary, tubular, glandular, or solid patterns. Endodermal sinus (yolk sac) tumor is composed of large clear cells forming a reticular pattern; it contains characteristic papillary structures (Schiller-Duval bodies) and hyaline globules. Choriocarcinoma is composed of both cytotrophoblastic and syncytiotrophoblastic elements. Mixtures of the various types are common in germ-cell tumors. For this reason, these tumors must be thoroughly sampled for microscopic examination. Small biopsy specimens of germ-cell tumors containing only undifferentiated malignant cells may be indistinguishable from lymphoma or thymoma.

Special Pathologic Techniques. Electron microscopy may be useful in characterizing seminoma. A battery of immunohistologic stains on paraffin sections can be useful in distinguishing malignant germ-cell tumors from lymphoma and thymoma; useful marker antigens include placental alkaline phosphatase, cytokeratin, AFP, HCG, and leukocyte-associated antigens (see Chap. 2).

Staging. Benign teratomas are usually well circumscribed. Seminomas are usually either well circumscribed or have only intrathoracic metastases, while the other germ-cell tumors often show extrathoracic spread at diagnosis. For nonseminomatous tumors, the serum AFP or HCG is an important marker for evaluation of remission status.

Treatment and Outcome. Treatment involves resection, if possible, followed by radiation or other adjuvant therapy. As in the testis, the prognosis varies among the different types, with mature teratoma usually being benign, seminoma potentially aggressive but responsive to radiation and chemotherapy, and nonseminomatous types being highly

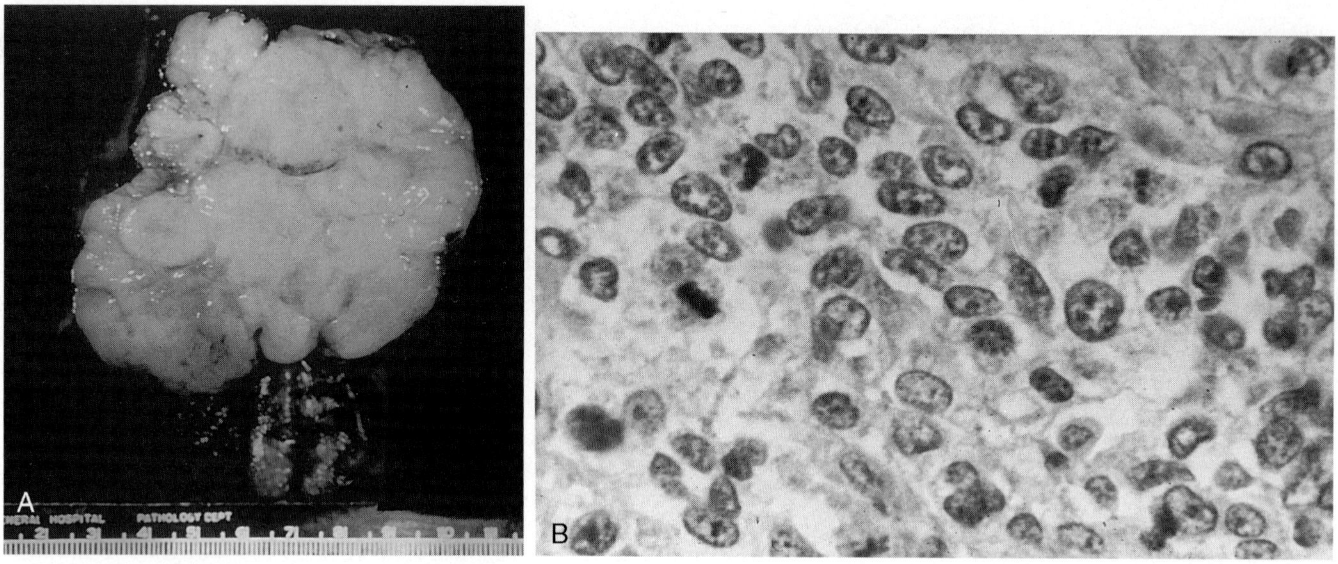

Figure 10–8. Mediastinal seminoma. *A,* Gross photograph showing a large encapsulated tumor. *B,* Photomicrograph showing large pale cells with prominent nucleoli; admixed lymphocytes may produce a resemblance to thymoma or lymphoma. The abundant pale cytoplasm and cohesive growth are useful in making the distinction from lymphoma, but the differential diagnosis can be difficult on small biopsy specimens or on frozen section.

aggressive, often disseminated, and relatively unresponsive to treatment. Resection may be a useful adjuvant to chemotherapy in patients with initially unresectable tumors. Since seminomas are sensitive to radiation, attempts to resect invasive tumors are not indicated.

Neurogenic Tumors

Clinical Features. Neurogenic tumors are about equal in overall frequency to thymoma and lymphoma and are by far the most common tumor in the posterior mediastinum.[1] There are three major categories: (1) tumors of peripheral nerve (neurilemoma, neurofibroma), which arise from the intercostal nerves, are most common in young adults, and may be associated with neurofibromatosis; (2) tumors of sympathetic nerves and ganglia (ganglioneuroma, ganglioneuroblastoma, neuroblastoma), which arise from the sympathetic ganglion chain and are more common in children; and (3) rare tumors of parasympathetic ganglion tissue (paraganglioma, pheochromocytoma), which occur in adults and may be associated with multiple endocrine neoplasia syndromes.

Neurilemoma (schwannoma), neurofibroma, and ganglioneuroma are often asymptomatic and discovered by chance on chest x-ray (Fig. 10–9). Neural tumors may be associated with back pain, dyspnea, or neurologic symptoms related to brachial or cervical plexus involvement or cord compression. The latter is seen in cases that extend into the spinal canal (so-called dumbbell tumors). Paragangliomas may occur either in the anterior and middle mediastinum, at the level of the aortic arch, or posteriorly in a paravertebral location[34]; because of their vascularity, they show contrast enhancement on CT.[1] Systemic manifestations may be associated with paragangliomas, ganglioneuroblastomas, and neuroblastomas due to catecholamine or peptide hormone production.

Gross Appearance. Neurilemomas (schwannomas) are well-circumscribed, firm, yellow-white nodules extending from an intercostal nerve. Neurofibromas appear as less well circumscribed, fusiform expansions of the nerve. Ganglioneuromas are also encapsulated and firm and may have areas of cystic degeneration.[35] Ganglioneuroblastomas and neuroblastomas have a softer, more fleshy appearance and are often poorly circumscribed and invasive. Paragangliomas are usually small and well circumscribed but tend to be very vascular.

Histopathology. Neurilemoma (schwannoma) is composed of bland spindle cells, which focally display a characteristic palisading pattern (Verocay bodies, Antoni type A) alternating with looser, edematous areas (Antoni type B). Bizarre nuclei may be present in some cases, but mitotic activity is sparse. Neurofibromas consist of more randomly oriented oval to spindle cells, which infiltrate between nerve fibers.[35] Rarely, both neurilemoma and neurofibroma may undergo malignant transformation, particularly in patients with neurofibromatosis.

Ganglioneuromas are composed of mature ganglion cells and neural tissue. The ganglion cells are very large cells with round nuclei, prominent nucleoli, and characteristically abundant eosinophilic cytoplasm (Fig. 10–9). They are usually scattered in a background of nerve fibers. Ganglioneuroblastomas contain a mixture of the aforementioned features with primitive neuroblasts: small, round cells with a high nuclear-cytoplasmic ratio and a high mitotic rate. Neuroblastoma is composed entirely of such blastic cells, often forming characteristic Homer Wright rosettes around masses of nerve filaments; the differential diagnosis includes other small round-cell tumors of childhood (in the chest, principally Ewing's sarcoma) and lymphoblastic lymphoma.

Paragangliomas are composed of medium-sized, polygonal cells with pale cytoplasm that form characteristic nests,

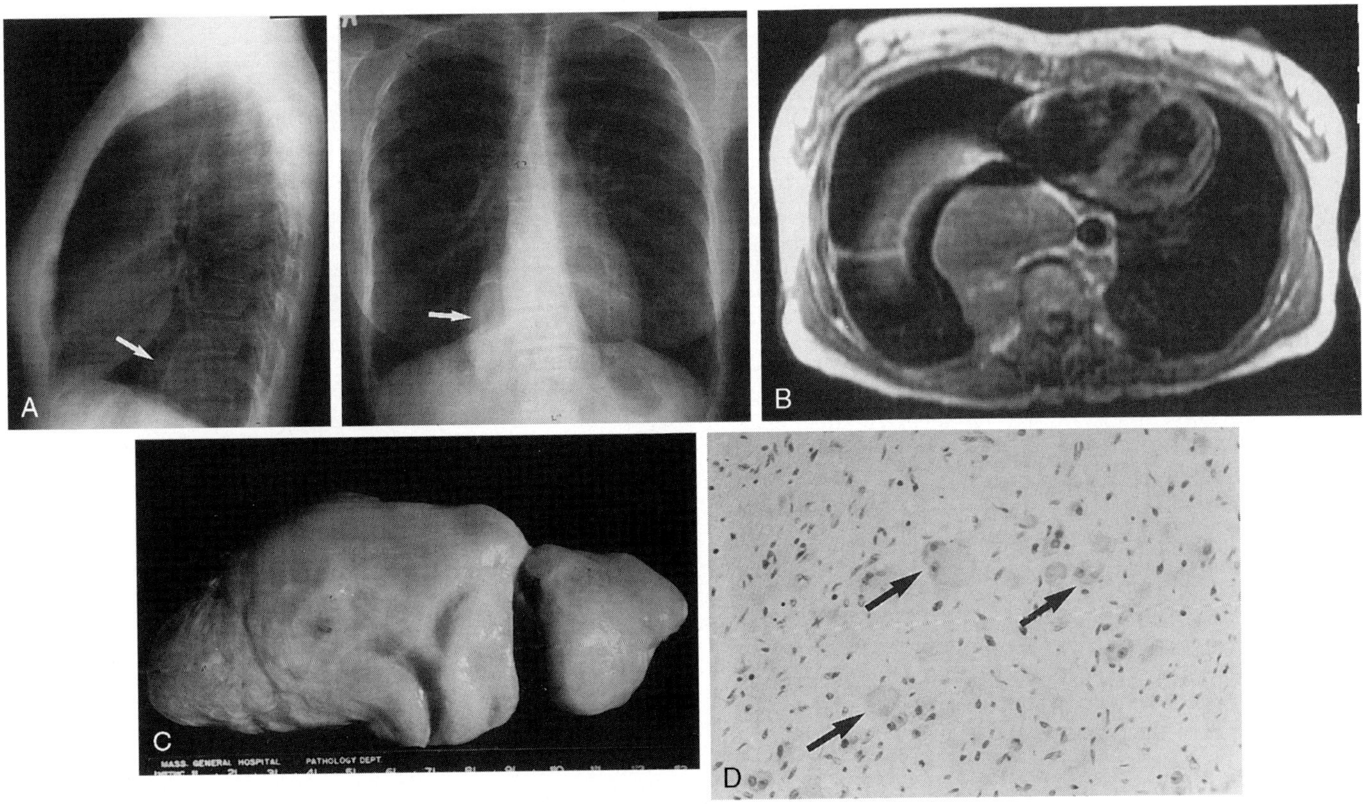

Figure 10–9. Ganglioneuroma of the posterior mediastinum. *A,* Chest x-rays showing a right posterior/paravertebral mediastinal mass. *B,* Computed tomography showing paravertebral location of the mass. *C,* Gross photograph showing lobulated, smooth-surfaced masses of firm white tissue. *D,* Photomicrograph showing mature ganglion cells *(arrows)* in a background of neural tissue.

or *"Zellballen,"* closely resembling normal paraganglia. Numerous small blood vessels are present in the intervening fibrous septa.[36]

Special Techniques. Electron microscopy is important in the differential diagnosis of small round-cell tumors of childhood. Immunoperoxidase stains for neurofilament protein or neuron-specific enolase may be useful (see Chap. 2).

Staging. Ganglioneuroblastoma and neuroblastoma are staged according to the extent of disease: stage 1, well-circumscribed; stage 2, local invasion only; stage 3, extension of tumor across the midline; stage 4, distant metastases.

Treatment and Outcome. Treatment is by excision for localized tumors, excision followed by radiation for invasive tumors, and chemotherapy with or without subsequent resection for widely metastatic blastic tumors. Neurilemomas, neurofibromas, and ganglioneuromas are benign tumors that are cured by excision, as are most paragangliomas. Paragangliomas are highly vascularized and may bleed excessively during attempts at removal. Ganglioneuroblastomas have some malignant potential, with the risk of metastasis depending on the degree of primitive neuroblast component. Neuroblastomas are highly malignant tumors that are usually metastatic at diagnosis. As with neuroblastomas of the retroperitoneum, very young children (less than 1 year of age) have a better prognosis (see Chap. 21).[1] Preoperative MRI or myelography should be done to rule out intraspinal extension by neurogenic tumor of the posterior mediastinum unless the tumor is clearly distinct from the intervertebral foramina on CT. The rare dumbbell neurogenic tumors require a combined neurosurgical and thoracic surgical approach for optimal one-stage removal.[1, 37]

CYSTS

Bronchogenic Cyst

Clinical Features. These are the most common mediastinal cysts (Table 10–4).[1] Patients may be children or adults, either asymptomatic or presenting with dyspnea, pain, cough, or respiratory compromise. Cysts are located most commonly in the middle or posterior mediastinum, at or above the carina.

Pathologic Features. The cysts are derived from the ventral foregut, during development of the tracheobronchial tree. They have a moderately thick wall, composed of all layers of the bronchial tree—smooth muscle, cartilage, and mucous glands—and they are lined by respiratory epithelium.[34]

Diagnosis. To confirm the cystic nature of the lesion and exclude the presence of malignant cells by cytopathologic examination, FNAB may be useful. The viscous nature of the fluid may prevent adequate aspiration. Pathologic examination of the resected specimen is required to confirm the diagnosis and exclude cystic malignancy.

Treatment and Outcome. Although these lesions are benign and nonprogressive, complete excision is advised to relieve symptoms and provide a definitive diagnosis as well as to prevent complicating infection within the cyst.

Pericardial Cyst

Clinical Features. These lesions are usually discovered on routine chest x-ray in asymptomatic adults and appear on CT as characteristic low-density masses. By far the most common location is the right cardiophrenic angle.[1]

Pathologic Features. Pericardial cysts arise from failure of fusion of the embryonic components of the pericardial sac. They are composed of a thin fibrous wall with a mesothelial lining.[34]

Diagnosis. The preferred method is FNAB, with fluid prepared for cytopathologic examination to exclude malignancy.

Treatment and Outcome. In a typical case, needle aspiration with total drainage may be sufficient treatment. If aspiration is unsuccessful, surgical excision may be indicated to exclude malignancy.

Enteric Cyst

Clinical Features. Enteric cysts are less common than bronchogenic or pericardial cysts; they are most common in children and are usually located in the posterior mediastinum, often attached to or embedded within the wall of the esophagus, where they cause symptoms of dysphagia. Compression of trachea or bronchi, with respiratory symptoms, may also occur.[1] Peptic ulceration caused by gastric-type mucosa may lead to perforation.

Pathologic Features. Enteric cysts arise from reduplication of the primitive foregut; they have a wall composed of smooth muscle, lined by esophageal, gastric, or intestinal epithelium.[34] They may show peptic ulceration.

Diagnosis. The diagnosis is usually suspected on clinical and radiologic grounds, and preoperative biopsy is not usually necessary.

Treatment and Outcome. Treatment consists of surgical excision for symptomatic relief.

Thymic Cyst

Clinical Features. These relatively uncommon lesions are similar in presentation to thymoma, with a mass effect in the anterosuperior mediastinum. They appear to occur with increased frequency in patients with a history of mediastinal tumors such as Hodgkin's disease and may be detected as residual masses after chemotherapy and/or radiation therapy.[38]

Pathologic Features. Thymic cysts are lined by either squamous or respiratory epithelium, which may be partially denuded. Residual thymic tissue is found within the wall (Fig. 10–10). Occasional thymomas and even thymic Hodgkin's disease may be predominantly cystic; therefore extensive histologic sectioning is required to exclude foci of thymoma within the wall of the cyst.[12]

Treatment and Outcome. Thymectomy is curative.

OTHER CONDITIONS

Castleman's Disease (Angiofollicular Lymph Node Hyperplasia)

Clinical Features. Mediastinal Castleman's disease (CD) is usually discovered on routine chest x-ray in an asymptomatic adult (see Chap. 17). Radiologic studies show a circumscribed mass in the anterosuperior or middle mediastinum corresponding to an enlarged lymph node or group of nodes. Small biopsy specimens (FNAB or mediastinoscopy) show only nonspecific reactive changes, and excision is usually required for the diagnosis in order to exclude a more threatening process.

Pathologic Features. The lesion consists of a large lymph node with an abundance of peculiar small follicles (involuted, "onionskin," or regressively transformed) surrounded by a broad mantle zone and penetrated by a small blood vessel. The interfollicular region is expanded by numerous proliferated small vessels of the high endothelial type. The combination of small follicles and a vascular interfollicular region can result in a gross appearance that resembles normal spleen. The histologic features of CD may be mimicked by reactions to a variety of stimuli, including partial nodal involvement by Hodgkin's disease or metastatic carcinoma.[39, 40] Therefore, a definite diagnosis of CD should never be made unless the entire mass has been excised and shown to consist entirely of this benign lymphoid proliferation.

Treatment and Outcome. The hyaline-vascular type of CD, which is typically found in the mediastinum, appears to be clinically benign and nonprogressive. Excision is usually required, however, to rule out more ominous conditions.

Granulomatous Lymphadenitis and Fibrosing Mediastinitis

Clinical Features. Mediastinal lymphadenopathy, usually paratracheal or hilar, can be produced by either sarcoidosis or infectious granulomas, particularly histoplasmosis. Patients with either disorder often have cough and may have pulmonary disease. Fibrosing or sclerosing mediastinitis is thought to be a delayed hypersensitivity reaction to antigens present in mediastinal lymph nodes, usually *Histoplasma capsulatum.* The mediastinal soft tissues are infiltrated and replaced by dense fibrous tissue, which surrounds major vessels and airways and mimics invasive malignancy of the anterosuperior mediastinum.[34] Patients may be adults or children and present with vascular or respiratory compromise. Chest x-ray shows mediastinal widening, often with a right-sided mass effect. Computed tomography reveals a cluster of matted nodes, usually subcarinal, often with calcification, and areas of fibrosis involving the SVC, trachea, or bronchi and even the esophagus. The CT findings of fibrosis and nodal calcification in the presence of an elevated erythrocyte sedimentation rate, a positive histoplasmic skin test, and a complement fixation titer for histoplasmosis in excess of 1:32 are said to be sufficient to establish the diagnosis of fibrosing mediastinitis.[41, 42] In the absence of these criteria, biopsy via mediastinoscopy or mediastinotomy is required for the diagnosis.

Pathologic Features. Sarcoidosis typically produces nonnecrotizing granulomas, although small areas of necrosis may occasionally be seen. Conversely, infectious granulomas are usually necrotizing and often caseous. There is sufficient overlap in clinical and histologic features that culture is

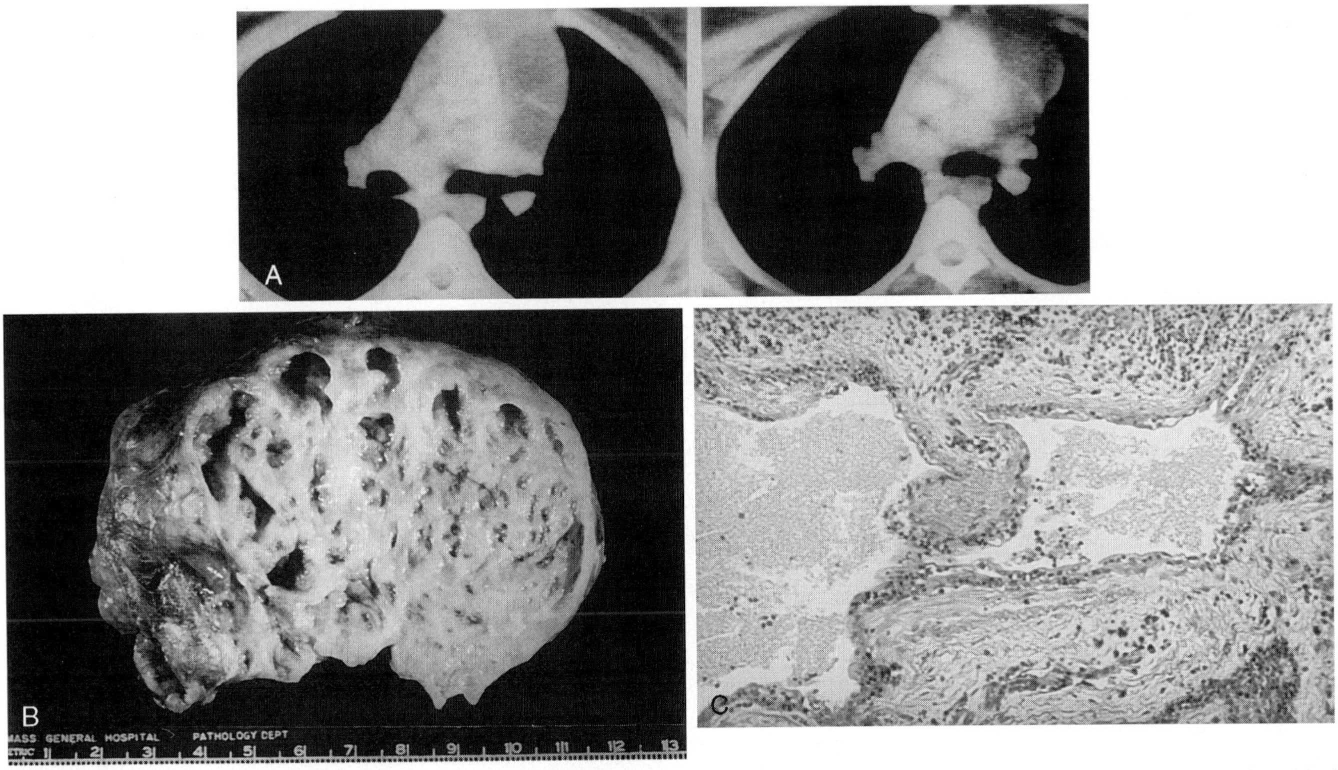

Figure 10–10. Thymic cyst in a patient with treated Hodgkin's disease. Persistence of a mass had led to the suspicion of residual lymphoma. *A,* Computed tomography views showing pretreatment study on the left and posttreatment study on the right. In retrospect, the lesion appears cystic on pre- as well as posttreatment studies. *B,* Gross photograph of the resected thymus showing a cystic lesion with a thick, trabeculated wall. *C,* Microscopic section showing only cystic thymic tissue, with no residual Hodgkin's disease.

mandatory if the intraoperative frozen section shows granulomas. Occasionally lymphomas, particularly Hodgkin's disease, may be associated with a granulomatous reaction indistinguishable from sarcoidosis (see "Pitfalls for the Pathologist"). Granulomas may be seen in uninvolved nodes as well as in nodes containing lymphoma. Sarcoidosis of lymph nodes is therefore a diagnosis of exclusion, after infections and neoplasms have been ruled out.

Chronic histoplasmic lymphadenitis may result in calcified granulomatous masses that can erode into the trachea or bronchi. Sclerosing mediastinitis produces a dense, white fibrous mass with a diffuse growth pattern.[34] Microscopic examination discloses bland fibrous tissue, often with foci of lymphocytic infiltration. In about half the cases, there is granulomatous inflammation, and approximately 50% of the cases are due to fungal infection, usually histoplasmosis[43]; some are associated with sarcoidosis, and the remainder are of unknown etiology.

Treatment and Outcome. Sarcoidosis is a chronic, progressive disorder, usually with predominance of pulmonary disease (see Chap. 11). Treatment is primarily with steroids. Mediastinal histoplasmosis requires treatment with antifungal agents; in chronic cases with erosion into bronchi, surgical resection of affected tissue and tracheobronchial reconstruction may be required. Sclerosing mediastinitis is usually a self-limited process not requiring treatment. However, some cases may progress to SVC syndrome or tracheobronchial obstruction. Early cases may respond to antifungal agents[42]; rarely, tracheobronchial resection or SVC bypass may be considered.[44, 45]

PITFALLS FOR THE SURGEON

1. *Biopsy of a vascular lesion.* This can lead to troublesome hemorrhage, particularly in the limited surgical field provided by cervical mediastinoscopy. Three rules to be followed should keep the surgeon out of trouble: (1) use intravenous contrast in CT imaging of any mediastinal tumor (except for the small, clearly localized anterior tumor), (2) use needle aspiration of the lesion prior to biopsy, and (3) ensure immediate availability of full thoracotomy equipment as a backup. Figure 10–11 illustrates a visceral compartment (middle mediastinum) tumor that proved to be an aneurysm of a right bronchial artery. Mediastinoscopic biopsy would have been inadvisable. Paravertebral tumors may have a generous arterial supply directly from the

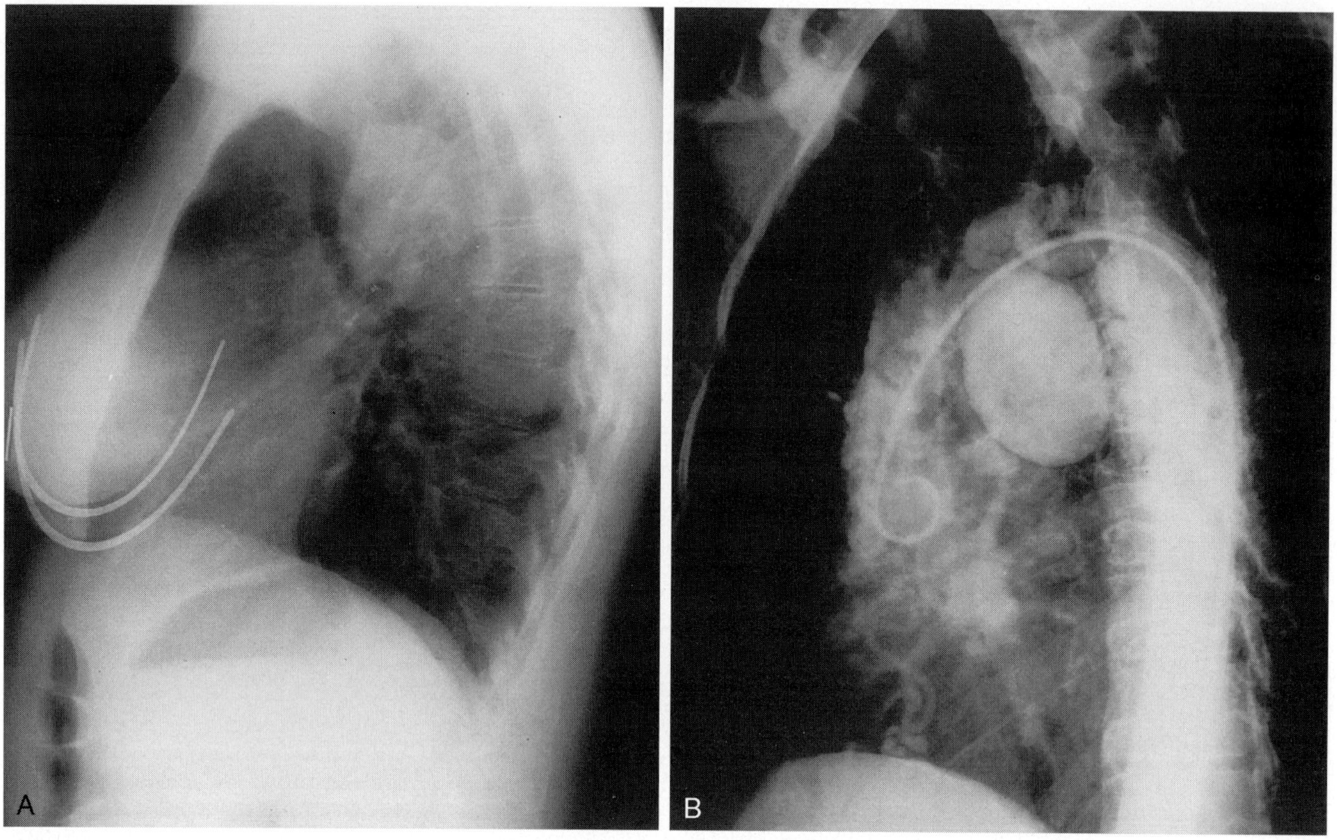

Figure 10–11. A pitfall for the surgeon: aneurysm of a right bronchial artery. Biopsy of vascular lesions is a major potential pitfall for the surgeon. On routine x-ray studies *(A),* the mass was interpreted as lymph nodes, whereas angiographic study *(B)* disclosed its vascular origin.

aorta, so that angiographic embolization of the feeding artery greatly facilitates subsequent surgical removal.

2. *The dumbbell neurogenic tumor.* Every paravertebral neurogenic tumor should be evaluated for enlargement of the intervertebral foramen, which would indicate extension of a neurofibroma within the spinal canal. Magnetic resonance imaging is especially helpful in identifying the so-called dumbbell or hourglass extension. If necessary, the ultimate diagnostic maneuver is metrizamide myelography to define the extent of intraspinous involvement. One-stage removal is advisable, utilizing a combined neurosurgical and thoracic surgical team approach.

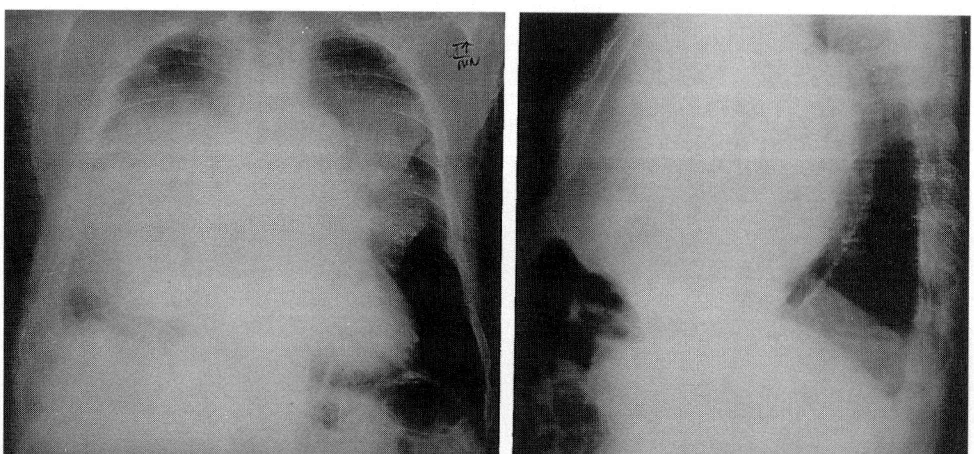

Figure 10–12. Another pitfall for the surgeon: massive tumor of the mediastinum. Although its radiologic appearance is daunting, this tumor proved to be a low-grade liposarcoma, which was encapsulated and completely resectable by median sternotomy. Anteroposterior chest x-ray *(left)*; lateral chest x-ray *(right)*.

Enucleation of the tumor from the intervertebral foramen by the thoracic surgeon alone risks paraplegia as a complication.

3. *The massive mediastinal tumor.* Unresectability cannot be reliably determined by size alone. Figure 10–12 illustrates a huge, biopsy-proven low-grade liposarcoma. Careful radiographic vascular evaluation indicated likely resectability, and a 512-g tumor was totally removed with median sternotomy. The pitfall here would have been not to operate on this patient with impending airway obstruction.
4. *Anesthesia in a patient with airway compromise.* Complete airway obstruction may develop in an anesthetized patient, with catastrophic consequences. Less severely compromised patients may have difficulty maintaining an airway postoperatively, requiring prolonged intubation. Prebiopsy consultation with the anesthesiologist is essential in a patient with a mediastinal mass and suspected airway compromise, particularly a small child.
5. *Failure to obtain cultures in granulomatous lymphadenitis.* The surgeon and the pathologist must agree on who will send material for microbial culture. A related pitfall is acceptance of a diagnosis of sarcoidosis in a patient with massively enlarged lymph nodes: in such a case, the biopsied lymph node showing granulomas may represent a reaction to a lymphomatous process not sampled.

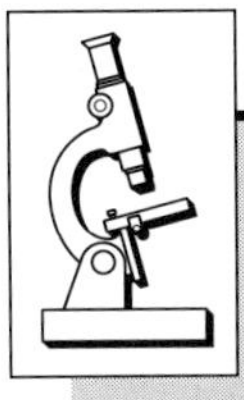

PITFALLS FOR THE PATHOLOGIST

1. *Determining adequacy of tissue for diagnosis.* A major indication for intraoperative consultation is to determine the adequacy of a biopsy specimen for diagnosis and special studies. The pathologist should make certain that sufficient abnormal tissue is present for both the frozen section (which can then be saved for immunologic and genetic studies) and permanent sections, and electron microscopy, microbial culture, and so on, as needed. The pathologist should not hesitate to tell the surgeon that the tissue is too fibrotic, necrotic, or small for a confident diagnosis. Remember, unless a confident diagnosis can be based on frozen section, there is no guarantee that the tissue will be sufficient for diagnosis. The need for additional surgery for diagnosis will be perceived unenthusiastically by patient and surgeon alike the next day.
2. *Failure to identify anatomic landmarks on a resected specimen.* In staging thymoma, it is imperative that the pathologist know what structures are present in the specimen—e.g., vena cava, pericardium, lung, pleura, nerve. If these are not identified by the surgeon, a phone call is necessary.
3. *Distinction between lymphoma, thymoma, and germ-cell tumor.* In this situation, lymphoma is the great imitator. When histologic indicators are mixed, it is likely lymphoma. This distinction should not as a rule be attempted on frozen section.
4. *Failure to save tissue for special studies to resolve critical differential diagnoses* (see Chap. 2).
5. *Failure to obtain or to recommend microbial cultures for granulomatous lymphadenitis.*
6. *Failure to recognize underlying lymphoma in lymph nodes showing granulomatous lymphadenitis.* Figure 10–13 illustrates a case of Hodgkin's disease with a prominent obscuring granulomatous component, on which a misdiagnosis of sarcoidosis was originally based.
7. *Diagnosis of Castleman's disease with biopsies smaller than excisional.* This may result in failure to identify malignancies inducing nodal reactions resembling Castleman's disease.
8. *Inadequate sampling of cysts and germ-cell tumors.* Small foci of malignancy or of higher-grade elements, respectively, can be missed in this way.

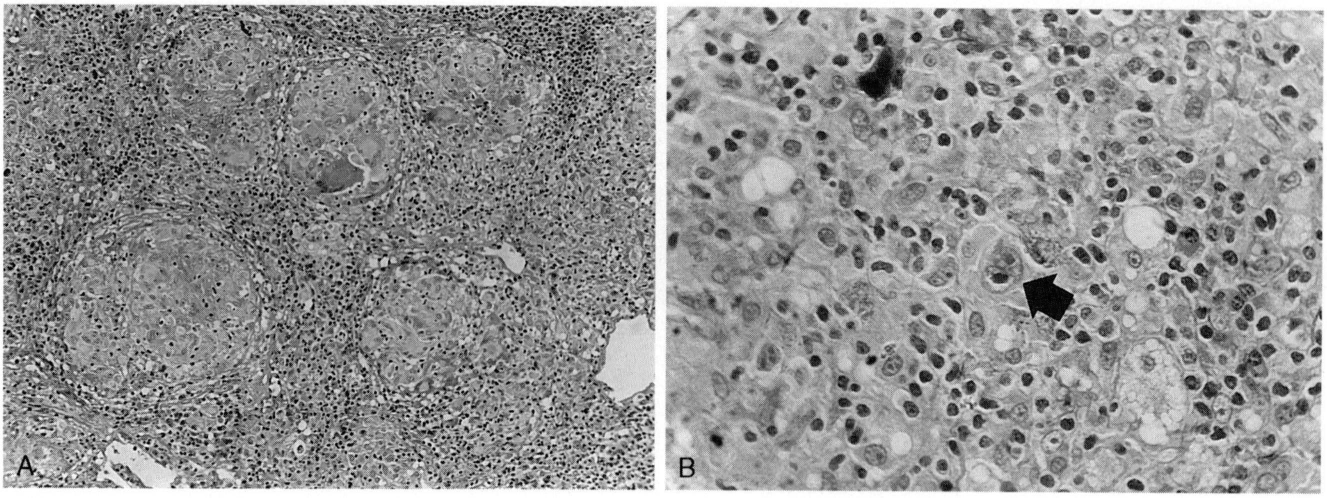

Figure 10–13. A pitfall for the pathologist: underdiagnosis of Hodgkin's disease. *A,* Low magnification of lymph node biopsy showing prominent noncaseating granulomas; a misdiagnosis of sarcoidosis was made. *B,* Higher magnification shows Reed-Sternberg cell *(arrow)* and variants, diagnostic of Hodgkin's disease.

FURTHER READING

Davis R, Sabiston D. The mediastinum. In: Sabiston D, ed. *Textbook of Surgery.* Philadelphia: Saunders; 1991:1771–1796.

Harris NL. The pathology of lymphomas: A practical approach to diagnosis and classification. *Surg Oncol Clin North Am.* 1993;2:167–206.

Quintanilla-Martinez L, Wilkins E, Choi N, et al. Thymoma: Histologic classification predicts clinical behavior. *Cancer.* 1994;74:606–617.

Shields TW. Thymic tumors. In: Shields TW, ed. *Mediastinal Surgery.* Philadelphia: Lea & Febiger; 1991:153–183.

Wick M. The mediastinum. In: Sternberg S, ed. *Textbook of Surgical Pathology.* New York: Raven Press; 1989:1135–1182.

REFERENCES

1. Davis R, Sabiston D. The mediastinum. In: Sabiston D, ed. *Textbook of Surgery.* Philadelphia: Saunders; 1991:1771–1796.
2. Dahlgren S, Nordenstrom B. *Transthoracic Needle Biopsy.* Stockholm: Almquist and Wiksell; 1966.
3. Pearson FG. An evaluation of mediastinoscopy in the management of presumably operable bronchial carcinoma. *J Thorac Cardiovasc Surg.* 1968;55:617–625.
4. Ginsberg RJ, Rice TW, Goldberg M, et al. Extended cervical mediastinoscopy. *J Thorac Cardiovasc Surg.* 1987;94:673–678.
5. McNeill TM, Chamberlain JM. Diagnostic anterior mediastinotomy. *Ann Thorac Surg.* 1966;2:532–539.
6. LoCicero J III. Mediastinotomy. In: Shields TW, ed. *Mediastinal Surgery.* Philadelphia: Lea & Febiger; 1991.
7. Sugarbaker DJ. Thoracoscopy in the management of anterior mediastinal masses. *Ann Thorac Surg.* 1993;56:654–656.
8. Shields TW. Thymic tumors. In: Shields TW, ed. *Mediastinal Surgery.* Philadelphia: Lea & Febiger; 1991:153–183.
9. Kirchner T, Müller-Hermelink H. New approaches to the diagnosis of thymic epithelial tumors. *Prog Surg Pathol.* 1989;10:167–189.
10. Quintanilla-Martinez L, Wilkins E, Choi N, et al. Thymoma: Histologic classification predicts clinical behavior. *Cancer.* 1994;74:606–617.
11. Quintanilla-Martinez L, Wilkins E, Ferry J, Harris N. Thymoma: Morphologic subclassification correlates with invasiveness and immunohistologic features: A study of 122 cases. *Hum Pathol.* 1993;24:958–969.
12. Rosai J, Levine G. Tumors of the thymus. In: Hartmann WH, ed. *Atlas of Tumor Pathology,* 2nd series. Fascicle 13. Washington, DC: Armed Forces Institute of Pathology; 1976.
13. Wilkins E Jr, Edmunds H Jr, Castleman B. Cases of thymoma at the Massachusetts General Hospital. *J Thorac Cardiovasc Surg.* 1966;52:322–330.
14. Wilkins E Jr, Castleman B. Thymoma: A continuing survey at the Massachusetts General Hospital. *Ann Thorac Surg.* 1978;28:252–256.
15. Marino M, Müller-Hermelink H. Thymoma and thymic carcinoma: Relation of thymoma epithelial cells to the cortical and medullary differentiation of thymus. *Virchows Arch Pathol Anat Histopathol.* 1985;407:119–149.
16. Kirchner T, Schalke B, Buchwald J, et al. Well-differentiated thymic carcinoma: An organotypical low-grade carcinoma with relationship to cortical thymoma. *Am J Surg Pathol.* 1992;16:1153–1160.
17. Snover D, Levine G, Rosai J. Thymic carcinoma: Five distinctive histological variants. *Am J Surg Pathol.* 1982;6:451–470.
18. Wick M, Weiland L, Scheithauer B, Bernatz P. Primary thymic carcinomas. *Am J Surg Pathol.* 1982;6:613–630.
19. Masaoka A, Monden Y, Nakahara K, Tanioka T. Follow-up study of thymomas with special reference to their clinical stages. *Cancer.* 1981;48:2485–2492.
20. Wilkins EW Jr, Grillo HC, Scannell JG, et al. Role of staging in prognosis and management of thymoma. *Ann Thorac Surg.* 1991;51:888–892.
21. Kersh C, Eisert D, Hazra T. Malignant thymoma: Role of radiation therapy in management. *Radiology.* 1985;156:207–209.
22. Kaplan H. *Hodgkin's Disease,* 2nd ed. Cambridge, MA: Harvard University Press; 1978.
23. Lukes R, Butler J, Hicks E. Natural history of Hodgkin's disease as related to its pathological picture. *Cancer.* 1966;19:317–344.
24. Levitt L, Aisenberg A, Harris N, et al. Primary non-Hodgkin's lymphoma of the mediastinum. *Cancer.* 1982;50:2486–2492.
25. Addis B, Isaacson P. Large cell lymphoma of the mediastinum: A B-cell tumor of probable thymic origin. *Histopathology.* 1986;10:379–390.
26. Jacobson J, Aisenberg A, Lamarre L, et al. Mediastinal large cell lymphoma: An uncommon subset of adult lymphoma curable with combined modality therapy. *Cancer.* 1988;62:1893–1898.
27. Lamarre L, Jacobson J, Aisenberg A, Harris N. Primary large cell lymphoma of the mediastinum. *Am J Surg Pathol.* 1989;13:730–739.
28. Moller P, Moldenhauer G, Momburg F, et al. Mediastinal lymphoma of clear cell type is a tumor corresponding to terminal steps of B cell differentiation. *Blood.* 1987;69:1087–1095.
29. Scarpa A, Bonetti F, Menestrina F. Mediastinal large cell lymphoma with sclerosis: Genotypic analysis establishes its B nature. *Virchows Arch.* 1987;412:17–21.
30. Yousem S, Weiss L, Warnke R. Primary mediastinal non-Hodgkins lymphomas: A morphologic and immunologic study of 19 cases. *Am J Clin Pathol.* 1985;83:676–680.
31. Nathwani B, Kim H, Rappaport H. Malignant lymphoma, lymphoblastic. *Cancer.* 1976;38:964–983.

32. Nathwani B, Diamond L, Winberg C, et al. Lymphoblastic lymphoma: a clinicopathologic study of 95 patients. *Cancer.* 1981;48:2347–2357.
33. Scully RE. Tumors of the ovary and maldeveloped gonad. In: Hartmann WH, ed. *Atlas of Tumor Pathology,* 2nd series. Fascicle 16. Washington, DC: Armed Forces Institute of Pathology; 1979.
34. Wick M. The mediastinum. In: Sternberg S, ed. *Textbook of Surgical Pathology.* New York: Raven Press; 1989:1135–1182.
35. Harkin JC, Reed RJ. Tumors of the peripheral nervous system. In: Firminger H, ed. *Atlas of Tumor Pathology,* 2nd series. Fascicle 3. Washington, DC: Armed Forces Institute of Pathology; 1969.
36. Glenner GG, Grimley PM. Tumors of the extra-adrenal paraganglion system (including chemoreceptors). In: Firminger H, ed. *Atlas of Tumor Pathology,* 2nd series. Fascicle 9. Washington, DC: Armed Forces Institute of Pathology; 1974.
37. Grillo HC, Ojemann RG, Scannell JG, Zervas N. Combined approach to ''dumbbell'' intrathoracic and intraspinal neurogenic tumors. *Ann Thorac Surg.* 1983;36:402–407.
38. Lindfors K, Meyer J, Dedrick C, et al. Thymic cysts in mediastinal Hodgkin's disease. *Radiology.* 1985;156:37–41.
39. Carey R, Harris NL. Case records of the Massachusetts General Hospital: Case 18-1982. *N Engl J Med.* 1982;306:1096–1102.
40. Pettit C, Ferry JA, Harris NL. Simultaneous occurrence of Hodgkin's disease and angiofollicular hyperplasia (Castleman's disease): Report of 3 cases. *Lab Invest.* 1991;62:81A.
41. Weinstein JG, Aronberg DG, Sagel SS. CT of fibrosing mediastinitis: Findings and their utility. *Am J Radiol.* 1983;141:247–251.
42. Urschel HC, Razzuk MD, Netto GJ, et al. Sclerosing mediastinitis: Improved management with histoplasmosis titer and ketoconazole. *Ann Thorac Surg.* 1990;50:215–225.
43. Weider S, Rabinowitz J. Fibrous mediastinitis: A late manifestation of mediastinal histoplasmosis. *Radiology.* 1977;125:305–312.
44. Mathisen DJ, Grillo HC. Clinical manifestation of mediastinal fibrosis and histoplasmosis. *Ann Thorac Surg.* 1992;54:1051–1058.
45. Doty DB. Bypass of superior vena cava. *J Thorac Cardiovasc Surg.* 1982;83:3326–3328.

11

The Lung and Pleura

Thomas V. Colby and Claude Deschamps

Definition

This chapter discusses pathologic conditions involving the alveoli, airways, and pleurae that a surgeon may encounter. By virtue of the role that the lungs play in gas exchange and hemodynamics, they are exposed to foreign material and infectious organisms via inspired air and to tumor metastases and emboli while filtering the bloodstream. Although some of the more common pulmonary conditions, such as asthma and pulmonary edema, are diagnosed and treated nonsurgically, the surgeon is indispensable in the management of many pulmonary diseases.

Diseases of the Lungs and Airways

BIOPSY TECHNIQUES

There are many ways to obtain lung cells and tissue for diagnostic purposes; each of these has different applications, depending on the clinical situation (Table 11–1).

Cytologic specimens provide single cells or groups of cells for microscopic evaluation. These techniques are particularly useful for diagnosis of infectious and neoplastic processes, but, since material shed into the airway is examined, they are most reliable for proximal lesions. Well-established cytologic criteria for malignancy include nuclear hyperchromatism, nuclear membrane irregularities, increased nuclear/cytoplasmic ratio, and (often) prominent nucleoli.[1]

Bronchial and transbronchial biopsies are often too small to evaluate pulmonary architecture, but, like cytology, they may be useful for the diagnosis of neoplasms and infection. In conjunction with bronchoalveolar lavage, these biopsy techniques can be more useful. If, however, pattern recognition is important for diagnosis, thoracoscopic or open lung biopsies may be required. An example of this is chronic interstitial pneumonia, in which the distribution and spatial relationship of cells within the lung are diagnostically important.

Regardless of the biopsy technique, the tissue sampled should represent the active disease process—neither the area least affected nor the area most affected. Biopsies from the tips of the lobes, especially the right middle lobe

Table 11–1. Biopsy Techniques[a]

Technique	Comment
Cytologic: Sputum, bronchial washing, bronchoalveolar lavage, fine needle aspiration biopsy	Small size of specimen Cannot discern architectural abnormalities Especially useful for tumors and infection
Bronchial wall biopsy	Small size of specimen Cannot discern architecture
Transbronchial biopsy samples alveolar parenchyma	Small size of specimen Cannot discern architecture
Transthoracic drill biopsy	Rarely used in North America
Thoracoscopic lung biopsy	Some problems with sampling (tissue cannot be fully palpated), traumatic distortion of specimen and sometimes small size relative to traditional open lung biopsy, but these are minor
Open lung biopsy/resection specimen	Excellent for pathologic evaluation

[a]*Note:* The morbidity of these techniques varies and the method(s) chosen must be tailored to each individual.

and the lingula, are of questionable value; however, these areas are readily accessible.[2, 3] If samples are at least 3 cm, even these areas may be adequate for diagnosis.

Although frozen sections can be done on virtually any tissue specimen, intraprocedural frozen sections are best reserved for the times when an immediate operative decision will be based on the findings. The reasons for this are threefold: first, inflammatory reactions may be mistaken for neoplasms on frozen section, leading to surgical treatment errors; second, tissue is "lost" (actually shaved away) during preparation for frozen section microscopy; and third, freezing introduces a tissue artifact that may confound final diagnosis. If a frozen section is needed, the pathologist can make *touch imprints* or *smear cytology* preparations from the fresh tissue before freezing it. These preparations may prove helpful in appreciating cytologic features otherwise obscured by frozen section artifacts.

If a pulmonary infection is suspected, microbial cultures are necessary. Depending on the routine in a particular institution, the surgeon may handle this in the operating room or send sterile tissue to the laboratory for the pathologist to allocate.

In addition to the usual histologic procedures, a number of special stains for organisms, mucin, iron, and other substances, as well as immunohistochemical stains, can be performed on biopsy material. These procedures can be done by most pathology laboratories. Sophisticated and experimental studies can also be performed on lung tissue if provisions are made prior to obtaining the tissue by consulting with the pathologist and the interested investigative laboratory.

LUNG MASSES

A mass in the lung is the most common problem presenting to the surgeon. Carcinoma of the lung is usually the first concern, although a metastasis or nonmalignant lesion can present in this fashion. Although carcinoma of the lung is extremely common, *the most common malignancies in the lung are metastases.*

The *solitary pulmonary nodule* is a relatively common problem. A number of factors such as age, smoking history, size, and radiographic features affect the probability of a given nodule being benign or malignant.[4] Small size, smooth contours, presence of calcification, radiologic stability over time, and occurrence in a nonsmoker favor a benign lesion. In the past, many benign cases came to resection for diagnosis; advances in computed tomography (CT) imaging and recognition of the features of benign nodules have greatly decreased the number of benign lesions coming to surgical resection.

Carcinoma of the Lung

Carcinoma of the lung is common and carries a poor prognosis; only a minority of patients qualify for surgical resection, effectively the only chance for cure. Adult smokers are most commonly affected, although passive exposure to cigarette smoke, radon, and asbestos are implicated as less common causes.[5, 6] Location, clinical behavior, and management are related to the histologic types: squamous-cell carcinoma, adenocarcinoma (including the subset called bronchioloalveolar carcinoma), small-cell carcinoma, and large-cell carcinoma.[1, 6–8] These histologic types are compared in Table 11–2 and illustrated in Figure 11–1.

Squamous-cell carcinomas are generally proximal bronchial (central) tumors that show differentiation toward squamous epithelium in the form of intercellular bridges or keratin production. Degree of differentiation is usually recognized in relation to how closely the tumors resemble normal squamous epithelium—i.e., well, moderately, and poorly differentiated squamous-cell carcinoma. Some squamous-cell carcinomas are in situ in the large airways and clinically occult, recognized only on the basis of abnormal cytology.

Adenocarcinomas tend to be parenchymal (peripheral) tumors that form tubules, glands, or papillae (mimicking glandular epithelium) or that secrete mucin identifiable with histochemical stains such as mucicarmine or digested periodic acid–Schiff (PAS) reagents. The latter are called solid adenocarcinomas with mucin production. Bronchioloalveolar carcinoma (also called alveolar-cell carcinoma) is a special form of well-differentiated adenocarcinoma that shows growth of tumor cells along alveolar walls with preservation of architecture. Mucinous and nonmucinous variants of bronchioloalveolar carcinoma are recognized (Fig. 11–2). Some cases present as a nodule and others as more widespread airspace-filling disease; sometimes they

Table 11–2. Comparison of Histologic Types of Carcinoma of the Lung

	Approx. Percent of Cases	Percent Smokers	Percent Central (Versus Peripheral)	Percent Localized at Presentation	All Comers: 5-Year Survival	Survival of Patients Undergoing Surgical Resection	
						Stage I	***Stage 2***
Squamous-cell	30%	98%	64%	21.5%	15.4%	≈50%	≈30%
Adenocarcinoma (bronchioloalveolar)	32%	82%	5%	22.2%	16.6% (42.1%)	≈45%	≈20%
Small-cell	18%	99%	74%	8.2%	4.6%	≈20%[a]	<10%[a]
Large-cell and rare subtypes	20%	93%	42%	15.2%	11.5%	[b]	[b]

[a]Surgical resections for small-cell carcinoma are very unusual.
[b]Adenocarcinoma and large-cell carcinoma included together.
Source: Compiled from references 6, 8, 11–13, 24–26.

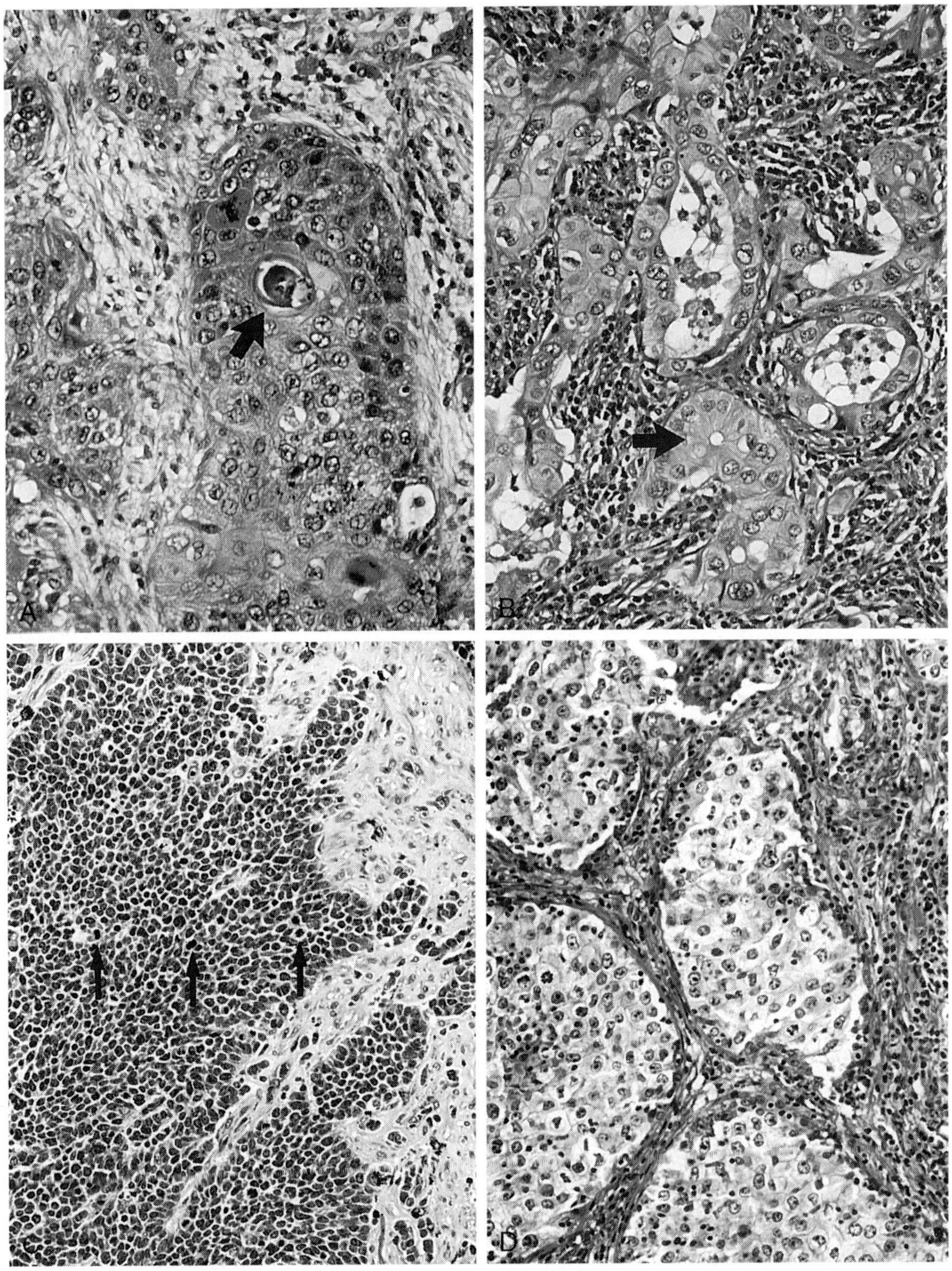

Figure 11–1. Microscopic appearances of the major histologic types of carcinoma of the lung. *A,* Squamous-cell carcinoma. There is a nest of malignant cells well demarcated from the surrounding fibrous stroma, which shows an inflammatory cell infiltrate. The cells become larger and have more abundant cytoplasm centrally, and there is keratin pearl formation *(arrow)*. *B,* Adenocarcinoma. Tumor cells form glands *(arrow)*, nests, and cords of cells, with surrounding stroma showing an inflammatory cell infiltrate. *C,* Small-cell carcinoma. Sheets of carcinoma cells are present, with numerous mitotic figures *(arrows)*. The cells show some palisading at the border with the stroma, which is hypocellular fibrous tissue. *D,* Large-cell carcinoma. Large carcinoma cells with some cytoplasmic clearing are present, but no glandular or squamous differentiation is seen. The stroma shows a moderate inflammatory cell infiltrate. All figures are taken at the same magnification. Hematoxylin and eosin, ×200.

involve a lobe (simulating lobar pneumonia), other times they present as diffuse bilateral lung disease.

Small-cell carcinomas lack squamous or glandular differentiation and are composed of small cells (approximately three times the size of an erythrocyte) with very little cytoplasm, a high mitotic rate, and extensive necrosis. They tend to be large, central, rapidly growing tumors and are the type of carcinoma most often associated with hormone production and paraneoplastic syndromes.

Large-cell carcinomas are composed of intermediate-to-large polygonal cells with relatively abundant cytoplasm and nuclei that usually have prominent nucleoli. Glandular and squamous differentiation are lacking.

The most important distinction between these subtypes

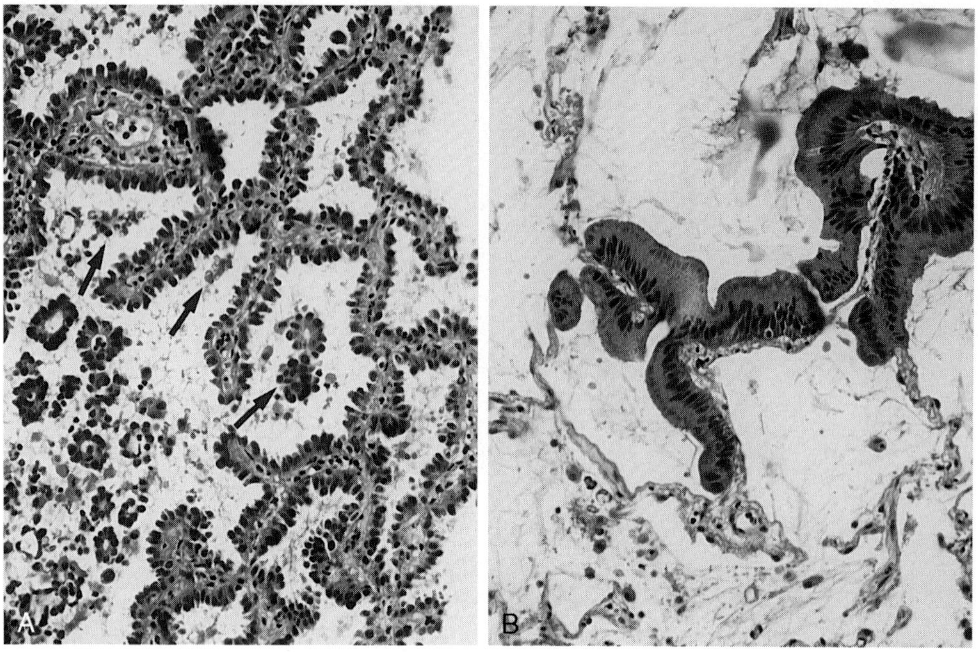

Figure 11–2. Bronchioloalveolar subtype of adenocarcinoma. *A,* The nonmucinous variant of bronchioloalveolar carcinoma is associated with a proliferation of atypical cells along alveolar walls. The cells have a somewhat hobnail appearance as they protrude from the alveolar walls. Some papillary groups have detached themselves and are present in alveolar spaces *(arrows). B,* Mucinous bronchioloalveolar carcinoma is seen as well-differentiated mucinous epithelium growing along alveolar walls *(center).* The surrounding alveoli show abundant strands of mucus in their lumens. Hematoxylin and eosin, ×200.

is the separation of small-cell carcinoma from the three other types; for this purpose, these three are often collectively termed ''non–small-cell carcinomas.''

Lung cancer is staged according to a standardized TNM staging system.[9–13] The T, N, and M factors are shown in Table 11–3. Clinical stage is assigned on the basis of T, N, and M factors (Table 11–4).[9] Determination of the TNM staging factors may be done on the basis of radiographic findings, but in patients who come to surgical exploration, the TNM stage is determined postsurgically on the basis of the pathologic findings in the lung and mediastinal lymph nodes.

Frozen section evaluation of tissues taken at the time of surgical staging (either at mediastinoscopy or thoracotomy) is useful, in some cases, to identify involved lymph node groups and thereby to determine operability. In resection specimens, frozen sections should be performed on bronchial margins when gross evaluation leaves any concern or doubt as to margin adequacy.

Carcinoid Tumor

Carcinoid tumors are low-grade neuroendocrine malignancies. Dense-core neurosecretory granules can be demonstrated in the cytoplasm of the cells,[14] and there is occasionally corresponding clinical evidence of hormone production. Such granules may be identified by electron microscopy or with special histochemical or immunohistochemical stains. They usually occur in adults and have no relationship to cigarette smoking. Carcinoid tumors are more commonly central than peripheral and may be endobronchial, covered by intact mucosa (Fig. 11–3). Grossly, on fresh sectioning, they are yellow or tan. Microscopically, they are made up of uniform nests or ribbons of cells with prominent, delicate vascularity. The cells are polygonal or somewhat fusiform, with central nuclei with a stippled ''salt and pepper'' chromatin and with eosinophilic or slightly basophilic cytoplasm (Fig. 11–4). Immunohistochemical stains for neurosecretory granules (e.g., chromogranin, synaptophysin) are usually positive (see Chap. 2). The prognosis with surgical resection is excellent, even in the presence of regional lymph node metastases (5-year overall survival, 90%).[14]

Atypical carcinoid tumors show neuroendocrine differentiation similar to carcinoid tumors but have increased mitotic activity, cytologic atypia, necrosis, and loss of architecture. The prognosis is less favorable than that for carcinoid tumors, with 5-year survival slightly better than 60%.[14]

Other low-grade malignant endobronchial tumors often grouped with carcinoid tumors are *mucoepidermoid carcinomas* and *adenoid cystic carcinomas.* Both are probably derived from salivary gland–type tissue that comprises the bronchial submucosal glands. In the past, these low-grade carcinomas were inappropriately termed ''bronchial adenomas.''

Benign Tumors of the Lung

Benign tumors of the lung are rare; a number have been described, including benign fibrous histiocytomas, lipomas, neurofibromas, schwannomas, hemangiomas, lymphangiomas, and others. One that is encountered with some frequency is the *pulmonary hamartoma,* a discrete nodular lesion usually composed of cartilage with variable amounts of fat, smooth muscle, or fibrous tissue. These tumors are lobulated, with clefts lined by bronchiolar epithelium. Some cases are sufficiently distinctive radiographically that biopsy is unnecessary. Cases that are resected are usually recognizable grossly based on their cartilaginous composition. *Inflammatory pseudotumor* is a term that has been applied to a variety of benign tumors, including plasma-cell granuloma (see subsequent discussion), fibroxanthoma, fibrous histiocytoma, and others.

Table 11–3. TNM Staging of Lung Carcinoma

T: Tumor (size or involvement)	
TX	Tumor proven by the presence of malignant cells in bronchopulmonry secretions but not visualized roentgenographically or bronchoscopically, or any tumor that cannot be assessed as in treatment staging.
T0	No evidence of primary tumor.
Tis	Carcinoma in situ.
T1	A tumor that is 3 cm or less in greatest dimension, surrounded by lung or visceral pleura, and without evidence of invasion proximal to a lobar bronchus at bronchoscopy. (Note: The uncommon superficial tumor of any size with its invasive component limited to the bronchial wall which may extend proximal to the main bronchus is also classified as T1.)
T2	A tumor more than 3.0 cm in greatest dimension or a tumor of any size that either invades the visceral pleura or has associated atelectasis or obstructive pneumonitis extending to the hilar region. At bronchoscopy, the proximal extent of demonstrable tumor must be within a lobar bronchus or at least 2.0 cm distal to the carcinoma. Any associated atelectasis or obstructive pneumonitis must involve less than an entire lung.
T3	A tumor of any size with direct extension into the chest wall (including superior sulcus tumors), diaphragm, or the mediastinal pleura or pericardium without involving the heart, great vessels, trachea, esophagus, or vertebral body, or a tumor in the main bronchus within 2 cm of the carina without involving the carina.
T4	A tumor of any size with invasion of the mediastinum or involving heart, great vessels, trachea, esophagus, vertebral body, or carina, or presence of malignant pleural effusion. [Note: Most pleural effusions associated with lung cancer are due to tumor. There are, however, a few patients in whom cytopathologic examination of pleural fluid (on more than one specimen) is negative for tumor, the fluid is nonbloody, and is not an exudate. In such cases where these elements and clinical judgment dictate that the effusion is not related to the tumor, the patient should be staged T1, T2, or T3, excluding effusion as a staging element.]
N: Nodes (status and extent of involvement)	
NX	Regional lymph nodes cannot be assessed.
N0	No demonstrable metastasis to regional lymph nodes.
N1	Metastasis to lymph nodes in the peribronchial or the ipsilateral hilar region, or both, including direct extension.
N2	Metastasis to ipsilateral mediastinal lymph nodes or subcarinal lymph nodes.
N3	Metastasis to contralateral mediastinal lymph nodes, contralateral hilar nodes, ipsilateral or contralateral scalene, or supraclavicular lymph nodes.
M: Metastasis (extent)	
MX	Presence of distant metastases cannot be assessed.
M0	No (known) distant metastasis.
M1	Distant metastasis present—specify site(s).

Source: From references 10, 12, and 13.

Miscellaneous Primary Lung Tumors

Lymphomas and sarcomas may arise in the lung. As is the case in other sites, there are various histologic types of lymphoma. In the case of a suspected lymphoma, it is critical that the pathologist allocate tissue specifically for lymphoid marker studies; biopsy of hilar lymph nodes is indicated for lymphoma staging. Sarcomas of the lung are rare and diverse in histologic type.

Metastatic Neoplasms

Tumor metastasis to the lung is extremely common; in most cases the histology of the metastasis recapitulates that of the primary site. The surgeon is often asked to confirm a diagnosis of metastatic carcinoma, and in patients with a history of a prior neoplasm, an effort should be made to obtain the prior slides to allow the pathologist comparison of the features of earlier disease with those of the current

Table 11–4. Clinical Stage Groupings According to TNM Subsets

Stage	Percent of Cases	T Factor	N Factor	M Factor	Consider Surgery?
Occult		TX	N0	M0	Yes
0		Tis	N0	M0	Yes
I	13	T1	N0	M0	Yes
		T2	N0	M0	Yes
II	10	T1	N1	M0	Yes
		T2	N1	M0	Yes
IIIA	22	T3	N0	M0	Yes
		T3	N1	M0	Yes
		T1–T3	N2	M0	Yes
IIIB	22	Any T	N3	M0	No
		T4	Any N	M0	No
IV	32	Any T	Any N	M1	No

Source: From references 9, 11, and 12.

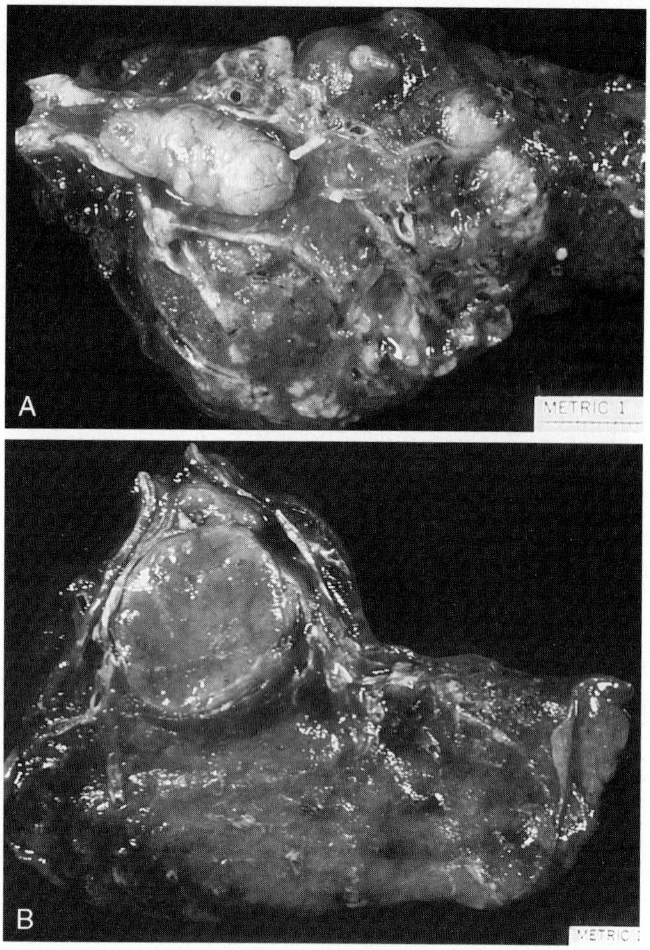

Figure 11–3. Carcinoid tumor (gross appearance). Carcinoid tumors may be endobronchial polypoid masses *(A)* or well-circumscribed nodules that compress bronchi *(B)*.

lung tumor (see Chap. 1, Case 1–1). For certain tumors, such as breast carcinoma, a panel of special stains often helps to distinguish a new primary from a metastasis (see Chap. 2). In some tumors (e.g., certain relatively indolent metastatic carcinomas and sarcomas), the surgeon is involved in the resection of lung tumors known to be metastases. Gross evaluation is usually sufficient to determine adequacy of margins, but if there is a question, intraoperative frozen section can be performed.

Anatomic patterns of metastatic carcinoma are diverse and include a single nodule, multiple nodules, localized infiltrates, diffuse lymphangitic involvement (with tumor cells in pulmonary lymphatics sometimes presenting as interstitial lung disease), intraarteriolar tumor emboli (sometimes with resultant acute or subacute *cor pulmonale*), and endobronchial lesions.

Metastatic carcinoma (and rarely sarcoma) from an occult primary site can produce a solitary mass that mimics primary neoplasm of the lung.

Focal Organizing Pneumonia

Some lung nodules suspected radiographically to be tumors are found instead to be composed of inflamed and organizing fibroblastic tissue; such a process is called *focal organizing pneumonia.* Such masses can be mistaken for neoplasms by both the surgeon and the pathologist. Only a minority of cases have an antecedent history of pneumonia. Pathologically, this is nonspecific repair reaction in the lungs.

Rounded Atelectasis

Rounded atelectasis is visualized as a ''lung nodule'' radiographically, sometimes with preceding history of a pleural effusion. It is thought to result from visceral pleural fibrosis, which retracts, causing focal parenchymal atelectasis. This appears as a nodule radiographically. Some cases are sufficiently distinctive in radiographic studies to allow recognition, but others come to resection as suspected neoplasms. In such instances, both the pathologist and the surgeon are amazed when gross dissection of the ''tumor'' reveals only lung tissue and thickened pleura.

Plasma-Cell Granuloma

Plasma-cell granuloma, also known as inflammatory pseudotumor, presents as a nodule or mass in children or adults. A small percentage of cases (especially in children) are locally invasive or may recur after excision. Histologically, they are composed of fibroblastic cells with clusters of interspersed numerous plasma cells.

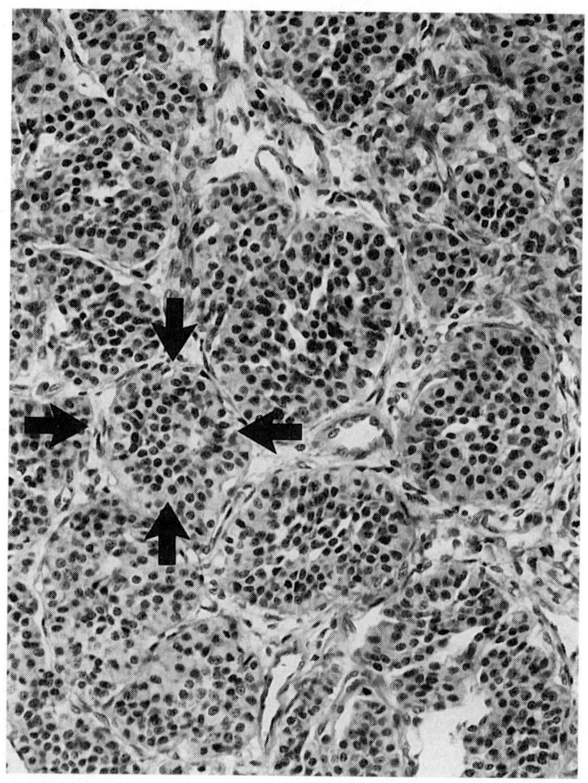

Figure 11–4. Carcinoid tumor (microscopic appearance). Typical carcinoid tumors are composed of nests of uniform cells with centrally placed nucleoli that have a salt-and-pepper chromatin pattern. The stroma shows prominent, delicate vascularity and surrounds the tumor cells, producing a ''cell ball'' appearance *(arrows)*. Hematoxylin and eosin, ×200.

Granulomatous Infection

Granulomatous infection may result in solitary nodules that mimic a neoplasm.

ACUTE DIFFUSE LUNG DISEASES

Acute pulmonary infiltrates, particularly in an immunosuppressed patient, can evolve very rapidly, engendering considerable concern on the part of the patient's primary physicians. Unless a diagnosis can be made rapidly by noninvasive means, some sort of more invasive procedure may be necessary (seemingly, more often than not, late on a Friday afternoon).

Bronchoalveolar lavage, sometimes with concomitant transbronchial biopsy, has largely replaced open biopsy in this setting, especially in immunosuppressed patients. The surgeon's role has thus decreased, although the advent of thoracoscopic biopsy may reverse this trend. In acute diffuse lung disease, an infection is usually the most important process to detect; one must be certain that appropriate microbial cultures are taken and that appropriate special stains are requested by the pathologist. Stains for microorganisms can be done on either frozen sections or tissue imprints if an immediate interpretation is necessary.

Many patients with acute diffuse lung disease, particularly those with the adult respiratory distress syndrome (ARDS), have *diffuse alveolar damage (DAD).* The DAD reaction pattern has a number of causes, including infections, chemotherapy, radiation, toxins, shock, and others. Early on, DAD shows edema in the alveoli and hyaline membranes lining the alveoli and alveolar ducts (Fig. 11–5). As the process organizes, type II alveolar lining cells repopulate the denuded alveolar walls and there may be interstitial fibrosis and granulation tissue in airspaces. Resolution may show either scarring or restoration of normal parenchymal architecture.

The majority of patients with acute diffuse lung disease are immunosuppressed, and the following are the main diagnoses encountered: infection, recurrence of the original disease process that necessitated immunosuppression (e.g., lymphoma, leukemia, vasculitis, connective tissue disease), and no specific diagnosis (usually diffuse alveolar damage); in many of these cases a drug, particularly of the cytotoxic type, is implicated.

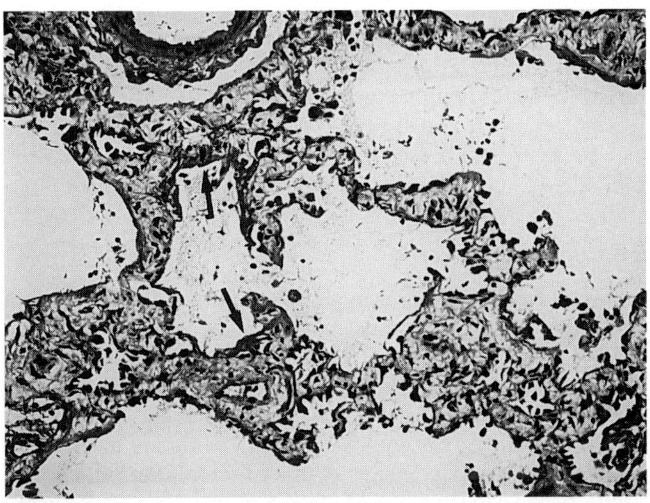

Figure 11–5. Diffuse alveolar damage. There is edema of the alveolar walls, which are partially lined by hyaline membranes *(arrows).* This pattern represents a nonspecific reaction to acute lung injury that can be seen with both infectious and noninfectious conditions. Hematoxylin and eosin, ×150.

In the setting of acute diffuse lung disease, *negative information (i.e., lack of identification of an organism or of the primary disease process) is useful information.* In addition, immunosuppressed patients may have more than one process, especially multiple infections. A battery of special stains is routinely performed by the pathologist on biopsies from immunosuppressed patients. This includes stains for fungi and *Pneumocystis carinii* (methenamine silver), bacteria (Gram), and mycobacteria (acid-fast). Immunohistochemical stains and other studies, such as in situ hybridization or even polymerase chain reaction, are also available to look for certain organisms when specifically implicated (see Chap. 2).

The *organ transplantation setting* presents other considerations in addition to infections (see Chap. 20). Epstein-Barr virus–associated post-transplant lymphoproliferations may present in the lung. These are usually seen as nodules grossly and resemble lymphomas microscopically. Acute rejection of a lung allograft shows perivenular lymphoid infiltrates. Chronic rejection includes the bronchiolitis obliterans syndrome, with progressive occlusion of small airways by fibrous tissue and concomitant progressive airflow obstruction as well as accelerated atherosclerosis in the graft vasculature. Bronchiolitis obliterans occurs in the setting of bone marrow transplantation as well.

Acute Pulmonary Infections

The following types of infection can occur in immunocompetent patients as well as in the immunosuppressed population.

Bacterial Infections. Acute consolidative pneumonia with neutrophils and fibrin in alveoli.

Viral Infections. Cytomegalovirus (CMV)-infected cells show large amphophilic intranuclear inclusions and often smaller basophilic cytoplasmic inclusions; herpes/varicella-infected cells show intranuclear eosinophilic inclusions, sometimes in multinucleated cells; adenovirus usually has a necrotizing bronchiolitis and the infected cells show smudgy change of the nucleus or intranuclear eosinophilic inclusions.

Fungal Infections. Histoplasmosis (small yeast forms), blastomycosis (thick-walled yeast forms), coccidioidomycosis (spherules with endospores), and cryptococcosis (yeast with mucicarmine-positive mucoid capsule) are all associated with granulomatous inflammation. In immunosuppressed patients, granuloma formation may not be prominent and neutrophils or sheets of histiocytes may predominate. *Candida* (small oval yeast), *Mucor* (thick nonseptate hyphae), and *Aspergillus* (septate hyphae branching at acute angles) typically infect immunosuppressed patients and are associated with necrosis, acute inflammation, and abundant organisms. *Mucor* and *Asper-*

gillus often invade pulmonary blood vessels, resulting in thrombosis, infarction, and hemorrhage.

Mycobacterial Infection. Necrotizing granulomatous inflammation is characteristic; however, typical granuloma formation may not be found in immunosuppressed patients. Acid-fast organisms may be very difficult to find even with special stains, and their absence does not exclude mycobacterial infection; cultures may ultimately be productive in such cases.

***Pneumocystis carinii* Pneumonia.** Methenamine silver–positive cyst forms are found within the foamy eosinophilic intraalveolar material. In current practice, at least 50% or more of cases of *Pneumocystis* do not have this foamy material and show nonspecific diffuse alveolar damage or mild alveolar injury. In any patient with acute (or even subacute) diffuse lung disease, special stains for *Pneumocystis* should be performed and carefully evaluated by the pathologist.

In immunosuppressed patients in whom the primary disease process is the cause of acute diffuse lung disease, the most common underlying diseases are lymphoma and leukemia. Cytologically, the tumor cells are similar to their counterparts in lymph nodes or bone marrow, but histologically they show a distinct pattern of infiltration of the lung: the neoplastic cells are found along bronchovascular structures and in the septa and pleurae; this distribution is common to nearly all hematolymphoid infiltrates in the lung.

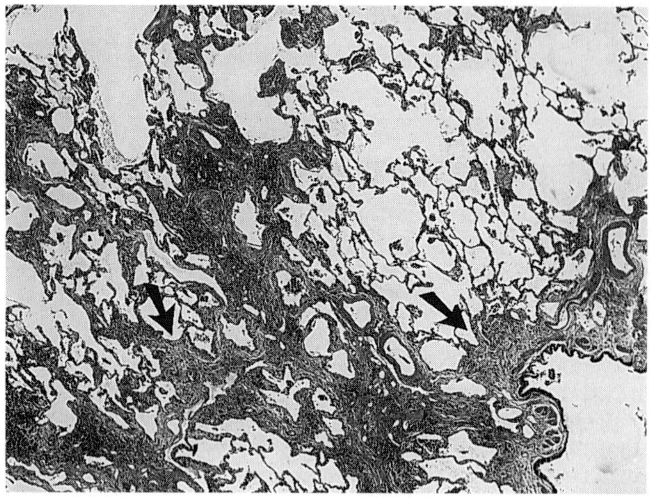

Figure 11–6. Idiopathic pulmonary fibrosis (usual interstitial pneumonia). There is patchy scarring of the lung tissue, with some foci in which the architecture is destroyed *(center, lower)* whereas elsewhere the alveoli are entirely normal. Active foci are seen as fibroblastic thickening of alveolar walls *(arrows)*. Hematoxylin and eosin, ×25.

SUBACUTE/CHRONIC DIFFUSE LUNG DISEASE

Subacute and chronic interstitial (also called infiltrative) lung diseases are characterized by gradually developing signs and symptoms. Characteristic features include cough, dyspnea, hypoxemia, restrictive pulmonary function deficit, and predominantly diffuse radiographic changes, although all these features are not present in every case. Many of these conditions require open or thoracoscopic biopsy, but some can be diagnosed on the basis of bronchoscopic biopsies (e.g., sarcoidosis) or bronchoalveolar lavage fluid examination (e.g., histiocytosis X).

There are many forms of interstitial lung disease; the pathologic features of the more commonly encountered types are summarized below.[15] The surgeon is generally involved in providing tissue for diagnosis in many of these conditions, since relatively large parenchymal samples are needed.

Idiopathic Pulmonary Fibrosis

Idiopathic pulmonary fibrosis (IPF) is usually seen in adults over the age of 50 who have progressive restrictive lung disease with diffuse radiographic infiltrates. Pathologists often prefer the term *usual interstitial pneumonia (UIP)*. Grossly, there is honeycombing, particularly in the periphery of the lung. The interstitial fibrosis often starts in alveoli adjacent to septa or in subpleural regions (Fig. 11–6). Active sites of disease are seen as interstitial proliferations of fibroblasts. Open lung biopsy is required for definitive diagnosis of IPF (although a presumptive clinical diagnosis is made in some cases on the basis of the clinical and radiographic findings); sampling should include active sites of disease and not only the honeycombed areas of advanced disease.

Idiopathic Bronchiolitis Obliterans with Organizing Pneumonia

This is also called cryptogenic organizing pneumonitis, and idiopathic bronchiolitis obliterans with organizing pneumonia (BOOP), and is a form of interstitial lung disease usually seen in adults. Chest radiographs generally show patchy airspace opacities or, less commonly, diffuse bilateral interstitial infiltrates. The main microscopic change is fibroblastic proliferation *within* airspaces associated with mild chronic inflammatory infiltrate in the adjacent alveoli (Fig. 11–7). The majority of cases are steroid-responsive. The diagnosis generally requires open lung biopsy, although suggestive changes of BOOP can be recognized with a transbronchial biopsy. A BOOP pattern can be seen in other conditions; thus, idiopathic BOOP is a diagnosis of exclusion.

Sarcoidosis

Sarcoidosis is the prototype of granulomatous interstitial pneumonia. Surgeons most commonly encounter intrathoracic sarcoidosis in lymph nodes biopsied from the mediastinum (see Chap. 10). In the lung, nonnecrotizing granulomas are found along bronchovascular structures, the septa, and the pleurae. Sarcoidosis forms confluent nodules of granulomas surrounded by dense eosinophilic lamellar fibrous tissue. The pathologic changes are best appreciated in open lung biopsies, although transbronchial biopsy showing the characteristic granulomas may allow a working diagnosis with the support of appropriate clinical and radiographic findings. Special stains for fungi and acid-

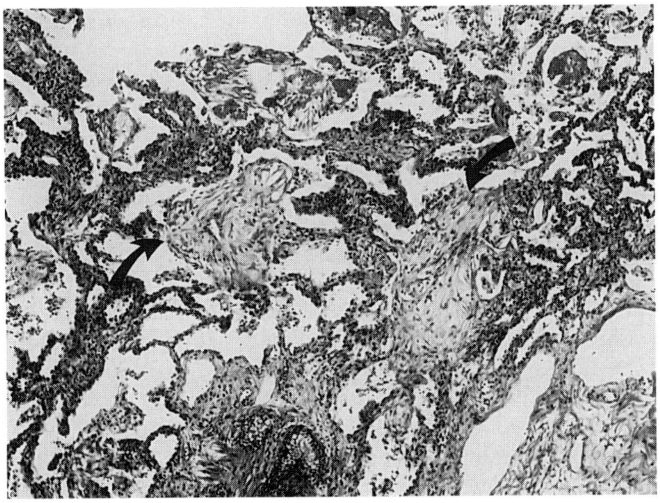

Figure 11–7. Idiopathic bronchiolitis obliterans with organizing pneumonia shows tufts of fibroblastic tissue within alveolar ducts *(arrows)*. The surrounding alveolar walls show a moderate inflammatory infiltrate. Hematoxylin and eosin, ×75.

fast organisms should always be performed to exclude an infectious process.

Collagen-Vascular Diseases

Pulmonary and pleural changes occur in many collagen-vascular diseases, most commonly rheumatoid arthritis. A number of disease manifestations may be encountered; interstitial pneumonia and rheumatoid nodules are the best known. Open lung biopsy is necessary for specific pattern recognition, although sometimes transbronchial biopsy suffices for management when clinical suspicion is high. Rheumatoid nodules in the lung resemble those in subcutaneous tissue; there is central fibrinoid degeneration surrounded by palisading histiocytes.

Vasculitides

Some forms of vasculitis present clinically as pulmonary disease,[16] and the surgeon is called on to perform a biopsy. Most cases manifest as multifocal nodules; however, in some cases, there is instead diffuse alveolar hemorrhage. In cases of suspected vasculitis, some of the most abnormal tissues should be included within the biopsy, and intraoperative frozen sections may be needed to confirm the adequacy of sampling of pathologic abnormalities. *Wegener's granulomatosis* is associated with necrosis and granulomatous inflammation in addition to vasculitis of medium-sized arteries and veins. Cases with extensive necrosis eventually cavitate and have an appearance similar to that of an infectious granuloma. *Churg-Strauss syndrome* (allergic granulomatosis) is very rare; most patients have a history of asthma, eosinophilia, and evidence of systemic vasculitis with multiple organ systems involved. The lung shows numerous foci of vasculitis, with marked eosinophilic infiltration of vessels, as well as necrotic granulomas containing degraded eosinophils and surrounded by a palisading histiocytic response.

Extrinsic Allergic Alveolitis (Hypersensitivity Pneumonitis)

Extrinsic allergic alveolitis can be induced by any one of a large number of inhaled organic antigenic substances. It consists of an immunologic reaction in the lung to the particular antigen to which the individual has become sensitized. Farmer's lung disease, caused by thermophilic species of actinomyces, is one of the best-known examples. Approximately three-quarters of the cases of extrinsic allergic alveolitis show a histologic triad of diffuse interstitial infiltration by lymphocytes and plasma cells, cellular bronchiolitis, and scattered small, nonnecrotizing granulomas (Fig. 11–8). The remainder of cases lack at least one of these three features, so that findings are considered nonspecific. Here again, transbronchial biopsy may be sufficient, but open biopsy provides a greater chance of definitive diagnosis.

Chronic Eosinophilic Pneumonia

Chronic eosinophilic pneumonia is classically associated with peripheral infiltrates on chest radiograph and peripheral blood eosinophilia. Pathologically, the major changes are accumulations of large numbers of eosinophils and histiocytes in the alveoli and a mild mononuclear inflammatory infiltrate in the interstitium. The features are distinctive and transbronchial biopsies are usually adequate. Bronchoalveolar lavage fluid showing large numbers of eosinophils suggests the diagnosis.

Pulmonary Histiocytosis X (Langerhans' Cell Granulomatosis)

Pulmonary histiocytosis X (HX) is caused by the proliferation of Langerhans' cells along small airways with associated inflammatory and fibrotic changes. A trend has de-

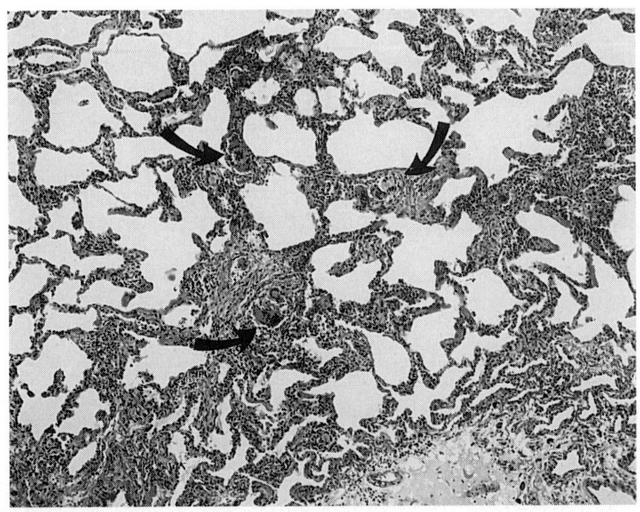

Figure 11–8. Extrinsic allergic alveolitis (hypersensitivity pneumonitis). There is prominent inflammation of alveolar walls, with granulomatous features including granulomas with giant cells *(arrows)*. Although the inflammatory infiltrate is prominent, there is little if any fibrosis; such a reaction can resolve without scarring. Hematoxylin and eosin, ×40.

veloped toward designating this process Langerhans' cell granulomatosis. The Langerhans' cell (HX cell) is now known to be a specialized accessory cell of the monocytic-histiocytic system which processes foreign antigens for cell-mediated immune recognition. Most patients are adult smokers; women are more frequently affected. Pathologically, one finds scattered fibrotic nodules containing HX cells, variable numbers of eosinophils, lymphocytes, and pigmented alveolar macrophages. The HX cell is recognizable by conventional microscopy as a histiocyte with pale cytoplasm and a distinctive nucleus with prominent nuclear folds. It can be definitively identified ultrastructurally based on the presence of Birbeck (Langerhans' cell) granules or immunohistochemically by demonstration of either S-100 protein or CD1 antigen (see Chap. 2). Such special studies may be necessary with small biopsies or with bronchoalveolar lavage. A presumptive diagnosis of HX can sometimes be made with high-resolution CT scans. Typical findings are scattered nodules with cystic change in adjacent lung parenchyma.

Lymphangioleiomyomatosis

This rare condition is seen only in women, usually of child-bearing age. Many patients have a history of repeated pneumothoraces. There is a multifocal proliferation of immature-appearing smooth muscle cells in the lung and thoracoabdominal lymphatics. In the lung, the cellular proliferation leads to widespread cystic change, recognizable with high-resolution CT scanning. The pathologic changes can often be appreciated in transbronchial as well as open lung biopsy; there are small fascicles of immature-appearing smooth muscle cells.

Pneumoconioses

Most pneumoconioses have diagnostic clinical-radiologic findings and rarely come to biopsy for diagnosis.[17] *Asbestosis* shows accumulations of iron-covered asbestos fibers (asbestos bodies) associated with interstitial fibrosis. *Silicosis* starts as clusters of macrophages containing birefringent silica and silicates; these are concentrated around small airways and along the lymphatics. They progress to fibrotic silicotic nodules.

MISCELLANEOUS CONDITIONS

The surgeon may be involved in the diagnosis and/or treatment of a variety of other miscellaneous conditions.

Granulomatous Infections

Solitary infectious granulomas may be resected for both diagnosis to exclude neoplasm and therapy (for removal of cavitary disease refractory to medical therapy). Histologically, one sees necrotizing granulomas; causative organisms may or may not be identified within the necrotic material even with special stains. The hilar or mediastinal nodes may also be involved and may even be the presenting finding.

The surgeon may also be involved in the management of sequelae of granulomatous infections. *Broncholithiasis* develops when the calcified necrotic center of an old infectious granuloma in a hilar lymph node erodes through the bronchial wall. The released material may be aspirated or expectorated; if it is saved, the pathologist may be able to identify organisms with special stains or even with molecular probes (see Chap. 2). *Sclerosing (fibrosing) mediastinitis* is an aggressive, often life-threatening fibrous proliferation occurring in the mediastinum with involvement of mediastinal structures such as pulmonary arteries and veins.[17] Surgical management is often on an emergent or semiemergent basis. The process consists of dense hyalinized fibrous tissue, sometimes with recognizable old necrotic granulomas within the center of the reaction. This process is thought to be an exaggerated response to an antigenic stimulus; histoplasmosis has frequently been implicated (see Chap. 10).[18]

Lung Abscesses

A lung abscess is a focus of purulent parenchymal necrosis with cavitation. Microscopically, the center is composed of degraded inflammatory cells and debris. The wall shows variable degrees of fibrosis and acute and chronic inflammation. Microorganisms may be identified microscopically in some cases; however, microbial culture is a more sensitive if slower method.

Aspergilloma (Mycetoma)

A pulmonary *mycetoma* is a saprophytic growth of fungus in an old cavity. *Aspergillus* is the most common organism, sometimes overgrowing an old tuberculous cavity, old sarcoidosis, or other conditions that structurally predispose to such colonization. Because aspergillomas are prone to life-threatening hemorrhage, the surgeon may be asked to resect such a lesion. Pathologically, there is a fibrous walled cavity lined by metaplastic epithelium, with underlying chronic inflammation. In the center is a tangle of grumous hyphal material that may be lost in pathologic dissection unless it is carefully retained for inspection.

Bullous Emphysema

Emphysema is characterized by the partial destruction of alveolar walls, with enlargement of airspaces. This is not associated with fibrosis or inflammatory activity.[19] Emphysema is classified according to the location of structural changes in the lung acini: centriacinar emphysema (typical of smokers), panacinar emphysema (typical of $alpha_1$-antitrypsin deficiency), distal acinar emphysema, and irregular emphysema. Distal acinar emphysema is associated with emphysematous changes adjacent to the septa and subpleural regions; it may result in bullous emphysema, with the formation of large subpleural air-filled sacs. When they are large, bullae may result in significant functional impairment. Bullae unassociated with surrounding emphysematous changes have narrow necks (Reid type I)[20] and are amenable to surgical resection. An improvement in respiratory status can be expected in such cases. By contrast, bullae with broad necks and those with associated attenu-

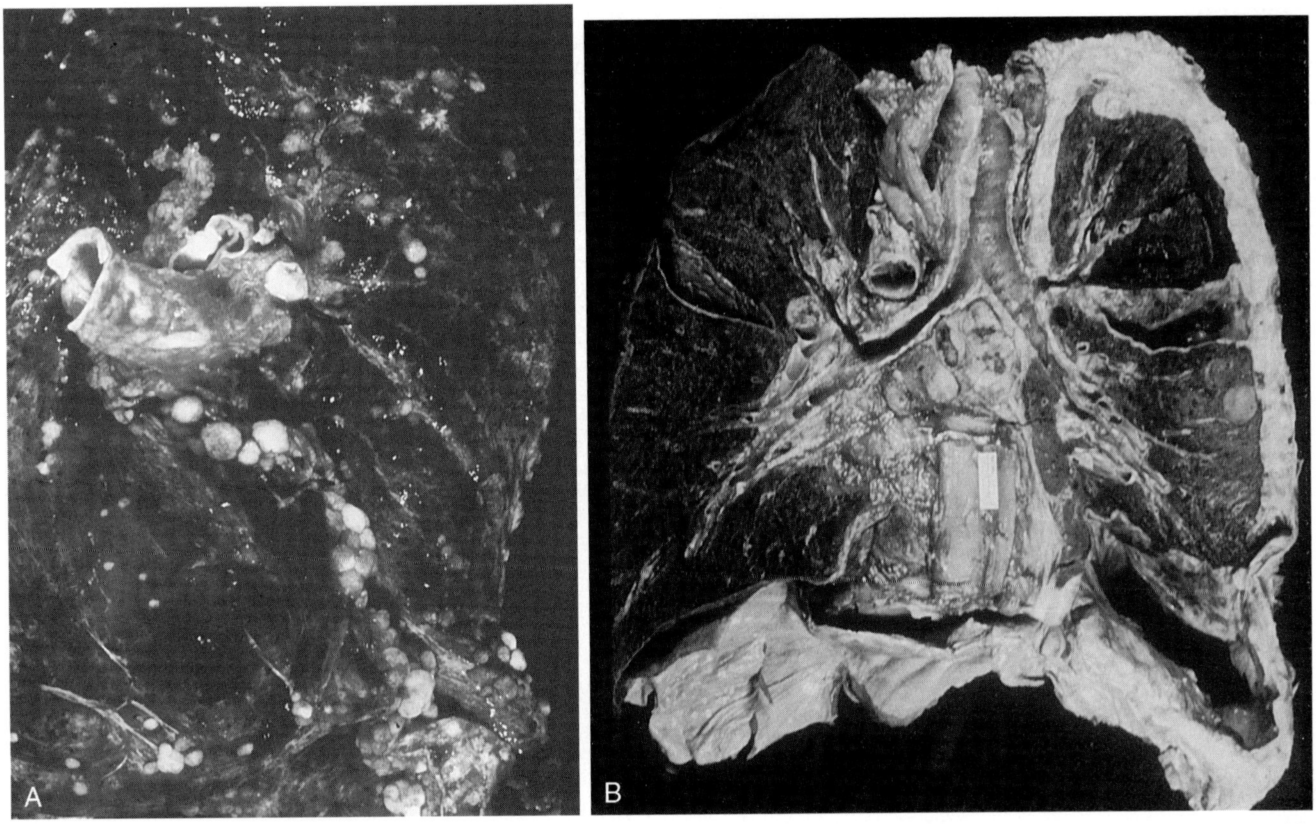

Figure 11–11. Diffuse malignant mesothelioma. Early in their course, diffuse malignant mesotheliomas may be seen as nodules studding the visceral pleural surface *(A)*, whereas late in their course, they form the classic rind surrounding the lung, sometimes extending into fissures *(B)*.

PITFALLS FOR THE SURGEON

1. Proceeding to surgery without sufficient clinical or radiographic data.
2. Inadequate sampling or selecting tissue that is too severely affected or too little affected by the pathologic process; missing focal lesions; obtaining biopsies less than 3 mm in greatest dimension, which may be too small to fully assess diffuse lung disease.
3. Lack of communication with the pathologist regarding clinical findings and expectations of the particular biopsy (i.e., differential diagnosis).

PITFALLS FOR THE PATHOLOGIST

1. Microscopic misinterpretation of inflammatory processes as malignant due to reparative atypia (particularly in intraoperative frozen sections).
2. Failure to apply an appropriate battery of special stains (e.g., for microorganisms).
3. Failure to detect ineffectiveness of special stains for microorganisms (most often in relation to *Pneumocystis carinii*). Careful attention to positive controls is constantly needed.
4. Lack of communication with clinicians, with resultant erroneous interpretation of slides due to an informational vacuum.

FURTHER READING

Colby TV, Koss M, Travis WT. Tumors of the lower respiratory tract. In: *Atlas of Tumor Pathology,* 3rd series. Fascicle 13. Washington, DC: Armed Forces Institute of Pathology; 1995.

Colby TV, Lombard C, Yousem SA, Kitaichi M. *Atlas of Pulmonary Surgical Pathology.* Philadelphia: Saunders; 1991.

Dail DH, Hammar SP. *Pulmonary Pathology,* 2nd ed. New York: Springer-Verlag; 1993.

Mackay B, Lukeman JM, Ordonez NG. *Tumors of the Lung.* Philadelphia: Saunders; 1991.

Thurlbeck WM. *Pathology of the Lung.* New York: Thieme Medical; 1988.

Thurlbeck WM, Miller RR, Müller NL, Rosenow EC. *Diffuse Diseases of the Lung: A Team Approach.* Philadelphia: Dekker; 1991.

REFERENCES

1. Matthews MJ, Mackay B, Lukeman J. Pathology of non-small cell carcinoma of the lung. *Semin Oncol.* 1983;10:34–55.
2. Miller RR, Nelems B, Müller NL, et al. Lingular and right middle lobe biopsy in the assessment of diffuse lung disease. *Ann Thorac Surg.* 1987;44:269–273.
3. Newman SL, Michel RP, Wang N-S. Lingular lung biopsy? Is it representative? *Am Rev Respir Dis.* 1985;132:1084–1086.
4. Swensen SJ, Jett JR, Payne WS, et al. An integrated approach to evaluation of the solitary pulmonary nodule. *Mayo Clin Proc.* 1990;65:173–186.
5. Minna JD, Pass H, Glatstein E, Ihde DC. Cancer of the lung. In: DeVita VT, Hellman S, Rosenberg SA, eds. *Cancer: Principles and Practice of Oncology.* Philadelphia: Lippincott; 1988:591–705.
6. Rosenow EC, Carr DT. Bronchogenic carcinoma. *Cancer J Clin.* 1979;29:233–245.
7. Gazdar AF, Linnoila RI. The pathology of lung cancer—Changing concepts and newer diagnostic techniques. *Semin Oncol.* 1988;15:215–225.
8. Travis WD, Travis LB, Percy C, Devesa SS. Lung cancer incidence and survival by histologic type. *Cancer.* (in press)
9. Bains MS. Surgical treatment of lung cancer. *Chest.* 1991;100:826–837.
10. Beahrs OH, Henson DE, Hutter RVP, Kennedy BJ. *Manual for Staging of Cancer,* 4th ed. American Joint Committee on Cancer (AJCC). Philadelphia: Lippincott; 1992:115–122.
11. Bülzebruck H, Bopp R, Drings P, et al. New aspects in the staging of lung cancer. *Cancer.* 1992;70:1102–1110.
12. Mountain CF. A new international staging system for lung cancer. *Chest.* 1986;89:225S–233S.
13. Mountain CF. Prognostic implications of the international staging system for lung cancer. *Semin Oncol.* 1988;15:236–245.
14. Travis WD, Linnoila RI, Tsokos MG, et al. Neuroendocrine tumors of the lung with proposed criteria for large-cell neuroendocrine carcinoma: An ultrastructural, immunohistochemical, and flow cytometric study of 35 cases. *Am J Surg Pathol.* 1991;15:529–553.
15. Colby TV. Interstitial lung disease. In: Thurlbeck WM, Churg A, eds. *Pathology of the Lung,* 2nd ed. New York: Thieme Medical; 1995:589–738.
16. Churg A, Churg J. *Systemic Vasculitides.* New York: Igaku-Shoin; 1991.
17. Churg A, Green FHY. *The Pathology of Occupational Lung Disease.* New York: Igaku-Shoin; 1988.
18. Deschamps C, Allen MS, Daly RC, et al. Histoplasmosis. *Chest Surg Clin North Am.* 1993;3:639–651.
19. Thurlbeck WM. *Chronic Airflow Obstruction in Lung Disease.* Philadelphia: Saunders; 1976.
20. Reid L. *The Pathology of Emphysema.* London: Lloyd-Luke; 1967:211–212.
21. Swensen SJ, Hartman TE, Williams DE. Computed tomographic diagnosis of *Mycobacterium avium-intracellulare* complex in patients with bronchiectasis. *Chest.* 1994;105:49–52.
22. Wagenvoort CA. Open lung biopsies in congenital heart disease for evaluation of pulmonary vascular disease: Predictive value with regard to corrective operability. *Histopathology.* 1985;9:417–436.
23. McCaughey WTE, Colby TV, Battifora H, et al. Diagnosis of diffuse malignant mesothelioma: experience of a US/Canadian panel. *Mod Pathol.* 1991;4:342–354.
24. Boring CC, Squires TS, Tong T. Cancer statistics, 1992. *CA Cancer J Clin.* 1992;42:19–38.
25. Cohen MH. Signs and symptoms of bronchogenic carcinoma. In: Strauss MJ, ed. *Lung Cancer: Clinical Diagnosis and Treatment,* 2nd ed. New York: Grune & Stratton; 1983:97–112.
26. Miller WE. Roentgenographic manifestations of lung cancer. In: Strauss MJ, ed. *Lung Cancer: Clinical Diagnosis and Treatment,* 2nd ed. New York: Grune & Stratton; 1983:175–184.

12

The Gastrointestinal Tract

Robert A. Wolber and Charles H. Scudamore

Definition

Diseases of the gastrointestinal (GI) tract represent 50% or more of the clinical practice of a general surgeon.[1] The heterogeneity of gross and microscopic anatomy within the GI tract, and the multiplicity of physiology and function, are mirrored by the diversity of inflammatory, mechanical, and neoplastic pathologic processes that affect this system. For the surgeon, recognition and understanding of these processes are essential to the diagnosis and management of GI diseases.

The GI tract begins at the level of the cricoid cartilage and ends at the anal margin. It includes the esophagus, stomach, small intestine, large intestine, vermiform appendix, and anal canal. The cross-sectional microanatomy of the GI tract can be divided into four layers: *mucosa, submucosa, muscularis propria*, and *serosa* (or adventitia). The mucosal type varies with the site, but three structural elements are maintained throughout: a regionally specialized *epithelium*, a connective tissue stroma known as *lamina propria*, and a thin layer of smooth muscle known as *muscularis mucosae*. The epithelial cell type of each region is defined herewith with progression from the esophagus to the anus.

Esophagus

The esophagus is approximately 25 cm in length in a normal-sized adult. All but the distal 2 cm are lined by stratified squamous epithelium. Endoscopically defined locations are usually measured from the incisors: the esophagus begins at 15 cm and extends to between 36 and 42 cm.[2]

DEVELOPMENTAL ABNORMALITIES

Developmental defects of the esophagus are uncommon. Because most result in regurgitation when feeding is initiated, they are usually discovered soon after birth. The most important developmental defects are various forms of atresia and tracheoesophageal fistula. Most commonly, the atretic segment is located at or near the tracheal bifurcation.[3]

VASCULAR, NEUROMUSCULAR, AND MECHANICAL DISORDERS

With cirrhosis of the liver or any other cause of portal hypertension, venous varicosities may form at sites of anastamosis between systemic and portal circulation. The most important of these is at the lower end of the esophagus.

Esophageal varices occur in about two thirds of cirrhotic patients. They are asymptomatic until the varices rupture spontaneously or following a bout of vomiting, resulting in massive hematemesis. Death occurs in 30 to 50% of patients following a first episode of upper GI hemorrhage from esophageal varices.[4] Management of actively bleeding varices includes the use of parenteral somatostatin analogues, balloon tamponade, endoscopic sclerotherapy, esophageal binding, or transvenous cannulation and obliteration of the coronary vein. A few surgeons still perform portal-systemic venous shunts for esophageal varices.

NEUROMUSCULAR DISORDERS

Abnormalities of esophageal motility are diagnosed by cineradiographic and manometric studies, thereby rarely coming to the attention of the pathologist.

A diminution or absence of myenteric plexus ganglion cells, with resultant esophageal dilatation, is implicated in several dysmotility disorders, including achalasia and Chagas's disease. *Achalasia* is characterized by an incomplete relaxation of the lower esophageal sphincter, a lack of effective peristalsis, and a reduction of ganglion cells in both the distal constricted and proximal dilated segments. The risk of development of squamous carcinoma in patients with achalasia remains controversial.[5, 6] *Chagas's disease* is a protozoan parasitic infection by *Trypanosoma cruzi*, endemic in tropical South America. Megaesophagus and megacolon may occur, owing to destruction of myenteric plexus cells. Chagas's disease is being seen with increasing frequency in North America in immigrant populations infected with *T. cruzi*.

MECHANICAL DISORDERS

Abnormalities due to the action of mechanical forces on the esophagus include hiatus hernia and spontaneous tears. The more common type of *hiatus hernia* is the ''sliding'' variety, often occurring in obese elderly individuals and pregnant women. The cardia and fundus are forced through the diaphragmatic hiatus. The less common paraesophageal type is due to a diaphragmatic defect. A sliding hiatus hernia may have the endoscopic appearance of tubular esophagus, causing misinterpretation of herniated gastric glandular mucosa as Barrett's esophagus. Gastroesophageal reflux and esophagitis are complications of hiatus hernia. When severe or chronic in duration, ulceration, stricture, or true Barrett's esophagus may occur. Most cases of chronic reflux esophagitis are found in individuals with demonstrable hiatus hernias.[7]

There are three recognized types of *spontaneous esophageal tears*. All are causally associated with severe vomiting, abdominal trauma, seizures, asthmatic attacks, parturition, or other sudden increases of intraabdominal pressure. Complete transmural rupture, resulting in bacterial mediastinitis, is referred to as Boerhaave's syndrome.[8] This is a life-threatening condition requiring antibiotic and surgical therapy. Mucosal tearing of the lower esophagus and gastric cardia, with massive hematemesis, is frequently associated with a history of chronic alcoholism and vomiting and is called the Mallory-Weiss syndrome.[9] Rare mucosal tears of the midesophagus, with mural dissection, have also been described. Although clinically alarming, superficial mucosal tears are usually not life-threatening.

INFLAMMATORY CONDITIONS

Esophagitis may occur due to a number of environmental insults, including ingestion of corrosive fluids, such as alkaline drain cleaners or bleach; drug ingestion; and irradiation therapy. The most common form of chemical injury is gastric acid reflux.

Infection is an uncommon cause of esophagitis in the immunocompetent host. Affected individuals usually have some form of immune defect. *Candida albicans* is responsible for most forms of fungal esophagitis. In the immunocompetent host, *Candida* is usually a commensal organism and may be found in the base of otherwise typical peptic-type ulcers. The presence of *Candida* in this clinical setting likely represents nonpathogenic colonization. Esophagitis due to *Candida* organisms may occur in individuals with diabetes mellitus. It may follow antibiotic therapy or nasogastric suction. At endoscopy, the lesions appear as white plaques on an erythematous or ulcerated mucosal background. Microscopic examination of biopsy specimens confirms the presence of fungal pseudohyphae and spores within inflammatory debris or intact epithelium.

Viral esophagitis is almost exclusively limited to herpes simplex virus (HSV) and cytomegalovirus (CMV) infection. Herpetic esophagitis may occur as a limited process in otherwise healthy adults or in patients with immunosuppression due to antineoplastic therapy, transplantation, or acquired immunodeficiency syndrome (AIDS). The disease occurs as a sudden onset of pain with swallowing. Endoscopically, the mucosa exhibits vesicles and shallow ulcers. Cytomegalovirus has a similar endoscopic appearance but occurs almost exclusively in the immunosuppressed. The diagnosis of both viral infections is usually made by histologic identification of characteristic nuclear inclusions. The inclusions of HSV are found within epithelial cells at the edge of an ulcer, whereas CMV inclusions are found in vascular endothelial cells and fibroblasts at an ulcer base. Hence, biopsies should be obtained from both sites in suspected cases. Both viral infections are amenable to specific antiviral therapy.

REFLUX ESOPHAGITIS AND BARRETT'S ESOPHAGUS

Approximately 36% of Americans experience symptomatic gastroesophageal (GE) reflux at least once per month, and 7% experience heartburn once per day.[10] Although a number of diagnostic tests for GE reflux have been developed, endoscopy with biopsy is the mainstay for documenting tissue injury from reflux. Endoscopic findings in affected patients range from normal-appearing mucosa to erythema, ulcers, strictures, and Barrett's esophagus. Histologic confirmation of reflux esophagitis is based upon the presence of acute inflammatory cells (neutrophils or eosinophils) within the squamous epithelium and/or evidence of epithelial regeneration manifested by increased thickness of the basal-cell layer.[11]

Biopsy of the esophagus can be technically demanding because of the narrowness of the lumen and possible stenosis at the site of interest. Biopsies should start distally and be taken in sequence superiorly, so that bleeding does not obscure the mucosal features. Larger specimens can be obtained using a rigid scope, but these are seldom necessary in order to obtain a diagnosis and have a higher risk of esophageal perforation.

Barrett's esophagus is estimated to occur as a complication of reflux esophagitis in approximately 10% of symptomatic individuals.[12] The term refers to the replacement of normal distal esophageal squamous epithelium by glandular epithelium. The extension of Barrett's esophagus proximally from the GE junction is usually continuous, endoscopically manifested by replacement of the normal tan or pink squamous mucosa by a velvety red glandular mucosa. Islands of residual squamous mucosa may be present in the affected segment.

Barrett's esophagus is described as exhibiting three epithelial types: gastric fundic, gastric cardiac, and intestinal.[13] The intestinal type is further divided into the complete and incomplete (specialized) varieties. The literature on Barrett's esophagus is complicated by two factors: first, hiatus hernia can resemble Barrett's esophagus endoscopically; second, the distal 2 cm of esophagus can normally be lined by gastric cardia-type mucosa.[14] Thus, esophageal biopsy specimens reported to contain gastric fundic mucosa may in fact represent hiatus hernia. By convention, those obtained from at least 2 cm proximal to the GE junction showing cardia-type mucosa are called Barrett's esophagus (hence the requirement that endoscopists state the level at which an esophageal biopsy was obtained). Nevertheless, it is the presence of *intestinalized epithelium* that allows a histologically specific diagnosis of Barrett's esophagus.

Accurate diagnosis of Barrett's esophagus is more than histologic hairsplitting. The risk for development of adenocarcinoma is estimated at thirty to forty times that of the background population.[15, 16] A progression of histologic changes from metaplasia through epithelial dysplasia to adenocarcinoma allows for endoscopic cancer surveillance of patients with Barrett's esophagus. Epithelial dysplasia is a histologic diagnosis based upon recognition of nuclear atypia and stratification in biopsy specimens. Unfortunately, this can be mimicked by cellular regeneration due to active mucosal inflammation. For this reason, a grading scheme for Barrett's esophageal biopsies has been devised that incorporates this ''uncertainty principle'': esophageal biopsy findings with Barrett's esophagus are classified as negative for dysplasia, positive for low- or high-grade dysplasia, or indefinite for dysplasia.[17]

There is no universally accepted protocol for the surveillance of patients with Barrett's esophagus. The following recommendations seem reasonable and prudent.[18–20] A patient with biopsy-proven Barrett's esophagus should undergo four quadrant biopsies at 2-cm intervals along the affected segment at 2-year intervals. Particular attention should be paid to ulcers, nodules, and strictures. Endoscopic biopsy surveillance is complemented but not replaced by brush cytologic examination. A diagnosis of low-grade dysplasia should lead to multiple-level rebiopsies to search for higher-grade lesions; if no high-grade dysplasia or carcinoma is found, follow-up with a shortened rebiopsy interval is indicated. An initial diagnosis of high-grade dysplasia warrants immediate review of the histology by another experienced pathologist and rebiopsy to look for carcinoma. If the diagnosis of high-grade dysplasia is confirmed, the patient and clinician are faced with the option of esophagectomy. Interpretation as ''indefinite for dysplasia'' should prompt rebiopsy following a period of intensified anti-inflammatory therapy.

NEOPLASMS

Benign tumors of the esophagus are rare and of limited clinical importance. The most common of these are leiomyomas.[21]

The majority of esophageal malignancies are either squamous carcinomas or adenocarcinomas. The absolute and relative incidence of these tumors varies dramatically with geographical location; high incidence areas are in Iran, Northern China, and Russia.[22] In North America, squamous carcinoma has accounted for up to 90% of esophageal malignancies and adenocarcinoma for 8%. The proportion of tumors diagnosed as adenocarcinoma has been increasing with time, however, and now is up to 30% of esophageal malignancies. This increase may be due in part to a trend toward classifying tumors straddling the GE junction as esophageal in origin.[23]

Grossly, esophageal carcinomas are most often located distally and may be polypoid, ulcerating, or diffusely infiltrative, or they may have a combination of these features (Fig. 12–1). The microscopic diagnosis is usually straightforward, with recognition of an infiltrative growth pattern and malignant nuclear features. Squamous differentiation consists of cellular keratinization and the presence of intercellular bridges, whereas adenocarcinomas exhibit gland formation and cytoplasmic mucin. Benign inflammatory processes can mimic carcinoma in small biopsy specimens. Most notably, benign ulcer beds may contain highly atypical reactive stromal, endothelial, and epithelial elements. The greatest degree of diagnostic accuracy can be obtained if the endoscopist provides multiple biopsy fragments and cytology brushings obtained from both the ulcer bed (if present) and intact mucosa at the ulcer edge.

Staging of esophageal carcinoma is critical for decisions in surgical management. After the histologic diagnosis is made, CT scanning is necessary for lymph node imaging. Endoscopic ultrasonography may accurately assess the depth of tumor penetration.

For the purposes of staging, the location of the cancer (cervical, upper thoracic, midthoracic, and lower thoracic portions of the esophagus), the depth of invasion, and the presence or absence of lymph node or distant metastases should be reported. The American Joint Committee on Cancer (AJCC) TNM system for the staging of esophageal carcinoma defines a stage I tumor as limited to the lamina propria or submucosa without nodal metastases, stage IIA

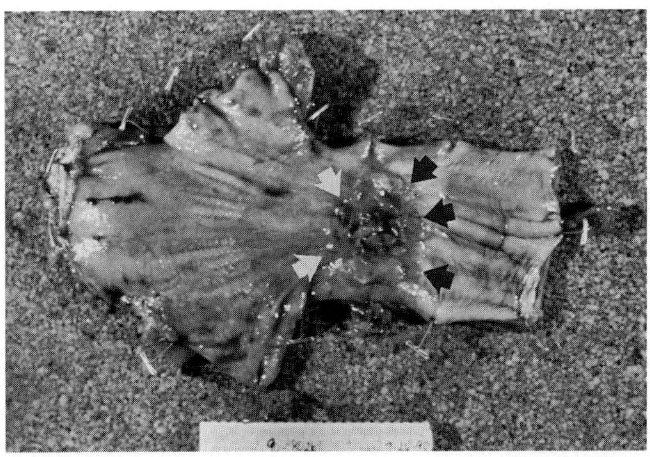

Figure 12–1. Semisessile, ulcerating adenocarcinoma *(white arrows)* of the esophagus. Resection specimen, including the proximal stomach, shows the neoplasm arising at the superior aspect of a short segment of Barrett's esophagus *(black arrows)*.

as invasive into or through the muscularis propria without nodal metastases, stage IIB as invasive into submucosa or muscularis propria with nodal metastases, stage III as invasive into adventitia with nodal metastases or any extension into adjacent thoracic structures, and stage IV as any tumor with distant metastases.[24]

Esophageal carcinoma has a poor prognosis: the 5-year survival for all patients is about 6%.[25] Only 60% of patients are considered operable at presentation. Direct extension through the esophageal wall into the mediastinum is present in 40% of surgical specimens, and metastases to cervical, mediastinal, and upper abdominal lymph nodes are found in up to 60% of resections.[26] Frequently, tumor cells spread longitudinally along submucosal lymphatics. Hence, intraoperative frozen section monitoring for adequacy of the resection margins is recommended. Special attention must be paid at the time of frozen section to the submucosal lymphatics. Some surgeons also request frozen section assessment of a celiac lymph node prior to even initiating a transhiatal esophagectomy.

Initially described in the Japanese and Chinese literature, ''superficial esophageal carcinoma'' refers to tumors invasive into the lamina propria or submucosa only.[27, 28] Some Japanese authors also include tumors with local nodal metastases in this group. Despite the potential for submucosal lymphatic spread, patients with superficial carcinomas have a more favorable overall 5-year survival, ranging from 46 to 90%. Occasionally, the endoscopist will biopsy a squamous carcinoma that does not yet invade the lamina propria (carcinoma in situ). Such lesions correspond endoscopically to subtle plaques or areas of granularity, the appearance of which is enhanced by Lugol's iodine. The detection of early esophageal carcinoma is uncommon in North America, usually occurring as the result of an adenocarcinoma screening program for patients with Barrett's esophagus.

Uncommon variants of esophageal carcinoma include the favorable verrucous carcinomas and polypoid biphasic spindle-cell carcinomas[29–31] as well as the clinically aggressive small-cell (neuroendocrine) carcinomas. Rare esophageal malignancies include adenoid cystic carcinoma, mucoepidermoid carcinoma, and malignant melanoma.[32–34]

Stomach

The gastric mucosa consists of three zones, roughly corresponding to the anatomic cardia, body or fundus, and antrum. The antral mucosal zone may extend up to 5 cm along the gastric lesser curvature. The cardia and antrum are lined by neutral mucin-secreting surface epithelium and glands, whereas the intervening fundic mucosa also contains glands specialized to secrete acid, intrinsic factor, and pepsin.

DEVELOPMENTAL ABNORMALITIES

With the exception of infantile hypertrophic pyloric stenosis, developmental abnormalities of the stomach are very rare. Adult pyloric hypertrophy with stenosis is a disease of male patients and is most commonly the result of pyloric inflammation and peptic ulcer disease.[35]

GASTRITIS

There is no single, well-accepted classification scheme for gastritis. Our understanding of the morphology, etiology, and clinical implications of gastritis is rapidly changing. In general, pathologists tend to classify gastritis on the basis of topographical location, histologic appearances, etiology (if known), and clinical correlations.

Acute Gastritis

This is also referred to as diffuse hemorrhagic or erosive gastritis. Acute gastritis is a pattern of mucosal damage of diverse etiologies, all having in common a loss of epithelial protection from acid gastric contents. Patients present with hematemesis or melena. Endoscopically, the mucosa is congested, with multiple bleeding erosions distributed throughout the stomach. Common clinical settings include patients who are critically ill following massive trauma or burns; those with systemic hypotension; those who have ingested caustic agents; alcoholic patients; patients who take nonsteroidal anti-inflammatory drugs (NSAIDs); those with bile reflux; patients who have uremia; and those with nasogastric intubation.[36] Microscopic examination of biopsy or resection specimens reveals subepithelial mucosal hemorrhage and superficial mucosal necrosis that generally does not penetrate the muscularis mucosae.

Chronic Gastritis

Chronic gastritis is characterized histologically by an inflammatory infiltrate of lymphocytes and plasma cells. The modifier ''active'' is applied when there is also neutrophilic infiltration of gastric epithelium. Chronic gastritis is often referred to as ''nonspecific gastritis''—a term that is best avoided. When a specific pathologic diagnosis cannot be given, it is best to provide a descriptive diagnosis, stating the possible etiologies (if known) as well as the entities not consistent with the histology (see ''Pitfalls'' section). Many authors also classify gastritis as ''superficial'' or ''atrophic.'' These designations are based upon the distribution of the inflammation in the superficial pit or deep glandular compartment of the mucosa and whether or not there is a numeric decrease of gastric glands.[37] This division is somewhat subjective, particularly in the gastric antrum, but is useful in suggesting possible etiologies for gastritis in the gastric body.

Helicobacter-associated chronic gastritis accounts for the majority of endoscopically biopsied chronic active gastritis cases.[38] The prevalence of *Helicobacter pylori* infection increases with age. In North America, serologic evidence of infection is uncommon prior to age 20 and reaches 50% by age 50.[39, 40] In nations with a lower standard of public sanitation, the prevalence in children as well as adults is much higher. Lesions very strongly associated with *H. pylori* infection include chronic active gastritis and duodenal ulcer. The association of gastric ulcer with *H. pylori* infection is not as pronounced, possibly being overshadowed by NSAID-associated ulcer disease.[41] Epidemiologic associations have also been demonstrated between serologic and histologic evidence of *H. pylori* infection and gastric carcinoma and lymphoma.[42–45]

The majority of patients with microscopically defined chronic gastritis are asymptomatic; when they are symptomatic, complaints include abdominal discomfort, belching, and bloating. Endoscopically, gastritis without ulcer may have the appearance of normal mucosa, erythema, erosion, gastric fold thickening, or atrophy. Hence, biopsy is required to establish the diagnosis. Most cases of *H. pylori*-associated gastritis are predominantly antral in distribution. Biopsy specimens reveal a superficial or panmucosal infiltrate of plasma cells and lymphocytes, usually with active neutrophilic inflammation of the epithelium. Secondary lymphoid follicles are frequently present. *H. pylori* organisms are usually identified in pit-associated mucus, without the requirement of special stains. A rapid, bedside urease test has also been developed to aid in detecting *H. pylori* in fresh gastric biopsy specimens.[46] Combined antibiotic and bismuth therapy to eradicate *H. pylori* infection has been advocated as an adjuvant to traditional pharmacologic therapy in the treatment of symptomatic gastritis and peptic ulcer disease in general.[47]

Chronic autoimmune gastritis, also referred to as fundic atrophic gastritis, is characterized by selective inflammation of the deep fundic glands with antral sparing. Clinically, it is associated with the presence of anti–parietal cell and anti–intrinsic factor antibodies in the patient's serum. These patients develop fundic gland atrophy, achlorhydria, vitamin B_{12} deficiency, and a macrocytic (''pernicious'') anemia.[48] The achlorhydria results in gastrin-cell hyperplasia in the antrum and a hypergastrinemic state. Elevated gastrin levels may cause hyperplasia of fundic endocrine cells, predisposing the patient to the development of multiple gastric carcinoid tumors.[49]

Chronic bile reflux, especially postgastrectomy, and the long-term use of NSAIDs have been associated with both acute and chronic gastritis.[50] The chronic gastritis is described as showing mucosal hyperplasia, scant eosinophilic inflammation, and marked epithelial regenerative changes on biopsy. The specificity of these microscopic changes is undetermined.

Diffuse varioliform gastritis is an endoscopically defined term for chronic erosive gastritis, which is characterized by diffuse thickening of the gastric folds and multiple small mucosal nodules topped by central erosions. Affected patients may have abdominal pain, weight loss, GI bleeding, and hypoproteinemia.[51] Biopsy specimens reveal a peculiar form of *lymphocytic gastritis*, characterized by infiltration of lymphocytes into the gastric epithelium, usually with accompanying mucosal hyperplasia. The etiology in most cases is undetermined, although some cases appear to be a gastric manifestation of gluten sensitivity.[52]

Intestinal metaplasia is encountered to a variable extent in virtually all forms of chronic gastritis. This may occur as a reparative response to chronic mucosal injury. Gastric adenocarcinoma is associated with intestinal metaplasia;[53] however, the finding of intestinal metaplasia in gastritis patients is so common as to be of no practical value as an indicator for regular screening endoscopy.

Phlegmonous gastritis is a rare, life-threatening infection of the gastric wall by pyogenic bacteria. If the responsible organism is gas-forming, emphysematous gastritis may result.[54] Rapid diagnosis and gastrectomy, with antibiotic therapy, can be lifesaving.

Once a diagnosis of mycobacterial infection has been ruled out, three potential forms of *granulomatous gastritis* must be considered: gastric involvement by Crohn's disease, systemic sarcoidosis, and isolated granulomatous gastritis.[55–57] The first two diagnoses are based upon identification of the disease elsewhere in the body, and the last is ultimately a diagnosis of exclusion.

POLYPS AND DIFFUSE ENLARGEMENT OF THE GASTRIC FOLDS

Localized expansions of gastric mucosa produce polyps, whereas diffuse expansions produce giant gastric folds. For this reason, distinction of a diffuse from a localized mucosal process requires clinicopathologic correlation (see ''Pitfalls'' section).

The most common gastric polyps are *focal foveolar hyperplasias* and *hyperplastic polyps.*[58] Focal foveolar hyperplasias are tiny (about 3 mm) sessile mucosal elevations often found near healing gastric ulcers and gastroenterostomy stomas. These nonneoplastic lesions consist of benign, elongated gastric pits with sparse chronic inflammation. Hyperplastic polyps are larger versions of the same lesion, often with a contributing component of proliferating smooth muscle. Hyperplastic polyps are often found in a background of chronic gastritis and are likely to occur secondary to inflammation and localized mechanical effects. These lesions are usually excised by endoscopic biopsy. Larger polypoid lesions, occurring at gastroenterostomy sites (Billroth I or II), are referred to as *polypoid mucosal prolapse* or *stomal polyps.*[59] Microscopically, these lesions resemble large hyperplastic polyps. There is also an increased risk for the development of gastric adenocarcinoma following surgery for peptic ulcer disease—approximately fourfold greater than for the background population.[60, 61] Since these neoplasms frequently occur at the gastroenterostomy site in association with a stomal polyp, mass lesions at a gastroenterostomy site should be viewed with suspicion and should be extensively biopsied to assess for dysplastic or malignant change.

Fundic gland polyps are small sessile nodules composed of cystically dilated parietal- and chief-cell glands that occur as multiple 1- to 5-mm lesions in the gastric body. These polyps are often present in patients with adenomatosis coli, although in most instances affected persons do not have this syndrome.[62] These polyps are probably a form of mucosal hamartoma.

Although diffuse expansions of the gastric folds may occur as the result of extensive mucosal or submucosal infiltration by inflammatory or neoplastic cells, the lesions characteristically associated with the endoscopic finding of giant gastric folds are the *hypertrophic gastropathies.*[58] Generally, these fall into two categories. *Zollinger-Ellison syndrome* is characterized by diffuse hyperplasia of the parietal-cell compartment of the gastric mucosa, secondary to a gastrin-secreting tumor of the pancreas or duodenum, with resultant acid hypersecretion and jejunal peptic ulceration. This condition is managed surgically by complete removal of the gastrin-secreting tumor if it is solitary, localizable, and not associated with multiple endocrine neoplasia type I. Total gastrectomy and vagotomy is indicated when the tumor is not localized or resectable. *Ménétrier's disease* corresponds to diffuse expansion of the gastric mucus-secreting compartment with cystic dilatation of gastric glands. It occurs as gastric hypochlorhydria and hypoproteinemia due to GI protein loss. The cause of this process is unknown, although some evidence suggests that some lesions initially diagnosed as Ménétrier's disease were actually lymphocytic gastritis.[63]

NEOPLASMS

Adenomas

Benign gastric neoplasms of epithelial origin are *adenomas*. Like their colonic counterparts, gastric adenomas are precursors of potential development of carcinoma.[64] However, gastric adenomas are relatively uncommon lesions. Hence, carcinomas arising from adenomas contribute relatively little to the total number of gastric carcinomas. Individuals with familial adenomatosis coli and hereditary nonpolyposis colorectal cancer syndromes are at a significantly increased risk for development of both adenomas and carcinomas of the stomach.[62, 65] Most gastric adenomas are asymptomatic lesions incidentally encountered at the time of gastroscopy. Ideally, all such tumors should be completely excised, usually by endoscopic means.

Adenocarcinomas

Gastric adenocarcinoma is a common malignancy worldwide. The incidence of gastric adenocarcinoma varies markedly with geographic location, with the highest incidence noted in Japan, South America, and Scandinavia.[66] Carcinomas arising in the distal stomach are decreasing in incidence in North America, paralleling a decline in the prevalence of chronic gastritis and intestinal metaplasia. Conversely, the incidence of carcinoma of the gastric cardia is increasing, possibly in relation to the same (undetermined) factors responsible for the higher prevalence of Barrett's esophagus.[67, 68]

Gastric adenocarcinomas occur most often in elderly individuals who present with abdominal pain and anemia. The gross or endoscopic appearance may be a polypoid mass, an ulcer with elevated margins, or a diffuse thickening of the gastric mucosa and wall. Gastric adenocarcinomas have two principal microscopic forms.[69] The more common intestinal type of adenocarcinoma most often arises in metaplastic epithelium of the antrum, pylorus, or cardia and resembles carcinoma of the large bowel. The less common diffusely spreading or signet ring–cell adenocarcinoma is thought to arise from nonmetaplastic gastric pit epithelium. It is composed of infiltrating single cells with abundant cytoplasmic mucin. With stromal infiltration, there is a striking fibroblastic response.

The biopsy-based diagnosis of gastric carcinoma relies upon adequate sampling of intact tumor. Polypoid lesions should be multiply sampled at the tumor apex and base. If an ulcer is identified by endoscopy, at least six biopsy specimens from the ulcer edge and at least one from the ulcer base should be submitted, along with cytology brushing specimens. Presurgical mapping of intramucosal tumor spread with multiple endoscopic biopsies is advocated but is not a common practice at most institutions.[70]

The prognosis of gastric adenocarcinoma is closely related to tumor stage. Depth of tumor invasion, status of mucosal margins, and regional lymph node or distant metastatic involvement are important criteria to be assessed in surgical resection specimens. Laparoscopy and biopsy have become important in the preoperative identification of transcoelomic, hepatic, and lymph node metastases, which may alter the surgical management of gastric carcinoma. *Early gastric cancer*, as defined in the Japanese literature, includes adenocarcinoma limited to the mucosa or submucosa regardless of regional lymph node status.[71] In Japan, where early gastric cancer is diagnosed in 30 to 50% of surgically resected cases of gastric carcinoma, reported 5-year survivals are up to 95%.[72–74] Invasion into the muscularis propria implies a 5-year survival of 60%. Patients with deeply invasive gastric carcinoma with positive lymph nodes, after curative resection, have a 5-year survival of about 10%.[74] The AJCC recommendations for staging of gastric carcinoma consider the Japanese survival figures for early gastric cancer.[24] Stage IA tumor is limited to invasion of the lamina propria or submucosa without lymph node metastasis, whereas stage IB tumor includes tumors invasive into muscularis propria or subserosa without nodal metastases as well as tumors invasive into submucosa only but with metastases in perigastric lymph nodes that are less than 3 cm from the main tumor. The distance of the tumor from the proximal resection margin also affects prognosis.[75] Tumors grossly less than 5 cm from the proximal margin have a reduced 5-year survival. This figure falls nearly to zero if the margin is microscopically positive for tumor cells. Therefore, gastric resection specimens for adenocarcinoma should be assessed intraoperatively. The pathologist should measure the distance of the gross tumor from the nearest (usually proximal) resection margin and report this to the surgeon. A frozen section of the proximal margin at the point of closest tumor approach should be performed when surgical extension of this margin is feasible.

Lymphomas

The GI tract is the most common extranodal site for presentation of lymphoma, and the stomach accounts for 50% of GI lesions.[76–78] The GI tract is also secondarily involved by lymph node–based lymphoma in up to 50% of advanced-stage disease. Involvement of regional lymph nodes associated with a GI site is considered to be localized spread of primary GI disease.

Malignant lymphomas of the stomach are most common in middle-aged individuals, and patients present with abdominal pain, obstruction, or a palpable mass. Endoscopically, gastric lymphomas may resemble carcinomas, and the diagnosis relies upon accurate microscopic assessment. In contrast to carcinomas, lymphomas vary greatly in respect to proper management—i.e., which modality or combination of modalities is indicated depends upon histologic classification.

In the stomach, the majority of lymphomas are of B-cell immunophenotype. T-cell lymphomas are uncommon, and gastric Hodgkin's disease is almost nonexistent.[79] Approximately two thirds of B-cell gastric lymphomas show microscopic features of mucosa-associated lymphoid tissue (MALT)—a monomorphic infiltrate of small lymphocytes with slightly angulated nuclei, an epithelial infiltration by these same cells, and a background of reactive lymphoid follicles and plasma cells. The majority of MALT-type lymphomas are low-grade (Fig. 12–2). A small proportion of these contain a higher-grade component of large-cell type. The remaining one third of gastric B-cell lymphomas are mostly of the unfavorable diffuse large-cell type. Five-year survival rates correlate with histologic subtype: 91% for low-grade MALT type, 73% for MALT type with a large-cell component, and 56% for de novo large-cell lymphoma.[80] Survival differences also correlate with tumor stage: patients with lymphomas limited to the gastric wall (stage IE, modified Ann Arbor system) have a significantly better survival than tumors involving regional lymph nodes (stage IIE). Grossly negative resection margins may also imply favorable survival.

The diagnostic approach to a patient with suspected gastric lymphoma should include physical examination for peripheral adenopathy, hepatosplenomegaly, and concurrent involvement of Waldeyer's ring. The diagnosis of lymphoma requires evaluation of the bone marrow. Endoscopic sampling of the gastric lesion should be generous, preferably using large forceps to minimize crush distortion of the specimens. Biopsy specimens should be submitted fresh on saline-soaked paper directly to the pathology laboratory, where they can be divided for purposes of conventional microscopy and special techniques for assessment of clonality. Assessment of clonality is an important consideration in the differential diagnosis of MALT lymphoma and florid lymphoid hyperplasia due to *H. pylori* infection. In previous years, these lesions were commonly grouped together as "gastric pseudolymphomas," a term that is no longer acceptable. Most or all of these lesions can be categorized as either neoplastic or reactive, based upon histologic, immunophenotypic, or molecular criteria.[81]

Treatment considerations for primary gastric lymphoma are currently in flux. These have included surgery with or without radiation or chemotherapy, radiation or chemotherapy alone, and, most recently, a trial of triple antibiotic therapy to eradicate gastric *H. pylori* infection in cases of early low-grade B-cell MALT lymphoma.[82] If a gastric resection is contemplated, complete removal of grossly apparent tumor should be attempted, but only if a debilitating procedure (total gastrectomy) can be avoided. Frozen section monitoring of resection margins is probably unnecessary and likely ineffective due to a high probability of multifocal mucosal disease.[83] Systemic chemotherapy can be relied upon to treat residual gross or microscopic lymphoma.[84] Resection specimens should be submitted to the pathology laboratory in the fresh state, along with a

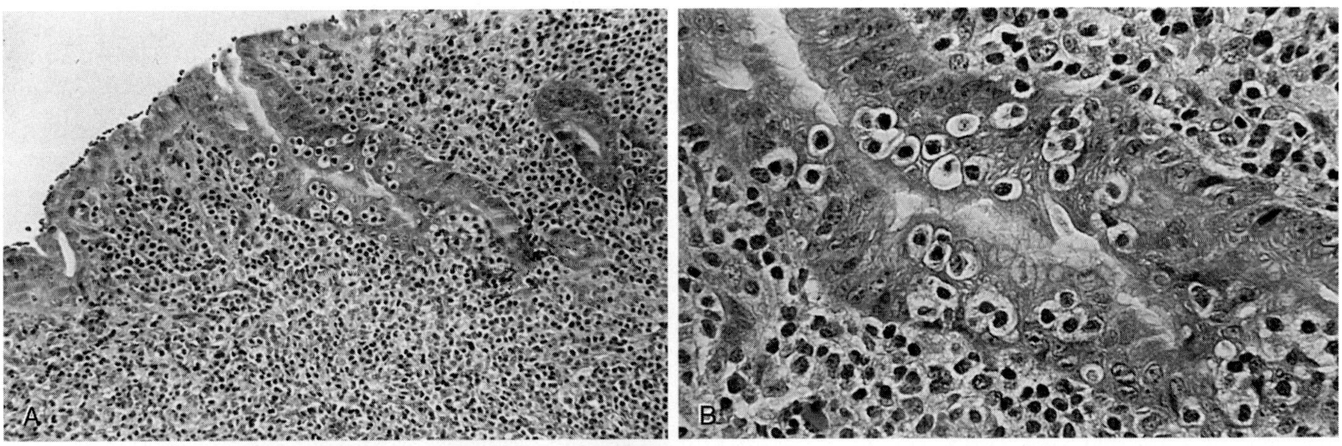

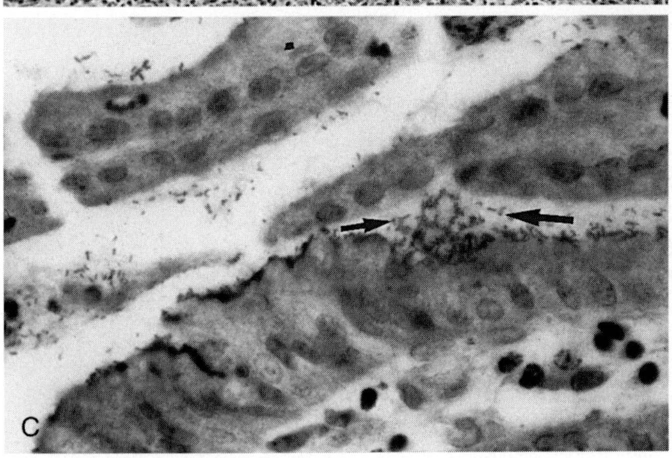

Figure 12–2. Photomicrograph of low-grade B-cell lymphoma of mucosa-associated lymphoid tissue (MALT). *A*, Low-magnification view of gastric mucosa reveals a monomorphic lymphoid infiltrate that displaces and infiltrates mucosal epithelium. Hematoxylin and eosin, ×10. *B*, Higher magnification shows a lymphoepithelial lesion specific for this type of lymphoma. Numerous neoplastic lymphocytes are present within glandular epithelium; ×40. *C*, Adjacent gastric mucosa with *Helicobacter pylori* organisms *(arrows)* in the overlying mucus. Warthin-Starry, ×100. (See also Chap. 17, Fig. 17–14.)

sampling of perigastric lymph nodes. A gross inspection of periaortic and abdominal lymph nodes may be carried out, but extensive lymph node sampling and splenectomy are unnecessary.

Stromal Tumors

The stomach is the most common site of involvement by GI stromal tumors. These tumors occur in patients of all ages, with a peak incidence in the sixth decade.[85] A small percentage occur in young female patients with associated pulmonary chondromas and extraadrenal paragangliomas (Carney's triad).[86] Gastric stromal tumors may be incidental findings or may occur with pain, GI blood loss, vomiting, or anorexia. Grossly, they have the appearance of either a submucosal nodule or a large, bulging mass with central ulceration. From the serosal aspect, attachment to the gastric wall can usually be demonstrated, and large lesions may directly invade adjacent organs. The cut surface is usually white or gray with a whorled texture, sometimes with hemorrhage or cavitation (Fig. 12–3). Microscopically, stromal tumors exhibit a spindled, epithelioid, or pleomorphic cellular appearance. They may exhibit ultrastructural and immunophenotypic evidence of smooth muscle or neural differentiation or neither.[87, 88]

Gastrointestinal stromal tumors are notorious for their unpredictable clinical behavior.[89] Irrefutable features of malignancy include histologically confirmed hematogenous metastases and direct invasion of adjacent organs. In the stomach, criteria indicating a high risk of recurrence or metastasis include size greater than 5.0 cm, infiltrative tumor margin, spontaneous coagulative tumor necrosis, marked nuclear pleomorphism, and mitotic rate of greater than 5 per 50 high-power microscopic fields.[90] These prognostic variables are not independent, and most malignant tumors show several of these features. Stromal tumors with two or more high-risk criteria are diagnosed as malignant stromal sarcomas.[91] The occasional tumors with only one high-risk feature may be designated as stromal tumors of uncertain malignant potential (STUMP). Gastric stromal tumors require grossly complete surgical resection and careful clinical follow-up, which should be longer than the usual 5 years.

Carcinoid Tumor. Solitary or multiple carcinoid tumors occur in the stomach, frequently in a background of gastric achlorhydria and hypergastrinemia with secondary fundic neuroendocrine cell hyperplasia. These tumors rarely metastasize when they are less than 1 cm in diameter and therefore can be managed conservatively with endoscopic surveillance.[92] Antrectomy to abolish compensatory hypergastrinemia in patients with autoimmune gastritis has also been proposed.

Duodenum and Small Intestine

The small bowel mucosa is expanded in absorptive surface area by permanent circumferential folds *(plicae)* and delicate fingerlike epithelial projections called *villi*. The villous epithelium contains absorptive cells and acid mucus–secreting *goblet cells*. Invaginations between villi, called *crypts*, also contain endocrine cells and lysozyme secreting *Paneth's cells*.

DEVELOPMENTAL ABNORMALITIES

There are several varieties of *intestinal malrotation* resulting from abnormalities of intestinal positioning during

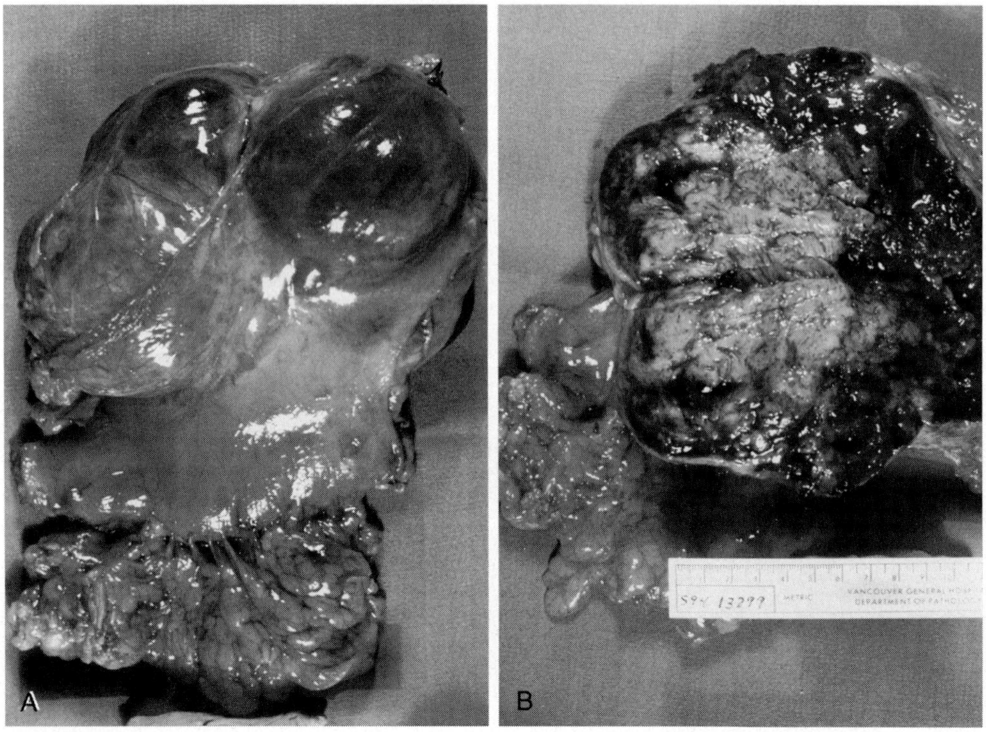

Figure 12–3. Malignant gastric stromal tumor. *A*, Multinodular tumor arises along the lesser curvature. *B*, The cut surface shows a whorled gray appearance with extensive hemorrhage. Both large size and hemorrhage suggest malignancy, confirmed by microscopy.

fetal life. These abnormalities predispose to intestinal obstruction or volvulus, which may present in infancy or adult life.[93] Treatment is surgical, with resection of any infarcted segments and visceropexy to prevent recurrence. Intestinal malrotation, atresia, duplication, and omphalocele are discussed elsewhere in this text.

INTUSSUSCEPTION

Invagination of an intestinal segment into a more distal segment, resulting in obstruction and, often, ischemic necrosis, is referred to as *intussusception*. It occurs predominantly in infants at the ileocecal junction, possibly caused by ileal lymphoid hyperplasia. In adults, a tumor is frequently found at the apex of the intussuscepted segment.[94] The treatment in adults is surgical resection of the involved bowel.

DIVERTICULA

Duodenal and jejunal diverticula occur as acquired malformations in association with local mechanical factors or disorders of intestinal smooth muscle or nerves. In the ileum, the more common *Meckel's diverticulum* occurs in 2% of individuals because of persistence of the vitelline duct. It occurs on the antimesenteric visceral border within 1 m of the ileocecal valve and ranges from 1 to 10 cm in length. About one half of Meckel's diverticula contain heterotopic tissue of gastric or pancreatic type. Up to half of affected patients develop symptoms in their lifetime; these include bleeding, obstruction, and ulceration secondary to heterotopic gastric acid secretion.[95] Surgical resection is indicated only for symptomatic lesions.

HETEROTOPIAS

Pancreatic hamartomas are found in the gastric antrum, duodenum, and jejunum. These may contain elements of ductal tissue, smooth muscle, exocrine glands, and islets.[96, 97] Larger lesions often have a central nipplelike duct apparent on endoscopic examination. When hamartomas occur in the duodenal papillae, they are referred to as adenomyomas. Clinically, they may appear as an ''ampullary mass'' and must be distinguished from adenocarcinoma.

PEPTIC ULCERATION AND DUODENITIS

The majority of peptic ulcers occur in the duodenum and stomach. Duodenal ulcers outnumber gastric ulcers by a ratio of 3:1, and approximately 30% of gastric ulcer patients have duodenal ulcers. Duodenal ulcers are strongly associated with gastric hyperchlorhydria and gastric colonization by *H. pylori*.[98, 99] They also occur in patients with renal failure, alcoholic cirrhosis, and chronic lung disease.[100–102] Gastric ulcers are associated with a variety of potential etiologic factors, including *H. pylori*, NSAIDs, and environmental parameters.[41]

Peptic ulcers most commonly occur with epigastric pain, often associated with meals. Massive bleeding occurs in about 5% of cases. At endoscopy, benign ulcers have a sharply circumscribed appearance. In contrast to malignancy-associated ulcers, undistorted mucosal folds extend to the ulcer edge, without elevation of the margin (Fig. 12–4). Benign ulcers are usually found in the antral lesser curvature, or the first portion of the duodenum. However, malignant ulcers may occur in any area of the stomach, may appear benign, and may even heal temporarily. Therefore, unequivocal proof of the benign nature of a nonhealing or recurrent ulcer requires endoscopic biopsy directed at the ulcer edge.[103] Biopsy specimens usually consist of ulcer slough, granulation tissue, and intact mucosa with varying degrees of inflammation. In the stomach, intestinal metaplasia may be evident; in the duodenum, gastric surface-cell metaplasia frequently accompanies chronic, active duodenitis.[104] The treatment for peptic ulceration is now primarily pharmacologic; hence, elective surgery for peptic ulcer has become rare. Indications for peptic ulcer surgery include free perforation, penetration into the pancreas, intractable bleeding, and gastric outlet obstruction, or the rare Zollinger-Ellison syndrome.[105]

SMALL INTESTINAL INFECTIONS

Historically, infections have been the most important diseases of the GI tract, and they remain so in many areas of the world today. Intestinal infections may be chronic and debilitating or sudden and life-threatening, depending on the agent and host factors. The specific diagnosis of infectious diarrhea is made by studying fecal specimens: direct examination for leukocytes and parasites, bacterial or viral culture, and identification of microbial antigens and toxins. In western countries, however, most patients with infectious diarrhea have a mild, self-limited course and neither stool culture nor specific treatment is required.

The normal intestinal microenvironment includes low concentrations of predominantly gram-positive facultative organisms in the proximal small bowel, changing to gram-negative bacteria in the ileum and colon. Conditions of mechanical small bowel stagnation—such as surgical blind loops, diverticula, strictures, fistulas, and motility abnormalities—may lead to bacterial overgrowth, altered bile salt metabolism, and fat malabsorption *(blind-loop syndrome)*. These effects may be surgically correctable or amenable to antibiotic therapy.[106]

Although there is considerable overlap, intestinal bacterial infections can be divided into those in the small intestine and those in the colon. Bacteria produce diarrhea by a number of mechanisms, including production of preformed and ingested toxins, enterotoxin or cytotoxin production following intestinal colonization, and direct bacterial invasion. The current discussion includes only those agents that colonize or invade the small intestine.

Pathogens that produce an acute self-limiting watery diarrheal illness include *Clostridium perfringens*, enterotoxigenic and enteropathogenic strains of *Escherichia coli, Vibrio cholerae*, and related vibrio species.[107] *Clostridium perfringens* has also been implicated in cases of antibiotic-associated diarrhea and of necrotizing enteritis in regions of endemic chronic malnutrition. *Salmonella* infections may produce mild symptoms, a choleralike diarrheal illness, or a dysenteric clinical picture with blood and pus in the

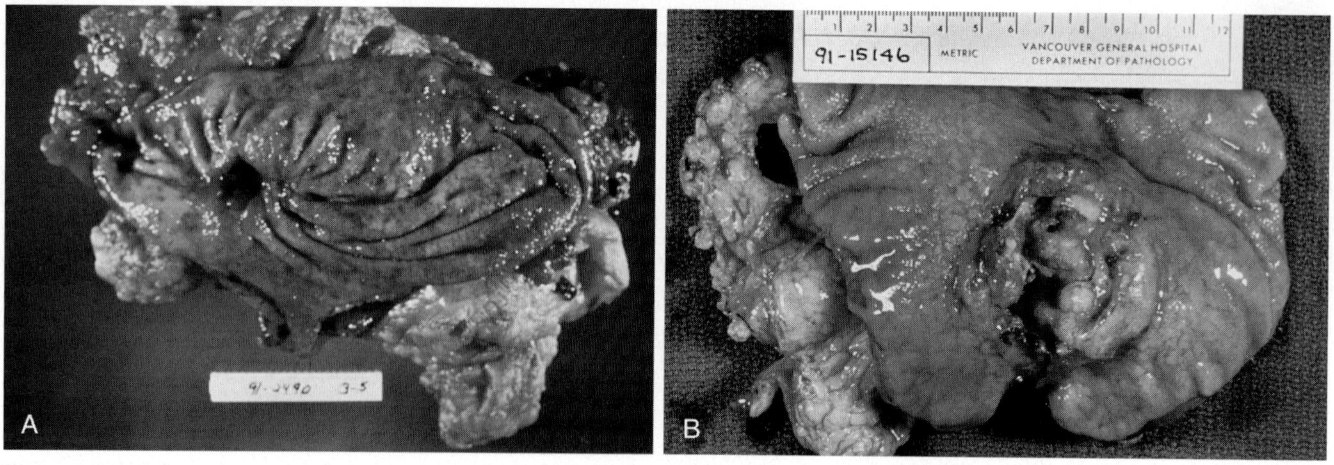

Figure 12–4. Comparative photographs of *(A)* benign gastric ulcer and *(B)* ulcerating gastric adenocarcinoma. The benign ulcer is sharply circumscribed, with undistorted mucosal folds extending to the ulcer edge. The gastric carcinoma has an elevated, ragged margin. Despite these differences, a diagnosis of benign versus malignant ulcer *requires* biopsy and microscopic verification.

stools. *Yersinia enterocolitica* and *Yersinia pseudotuberculosis* produce an intestinal illness predominantly in children.[108] These patients present with diarrhea and pain localized to the right lower quadrant, so closely mimicking acute appendicitis that an appendectomy may be performed. The illness tends to be self-limited, although young patients may develop severe hemorrhagic enterocolitis and mesenteritis.

Proper collection and preservation of fecal or gastric washing specimens are frequently neglected requirements for identification of microorganisms responsible for intestinal disease. Specimens should be submitted immediately, at body temperature, to the microbiology laboratory in a sterile, screw-topped container in order to prevent changes in pH that may kill intestinal pathogens such as *Shigella* and *Salmonella*. A second specimen preserved in fixative (such as phosphate buffer and glycerol) should also be sent.

The majority of small intestinal parasites are diagnosed by stool examination for ova and parasites and rarely come to the attention of the surgeon. Exceptions include parasites that produce perforation or obstruction, such as *Entamoeba histolytica, Anisakis*, or *Ascaris* organisms or parasitic infections that occur in immunodeficient patients.

Infections in the Immunocompromised Host. Specific infections are characteristic in patients with AIDS or those who are receiving immunosuppressive therapy.[109–111]

Cytomegalovirus (CMV) infection is common in AIDS patients and in bone marrow or solid organ transplant recipients. In most, this represents reactivation of latent virus. Individuals receiving systemic steroids for inflammatory diseases are also at risk for CMV disease. The diagnosis is made by endoscopy and biopsy. Ulceration due to CMV is an infrequent cause of intestinal perforation.

Gastrointestinal mycobacterial infections are encountered with increasing frequency in AIDS patients.[112] These are most commonly due to *Mycobacterium avium-intracellulare* but may also be due to disseminated *Mycobacterium tuberculosis*. Biopsy specimens may exhibit only subtle evidence of mycobacterial infection with infiltration of the intestinal lamina propria by histiocytes. Acid-fast stains are diagnostic and should be routinely performed on intestinal biopsies from HIV-positive patients.

Patients with AIDS are at risk for development of a therapy-resistant form of *cryptosporidiosis*. This small intestinal coccidian parasite causes an acute, self-limited diarrheal disease in the immunocompetent host,[113] but in AIDS patients the disease may be life-threatening. Diagnosis is by identification of acid-fast cysts in stool specimens or attached to the small intestinal epithelial brush border in biopsy specimens. Other coccidian parasites commonly found in the immunosuppressed include *Isospora belli*, usually diagnosed on stool examination, and Microsporidia genera, the developmental forms of which are occasionally seen on close microscopic examination of small-intestinal epithelium.[114]

The roundworm *Strongyloides stercoralis* produces a chronic small intestinal infection in the immunocompetent patient that may manifest as mild anemia. Radical alteration of the host's immunologic status, including organ transplantation and initiation of antineoplastic chemotherapy or radiotherapy, may result in an overwhelming and a life-threatening intestinal autoinfection.[115] Serologic assay and stool examination for *Strongyloides* organisms are suggested prior to institution of immunosuppressive therapy in endemic areas.

CELIAC SPRUE

Celiac sprue is a malabsorptive, frequently diarrheal disease resulting from an immunologic reaction to the alcohol-soluble alpha-gliadin fraction of gluten, a protein found in cereal grains including wheat, barley, rye, and oats.[116] Etiologically, gluten sensitivity may be related to early infection with *Adenovirus serotype 12* in persons with HLA-related genetic susceptibility.[117] In North America, the disease symptomatically affects between 1 in 10,000 and 1 in 3,000 individuals, although screening studies for serum antigliadin antibodies suggest that a large subclinical, gluten-sensitive population may exist.[118]

Although upper GI radiologic studies and the presence

of serum antigliadin antibodies may suggest a diagnosis of celiac sprue, the diagnosis is still established by small-intestinal mucosal biopsy. The characteristic microscopic findings include blunting or flattening of the mucosal villi, lamina propria inflammation, crypt hyperplasia, and superficial epithelial lymphocytosis (Fig. 12–5).[52] This last feature lends histologic specificity to the diagnosis of celiac sprue, and in North America the majority of individuals with malabsorption and these features on mucosal biopsy have gluten sensitivity. The mucosal changes of celiac disease are usually most pronounced in the proximal duodenum, although biopsy samples are usually obtained from the distal duodenum or proximal jejunum in order to avoid confusion with peptic duodenitis. Clinical improvement on a gluten-free diet is usually rapid. Rebiopsy of intestinal mucosa to confirm histologic improvement with gluten withdrawal is frequently recommended in the literature but in our experience is rarely carried out.

Approximately 15% of individuals with long-term celiac sprue will develop a malignancy, most often a small intestinal T-cell lymphoma. Clinically, patients with this complication present with obstructive symptoms or sudden weight loss and are physiologically stable. Later studies on the relationship of diet and malignancy to celiac disease suggest that strict adherence to gluten avoidance significantly reduces the risk of malignancy.[119]

OTHER CAUSES OF MALABSORPTION

Common variable immune deficiency (CVID) is a group of disorders characterized by defective differentiation of B lymphocytes into plasma cells. Patients present in the second or third decade with recurrent respiratory infections or malabsorptive diarrhea and intestinal colonization by *Giardia lamblia*.[120]

The GI tract is a potential site of involvement by *systemic amyloidosis*, resulting in symptoms of malabsorptive diarrhea or, alternatively, constipation due to intestinal dysmotility.[121] Duodenal and rectal endoscopic biopsies are commonly used to demonstrate amyloid deposition within the mucosal lamina propria or submucosal vessels. Congo red staining of amyloid deposits with apple-green birefringence in polarized microscopy is diagnostic.

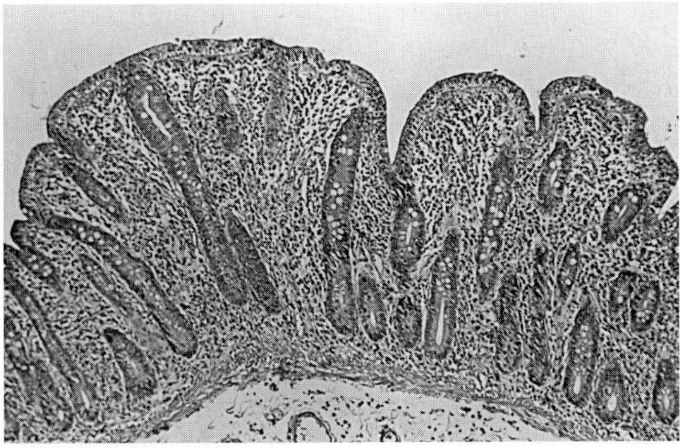

Figure 12–5. Photomicrograph of small-intestinal mucosa from a patient with untreated celiac sprue. Total villous atrophy, crypt hyperplasia, inflammation, and epithelial lymphocytosis are evident. Hematoxylin and eosin, ×10.

Whipple's disease, although a bacterial infection, occurs as a chronic systemic illness, characterized clinically by malabsorptive diarrhea, arthritis, lymphadenopathy, and central nervous system disease.[122] Small-intestinal mucosal biopsy reveals infiltration of the lamina propria by foamy macrophages containing numerous periodic acid-Schiff (PAS)-positive bacilli. This potentially fatal disease responds rapidly to antibiotic therapy.

Iatrogenic causes of malabsorptive diarrhea include drug ingestion (such as colchicine or cholestyramine), radiation enterocolitis, short bowel syndrome secondary to extensive small intestinal resection, and intestinal involvement by graft-versus-host disease (GVHD). Endoscopic biopsy is useful in the diagnosis of radiation enterocolitis and GVHD. Intestinal GVHD following allogeneic bone marrow transplantation is characterized by crypt epithelial cell necrosis (apoptosis) and neutrophilic inflammation. Early changes of GVHD may be indistinguishable from the direct toxic effects of systemic chemotherapy. A rash and jaundice, if present, are supportive of a diagnosis of GVHD.[123] The clinical differential diagnosis often includes CMV disease; concurrent GI involvement by both GVHD and CMV is not uncommon.

POLYPS

Polyps of the small intestine are uncommon and include hamartomas and neoplasms. Hamartomas of the small intestine usually occur as part of a polyposis syndrome, of which there are several. The two most important are *juvenile polyposis* and *Peutz-Jeghers syndrome*.[124, 125]

NEOPLASMS

Adenomas

Small intestinal adenomas occur most commonly in the duodenum and are often found in patients with familial adenomatous polyposis of the colon and other forms of hereditary colorectal carcinoma.[126, 127] Most small intestinal adenomas are asymptomatic lesions discovered incidentally or upon subsequent development of adenocarcinoma, which is present in up to 65% of biopsied or resected lesions.[128] Microscopically, they are identical to their colonic counterparts.

Adenomas arising in the region of the duodenal papilla may produce symptoms of pancreatic or biliary obstruction. They are usually less than 2 cm in diameter when discovered and frequently have a villiform architecture.[129] Lesions with a superficial adenomatous component may harbor an underlying invasive carcinoma that may be missed by endoscopic biopsy (Fig. 12–6). From a surgical standpoint, this distinction may not be critical. In our experience, the majority of adenomas of the duodenal papilla occurring with obstructive symptoms have proved upon resection to contain carcinoma, often minimally invasive. When clinically feasible, even benign lesions are optimally treated by pancreaticoduodenectomy, in order to relieve symptoms and remove a potentially malignant tumor. In surgically

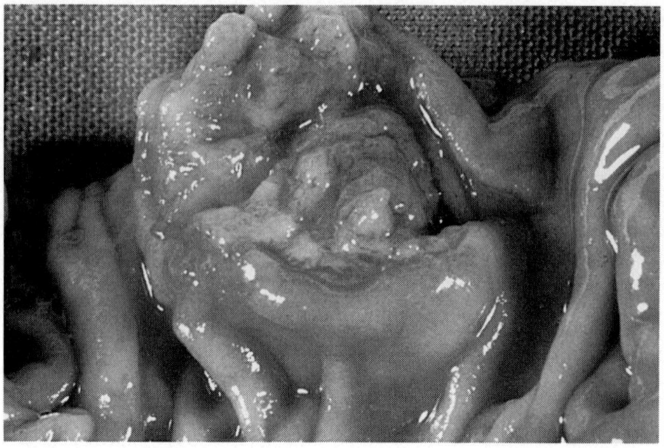

Figure 12–6. Adenoma arising from the duodenal papilla with extension into a dilated ampullary orifice. Microscopic examination revealed an underlying, minimally invasive adenocarcinomatous component. The lesion was completely resected by a Whipple procedure.

high-risk patients, local excision has been performed with good long-term results.

Adenocarcinomas

Adenocarcinomas of the small intestine occur much less commonly than those of the large intestine. Approximately 40% are in the duodenum. Predisposing conditions include intestinal polyposis syndromes, Crohn's disease, and celiac sprue.[130, 131] Clinically, patients present with obstruction and occult bleeding or, less commonly, jaundice if the tumor is periampullary. At the time of surgery, a constrictive growth pattern with kinking of the bowel is a frequent finding. Microscopically, small-intestinal adenocarcinoma resembles adenocarcinoma of the colon. Because patients with small-intestinal adenocarcinomas usually present with advanced-stage disease, they have a poor prognosis, with 5-year survival between 10 and 20%.[132] Adenocarcinomas of the duodenal papillary region may give a better prognosis than those arising elsewhere in the small intestine, possibly due to an earlier presentation with biliary obstructive symptoms. Jejunal and all but the most distal ileal lesions are usually resected with 10-cm flanking margins of normal intestine and a wedge of mesentery. Mesenteric lymph node metastasis is a predictor of poor outcome. Duodenal carcinomas are treated by pancreaticoduodenectomy in patients who can tolerate the procedure. The operative approach is often similar, whether the intent is curative or palliative. Bypass or diverticularization is employed for nonresectable lesions.

Carcinoid Tumors

The second most common small-intestinal malignancies are carcinoid tumors. The majority are located in the ileum. Up to 70% of small-intestinal carcinoids are asymptomatic lesions discovered incidentally at the time of endoscopy, laparotomy, or autopsy. Symptomatic lesions produce intestinal obstruction due to infiltrative growth. Only 10% of patients with symptomatic small-intestinal carcinoids develop carcinoid syndrome (flushing, diarrhea, abdominal pain, and endocardial lesions), usually indicating hepatic metastases.[133] Elevated urinary 5-hydroxyindoleacetic acid (5-HIAA) levels may aid in the preoperative evaluation for carcinoid.

At the time of surgery for carcinoid tumors, intestinal stricture, kinking, or localized ischemic necrosis due to a characteristically florid stromal response to the tumor is often seen (Fig. 12–7). Multiple tumors occur in up to 40% of patients with small-intestinal carcinoids, mandating operative inspection of the entire bowel.[134] The cut surface of the tumor reveals a hard, yellow-tan mural nodule up to 4 cm in diameter. Microscopically, the tumors are composed of infiltrating nests, tubules, or trabeculae of cytologically bland epithelial cells with clear or eosinophilic cytoplasm. The neuroendocrine nature of the cells is confirmed by histochemical or immunohistochemical staining of routinely fixed tissues.

All small-intestinal carcinoid tumors are potentially malignant. The risk of metastasis increases with tumor size. In the Mayo Clinic series, lesions less than 0.5 cm in diameter did not metastasize. However, 15% of tumors 0.5 to 0.9 cm, 61% of tumors 1.0 to 1.5 cm, 84% of tumors 1.5 to 1.9 cm, and 94% of tumors over 2 cm metastasized to regional lymph nodes and liver.[135] Treatment with curative intent for small-intestinal carcinoids includes ileocecal resection and lymph node dissection for terminal ileal lesions, wide local excision with a mesenteric wedge for proximal ileal and jejunal lesions, and Whipple's resection for duodenal lesions. Tumors less than 1 cm in diameter are amenable to local excision. Carcinoids are slow-growing tumors, and the carcinoid syndrome can be clinically debilitating; hence, aggressive surgical resection or debulking is indicated for patients with a solitary hepatic metastasis or multiple symptomatic metastases. Pharmacologic control of carcinoid syndrome with somatostatin analogues has been advocated.[136] The overall 5-year survival for patients with small-bowel carcinoids is 54%. Complete surgical resection is associated with a 5-year survival of 75%,

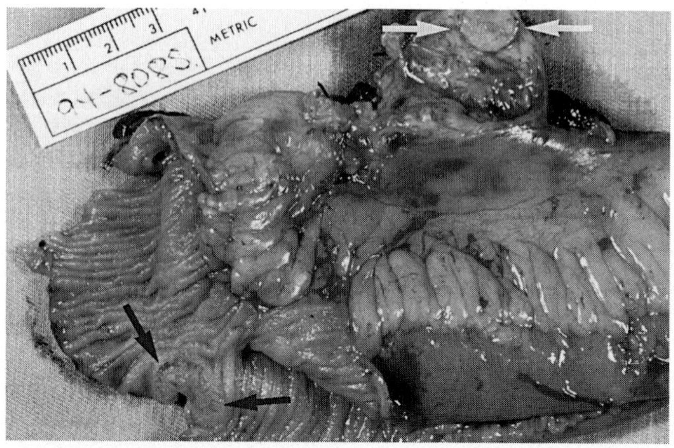

Figure 12–7. Small-bowel resection specimen containing a carcinoid tumor. The intestinal primary *(black arrows)* has produced kinking of the involved segment. A metastasis to a mesenteric lymph node is evident *(white arrows).*

whereas 20% of patients with distant metastases at the time of diagnosis will be alive 5 years later.[137]

Lymphomas

Primary lymphoma is the third most common small intestinal malignancy and accounts for up to 30% of primary GI lymphomas in North America. Essentially all are of the non-Hodgkin's type. In contrast to the stomach, lymphomas of T-cell type are common in the small intestine, accounting for one third of cases. Half of these occur in association with long-standing celiac sprue.[138] Similar to other small intestinal malignancies, lymphomas occur with intussusception, obstruction, and bleeding, but they are prone to produce marked weight loss and perforation.

Up to 80% of B-cell lymphomas of the small intestine in North America are of the diffuse large-cell type. The remaining 20% include the highly aggressive Burkitt's and lymphoblastic lymphomas of the ileum, low-grade B-cell lymphomas of MALT, and mantle-cell lymphomas. This last entity produces multiple polypoid lesions of the small and large intestines *(multiple lymphomatous polyposis)*.[139] The prognosis of small-intestinal B-cell lymphomas, like that of gastric lymphomas, depends on histologic type and tumor stage. Low-grade lesions have a 5-year survival of 75%, whereas higher-grade large-cell lesions have a 5-year survival of 40%. The absence of mesenteric lymph node involvement implies a better prognosis.[138]

Stromal Tumors

Spindle-cell mesenchymal neoplasms of the small intestine, analogous to benign and malignant stromal tumors of the stomach, occur primarily in the jejunum and proximal ileum. When symptomatic, they cause intestinal obstruction and bleeding. Gross, microscopic, and immunohistochemical features are similar to the corresponding gastric lesions. Criteria for malignancy, however, are even more complicated. The criteria presented previously for gastric stromal tumors are advocated, with the following modifications: size greater than 3 cm in diameter and any mitotic activity are considered features highly suggestive of malignancy.[91] For practical purposes, stromal tumors occurring as obstructive or bleeding intestinal masses are usually considered malignant or of undetermined malignant potential, whereas small stromal tumors encountered incidentally at the time of surgery usually are benign.

A variety of benign and malignant vascular tumors involve the small intestine. Hemangiomas account for 10% of benign small-intestinal tumors, occurring predominantly in the jejunum and ileum.[140] Malignant vascular tumors of the GI tract are rare, with the increasingly common exception of *Kaposi's sarcoma* in patients with AIDS. Gastrointestinal involvement by Kaposi's sarcoma is present in up to 50% of AIDS patients, although only a minority of affected individuals have symptoms attributable to intestinal tumor.[141] Symptomatic GI involvement by Kaposi's sarcoma is responsive to localized laser ablation, radiotherapy, and chemotherapy.

The small intestine is a common site for metastasis of a tumor arising outside of the GI tract, mimicking a primary GI tumor. Disseminated malignant melanoma has a high frequency of intestinal involvement, and there is often a prolonged interval between the diagnosis of the primary skin or ocular lesion and the subsequent presentation of intestinal metastases. These are often polypoid, submucosal, and nonpigmented. Carcinomas of prostatic, bladder and gynecologic origin may involve the intestines by either direct extension or peritoneal dissemination. Gastrointestinal involvement by leukemic infiltrates is common.

Ileocecal Region and Large Intestine

The large-intestinal (and appendiceal) mucosa is made up of numerous test-tube–shaped crypts lined by absorptive, mucus-secreting, and endocrine cells.

BENIGN NONINFLAMMATORY DISORDERS

Irritable Bowel Syndrome

The most common disorder of colonic motility in North America is irritable bowel syndrome.[142] Other terms for this syndrome, such as ''spastic'' or ''nonulcerative'' colitis, should be avoided. By definition, there is no inflammation of the bowel.[143] The diagnosis is based upon the presence of altered bowel frequency (ranging from constipation to diarrhea), abdominal distention, and pain. Structural or mucosal abnormalities in the bowel are absent and mucosal histology is normal.

Intestinal Pseudoobstruction

Pseudoobstruction exists when a patient has symptoms of intestinal obstruction without a detectable structural lesion. Acute colonic pseudoobstruction is referred to as *Ogilvie's syndrome* and is characterized clinically by abdominal distension, pain, anorexia, and respiratory compromise. Radiography reveals colonic distension. Bowel perforation is an uncommon but life-threatening complication. Predisposing conditions include recent surgery, chronic obstructive pulmonary disease, metabolic disturbances, neurologic disorders, cardiac insufficiency, and serious infections.[144] Other causes of acute megacolon, such as inflammatory bowel disease, should be ruled out. Therapeutic management is conservative, although a minority of affected individuals will eventually undergo colectomy. Pathologic findings are either nonspecific or absent altogether.

Chronic intestinal pseudoobstruction may occur secondary to a number of systemic diseases, which may or may not produce histologic lesions within the large intestine. Examples include diabetes mellitus, hypothyroidism, hypoparathyroidism, Parkinson's disease, collagen-vascular disease, neuroactive drug therapy, chemotherapy with nerve-blocking agents such as vincristine and vinblastine, and pregnancy.[145] Intestinal pseudoobstruction due to primary changes in the GI tract include Hirschsprung's disease, visceral myopathies and neuropathies, and *cathartic colon*. Cathartic colon is the end stage of chronic constipation.

The bowel is flaccid, with a thin muscularis propria and a decreased number of neurons in Auerbach's plexus. The mucosa exhibits *melanosis coli*, a deep-brown pigmentation due to the presence of a lipofuscinlike pigment concentrated by histiocytes of the lamina propria.[146] Melanosis coli is also associated with a history of laxative abuse, specifically with agents of the anthraquinone group (cascara sagrada, aloe, rhubarb, senna, and frangula).

Volvulus

The cecum and sigmoid colon are at risk for torsion and vascular occlusion, especially in elderly patients. The clinical presentation is sudden onset of pain, abdominal distension, and palpable mass. Plain abdominal films are often diagnostic. Early volvulus can be managed endoscopically. When obstruction is complete, the risk of ischemia and perforation is high.[147] Surgical resection of involved segments reveals mucosal or transmural changes of ischemic colitis (see subsequent discussion).

Angiodysplasia

Colonic angiodysplasia is the commonest cause of severe, recurrent lower-GI hemorrhage in the elderly.[148] Angiodysplastic lesions are collections of multiple, thin-walled, ectatic veins in the mucosa and submucosa, most commonly in the cecum and ascending colon. The etiology is undetermined, although associated clinical conditions include aortic valvular stenosis and von Willebrand's disease.[149, 150] The commonest clinical presentation is recurrent low-grade bleeding, but massive hemorrhage occurs in 15% of cases. Colonic lesions may be diagnosed by endoscopy or angiography.[151] Radioactively tagged red-cell scans are only rarely useful as guides to the bleeding site location. Endoscopically, the lesions are small, flat, red, and stellate, with a visible draining vein. Therapeutically, lesions producing low-grade hemorrhage are managed with iron replacement and endoscopic electrocautery or laser coagulation. Recurrence is due to the high frequency of multiple lesions. Severe acute or chronic transfusion-dependent hemorrhage is managed with right hemicolectomy.[152] Demonstration of the collapsed vascular lesions in resection specimens is notoriously difficult by standard pathology techniques.

Pneumatosis Cystoides Intestinalis

Pneumatosis cystoides intestinalis (PCI) is an uncommon lesion that may occur throughout the GI tract but most commonly is recognized in the distal large intestine.[153] It consists of multiple gas-filled submucosal cysts lined by stromal cells and foreign-body giant cells. When it occurs in adults, PCI is most likely due to an intestinal mucosal tear or defect induced by inflammation or increased luminal pressure. Thus, PCI is encountered in patients with emphysema, abdominal trauma, diverticular disease, volvulus, Crohn's disease, appendicitis, or prior surgery. It is most often an incidental finding on radiographic or endoscopic examination. Microscopically, the lesions must be distinguished from the artifactual entity of ''pseudolipomatosis,'' which consists of mucosal air cysts that resemble fat cells; these are iatrogenically introduced by excessive air inflation during colonoscopy. Adult PCI must be distinguished from fulminant pneumatosis intestinalis of infancy due to necrotizing enterocolitis.

INFLAMMATORY BOWEL DISEASE

Idiopathic inflammatory bowel disease (IBD) includes *ulcerative colitis* (UC) and *Crohn's disease* (CD). These are chronic inflammatory processes of unknown etiology, diagnosed on the basis of combined clinical, endoscopic, and histologic features. Both UC and CD are most common among white populations of Northern European ancestry, among whom the prevalence is 1 in 1,000 persons.[154] The age of onset for both diseases peaks at 15 to 25 years, with a second peak at 55 to 65 years. Approximately 15% of patients with IBD have an affected first-degree relative.

Ulcerative Colitis

A patient with ulcerative colitis initially presents with diarrhea, frequently bloody. Additional symptoms include fever, abdominal pain, weight loss, and rectal pain.[155] Endoscopic examination is required at the time of presentation to establish the diagnosis and to determine the extent of disease. Ulcerative colitis is normally limited to the large-intestinal mucosa and extends continuously from the rectum to more proximal regions. At initial presentation, 75% of patients will have disease limited to the rectum and sigmoid colon.[156] About 20% will have disease extending to the cecum. Occasionally, pancolonic involvement will extend for a few centimeters into the terminal ileum, a condition referred to as ''backwash ileitis.'' Endoscopic mucosal appearances vary with disease intensity. Ulcerative colitis with mild activity has an erythematous and edematous mucosa that may bleed when touched. With more severe involvement, the mucosa bleeds spontaneously and is coated with a purulent exudate, with areas of ulceration.

About 90% of UC patients will have a period of clinical quiescence following their initial attack. Over the long term, nearly all will have periodic recurrent attacks.[156] Colonoscopic examination of long-standing disease often reveals large-bowel foreshortening due to muscular spasm, atrophy of the mucosal folds, and ulceration and regenerative hyperplasia of nonulcerated mucosa, which produces inflammatory pseudopolyps. Colonoscopic biopsy, when correlated with clinical and endoscopic findings, is usually diagnostic in both active and quiescent disease. Specimens submitted for histology should include a description of the distribution of inflammatory changes. Biopsy specimens should be taken from multiple levels, including grossly involved and uninvolved segments, and submitted in separate containers labeled with the site of origin. Mucosal biopsy findings of active UC show diffuse expansion of the lamina propria by inflammatory cells, with sheets of plasma cells extending to the mucosal base, distortion of the crypt architecture, and active crypt inflammation by acute inflammatory cells. Without the histologic features of chronicity (crypt distortion and basal plasmacytosis), a

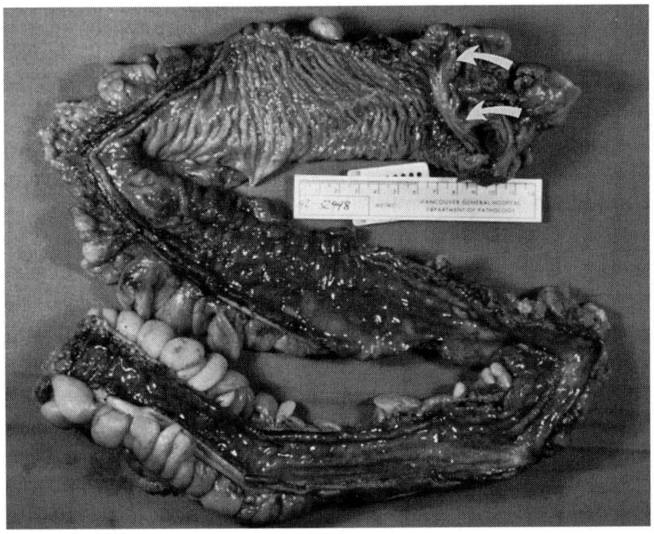

Figure 12–8. Ulcerative colitis with active disease of the distal transverse, descending, and sigmoid segments *(white arrows show ileocecal valve).*

diagnosis of IBD cannot be confirmed and acute self-limiting (infectious) colitis must be considered.[157, 158] These features are usually retained even during a clinically quiescent phase. The distinction of UC from CD requires microscopic verification of a diffuse, left-sided or pancolonic distribution of inflammation without skip lesions and without mucosal granulomas.

The early complications of UC include perforation and toxic megacolon. Although perforation often occurs as the result of toxic megacolon, it may occur during severe episodes of colitis without massive colonic dilatation. *Toxic megacolon* specifically refers to extension of the inflammatory process into the muscularis propria, with resultant colonic dilatation, fever, neutrophilia, hypotension, and dehydration.[159] Toxic megacolon most often occurs early in the course of UC in patients with pancolonic involvement. Toxic megacolon may be precipitated by the administration of anticholinergic and antidiarrheal drugs in patients with highly active disease. The most important long-term complication of UC is the development of adenocarcinoma (see subsequent discussion).

Crohn's disease is complex because of the variety of anatomic sites that may be involved. Approximately 70% of patients present with disease in the ileum or ileum plus cecum, whereas up to 25% present with colonic involvement only.[160] Five percent of patients present with more proximal GI involvement, including mouth, esophagus, stomach, and proximal small intestine. The onset of CD is often indolent, with intermittent diarrhea, crampy abdominal pain, anemia, and moderate weight loss. The pain is often localized to the right lower quadrant, and weight loss may be malabsorptive or due to a diminished caloric intake. Physical examination may reveal a tender right-lower-quadrant abdominal mass.

The endoscopic appearances of CD are diverse. The earliest visible manifestation is the aphthous ulcer: a discrete, often multifocal lesion measuring a few millimeters in diameter, with a thin red mucosal halo. Multiple lesions may coalesce into stellate, linear, or serpiginous ulcers. Longitudinal and transverse ulcers may intersect, resulting in a cobblestonelike mucosal appearance. Typically, right-colonic and ileal involvement predominates. Even with extensive colonic and rectal involvement, segments of mucosal sparing are characteristic.

The salient microscopic features of CD are ileal involvement, the predominantly right-sided colonic distribution of the inflammation, the marked variability of the inflammation between biopsy fragments from various levels or even with individual biopsy fragments, and the presence of granulomas. Despite these differences, UC and CD cannot be distinguished in up to 15% of cases. In such instances, the process must be designated as "chronic inflammatory bowel disease, type indeterminate."[161]

Complications of CD include abdominal abscesses, fistulas (enteroenteric, enterocutaneous, enterovesical, enterovaginal), strictures, perianal inflammation, and malabsorption. There is also an increased risk of small-intestinal and colonic adenocarcinoma in CD patients.[162]

The treatment of chronic inflammatory bowel disease includes enteric or parenteral nutritional support; medical management of pain, bowel frequency, and inflammation; and surgery. Anti-inflammatory therapy usually involves sulfasalazine or other salicylate-containing compounds and local or systemic corticosteroids. About 25% of patients with UC eventually undergo total colectomy, because of poor disease control with medical therapy, fulminant colitis with toxic megacolon, severe hemorrhage, perforation, or development of mucosal dysplasia or carcinoma.[163] Specimens resected for severe UC show extensive mucosal ulceration and hemorrhage (Fig. 12–8). If toxic megacolon is present, the bowel wall is thinned and prone to rupture with manipulation. Colectomy specimens from patients with long-standing UC may show mucosal atrophy or multiple inflammatory pseudopolyps. If the patient has been treated with corticosteroid enemas, relative rectal sparing may be grossly evident.

Surgical intervention in CD is most often for strictures, abscesses, fistulas, or bleeding. The specimen most commonly received in the pathology laboratory consists of terminal ileum and right colon (Fig. 12–9). Grossly, the

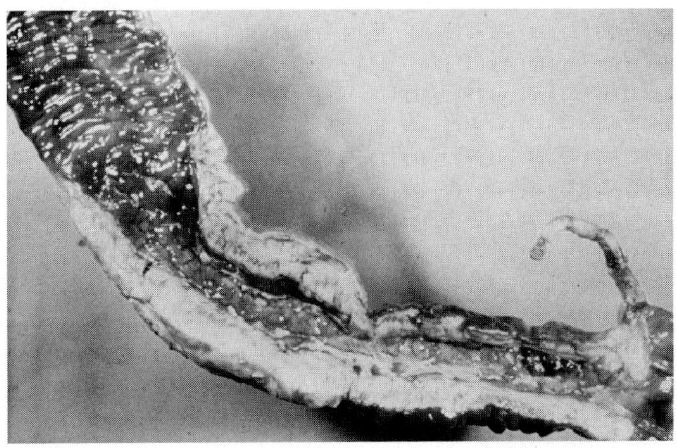

Figure 12–9. Crohn's disease of the terminal ileum. Resection specimen with mucosal ulceration, and luminal narrowing due to marked thickening of the ileal wall.

specimens exhibit segmental and transmural inflammatory changes: mucosal ulceration, mural thickening and fibrosis, serosal fat wrapping, and peritonitis if an abscess or a fistula is present. Histologically, transmural clefting ulceration and chronic inflammation of all levels of the bowel thickness, with or without granulomas, are seen. Surgical resections in CD should attempt to remove all grossly abnormal bowel based upon inspection and palpation. *There is no role for intraoperative frozen section microscopic examination of resection margins in Crohn's disease.*

Both UC and CD may occur as a part of a systemic inflammatory process.[164–166] Associated processes include both a migratory "colitic" arthritis of limb joints and ankylosing spondylitis. Hepatobiliary manifestations of inflammatory bowel disease include fatty liver, chronic active hepatitis, gallstones, and sclerosing cholangitis. Ocular complications are uveitis and episcleritis, whereas cutaneous manifestations are pyoderma gangrenosum and erythema nodosum.

Ulcerative Colitis and Carcinoma

Long-term UC is associated with an increased risk for development of large-bowel carcinoma. The likelihood of malignancy depends upon the duration and extent of disease but not upon disease severity.[167] For patients with ulcerative pancolitis, the risk is approximately 10% at 8 to 10 years. It increases by 0.5 to 2.0% each year thereafter. Patients with disease distal to the splenic flexure have no greater risk for development of carcinoma than the background population. The tumors that occur in UC patients appear at a younger age, are more commonly proximal, and are more frequently multifocal than those in the noncolitic population.[168]

The risk for carcinoma in UC patients is high enough after 10 years of pancolonic disease (and, debatably, after 15 to 20 years of left-sided disease) to warrant surveillance colonoscopy with multiple biopsies in order to identify dysplasia before development of invasive neoplasm. The surveillance protocol should include full colonoscopy with at least one biopsy specimen for each 10-cm interval throughout the large intestine. Initial surveillance should be at 3-year intervals, with shortening of this interval as the duration of disease increases.[169] Biopsy specimens should be labeled for site, with particular attention paid to masses, strictures, plaque lesions, or unusual polyps. Inflammatory pseudopolyps are not sites of preferential risk for development of malignancy, hence they do not require surgical removal. Biopsy specimens are assessed for dysplasia, which is quantified as low- or high-grade.[170] If the biopsy findings are negative for dysplasia, colonoscopy should be repeated at a 1- to 3-year intervals. If the specimens show an actively inflamed mucosa with epithelial-cell atypia that cannot be reliably classified as either reactive or dysplastic, a diagnosis of "indefinite for dysplasia" is given. The patient should undergo rebiopsy within a few months following a course of intensified anti-inflammatory therapy, in order to document the regression of the atypical changes or to confirm a diagnosis of dysplasia.

If a diagnosis of dysplasia is made, it is generally accepted that the case should be reviewed by a second pathologist experienced in the identification of dysplasia in UC. The presence of any grade of dysplasia found in a biopsy from an endoscopically defined mass, stricture, or plaque is an indication for consideration of colectomy. Up to 50% of dysplasia-associated lesions or masses contain invasive carcinoma.[171] The identification of low-grade dysplasia in flat, nonlesional mucosa should be followed by repeat colonoscopy with biopsies at 6-month intervals or less. If high-grade dysplasia is diagnosed in nonlesional mucosa and confirmed by a second experienced pathologist, colectomy should be considered. In our experience, the majority of UC patients who develop unequivocal dysplasia ultimately undergo colectomy, usually sooner rather than later.

Patients with CD are also at increased risk for development of large- and small-bowel carcinoma, but significantly less so than patients with UC.[172] There are currently no widely accepted recommendations for routine surveillance in CD.

POSTCOLECTOMY INFLAMMATORY DISEASE

Depending upon the type of procedure performed, the postcolectomy patient may have an ileostomy with or without a diverted large-intestinal segment, an ileorectal anastomosis, or an ileoanal anastomosis with formation of an ileal pouch. Each procedure may be associated with postsurgical inflammatory complications.

Diversion colitis and enteritis occur when a segment of distal colon or small intestine has been surgically diverted from the normal fecal stream. The etiology is undetermined but may be related to mucosal nutritional deprivation of short-chain fatty acids.[173] Diversion colitis may occur months to years following the procedure, with symptoms of bloody or purulent anal discharge. Microscopically, the mucosal inflammatory changes suggest inflammatory bowel disease; however, florid nodular lymphoid hyperplasia is frequently present and supports a diagnosis of diversion colitis. Symptoms resolve with reanastomosis of the diverted segment.

Ileal pouchitis occurs in a pouch constructed as part of an ileostomy or ileoanal anastomosis. The etiology is undetermined. The possibility of bacterial overgrowth in the pouch lumen has been suggested.[174] Ileal pouchitis has a higher frequency following colectomy for UC than for familial polyposis.[175] The presence of "backwash ileitis" in the terminal ileum at the time of colectomy is not a predisposing factor for postsurgical pouchitis. Microscopic evaluation of biopsy findings from affected ileal pouches reveals an inflammatory pattern that may mimic UC. Most patients respond dramatically to antimicrobial therapy.[174]

Patients who undergo colectomy with ileorectal or ileoanal anastomosis for UC or familial polyposis remain at risk (albeit small) for development of carcinoma within the residual rectal mucosa that remains with both procedures. Regular surveillance with inspection of this limited mucosal segment is required.

INFECTIOUS COLITIS

Important large-intestinal bacterial pathogens include *Shigella* and *Campylobacter* species, *C. difficile*, and pathogenic *E. coli. Shigella*, enterotoxigenic *E. coli*, and *Campylobacter* produce an acute, self-limited colitis, characterized clinically by abdominal pain and bloody, mucousy stools. Endoscopically, the mucosa shows diffuse erythema, edema, and purulent exudate. Mucosal biopsy specimens show an active colitis with a predominantly superficial inflammatory infiltrate and preservation of crypt architecture. These histologic features help distinguish acute self-limited colitis from inflammatory bowel disease.[157] Stool cultures are diagnostic for specific organisms.

Clostridium difficile is the major causative agent of *antibiotic-associated colitis*.[176] *C. difficile* cannot prevail over the normal large-intestinal microflora without antibiotic therapy. The organisms produce potent toxins that are responsible for the intestinal inflammation and are the basis for diagnostic assays. Clinically, patients present with abdominal pain, diarrhea, fever, and dehydration following a recent course of antibiotics. Colonoscopically, severe disease is characterized by raised yellow-white mucosal plaques or confluent pseudomembranes (Fig. 12–10). Histologically, *pseudomembranous colitis* exhibits patchy, superficial mucosal necrosis with adherent mucus, neutrophils, and necrotic epithelial cells over the mucosal surface. Definitive diagnosis relies on the identification of *cytotoxin B* in stool specimens. Treatment is oral vancomycin or metronidazole unless full-thickness colitis requiring resection is recognized.

A clinical syndrome characterized by a severe hemorrhagic colitis is due to *E. coli serotype* 0157:H7.[177, 178] It is associated with consumption of undercooked beef (''hamburger disease''). The organism produces toxins similar to those produced by *Shigella* species and may precipitate a hemolytic-uremic syndrome. Endoscopically, the colitis frequently has a right-sided predominance with a hemorrhagic mucosa. Microscopically, enterohemorrhagic *E. coli* colitis resembles ischemic and pseudomembranous colitis. The correct diagnosis is suggested by the clinical history and endoscopic distribution of the disease. Specific stool culture and immunologic typing assay are diagnostic.

Many large intestinal parasites, such as *Enterobius vermicularis* and *Trichuris trichiura*, are commonly identified clinically, but only infrequently do they come to the attention of the surgeon. One important exception is *Entamoeba histolytica*, an amebic parasite of worldwide distribution, acquired by fecal-oral contamination. The infected state may be asymptomatic or manifest clinically as dysentery. Colonoscopic examination reveals predominantly cecal or ascending colonic ulceration. An amebic abscess may manifest as a right-sided pericolonic mass. This may, in turn, disseminate to liver and lung. *Amebic colitis* may mimic inflammatory bowel disease both clinically and histologically.[179] Severe untreated disease may result in large-bowel perforation and death. The diagnosis is made by stool ova and parasite examination or by microscopic examination of biopsy specimens.

As previously noted, the intestines are a major site of opportunistic disease in patients with AIDS. However, individuals practicing receptive anal sex, regardless of immune status, are at risk for direct rectal mucosal trauma and for venereally acquired proctitis. Most patients present with tenesmus and bleeding. The mucosal appearance may range from diffuse inflammation to localized ulceration. Causative organisms include bacteria *(Treponema pallidum, Neisseria gonorrhoeae), Chlamydia* (lymphogranuloma venereum), and herpes simplex virus.[180]

DIVERTICULAR DISEASE

The lifetime risk of developing large-bowel diverticula in North America is estimated at 50%.[181] Diverticular disease occurs in populations with low dietary fiber intake and high levels of meat consumption. Reduced fecal bulk predisposes patients to increased intraluminal pressure, forcing colonic mucosa to herniate through points of vascular penetration of the muscularis propria. The sigmoid colon is the most commonly affected site. It is usual to find two rows of diverticula between the mesenteric and antimesenteric taeniae. About 70% of patients with diver-

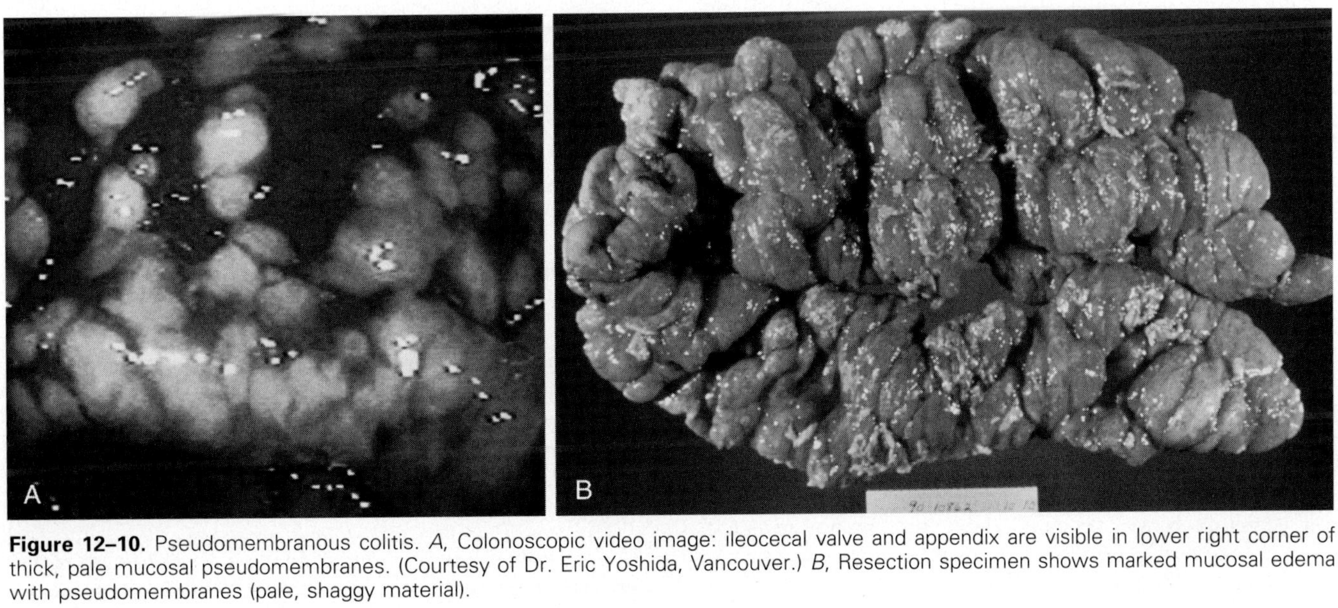

Figure 12–10. Pseudomembranous colitis. *A*, Colonoscopic video image: ileocecal valve and appendix are visible in lower right corner of thick, pale mucosal pseudomembranes. (Courtesy of Dr. Eric Yoshida, Vancouver.) *B*, Resection specimen shows marked mucosal edema with pseudomembranes (pale, shaggy material).

ticula have no symptoms.[182] Occasional patients will experience colicky abdominal pain or self-limited hemorrhage due to vascular erosion by fecal contents within a diverticulum. Patients with diverticular inflammation due to diverticular obstruction and bacterial overgrowth present with abdominal pain, nausea, vomiting, fever, ileus, and occasionally a mass on rectal examination. Episodes of inflammation may subside or progress to abscess formation, perforation, or obstruction. Surgical management, consisting of sigmoid colectomy, is required in up to 30% of symptomatic patients.[181] Resection specimens reveal multiple flask-shaped pouches protruding through the muscle wall, often containing impacted feces. If abscess formation or perforation has occurred, peritonitis may be evident and a mass, grossly resembling a neoplasm, may be present.

ISCHEMIA

In the adult patient, causes of intestinal ischemia include arteriosclerosis; mesenteric arterial or venous thrombosis (due to arterial atherosclerotic narrowing or hypercoagulable states such as polycythemia rubra vera, dehydration, disseminated malignancy, and antithrombin III or tissue plasminogen activator deficiency); emboli originating from the heart, often in a setting of atrial fibrillation; intestinal strangulation due to volvulus, hernia, or obstruction; systemic hypotension with intestinal vasoconstriction; iatrogenic interruptions of the arterial supply; and, rarely, vasculitis. The clinical picture is dominated by abdominal pain and marked hypovolemia due to intestinal edema and hemorrhage.

Ischemia limited to the colon is much more likely due to decreased perfusion pressure secondary to atherosclerosis or hypotensive vasoconstriction than to arterial embolism or thrombosis.[183] The most common cause of acute ischemic colitis is inferior mesenteric artery compromise during aortic surgery. The sites of the most peripheral collateral blood supply to the colon are at greatest risk for ischemic damage. These include the splenic flexure and adjacent transverse and descending colon. The clinical symptoms are abdominal pain, fever, and bloody diarrhea. A reversible ischemic process shows a ''thumbprinting'' pattern on barium enema examination. Endoscopy reveals an edematous, hemorrhagic, and frequently ulcerated mucosa in the affected segment. The mucosal edema may be prominent enough to suggest a tumor. Biopsy specimens from acute lesions show superficial mucosal necrosis with deep crypt sparing, vascular ectasia, paucity of mucosal inflammatory cells, and often pseudomembrane formation. This ''ischemic pattern'' may be indistinguishable from the mucosal changes of colitis associated with *C. difficile* and *E. coli* 0157:H7 (see previous discussion).[184] The clinical history, patient age, endoscopic appearance, and appropriate stool culture and toxin assay findings should distinguish these diagnostic possibilities. Ischemic colitis, if severe and prolonged, will result in transmural necrosis, perforation, and peritonitis. Surgical resection of the affected segment with grossly viable margins is required. If the ischemic bowel remains viable and is not resected, clinical recovery from the acute insult may be complicated by stricture formation.

DRUG-INDUCED COLITIS

A number of therapeutic agents are associated with a direct toxic effect on the large-bowel mucosa. Up to 70% of patients receiving combinations of chemotherapeutic agents that include cytosine arabinoside develop colonic ulceration.[185] Cyclophosphamide and fluorouracil are associated with development of hemorrhagic colitis.[186] Colitis has also been reported in patients receiving methotrexate for malignant disease or psoriasis.[187] Parenteral and oral gold therapy for rheumatoid arthritis is associated with a syndrome resembling ulcerative colitis, and acute colitis has been reported in patients receiving methyldopa and isotretinoin.[188, 189] Abnormal bowel function and colitis occur as a direct irritant effect of soap enemas. Prepackaged enemas, bisacodyl, and hypertonic saline all may induce microscopic changes that mimic acute colitis. These agents should be avoided during bowel preparation for endoscopic evaluation.

RECTAL INFLAMMATION DUE TO ABNORMAL DEFECATION

Stercoral ulceration of the rectum and sigmoid colon occurs in the setting of chronic constipation and fecal impaction due to a variety of causes, including the use of anticholinergic agents, antidepressants, and tranquilizers. Stercoral ulcers may uncommonly be complicated by spontaneous perforation and peritonitis.[190]

Solitary rectal ulcer is an inflammatory condition of the anterior rectal wall, about 7 to 10 cm from the anal verge, associated with prolonged straining at stool.[191] The lesion usually presents in young adults with anorectal pain and passage of blood and mucus. Although single or multiple discrete ulcers less than 1 cm in diameter are the usual endoscopic findings, the lesion may appear as an erythematous nodule. Biopsy specimens reveal superficial mucosal erosion, smooth muscle proliferation, and *colitis cystica profunda* (the displacement of benign colonic crypts beneath the muscularis mucosa).[192] These histologic features suggest an etiology of localized mucosal prolapse during defecation. Conservative treatment, with a high-fiber diet and limited laxatives, is aimed at eliminating straining at stool.

LYMPHOCYTIC AND COLLAGENOUS COLITIS

These inflammatory diseases of the large bowel are characterized clinically by chronic, watery, usually painless diarrhea and colonoscopically by absence of abnormalities.[193] The diagnosis of both conditions is established by microscopic examination of colonoscopic biopsy samples, accounting for the previously used terminology of ''microscopic colitis.'' The therapeutic approach to both diseases is similar. Sulfasalazine or oral 5-aminosalicylate is the usual agent of choice.[194]

POLYPS AND NEOPLASMS

Polyps

Large-bowel polyps are classified as hamartomatous, inflammatory, hyperplastic, and neoplastic. Intestinal hamartomas are discussed previously in relation to the small intestine. Inflammatory pseudopolyps are part of the spectrum of inflammatory bowel disease.

Hyperplastic polyps are sessile, smooth mucosal polyps, usually less than 5 mm in diameter, present in up to 80% of large bowels examined grossly or endoscopically.[195] They occur most often in the left colon. Hyperplastic polyps are not neoplasms but rather localized areas of defective epithelial-cell exfoliation. Microscopically, they exhibit a distinctive serrated-edge contour of the crypts and excessive accumulation of goblet-cell mucin. No histologic correlate to the large intestinal hyperplastic polyp is found elsewhere in the GI tract.

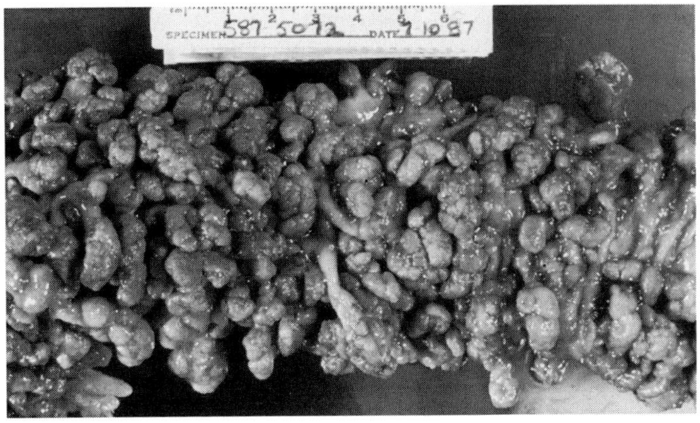

Figure 12–11. Colectomy specimen, familial adenomatous polyposis.

Adenomas

Benign epithelial neoplasms of the large intestine are called *adenomas*. Although only a minority of large-intestinal adenomas progress to carcinomas, the majority of large-intestinal carcinomas are believed to arise from either precursor adenomas or the flat dysplasia of UC.[196] Large intestinal adenomas and carcinomas occur most commonly in populations with a low-fiber, high-fat diet, usually in individuals over age 40. Approximately 50% of adenomas and carcinomas are in the rectum and sigmoid colon.[197] Carcinoma is present in about 5% of resected adenomas, and most well-sampled carcinomas have a demonstrable precursor adenoma component. The risk of carcinoma arising in an adenoma is related directly to tumor size.[198] Adenomas less than 1 cm in diameter (accounting for three fourths of resected specimens) contain carcinoma in 1% of lesions. Some 6.5% of adenomas 1 to 2 cm in diameter and 35% of adenomas greater than 2 cm in diameter contain carcinoma. Increasing adenoma size also correlates with the accumulation of genetic deletions and mutations within tumor cells that are characteristically found in large-intestinal carcinomas.[196]

Large-intestinal adenomas occur in three clinical settings. The least common of these, *familial adenomatous polyposis* (FAP), accounts for about 1% of large-intestinal carcinomas. This condition is inherited as an autosomal dominant trait due to a mutation of the adenomatous polyposis coli (APC) gene on the long arm of chromosome 5.[199] Up to one third of affected individuals lack a family history of FAP and appear to have a de novo mutation. Familial adenomatous polyposis is characterized by the development of at least 100 and usually thousands of adenomas in the large intestine as well as by the frequent occurrence of adenomas in the small intestine and stomach. In 80% of individuals, adenomas are present at puberty, and the risk of carcinoma becomes appreciable by age 18.[200] The lifetime risk of large-intestinal carcinoma in FAP patients is 100%. The management of this condition is relatively straightforward. A diagnosis of FAP requires colonoscopic identification of innumerable polyps (Fig. 12–11), with histologic confirmation that the multiple polyps are adenomas.

The recommended therapy is total proctocolectomy with ileoanal pouch anastomosis or colectomy with rectal mucosal stripping and ileorectal anastomosis.[201, 202] Follow-up consists of visual surveillance of any residual rectal mucosa at the ileal anastomosis site and periodic upper-GI endoscopy to monitor for gastric or duodenal neoplasms. All first-degree relatives should undergo screening by colonoscopy after puberty.

The second clinical setting for the development of large-intestinal adenomas and carcinomas includes the two forms of *hereditary nonpolyposis colorectal cancer* (HNPCC), also referred to as the *Lynch's syndromes type I* and *II*.[203] Both are autosomal dominant conditions. Some 90% of cases can be accounted for by defects in one of two genes, located on chromosomes 2 and 3, that normally function to prevent genetic instability during cell replication.[204, 205] These defects may account for 13% of large-intestinal carcinomas in North America. Lynch's syndrome type I is characterized by the early onset (mean, 44 years) of right-sided colonic adenomas and carcinomas, with an excess of multiple tumors. Lynch's syndrome type II has the same features, plus frequent carcinomas of the endometrium, ovary, ureter, stomach, small intestine, and pancreaticobiliary ducts.[203] Diagnostic criteria require at least three relatives with large-intestinal carcinoma in at least two successive generations, with at least one individual diagnosed at age 50 or less. Individuals from an HNPCC family should enter a full colonoscopic screening program at age 25, or 5 years earlier than the earliest diagnosis of large-intestinal carcinoma in the kindred. The appearance of large-intestinal carcinoma warrants at least subtotal colectomy. Affected women also require regular gynecologic examination.

The third and most common setting for the occurrence of large-intestinal adenomas and carcinomas is sporadic (i.e., in the absence of any identified syndrome). The prevalence of sporadic adenomas varies with age and geographic location; it ranges up to 69% in men aged 40 to 59.[206, 207] The contribution that genetic factors make in the occurrence of sporadic large-intestinal neoplasms is unknown. The incidence of large-intestinal carcinoma among first-degree relatives of affected patients is fourfold greater than that in the background population.[208] One third to one half of individuals with rectal adenomas or carcinomas will have adenomas in the remaining colon, and about the same proportion will have new adenomas in the next 5 years.[209]

The clinical implications of the discovery of a large-intestinal adenoma are clear. The patient should have a careful family history taken. Full colonoscopy should be performed. Follow-up colonoscopy, possibly on a 3-year periodic basis, is suggested.[210]

Most patients with large-intestinal adenomas are asymptomatic. Symptomatic lesions tend to be large and result in gross or occult rectal bleeding, change in bowel habits, and abdominal pain. Lesions are detected by digital examination, barium enema, or colonoscopic examination. The colonoscopic appearance ranges from a small mucosal plaque to a pedunculated polyp to a broad-based (sessile) growth. Biopsy or polypectomy of all suspected adenomas should be performed for diagnostic microscopic examination and for therapy.

Microscopically, large-intestinal adenomas are classified as tubular, villous, or tubulovillous, based upon architecture. The more important histologic considerations are confirmation that the lesion is an adenoma, examination for invasive carcinoma, and assessment for completeness of excision. Confirmation that the lesion is an adenoma requires identification of epithelial dysplasia (a pathologic diagnosis of ''adenoma with/without dysplasia'' is meaningless). Invasive carcinoma is identified when there is growth of malignant epithelium below the muscularis mucosae with desmoplastic stromal response. The term ''carcinoma in situ'' should not be applied to large-intestinal neoplasms, since, in the absence of invasion, the cytologic features of carcinomatous and highly dysplastic epithelium are indistinguishable. Occasional adenomas contain *intramucosal carcinoma*. This is recognized when there is definite invasion of the mucosal lamina propria that does not extend below the muscularis mucosae. When the lesion is completely excised, an adenoma with intramucosal carcinoma carries essentially no risk for metastasis.[211]

Pathologic evaluation of the completeness of excision of a GI adenoma is in part dependent upon the architecture of the lesion. Diminutive polyps removed by ''hot biopsy forceps'' cannot be assessed for completeness of excision, although it can be hoped that electrocoagulation of the surrounding mucosa will destroy any residual dysplastic epithelium. Larger pedunculated adenomas are usually removed by snare polypectomy with electrocautery. If a significant stalk is present and if the specimen is properly oriented and sectioned by the pathologist, it is usually possible to identify cautery artifact transecting the nondysplastic polyp stalk, thus assuring complete excision. Impaling the polyp stalk on a toothpick at the time of polypectomy may help the pathologist to identify the stalk in the fixed specimen. Larger sessile lesions removed piecemeal cannot be assessed for completeness of excision. Low-rectal sessile adenomas are frequently removed by deep submucosal surgical excision. These specimens should be submitted with a suture tag to indicate the proximal or distal mucosal margin. This allows the pathologist to provide a precise location of any histologically positive mucosal margin.

Occasional large intestinal adenomas will contain displaced neoplastic mucosa below the muscularis mucosae. This condition is referred to as *stalk pseudoinvasion* and is due to mechanical trauma and hemorrhage into the polyp. Pseudoinvasion is distinguished from invasive carcinoma by the lack of infiltrative growth pattern, the presence of lamina propria around the misplaced epithelium, and the stromal accumulation of hemorrhage and hemosiderin.[212]

The presence of invasive carcinoma within a colonoscopically excised adenoma is no longer considered a justification for colectomy.[213] The criteria for colectomy must include the relative risks of metastasis and operative mortality. If a pedunculated or broad-based adenoma contains a focus of invasive carcinoma with no evidence of lymphatic or venous invasion and if the carcinomatous component is verified microscopically as completely excised, no further treatment is necessary. Exceptions to this approach are adenomas that contain a poorly differentiated invasive carcinomatous component and sessile adenomas in which the carcinomatous component invades to a depth equivalent to the submucosal level of the surrounding mucosa.[214, 215]

Adenocarcinomas

In the United States, large-intestinal carcinoma accounts for 14% of all diagnosed malignancies (excluding nonmelanoma skin cancers) and causes 11% of all cancer deaths.[216] The median age at diagnosis is 62 years, with an equal sex distribution.

Large-intestinal carcinomas uncommonly produce symptoms in their early stage. Most early large-intestinal carcinomas are discovered during a colonoscopic screening procedure. Occasional early tumors will produce sufficient gross or occult bleeding to bring the patient to the attention of a physician. Symptoms correlating with advanced-stage disease are obstruction, perforation, and cachexia.[217] Symptomatic patients require full colonoscopic evaluation with biopsy to establish a diagnosis of carcinoma and to find the additional synchronous large-intestinal carcinoma that will be present in up to 6% of carcinoma cases.[218] Typically, carcinomas have an elevated peripheral edge and a central ulcer (Fig. 12–12). When the tumor has extended circumferentially around the intestinal lumen, a constricted ''apple-core'' lesion is produced. This growth configuration is more common in the sigmoid colon. Cecal and ascending colonic carcinomas are more often flat or polypoid.

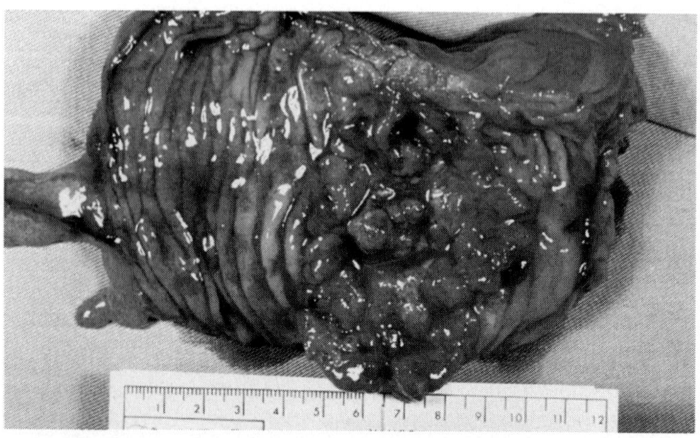

Figure 12–12. Colectomy specimen, locally advanced stage (Dukes' B) adenocarcinoma.

The overwhelming majority of colonic and rectal carcinomas are intestinal-type adenocarcinomas. Most are well- to moderately differentiated. A minority show little or no glandular differentiation and are therefore classified as poorly differentiated. Although focal extracellular mucin production is a component of most large-intestinal adenocarcinomas, about 15% will exhibit marked mucin production, with the formation of mucin pools that dissect between tissue planes. These ''colloid carcinomas'' often occur in younger patients and may behave in a slightly more aggressive fashion than do typical adenocarcinomas.[219, 220] Other, less common varieties of large-intestinal carcinomas include primary signet ring–cell carcinoma and small-cell neuroendocrine carcinoma, which are associated with very poor prognoses.[221, 222]

The primary treatment for large-intestinal carcinoma is wide local resection of the tumor with a minimum mucosal margin of 5 cm and resection of regional lymph nodes. Gross evaluation of the mucosal resection margin is usually adequate with the exception of rectal lesions, which are sometimes excised with a very limited distal margin. If the tumor is grossly less than 1 cm from the margin, intraoperative frozen section monitoring of the margin is appropriate. At the time of surgery, the liver should be examined for gross evidence of metastases. Right colonic tumors are removed by right hemicolectomy with ileocolonic anastomosis. Descending and sigmoid colonic lesions are segmentally resected with end-to-end colonic anastomosis. For rectal lesions, a low anterior resection is preferred, if feasible, to avoid the need for a colostomy. About 70% of large-intestinal resections for carcinoma have a curative intent, although one third of these tumors will recur.[223] The prognosis of a patient with resected large-intestinal carcinoma is best predicted by tumor stage. Dukes' originally proposed classification scheme was published in 1932, and modified versions are still widely used today.[224–226] Dukes' stage A tumors are confined to the intestinal wall (invasion to the submucosa or muscularis propria); Dukes' stage B tumors penetrate through the muscularis propria into pericolonic adipose tissue; and Dukes' stage C tumors have metastasized to regional lymph nodes. Current actuarial survival rates at 5 years using this system are 99, 85, and 67%, respectively.[223] Up to 30% of large-intestinal carcinomas will have distant metastases at the time of diagnosis, usually within the liver. The survival at 5 years in these cases is 14%.

The AJCC system for TNM staging of colorectal carcinoma is widely utilized and roughly correlates with Dukes' staging system.[24] An AJCC stage 0 tumor consists of intramucosal carcinoma only. Stage I includes tumors invasive into submucosa or muscularis propria only, without lymph node metastases. Stage II tumors are invasive into pericolic or perirectal tissues or into adjacent organs. Stage III includes all tumors with lymph node metastases but without distant metastases. Stage IV tumors have distant metastases. The AJCC system also distinguishes tumors with metastases to one lymph node, to less than four nodes, or to apical lymph nodes, although all are considered stage III disease.

Postoperative management of the patient may be aided by serial measurements of serum carcinoembryonic antigen (CEA), including a preoperative baseline sample.[227] Adjuvant chemotherapy using levamisole and 5-fluorouracil provided a significantly improved survival at 5 years in patients with stage C disease in one study.[228] Follow-up colonoscopy should be performed 6 months postoperatively to detect anastomotic recurrences.

Carcinoid Tumors

Carcinoids account for less than 1% of large intestinal neoplasms. The peak age of incidence is the sixth decade.[229] Colonic carcinoids are found most commonly in the cecum, tend to be large (5 cm), and are usually Dukes' stage B or C at the time of diagnosis. These usually require colectomy and regional lymph node resection. The 5-year survival for colonic carcinoids is 37%.

Rectal carcinoids are more likely to be diagnosed when they are small, nodular, or polypoid lesions. For tumors less than 1 cm in diameter, an endoscopic polypectomy resection with a clear cautery line is sufficient treatment. Tumors 1 to 2 cm in diameter have a 10% metastatic rate; hence, wide local excision with careful evaluation of the resection margins is recommended. If a histologically negative resection margin cannot be obtained by this method, abdominoperineal resection should be considered. Rectal carcinoids greater than 2 cm in diameter require an abdominoperineal resection in consideration of a nodal metastasis rate of 82%.[135]

Lymphomas

Lymphomas account for less than 1% of large intestinal malignancies. Most patients are diagnosed in the sixth decade. The cecum and rectum are the most commonly involved sites.[76] An association between large-intestinal lymphoma and autoimmune and immunodeficiency disease is recognized, including AIDS.[230] The clinical presentation of large-intestinal lymphoma is similar to that of carcinoma.

Stromal Tumors

Stromal neoplasms of the large intestine are clinically, histologically, and prognostically similar to stromal tumors of the small intestine but are less common.[231] Small tumors encountered incidentally at endoscopy should be considered benign. Most tumors with obstruction or bleeding are large and behave as sarcomas.

Appendix

CONGENITAL ABNORMALITIES

Congenital abnormalities are rare and may be associated with cecal deformities. Congenital duplication and congenital diverticula have been reported.[232] Acquired diverticula are occasionally noted in appendectomy specimens, usually in association with conditions of appendiceal luminal obstruction.[233]

ACUTE APPENDICITIS

This is an extremely common inflammatory condition resulting from appendiceal obstruction, proliferation of endogenous bacteria, and ischemia. Acute appendicitis may occur at any age, but is most common in the second and third decades. The typical history consists of midabdominal pain shifting to the right lower quadrant, nausea, vomiting, and fever. Physical examination reveals signs of peritoneal irritation. Laboratory analyses should include white blood cell count with differential, urinalysis, and, if the patient is female, serum beta-HCG.

Appendiceal resection specimens for acute appendicitis reveal serosal erythema and often a purulent exudate, dilatation, mural hemorrhagic necrosis, and occasionally perforation. The cause of appendiceal obstruction may be obvious, in the form of a fecalith.[234] If perforation has remained unrecognized for a prolonged period, the appendix may be surrounded or replaced by an abscess. Histologic findings vary from focal acute mucosal inflammation to transmural suppurative necrosis. Although bacterial cultures usually demonstrate normal cecal flora, occasional cases of acute appendicitis may be attributable to *Yersinia enterocolitica, Actinomyces israelii*, measles, or adenovirus. There is no convincing pathologic evidence for the existence of a ''chronic appendicitis.''

Luminal *fibrous obliteration* of the appendix is a common incidental finding in resection specimens. This may occur as part of the normal aging process. Typically, fibrous obliteration begins in the appendiceal tip and progresses proximally. The lumen is replaced by fibrous tissue, Schwann cells, and neuroendocrine cells.[235] This is a noninvasive neuroendocrine cell hyperplasia and should not be overinterpreted as invasive carcinoid.

Serosal appendiceal inflammation (periappendicitis) in the absence of mucosal inflammation is a histologically identified change indicative of inflammation elsewhere in the abdominal cavity or pelvis. The surgeon should be alerted by this diagnosis and immediately consider other sources of inflammation, including pelvic inflammatory disease, diverticulitis, and inflammatory bowel disease.

Granulomatous appendicitis may result from a number of causes. Parasitic infection may be associated with appendiceal granuloma formation, although it is unclear whether these organisms can cause a clinically evident appendicitis.[236, 237] Appendiceal tuberculosis is usually associated with obvious intestinal disease. The appendix is involved in about 25% of patients with Crohn's disease. Occasionally, a patient undergoing surgery for acute appendicitis is found to have a fibrotic, thickened appendix with granulomatous inflammation on microscopic examination. At the time of surgery, no evidence of small intestinal Crohn's disease is seen, and study results for mycobacterial and fungal organisms are negative. Such cases are appropriately designated ''isolated granulomatous appendicitis,'' since the majority have no subsequent evidence of systemic Crohn's disease.[238]

NEOPLASMS

The term ''mucocele'' refers to any dilatation of the appendix due to accumulation of mucus. It is frequently and incorrectly used as a synonym for ''appendiceal neoplasm.'' Neoplastic mucoceles are caused by mucosal *adenoma* or *adenocarcinoma*. Clinically, appendiceal mucosal neoplasms occur with symptoms and signs of acute appendicitis in 75% of cases. Adenomas may have a polypoid architecture or grow circumferentially around a dilated, mucus-filled appendiceal lumen *(cystadenoma)*.[239] Cystadenomas may dissect through the appendiceal wall and be difficult to differentiate from the infiltrative growth of appendiceal carcinoma. Simple appendectomy with a negative resection margin is curative for unruptured appendiceal adenomas.

Appendiceal adenocarcinomas, like large intestinal colloid carcinomas, usually secrete abundant mucus. The diagnosis of carcinoma relies upon the identification of infiltrative tumor cell growth.[240] The tumor spreads by direct extension into adjacent structures, regional lymph node metastasis, or peritoneal dissemination, if the appendix ruptures. The surgical treatment is right hemicolectomy and lymph node dissection. In women, the ovaries should be examined intraoperatively because of the high frequency of their simultaneous involvement.[241]

Pseudomyxoma Peritonei

Pseudomyxoma peritonei occurs when mucus spills into the peritoneal cavity, usually from a ruptured appendiceal or ovarian mucinous neoplasm. Mucus may accumulate in the right lower quadrant or may diffusely involve peritoneal surfaces. Neoplastic epithelial cells may or may not be identified in the mucus. If the adenomatous epithelium derives from a mucinous cystadenoma and lacks invasive capabilities, the spread of mucus-secreting cells and the accumulation of mucus tend to remain localized. If the appendiceal adenoma, epithelial implant, and mucin are removed, pseudomyxoma peritonei localized to the right lower quadrant does not usually progress to widespread peritoneal spread and death.[240] Conversely, diffuse pseudomyxoma peritonei has a 5-year survival rate of 69% and is much more likely to be derived from a mucinous cystadenocarcinoma.

Carcinoid Tumors

Carcinoid tumors account for one half of all diagnosed appendiceal neoplasms and are found in 0.3% of surgically resected appendices. Carcinoids are most often an incidental finding in the distal portion of appendices removed for appendicitis. Microscopically, they resemble carcinoid tumors of the small intestine. The majority of appendiceal carcinoids are less than 2.0 cm in diameter and are clinically benign.[242] Carcinoid tumors greater than 2.0 cm in diameter are probably best treated by right hemicolectomy unless the affected patient has a high operative risk.

The Anus

The anal canal is lined by colonic-type mucosa proximally and squamous mucosa distally. The intervening portion is lined by a specialized transitional epithelium.

Congenital Abnormalities

Congenital abnormalities of the anal canal are uncommon and include stenosis, imperforate anus, duplications, and cysts. These are discussed elsewhere in this text.

Hemorrhoids

Hemorrhoids are dilated and prolapsed veins of the submucosal hemorrhoidal plexus located in the lower rectum and anus. Internal hemorrhoids are derived from superior hemorrhoidal veins located superior to the junction of squamous and transitional epithelium; external ones are derived from inferior hemorrhoidal veins and overlaid by squamous mucosa. Hemorrhoids in no way indicate the presence of portal hypertension, as hemorrhoidal veins are not directly connected with the portal venous system.[243] However, cirrhotic patients may develop massive bleeding from anorectal varices, which may be difficult to distinguish from hemorrhoids, and of course hemorrhoids may occur in patients with portal hypertension. Anorectal varices are described as discrete, serpentine, and compressible; they are usually accompanied by other signs of portal hypertension.[244] From a surgical standpoint, it is important to recognize portal hypertension in a patient with either anorectal varices or hemorrhoids. These patients frequently have coagulation defects and cannot be treated on an outpatient basis due to the risk of massive hemorrhage.

Individuals with hemorrhoids typically complain of bleeding. Pain usually indicates hemorrhoidal strangulation or thrombosis. Therapy includes dietary modification, topical anti-inflammatory agents, ligation, coagulation, and hemorrhoidectomy.

Microscopic examination of excised hemorrhoids reveals dilated submucosal vessels, often with thrombosis, and occasionally ulceration of the overlying epithelium. Histologic examination of all resected hemorrhoids is strongly recommended, due to the infrequent but potentially lifesaving discovery of a malignant neoplasm in a lesion clinically diagnosed as a hemorrhoid.

Fissures

Anal fissures are linear ulcers of the anal canal; they are usually found in the posterior midline in young adults. Occasionally they occur as an anal manifestation of inflammatory bowel disease. The clinical presentation is severe pain and scant bleeding with defecation. Upon examination, a fibrotic polyp, referred to as a "sentinel pile," is often discovered at the anal verge. Anal fissures are believed to result from traumatic passage of fecal boluses.[245] Initial conservative therapy is dietary modification. Chronic fissures require surgical sphincterotomy.

Abscesses

Anorectal abscesses and *fistulas* result from suppurative inflammation and require prompt surgical intervention. Both are believed to be caused by infection of the anal glands located at the level of the crypts of Morgagni.[246] The most common wound isolates are polymicrobial colonic flora. *Mycobacterium tuberculosis* along with lymphogranuloma venereum may also occur as an anorectal infection. Neutropenic patients with hematologic malignancies are particularly susceptible to anorectal infections, which, if left untreated, carry a high mortality. Anorectal abscesses and fistulas are classified by anatomic site and pathway of extension, criteria that guide surgical management.[247]

Polyps

Inflammatory cloacogenic polyps are benign, nonneoplastic lesions that occur near the anal transitional zone. The clinical presentation and appearance are similar to those of hemorrhoids. Microscopically, they are composed of colonic, transitional, or squamous mucosa or a combination of the three. Smooth muscle proliferates into the mucosa and displaces crypt epithelium into the submucosa. Both of these features suggest that these polyps arise from mucosal prolapse.[248] Simple resection is curative.

Benign, hyperplastic lymphoid tissue in the rectum and upper anal canal may manifest clinically as a polyp. Florid anorectal lymphoid hyperplasia occurs more frequently in children than adults. The etiology is undetermined.

HUMAN PAPILLOMAVIRUS INFECTION OF THE ANUS

Venereally transmitted infections with human papillomavirus (HPV) occur in the anal canal and perianal skin. These infections are associated with receptive anal intercourse and genital HPV infections in both sexes.[249, 250] The spectrum of anal HPV disease is analogous to that in the genital organs.[251]

The clinical management of anal HPV-associated lesions is difficult. There is no therapy that specifically inhibits HPV replication other than ablation of the affected epithelium. Lesions tend to be multiple and recurrence is frequent, probably due to both reinfection and reservoirs of HPV in nonlesional epithelium. The treatment of lesions at the anal verge should include full anoscopic examination in order to visualize and clear areas of high anal involvement. Women should undergo cervical cytologic examination to assess for gynecologic involvement.

MALIGNANT NEOPLASMS

The majority of anal canal malignancies are derived from squamous epithelium and epithelium of the anal transitional zone. Anal canal carcinomas are found in adults of all ages, with a peak incidence in the fifth and sixth decades and a 3:1 female:male ratio.[252] Carcinomas of the anal verge and perianal skin are more common in men. Carcinomas at both sites are associated with anal and genital HPV infections. Other predisposing factors include Crohn's disease.[253] Patients with anal carcinomas present clinically with anal bleeding, pain, and occasionally the sensation of a mass. Lesions may be polypoid or ulcerating. Biopsy specimens reveal a typical *squamous carcinoma* in 70% of cases, and a *basaloid* ("transitional") microscopic appearance in over 20% of cases. Stage for stage, these common variants of squamous and basaloid carcinoma have the same prognosis. Rare variants of anal carcinoma include anal duct carcinoma, mucoepidermoid carcinoma, adenoid cystic carcinoma, and high-grade small-cell neuroendocrine carcinoma.[254]

At diagnosis, up to 30% of patients with carcinoma of the anal canal have metastases to pelvic or inguinal lymph nodes, and 10% have distant tumor spread.[254] Carcinomas of the anal margin tend to have a well-differentiated, noninfiltrative morphology and are probably diagnosed earlier; hence, these tumors are associated with a better prognosis. Treatment for small anal carcinomas is wide local excision with an attempt to preserve normal anal function. More extensive lesions are treated with combination chemotherapy and radiation *or* radiation.[255] Rarely, for advanced tumors, abdominal perineal resection with lymph node dissection may be required.

Extramammary Paget's disease may affect the perianal skin and anal margin. This is a form of intraepidermal mucinous *adenocarcinoma* that produces symptoms of itching and induration of the involved skin. The typical patient is elderly, with symptoms that may have been present for years prior to diagnosis. A large proportion of patients with perianal Paget's disease are subsequently discovered to have carcinoma of the low rectum or perianal ducts. The remaining cases are believed to be of primary cutaneous origin.[256] Microscopic examination of biopsy specimens reveals cytologically malignant Paget's cells infiltrating through inflamed and hyperplastic squamous epithelium.

Perianal Paget's disease requires investigation for rectal or anal gland carcinoma, followed by wide local excision or laser excision. Areas of cutaneous involvement may be inapparent on visual inspection–hence, frozen section intraoperative monitoring of resection margins is sometimes requested. This approach is not reasonable, due to the multifocal distribution of Paget's disease and the potential difficulty of recognizing sparsely distributed Paget's cells by frozen section histology. A better approach is the preoperative mapping of Paget's disease by multiple biopsies.

Anal melanomas are rare tumors, accounting for 1% of anal malignancies. The mean age at diagnosis is 58 years. Anal melanomas manifest as bleeding masses, often mistaken for hemorrhoids, or are discovered subsequent to the diagnosis of a metastasis. Most lesions are polypoid, and they may prolapse through the anal orifice. About two thirds are grossly pigmented. The prognosis of anal melanoma is poor.[257] Long-term survival of patients with tumors with a vertical thickness greater than 1.7 cm is rare. Studies indicate that radical abdominal-perineal resection may provide no prognostic advantage over local excision.[258]

PITFALLS FOR THE SURGEON

Obtaining Endoscopic Specimens

1. Inadequate endoscopic biopsies. The informational value of endoscopic biopsies is, in many cases, directly proportional to the amount of tissue obtained. Adequate mucosal sampling may be difficult, particularly in an area of a narrowed lumen, such as the esophagus or a stricture site. The ideal endoscopic biopsies should be large, deep, and multiple.
2. Placing endoscopic biopsies from separate sites in the same container. Always place biopsies from separate sites in separate containers and clearly label each container with the precise site of origin (example: "esophagus at 32 cm" or "splenic flexure," not "colon" or "biopsy #3").
3. Using the wrong fixatives. Specimens are best fixed immediately in 10% buffered formalin. Bouin's or Hollande's fixatives are frequently recommended for endoscopic biopsies due to a putative improvement in tissue morphology. However, preference for such subtle differences in histology is entirely subjective. More importantly, Bouin's and Hollande's solutions provide poor results when used for diagnostic immunohistochemical studies and do not preserve DNA for molecular assays.
4. Sending lymphoma biopsies in fixative. It is preferable to contact the pathologist prior to or during the procedure to discuss the strategy for tissue handling of a suspected lymphoma. Most pathologists will request that the tissue be sent fresh on a saline-soaked towel for immediate freezing and fixation.
5. Requesting frozen section interpretation of endoscopic biopsy specimens. A frozen section diagnosis is usually less informative than the corresponding fixed, permanent section biopsy. In addition, the frozen biopsy is suboptimal for standard histology after it has been thawed and fixed. A frozen section should be reserved for cases when an intraprocedural therapeutic decision is required and when another sample can be obtained for fixation and standard histology.

6. Failing to provide the pathologist with adequate endoscopic information. The endoscopist is the "gross pathologist" for the GI histologist. Pathologists rely on both the gross and microscopic appearances of lesions to make a diagnosis. All endoscopic biopsy specimens should be accompanied by a brief summary of pertinent clinical data and a description of the distribution, severity, extent, and character of endoscopic changes. Specific diagnostic questions should be asked on the requisition.

Surgical Specimens

1. Allowing a resected viscus to languish, unopened and unfixed, on a shelf in a refrigerator overnight. Similarly, specimens should not be dropped unopened into a container of fixative. Unfixed GI mucosa autolyses rapidly. Gastrointestinal resection specimens should be sent fresh, unopened, to the pathology laboratory for immediate opening and fixation. If opened in the operating room, the specimen should be cut longitudinally with scissors, along the antimesenteric border, avoiding the lesion of interest. The specimen should then be completely immersed in 10% buffered formalin. Labeling of the proximal and distal resection margins, sites of potential side wall invasion, or areas of potential neoplastic adhesion to a contiguous organ is helpful to the pathologist and easily accomplished with sutures.
2. Ignoring what constitutes an adequate resection margin for specific malignancies. A *microscopically* negative mucosal resection margin is important for surgical therapy of carcinomas. A slight prognostic advantage may be provided by *gross* total removal of lymphomas and stromal tumors, but a debilitating procedure (such as total gastrectomy) should generally be avoided when dealing with these latter tumors.
3. Failing to label separately submitted lymph nodes from a mesenteric node dissection with the site of origin. Prognostic implications of nodal involvement vary according to distance from the primary lesion and proximity to mesenteric margin.

PITFALLS FOR THE PATHOLOGIST

1. Failure to use standard terminology when describing a histologic finding ("chronic, active"; "low-grade dysplasia").
2. Failure to contact the clinician if there are any questions with regard to clinical, endoscopic, or surgical findings or with regard to the histologic diagnosis.
3. Unwillingness to diagnose a specimen as normal. If a specimen is grossly and histologically without abnormality, say so.
4. Habitual diagnosis of a mucosal inflammatory process as "nonspecific." This tells the clinician nothing and gives license for just about anything. Be as specific as possible in describing the histologic changes, stating which diagnostic possibilities could include the histologic changes and which are ruled out or unsupported.
5. *Incorrect orientation of tissue sections for histology.* In the gross pathology room, always cut *longitudinally.* Never transect the base of a polyp stalk horizontally and submit it as a margin. Ink the base and bread-loaf the polyp along axial planes. Always take longitudinal, not circumferential, sections of a resected viscus: the specimen remains intact for a second gross examination and mucosal resection margins are always best monitored using ink and sections perpendicular to the line of resection. One exception is frozen section monitoring of the proximal margin of an esophagectomy specimen removed for carcinoma: here, the circumferential margin should be completely sampled. If tumor approaches the margin to within the thickness of a frozen tissue block, it should be considered positive.

FURTHER READING

Appelman HD, ed. *Pathology of the Esophagus, Stomach and Duodenum.* New York: Churchill Livingstone; 1984.

Lewin KJ, Riddell RH, Weinstein WM. *Gastrointestinal Pathology and Its Clinical Implications.* New York: Igaku-Shoin; 1992.

Norris HT, ed. *Pathology of the Colon, Small Intestine and Anus.* New York: Churchill Livingstone; 1991.

REFERENCES

1. Pezim MA. Personal communication.
2. Strobel CT, Byrne WJ, Ament ME, et al. Correlation of esophageal lengths with height: Application of the Tuttle test without prior esophageal manometry. *J Pediatr.* 1979;94:81.
3. Manning PB, Morgan RA, Coran AG, et al. Fifty years' experience with esophageal atresia and tracheoesophageal fistula. *Ann Surg.* 1986;204:446.
4. Graham DY, Smith JL. The course of patients after variceal hemorrhage. *Gastroenterology.* 1981;80:800.
5. Cassella RR, Brown AL, Sayre GP, Ellis F. Achalasia of the esophagus: Pathologic and etiologic considerations. *Ann Surg.* 1964;160:474.
6. Chuong JJH, Du Bovile S, McCallum RW. Achalasia as a risk for esophageal carcinoma: A reappraisal. *Dig Dis Sci.* 1984;29:1105.
7. Dodds WJ. Current concepts of esophageal motor function: Clinical implications of radiology. *Am J Roentgenol.* 1977;128:549.
8. Flynn AE, Verrier ED, Way LW, et al. Esophageal perforation. *Arch Surg.* 1989;124:1211.
9. Michel L, Serrano A, Malt RA. Mallory-Weiss syndrome: Evolution of diagnostic and therapeutic patterns over two decades. *Ann Surg.* 1980;192:716.
10. Nebel OT, Fornes MF, Castell DO. Symptomatic gastroesophageal reflux: Incidence and precipitating factors. *Am J Dig Dis.* 1976;21:953.
11. Mitros FA. Inflammatory and neoplastic diseases of the esophagus. In: Appelman HD, ed. *Pathology of the Esophagus, Stomach and Duodenum.* London: Churchill Livingstone; 1984:1.
12. Winters CJ, Spurling TJ, Chabanion SJ, et al. Barrett's esophagus: A prevalent, occult complication of gastroesophageal reflux disease. *Gastroenterology.* 1987;92:118.
13. Paull A, Trier JS, Dalton MD, et al. The histologic spectrum of Barrett's esophagus. *N Engl J Med.* 1976;295:476.
14. Hayward J. The lower end of the oesophagus. *Thorax.* 1961;16:36.
15. Cameron AJ, Ott BJ, Payne WS. The incidence of adenocarcinoma in columnar-lined (Barrett's) esophagus. *N Engl J Med.* 1985;313:857.
16. Spechler SJ, Goyal RK. Barrett's esophagus. *N Engl J Med.* 1986;315:362.
17. Schmidt HG, Riddell RH, Walther B, et al. Dysplasia in Barrett's esophagus. *J Cancer Res Clin Oncol.* 1985;110:145.
18. Hamilton SR, Smith RRL. The relationship between columnar epithelial dysplasia and invasive adenocarcinoma arising in Barrett's esophagus. *Am J Clin Pathol.* 1987;87:301.
19. Reid BJ, Weinstein WM, Lewin KJ, et al. Endoscopic biopsy can detect high-grade dysplasia or early adenocarcinoma in Barrett's esophagus without grossly recognizable neoplastic lesions. *Gastroenterology* 1988;94:81.
20. Reid BJ, Haggit RC, Rubin CE. *Barrett's Esophagus: Medical and Surgical Management.* Philadelphia: Saunders, 1988:157.
21. Seremetic MG, Lyons WS, DeGuzman VC, et al. Leiomyomata of the esophagus: An analysis of 838 cases. *Cancer.* 1976;38:2166.
22. Day NE, Munoz N: Esophagus. In: Schottefeld D, Fraumeni JF, eds. *Cancer Epidemiology and Prevention.* Philadelphia: Saunders, 1982:596.
23. Wong HH, Antonioli DA, Goldman H. Comparative features of esophageal and gastric adenocarcinoma: Recent changes in type and frequency. *Hum Pathol.* 1986;17:482.
24. Beahrs OH, Henson DE, Hutter RVP, Kennedy BJ, eds. *Manual for Staging of Cancer*, 4th ed. Philadelphia: Lippincott, 1992.
25. Galandiuk S, Hermann RE, Cosgrove DM, et al. Cancer of the esophagus: The Cleveland Clinic experience. *Ann Surg.* 1986;201:101.
26. Akiyama H, Tsurumaru M, Kawamura T, et al. Principles of surgical treatment for carcinoma of the esophagus: Analysis of lymph node involvement. *Ann Surg.* 1981;194:438.
27. Huang GJ. Recognition and treatment of the early lesion. In: Delarve NC, Wilkins EW, Wong J, eds. *International Trends in General Surgery.* Vol. 4. *Esophageal Cancer.* St. Louis: Mosby; 1988:149.
28. Mountain CF. Rationale in staging of cancer of the esophagus. In: Delarve NC, Wilkins EW, Wong J, eds. *International Trends in General Surgery.* Vol. 4. *Esophageal Cancer.* St. Louis: Mosby; 1988:73.
29. Zarbo RJ, Crissman JD, Venkat H, et al. Spindle cell carcinoma of the upper aerodigestive tract mucosa: An immunohistochemical and ultrastructural study of 18 biphasic tumors and comparison with seven monophasic tumors. *Am J Surg Pathol.* 1986;10:741.
30. Agha FP, Weatherbee L, Sams JS. Verrucous carcinoma of the esophagus. *Am J Gastroenterol.* 1984;79:844.
31. Sabanathan S, Graham GP, Salama FD. Primary oat cell carcinoma of the oesophagus. *Thorax.* 1986;41:318.
32. Epstein JI, Sears DL, Tucker RS, et al. Carcinoma of the esophagus with adenoid cystic differentiation. *Cancer.* 1984;53:1131.
33. Kuwano H, Ueo H, Sugimachi K, et al. Glandular or mucus-secreting components in squamous cell carcinoma of the esophagus. *Cancer.* 1985;56:514.
34. DiCostanzo DP, Urmacher C. Primary malignant melanoma of the esophagus. *Am J Surg Pathol.* 1987;11:46.
35. Eastwood GL. Stomach: Anatomy and structural abnormalities. In: Yamada T, Alpers DH, Owyong C, et al., eds. *Textbook of Gastroenterology.* Philadelphia: Lippincott; 1991:1198.
36. Marrone GC, Silen W. Pathogenesis, diagnosis and treatment of acute gastric mucosal lesions. *Clin Gastroenterol.* 1984;13:635.
37. Owen DA. Stomach. In: Steinberg SS, ed. *Diagnostic Surgical Pathology.* New York: Raven; 1989:937.
38. Bayerdorffer E, Oertel H, Lehn N, et al. Topographic association between active gastritis and *Campylobacter pylori* colonization. *J Clin Pathol.* 1989; 42:834.
39. Blaser MJ. Epidemiology and pathophysiology of *Campylobacter pylori* infections. *Rev Infect Dis.* 1990; 12:599.
40. Megraud F, Brossens-Rabbe MP, Denis F, et al. Seroepidemiology of *Campylobacter pylori* infections in various populations. *J Clin Microbiol.* 1989; 27:1870.
41. Laine L, Marin-Sorensen M, Weinstein WM. Is *Campylobacter pylori* (CP) prevalence lower in gastric ulcers (GU's) because of nonsteroidal anti-inflammatory drug (NSAID) use? A prospective evaluation (abstr). *Gastroenterology.* 1989; 96:A282.
42. Nomura A, Stemmermann GN, Chyou P-H, et al. *Helicobacter pylori* infection and gastric carcinoma among Japanese Americans in Hawaii. *N Engl J Med.* 1991;325:1132.
43. Parsonnet J, Friedman GD, Vandersteen DP, et al. *Helicobacter pylori* infection and the risk of gastric carcinoma. *N Engl J Med.* 1991;325:1127.
44. Wotherspoon AC, Ortiz-Hidalgo C, Falzon MR, et al. *Helicobacter pylori*–associated gastritis and primary B-cell gastric lymphoma. *Lancet.* 1991;338:1175.
45. Parsonnet J, Hansen S, Rodriguez L, et al. *Helicobacter pylori* infection and gastric lymphoma. *N Engl J Med.* 1994; 330:1267.
46. Barthel JS, Everett ED. Diagnosis of *Campylobacter pylori* infections: The "gold standard" and the alternatives. *Rev Infect Dis.* 1990;12:5107.
47. Tytgat GN, Rauws EA. *Campylobacter pylori* and its risk in peptic ulcer disease. *Gastroenterol Clin North Am.* 1990;19:183.
48. Borch K, Renvall H, Liedberg G. Prevalence and incidence of pernicious anemia: An evaluation for gastric screening. *Scand J Gastroenterol.* 1984;19:154.
49. Borch K, Renvall H, Liedberg G. Gastric endocrine cell hyperplasia and carcinoid tumors in pernicious anemia. *Gastroenterology.* 1985;88:638.
50. Dixon MF, O'Connor HJ, Axon ATR, et al. Reflux gastritis—Distinct histological entity? *J Clin Pathol.* 1986;39:524.
51. Haot J, Hamichi L, Wallez L, et al. Lymphocytic gastritis: A newly described entity: A retrospective endoscopic and histological study. *Gut.* 1988;29:1298.
52. Wolber R, Owen D, Del Buono L, et al. Lymphocytic gastritis in patients with celiac sprue or sprue-like intestinal disease. *Gastroenterology.* 1990;98:310.

53. Rothery GA, Day DW. Intestinal metaplasia in endoscopic biopsy specimens of gastric mucosa. *J Clin Pathol.* 1985;38:613.
54. Lifton LJ, Schlossberg D. Phlegmonous gastritis after endoscopic polypectomy. *Ann Intern Med.* 1982;97:373.
55. Rutgaerts P, Onette E, Vantrappen G, et al. Crohn's disease of the stomach and duodenum: A clinical study with emphasis on the value of endoscopy and endoscopic biopsy. *Endoscopy.* 1980;12:288.
56. Chinitz MA, Brandt LJ, Frank MS, et al. Symptomatic sarcoidosis of the stomach. *Dig Dis Sci.* 1985;30:682.
57. Fahimi HD, Deren JJ, Gottlieb MD, et al. Isolated granulomatous gastritis: Its relationship to disseminated sarcoidosis and regional enteritis. *Gastroenterology.* 1963;45:161.
58. Appelman HD. Localized and extensive expansions of the gastric mucosa: Mucosal polyps and giant folds. In: Appelman HD, ed. *Pathology of the Esophagus, Stomach and Duodenum.* New York: Churchill Livingstone; 1984:79.
59. Jablokow VR, Aranha GV, Reyes CV. Gastric stomal polypoid hyperplasia: Report of four cases. *J Surg Oncol.* 1982;19:106.
60. Lundegarth G, Adami HO, Helmick C, et al. Stomach cancer after partial gastrectomy for benign ulcer disease. *N Engl J Med.* 1988;319:195.
61. Offerhaus GJA, Tersmette AC, Huigbretse K, et al. Mortality caused by stomach cancer after remote partial gastrectomy for benign conditions: 40 years follow-up of an Amsterdam cohort or 2633 postgastrectomy patients. *Gut.* 1988;29:1588.
62. Watanabe H, Enjoji M, Yao T, et al. Gastric lesions in familial adenomatosis coli. *Hum Pathol.* 1978;9:269.
63. Wolfsen HC, Carpenter HA, Talley NH. Menetrier's disease: A form of hypertrophic gastropathy or gastritis? *Gastroenterology.* 1993;104:1310.
64. Laxen F, Sipponen P, Ihamaki T, et al. Gastric polyps: Their morphological and endoscopical characteristics and relation to gastric carcinoma. *Acta Pathol Microbiol Immunol Scand.* 1982;90:221.
65. Lynch HT, Smyrk TC, Watson P, et al. Genetics, natural history, tumor spectrum, and pathology of hereditary nonpolyposis colorectal cancer: An updated review. *Gastroenterology.* 1993;104:1535.
66. Parkin DM, Laara E, Muir CS. Estimates of the worldwide frequency of sixteen major cancers in 1980. *Int J Cancer.* 1988;41:184.
67. Antonioli DA, Goldman H. Changes in the location and type of gastric adenocarcinoma. *Cancer.* 1982;50:775.
68. Wong HH, Antonioli DA, Goldman H. Comparative features of esophageal and gastric adenocarcinomas: Recent changes in type and frequency. *Hum Pathol.* 1986;17:482.
69. Lauren P. The two histological main types of gastric carcinoma: diffuse and so-called intestinal-type carcinoma. *Acta Pathol Microbiol Scand.* 1965;64:31.
70. Lewin KJ, Riddell RH, Weinstein WM. Gastrointestinal pathology and its clinical implications. Vol. 1. Igaku-Shoin: New York; 1992:647.
71. Murakami T. Pathomorphological diagnosis. Definition and gross classification of early gastric cancer. In: *Early Gastric Cancer, Gann Monograph on Cancer Research No. 11.* Tokyo: University of Tokyo Press; 1972:53.
72. Ohta H, Noguchi Y, Takagi K, et al. Early gastric carcinoma with special reference to macroscopic classification. *Cancer.* 1987;60:1099.
73. Antonioli DA. Precursors of gastric carcinoma: A critical review with a brief description of early (curable) gastric cancer. *Hum Pathol.* 1994;25:994.
74. Hisamichi S, Sugawara N. Mass screening for gastric cancer by x-ray examination. *Jpn J Clin Oncol.* 1984;14:211.
75. Horning D, Hermanek P, Gall FP. The significance of the extent of proximal margins of clearance in gastric cancer surgery. *Scand J Gastroenterol.* 1987;22(suppl 133):69.
76. Lewin KJ, Ranchod M, Dorfman RF. Lymphomas of the gastrointestinal tract: A study of 117 cases presenting with gastrointestinal disease. *Cancer.* 1978;42:693.
77. Contreary K, Nance FC, Becker WF. Primary lymphoma of the gastrointestinal tract. *Ann Surg.* 1980;191:593.
78. Gray GM, Rosenberg SA, Cooper AD, et al. Lymphomas involving the gastrointestinal tract. *Gastroenterology.* 1982;82:143.
79. Devaney K, Jaffe ES. The surgical pathology of gastrointestinal Hodgkin's disease. *Am J Clin Pathol.* 1991;95:794.
80. Cogliatti SB, Schmid U, Schumacher U, et al. Primary B-cell gastric lymphoma: A clinicopathological study of 145 patients. *Gastroenterology.* 1991;101:1159.
81. Zukerberg L, Ferry J, Southern J, et al. Lymphoid infiltrates of the stomach: Evaluation of histologic criteria for the diagnosis of low-grade gastric lymphoma on endoscopic biopsy specimens. *Am J Surg Pathol.* 1991;15:819.
82. Wotherspoon AC, Doglioni C, Diss TC, et al. Regression of primary low grade B-cell gastric lymphoma of mucosa associated lymphoid tissue type after eradication of *Helicobacter pylori. Lancet.* 1993;342:575.
83. Wotherspoon AC, Doglioni C, Isaacson PG. Low-grade gastric B-cell lymphoma of mucosa-associated lymphoid tissue (MALT): a multifocal disease. *Histopathology.* 1992;20:29–34.
84. Ruskone-Fourmestraux A, Aegerter P, Delmer A, et al. Primary digestive tract lymphoma: A prospective multicentric study of 91 patients. *Gastroenterology.* 1993;105:1662.
85. Ranchod M, Kempson RL. Smooth muscle tumors of the gastrointestinal tract and retroperitoneum. *Cancer.* 1977;39:255.
86. Carney JA. The triad of gastric epithelioid leiomyosarcoma, pulmonary chondroma and functioning extra-adrenal paraganglioma: A 5 year review. *Medicine.* 1983;62:159.
87. Pike AM, Lloyd RV, Appelman HD. Cell markers in gastrointestinal stromal tumors. *Hum Pathol.* 1988;19:830.
88. Hjermstead BM. Stromal tumors of the gastrointestinal tract: Myogenic or neurogenic? *Am J Surg Pathol.* 1987;11:383.
89. Evans HL. Smooth muscle tumors of the gastrointestinal tract. A study of 56 cases followed for a minimum of 10 years. *Cancer.* 1985;56:2242.
90. Appelman HD. Stromal tumors of the esophagus, stomach, and duodenum. In: Appelman HD, ed. *Pathology of the Esophagus, Stomach and Duodenum.* New York: Churchill Livingstone; 1984:195.
91. Lewin KJ, Riddell RH, Weinstein WM. Mesenchymal tumors. In: *Gastrointestinal Pathology and Its Clinical Implications.* New York: Igaku-Shoin; 1992:284.
92. Borch K, Renvall H, Kullman E, et al. Gastric carcinoid associated with the syndrome of hypergastrinemic atrophic gastritis. *Am J Surg Pathol.* 1987;11:435.
93. Rubin W. Small intestine: Anatomy and structural anomalies. In: Yamada T, ed. *Textbook of Gastroenterology.* Vol II. New York: Lippincott; 1991:1409.
94. Stubenbord WT, Thorbjarnarson B. Intussusception in adults. *Ann Surg.* 1970;172:306.
95. Leijonmarck CE, Bonman-Sondelin K, Frisell J, et al. Meckel's diverticulum in the adult. *Br J Surg.* 1986;73:146.
96. Zarling EJ. Gastric adenomyoma with coincidental pancreatic rest: A care report. *Gastrointest Endosc.* 1981;27:175.
97. Ulich TR, Kollin M, Simmons GE, et al. Adenomyoma of the ampulla of Vater. *Arch Pathol Lab Med.* 1987;111:388.
98. Coghlan JG, Gilligan D, Humphries H, et al. *Campylobacter pylori* and recurrence of duodenal ulcers—A 12 month follow-up study. *Lancet.* 1987;2:1109.
99. Blaser MJ. Gastric *Campylobacter*-like organism, gastritis, and peptic ulcer disease. *Gastroenterology.* 1987;93:371.
100. Langman MJS, Cooke AR. Gastric and duodenal ulcer and their associated diseases. *Lancet.* 1976;1:680.
101. Kirk AP, Dooley JS, Hunt RH. Peptic ulceration in patients with chronic liver disease. *Dig Dis Sci.* 1980;25:10.
102. Kang JY, Wu AYT, Sutherland IH, et al. Prevalence of peptic ulcer in patients undergoing maintenance hemodialysis. *Dig Dis Sci.* 1988;33:774.
103. Farini R, Farinati F, Cardin F, et al. Evidence of gastric carcinoma during follow-up of apparently benign gastric ulcer. *Gut.* 1983;24:A486.
104. Hui WM, Lam SK, Chau PY, et al. Persistence of *Campylobacter pylori* despite healing of duodenal ulcer and improvement of accompanying duodenitis and gastritis. *Dig Dis Sci.* 1987;32:1255.
105. Debas HT, Orloff SL. Surgery for peptic ulcer disease. In: Yamada T, ed. *Textbook of Gastroenterology.* New York: Lippincott; 1991:1379.
106. King CE, Toskes PP. Small intestinal bacterial overgrowth. *Gastroenterology.* 1979;76:1035.
107. Miranda AG, Dupont HL. Small intestine: Infections with common

bacterial and viral pathogens. In: Yamada T, ed. *Textbook of Gastroenterology*. New York: Lippincott; 1991:1447.
108. Cover TL, Aber RC. *Yersinia enterocolitica. N Engl J Med.* 1989;321:16.
109. McDonald GB, Shulman HM, Sullivan KM, et al. Intestinal and hepatic complications of human bone marrow transplantation: Part II. *Gastroenterology*. 1986;90:770.
110. Komorowski RA, Cohen EB, Kauffman HM, et al. Gastrointestinal complications in renal transplant recipients. *Am J Clin Pathol.* 1986;86:161.
111. Francis ND, Boylston AW, Roberts AH, et al. Cytomegalovirus infection in gastrointestinal tracts of patients infected with HIV-1 or AIDS. *J Clin Pathol.* 1989;42:1055.
112. Young LS, Interlied CB, Berlin OG, et al. Mycobacterial infections in AIDS patients, with an emphasis on the *Mycobacterium avium* complex. *Rev Infect Dis.* 1986;6:1024.
113. Navin TR, Juranek DD. Cryptosporidiosis: Clinical, epidemiologic and parasitologic review. *Rev Infect Dis.* 1984;6:313.
114. Orenstein J, Chiang J, Steinberg W, et al. Intestinal microsporidiosis as a cause of diarrhea in HIV-infected patients: A report of 20 cases. *Hum Pathol.* 1990;21:475.
115. Morgan JS, Schaffner W, Stone WJ. Opportunistic strongyloidiasis in renal transplant recipients. *Transplantation.* 1986;42:518.
116. Ciclitira PJ, Evans DJ, Fagg NLK, et al. Clinical testing of gliadin fractions in celiac patients. *Clin Sci.* 1984;66:357.
117. Kagnoff MF, Paterson YJ, Kumar PJ, et al. Possible role for a human adenovirus in the pathogenesis of celiac disease. *Gut.* 1987;28:995.
118. Arranz E, Ferguson A. Intestinal antibody pattern of celiac disease: Occurrence in patients with normal jejunal biopsy histology. *Gastroenterology.* 1993;104:1263.
119. Holmes GKT, Prior P, Lane MR, et al. Malignancy in coeliac disease—Effect of a gluten-free diet. *Gut.* 1989;30:333.
120. Cunningham-Rundles C. Clinical and immunologic analyses of 103 patients with common variable immunodeficiency. *J Clin Immunol.* 1989;9:22.
121. Kyle RA, Greippo PR, Garton JP, et al. Primary systemic amyloidosis. *Am J Med.* 1985;79:708.
122. Dobbins WO III. *Whipple's Disease*. Springfield, IL: Charles C Thomas; 1987.
123. Sale GE, Shulman HM, McDonald GB, et al. Gastrointestinal graft versus host disease in man: A clinicopathologic study of the rectal biopsy. *Am J Surg Pathol.* 1979;3:291.
124. Haggit RC, Reed BJ. Hereditary gastrointestinal polyposis syndromes. *Am J Surg Pathol.* 1986;12:871.
125. Jeghers H, McKusick VA, Katz KH. The syndrome of generalized intestinal polyposis and melanin spots of the oral mucosa, lips and digits. *Ciba Clin Symp.* 1980;2:199.
126. Kurtz RC, Sternberg SS, Miller HH, et al. Upper gastrointestinal neoplasia in familial polyposis. *Dig Dis Sci.* 1987;32:459.
127. Lynch HT, Smyrk TC, Lynch RM, et al. Adenocarcinoma of the small bowel in Lynch syndrome II. *Cancer.* 1989;64:2178.
128. Perzin KH, Bridge MF. Adenomas of the small intestine: A clinicopathologic review of 51 cases and a study of their relationship to carcinoma. *Cancer.* 1981;48:799.
129. Galandiuk S, Hermann RE, Jagelman DG, et al. Villous tumors of the duodenum. *Ann Surg.* 1988;207:234.
130. Swinson CM, Slavin G, Coles EC, et al. Coeliac disease and malignancy. *Lancet.* 1983;1:111.
131. Petras RE, Mir-Madjlessi SH, Farmer RG. Crohn's disease and intestinal carcinoma. *Gastroenterology.* 1987;93:1307.
132. Sindelar WF. Cancer of the small intestine. In: Devita VT, Hellman S, Rosenberg SA, eds. *Cancer: Principles and Practice of Oncology*, 3rd ed. Philadelphia: Lippincott; 1989:875.
133. Creutzfeld W, Stockman F. Carcinoids and carcinoid syndrome. *Am J Med.* 1987;82:4.
134. Norheim I, Oberg K, Theodorsson-Norheim E, et al. Malignant carcinoid tumors: An analysis of 103 patients with regard to tumor localization, hormone production, and survival. *Ann Surg.* 1987;206:115.
135. Moertel CG. An odyssey in the land of small intestinal tumors. *J Clin Oncol.* 1987;5:1503.
136. Gorden P, Comi RJ, Maton PN, et al. Somatostatin and somatostatin analogue (SMS 201–995) in treatment of hormone secreting tumors of the pituitary and gastrointestinal tract and non-neoplastic diseases of the gut. *Ann Intern Med.* 1989;110:35.
137. Godwin DJ. Carcinoid tumors: An analysis of 2,837 cases. *Cancer.* 1975;36:560.
138. Domizio P, Owen RA, Shepherd NA, et al. Primary lymphoma of the small intestine: A clinicopathological study of 119 cases. *Am J Surg Pathol.* 1993;17:429.
139. O'Brian DS, Kennedy MJ, Daly PA, et al. Multiple lymphomatous polyposis of the gastrointestinal tract: A clinicopathologically distinctive form of non-Hodgkin's lymphoma of B-cell centrocytic type. *Am J Surg Pathol.* 1989;13:691.
140. Allred HW, Spencer RJ. Hemangiomas of the colon, rectum and anus. *Mayo Clin Proc.* 1974;49:739.
141. Friedman SL, Wright TL, Altman DF. Gastrointestinal Kaposi's sarcoma in patients with acquired immune deficiency syndrome: Endoscopic and autopsy findings. *Gastroenterology.* 1985;89:102.
142. Mendeloff AI. Epidemiology of the irritable bowel syndrome. *Pract Gastroenterol.* 1979;3:12.
143. Drossman DA. Irritable bowel syndrome. *Am Fam Phys.* 1989;39:159.
144. Fausel CS, Goff JS. Non-operative management of acute idiopathic colonic pseudoobstruction (Ogilvie's syndrome). *West J Med.* 1985;143:50.
145. Stanghelli V, Malagelada JR. Chronic idiopathic intestinal pseudo-obstruction: Clinical and intestinal manometric findings. *Gut.* 1987;28:5.
146. Badiali D, Marcheggiano A, Pallone F, et al. Melanosis of the rectum in patients with chronic constipation. *Dis Colon Rectum.* 1985;28:241.
147. Sarr MG, Balkley GB, Zuidema GD. Preoperative recognition of intestinal strangulation obstruction: Prospective evaluation of diagnostic capability. *Am J Surg.* 1983;145:176.
148. Boley SJ, Di Biase A, Brandt LJ, et al. Lower intestinal bleeding in the elderly. *Am J Surg.* 1979;137:57.
149. Imperiale TF, Ransohoff DF. Aortic stenosis, idiopathic gastrointestinal bleeding, and angiodysplasia: Is there an association? *Gastroenterology.* 1988;95:1670.
150. Duray PH, Marcal JM, LiVolsi VA, et al. Gastrointestinal angiodysplasia: A possible component of von Willebrand's disease. *Hum Pathol.* 1984;15:539.
151. Salem RR, Wood CB, Rees HC, et al. A comparison of colonoscopy and selective visceral angiography in the diagnosis of colonic angiodysplasia. *Ann R Coll Surg Engl.* 1985;67:225.
152. Hutcheon DF, Kabelin J, Bulkley GB, et al. Effect of therapy on bleeding rates in gastrointestinal angiodysplasia. *Am Surg.* 1987;53:6.
153. Galandiuk S, Fazio VW. Pneumatosis cystoides intestinalis: A review of the literature. *Dis Colon Rectum.* 1986;29:358.
154. Calkins BM, Lilienfeld AM, Garland CF, et al. Trends in the incidence rates of ulcerative colitis and Crohn's disease. *Dig Dis Sci.* 1984;29:913.
155. Both H, Torp-Pedersen K, Kreiner S, et al. Clinical appearance at diagnosis of ulcerative colitis and Crohn's disease in a regional patient group. *Scand J Gastroenterol.* 1983;18:987.
156. Sinclair TS, Brunt PW, Mowat NAG. Nonspecific proctocolitis in northeastern Scotland: A community study. *Gastroenterology.* 1983;85:1.
157. Nostrant TT, Kumar NB, Appelman HD. Histopathology differentiates acute self-limited colitis from ulcerative colitis. *Gastroenterology.* 1987;92:318.
158. Surawicz CM, Belic L. Rectal biopsy helps to distinguish acute self-limited colitis from idiopathic inflammatory bowel disease. *Gastroenterology.* 1984;86:104.
159. Jalan KN, Sircus W, Card WI, et al. An experience of ulcerative colitis: I. Toxic dilatation in 55 cases. *Gastroenterology.* 1969;57:68.
160. Farmer RG, Hawk WA, Turnbull RB. Clinical patterns in Crohn's disease: A statistical study of 615 cases. *Gastroenterology.* 1975;68:627.
161. Price AB. Overlap in the spectrum of nonspecific inflammatory bowel disease—"Colitis indeterminate." *J Clin Pathol.* 1971;31:567.
162. Gyde SN, Prior P, Macartney JC, et al. Malignancy in Crohn's *disease. Gut.* 1980;21:1024.
163. Ritchie JK, Powell-Tuck J, Lennard-Jones JE. Clinical outcome

of the first ten years of ulcerative colitis and proctitis. *Lancet.* 1978;1:1140.
164. Miller MM. Ankylosing spondylitis, Reiter's syndrome, psoriatic arthritis and arthritis of inflammatory bowel disease. *Primary Care.* 1984;11:271.
165. Christophi C, Hughes ER. Hepatobiliary disorders in inflammatory bowel disease. *Surg Gynecol Obstet.* 1985;160:187.
166. Somitz MH. Skin complications of ulcerative colitis and Crohn's disease. *Cutis.* 1973;16:533.
167. Lennard-Jones JE, Mellville DM, Morson BC, et al. Precancer and cancer in extensive ulcerative colitis: Findings among 401 patients over 22 years. *Gut.* 1990;31:800.
168. Rosenstock E, Farmer RG, Petras R, et al. Surveillance for colonic carcinoma in ulcerative colitis. *Gastroenterology.* 1985;89:1342.
169. Lashner BA, Hanover SB, Silverstein MD. Optimal timing of colonoscopy to screen for cancer in ulcerative colitis. *Ann Intern Med.* 1988;108:274.
170. Riddell RH, Goldman H, Ransohoff DF, et al. Dysplasia in inflammatory bowel disease: Standardized classification with provisional clinical applications. *Hum Pathol.* 1983;14:931.
171. Blackstone MD, Riddell RH, Rogers BHG, et al. Dysplasia associated lesion or mass (DALM) detected by colonoscopy in longstanding ulcerative colitis: An indication for colectomy. *Gastroenterology.* 1981;80:366.
172. Greenstein AJ, Sachor DB, Smith H, et al. A comparison of cancer risk in Crohn's disease and ulcerative colitis. *Cancer.* 1981;48:2742.
173. Glotzer DJ, Glick ME, Goldman H. Proctitis and colitis following diversion of the fecal stream. *Gastroenterology.* 1981;80:438.
174. Hulten L, Svaninger G. Facts about the Koch continent ileostomy. *Dis Colon Rectum.* 1984;27:553.
175. Moskowitz RL, Shepherd NA, Nicholls RJ. An assessment of inflammation in the reservoir after restorative proctocolectomy with ileoanal ileal reservoir. *Colorect Dis.* 1986;1:167.
176. Bartlett JG, Chang TW, Gurwith M, et al. Antibiotic associated pseudomembranous colitis due to toxin producing clostridia. *N Engl J Med.* 1978;298:531.
177. Kelly J, Oryshak A, Wenetsek M, et al. The colonic pathology of *Escherichia coli* 0157:HZ infection. *Am J Surg Pathol.* 1990;14:87.
178. Sack RB. Enterohemorrhagic *Escherichia coli. N Engl J Med.* 1987;317:1535.
179. Pittman FE, El-Hashimi WK, Pittman JC. Studies of human amebiasis: I. Clinical and laboratory findings in eight cases of acute amebic colitis. *Gastroenterology.* 1973;65:581.
180. Quinn TC, Corey L, Chaffee RG, et al. The etiology of anorectal infections in homosexual men. *Am J Med.* 1981;71:395.
181. Parks TG. Natural history of diverticular disease of the colon. *Clin Gastroenterol.* 1975;4:53.
182. Thompson WG. Do colonic diverticula cause symptoms? *Gastroenterology.* 1986;81:613.
183. Johnson WC, Nasbeth DC. Visceral infarction following aortic surgery. *Ann Surg.* 1974;180:312.
184. Norris HT. Re-examination of the spectrum of ischemic bowel disease. In: HT Norris, ed. *Pathology of the Colon, Small Intestine and Anus.* New York: Churchill Livingstone; 1991:121.
185. Slavin RE, Dias MA, Sarol R. Cytosine arabinoside induced gastrointestinal toxic alterations in sequential chemotherapeutic protocols. *Cancer.* 1978;42:1747.
186. Mehcotra TN. Hemorrhagic colitis after cyclophosphamide. *Lancet.* 1966;2:345.
187. Atherton LD, Leib E, Kaye MD. Toxic megacolon associated with methotrexate therapy. *Gastroenterology.* 1984;86:1583.
188. Graham CF, Gallager K, Jones JK. Acute colitis with methyldopa. *N Engl J Med.* 1981;304:1044.
189. Martin P, Marley PN, De Pew WT, et al. Isotretinoin-associated proctosigmoiditis. *Gastroenterology.* 1987;93:606.
190. Gekas P, Schuster MM. Stercoral perforation of the colon: Case report and review of the literature. *Gastroenterology.* 1981;80:1054.
191. Rutter KRP, Riddell RH. The solitary ulcer syndrome of the rectum. *Clin Gastroenterol.* 1975;4:505.
192. Levine DS. ''Solitary'' rectal ulcer syndrome: Are ''solitary'' rectal ulcer syndrome and ''localized'' colitis cystica profunda analogous syndromes caused by rectal prolapse? *Gastroenterology.* 1987;92:243.
193. Giardiello FM, Lazenby AJ, Bayless TM, et al. Lymphocytic (microscopic) colitis: Clinicopathologic study of 18 patients and comparison to collagenous colitis. *Dig Dis Sci.* 1989;34:1730.
194. Fasoll RA, Hewell DP. Short-term response to treatment in microscopic colitis. *Gut.* 1989;30:1481.
195. Stemmermann GM, Yatani R. Diverticulosis and polyps of the large intestine: A microscopic study of Hawaii Japanese. *Cancer.* 1973;31:1260.
196. Vogelstein B, Fearon ER, Hamilton ST, et al. Genetic alterations during colorectal tumor development. *N Engl J Med.* 1988;319:525.
197. Halvorsen TB. Site distribution of colorectal adenocarcinomas. *Scand J Gastroenterol.* 1986;21:973.
198. Muto T, Bussey HJR, Morson BC. The evolution of cancer of the colon and rectum. *Cancer.* 1975;36:2251.
199. Groden J, Thliveris A, Samowitz W, et al. Identification and characterization of the familial adenomatous polyposis gene. *Cell.* 1991;66:589.
200. Bussey HJR. *Familial Polyposis Coli: Family Studies, Histopathology, Differential Diagnosis and Results of Treatment.* Baltimore: Johns Hopkins University Press; 1975.
201. Sarre RG, Jagelman DG, Beck GJ, et al. Colectomy with ileorectal anastamosis for familial adenomatous polyposis: The risk of rectal cancer. *Surgery.* 1987;101:20.
202. Hrabovsky EE, Watne AL, Carrier JM. Changing management in familial polyposis: Role of ileoanal endorectal pull-through. *Am J Surg.* 1984;147:130.
203. Lynch HT, Smyrk TC, Watson P, et al. Genetics, natural history, tumor spectrum, and pathology of hereditary nonpolyposis colorectal cancer: An updated review. *Gastroenterology.* 1993;104:1535.
204. Aaltonen LA, Peltomaki P, Leach FS, et al. Clues to the pathogenesis of familial colorectal cancer. *Science.* 1993;260:812.
205. Papadopoulos N, Nicolaides NC, Wei YF, et al. Mutation of *mut*L homolog in hereditary colon cancer. *Science.* 1994;263:1625.
206. Correa P, Strong JP, Reif A, et al. The epidemiology of colorectal polyps: Prevalence in New Orleans and international comparisons. *Cancer.* 1977;38:2258.
207. Correa P, Haenszel W. The epidemiology of large bowel cancer. *Adv Cancer Res.* 1978;26:1.
208. Bonelli L, Martines H, Conio M, et al. Family history of colorectal cancer as a risk factor for benign and malignant tumors of the large bowel: A case-control study. *Int J Cancer.* 1988;41:513.
209. Nava H, Carlsson G, Petrelli NJ, et al. Follow-up colonoscopy in patients with colorectal adenomatous polyps. *Dis Colon Rectum.* 1987;30:465.
210. Williams CB, Macrae FA. The St. Marks neoplastic polyp follow-up study. *Front Gastrointest Res.* 1986;10:226.
211. Fenoglio CM, Kaye GI, Lane N. Distribution of human colonic lymphatics in normal, hyperplastic, and adenomatous tissue: Its relationship to metastasis from small carcinomas in pedunculated adenomas, with two case reports. *Gastroenterology.* 1973;64:51.
212. Quizilbash AH, Meghji M, Castelli M. Pseudo-carcinomatous invasion in adenomas of the colon and rectum. *Dis Colon Rectum.* 1980;23:529.
213. Lewin KJ, Riddell RH, Weinstein WM. Large bowel polyps and tumors. In: *Gastrointestinal Pathology and Its Clinical Implications.* New York: Igaku-Shoin; 1992:1198.
214. Haggit RC, Glatzbach RE, Soffer EE, et al. Prognostic factors in colorectal carcinomas arising in adenomas: Implications for lesions removed by endoscopic polypectomy. *Gastroenterology.* 1985;89:328.
215. Riddell RH. Hands off ''cancerous'' large bowel polyps. *Gastroenterology.* 1985;89:432.
216. American Cancer Society. Cancer statistics 1987. *CA.* 1987;35:19.
217. Steinberg SM, Barkin JS, Kaplan RS, et al. Prognostic indicators of colon tumors: The gastrointestinal tumor study group experience. *Cancer.* 1986;57:1866.
218. Welch JP. Multiple colorectal tumors: An appraisal of natural history and therapeutic options. *Am J Surg.* 1981;142:274.
219. Mills SE, Allen MS. Colorectal carcinoma in the first three decades of life. *Am J Surg Pathol.* 1979;3:443.
220. Symonds DA, Vickery AL Jr. Mucinous carcinoma of the colon and rectum. *Cancer.* 1976;37:1891.
221. Sasaki O, Atkin WS, Jass JR. Mucinous carcinoma of the rectum. *Histopathology.* 1987;11:259.

222. Schwartz AM, Orenstein JM. Small cell undifferentiated carcinoma of the rectosigmoid colon. *Arch Pathol Lab Med.* 1985;109:629.
223. Boland CR. Malignant tumors of the colon. In: Yamada T, ed. *Textbook of Gastroenterology.* Vol. II. Philadelphia: Lippincott; 1991:1768.
224. Dukes CE. The classification of cancer of the rectum. *J Pathol Bacteriol.* 1932;35:323.
225. Turnbull RB. The no-touch isolation technique of resection. *JAMA.* 1975;231:1181.
226. Hutter RVP, Sobin LH. A universal staging system for cancer of the colon and rectum. *Arch Pathol Lab Med.* 1986;110:367.
227. Fletcher RH. Carcinoembryonic antigen. *Ann Intern Med.* 1986;104:66.
228. Laurie JA, Moertel CG, Fleming TR, et al. Surgical adjuvant therapy of large bowel carcinoma: An evaluation of levamisole and the combination of levamisole and fluorouracil. *J Clin Oncol* 1989;7:1447.
229. Berardi RS. Carcinoid tumors of the colon (exclusive of the rectum): Review of the literature. *Dis Colon Rectum.* 1972;15:383.
230. Haber DA, Mayer RJ. Primary gastrointestinal lymphoma. *Semin Oncol.* 1988;15:154.
231. Moyana TN, Friesen R, Tan LK. Colorectal smooth-muscle tumors: A pathobiologic study with immunohistochemistry and histomorphometry. *Arch Pathol Lab Med.* 1991;115:1016.
232. Collins DC. A study of 50,000 specimens of the human vermiform appendix. *Surg Gynecol Obstet.* 1955;101:437.
233. Trollope ML, Lindenauer SM. Diverticulosis of the appendix: A collective review. *Dis Colon Rectum.* 1974;17:200.
234. Butler C. Surgical pathology of acute appendicitis. *Hum Pathol.* 1981;12:870.
235. Stanley MW, Cherwitz D, Hagen K, et al. Neuromas of the appendix: A light microscopic, immunohistochemical and electron microscopic study of 20 cases. *Am J Surg Pathol.* 1986;10:801.
236. Chan W, Foo KH. Value of routine histopathological examination of appendices in Hong Kong. *J Clin Pathol.* 1987;40:429.
237. Gupta SC, Gupta AK, Keswani NK, et al. Pathology of tropical appendicitis. *J Clin Pathol.* 1989;42:1169.
238. Ariel I, Vinograd I, Hershlag A, et al. Crohn's disease isolated to the appendix: Truths and fallacies. *Hum Pathol.* 1986;17:1116.
239. Higa E, Rosai J, Pizzimbono CA, et al. Mucosal hyperplasia, mucinous cystadenoma and mucinous cystadenocarcinoma of the appendix. *Cancer.* 1973;32:1525.
240. Appelman HD. Epithelial neoplasia of the appendix. In: Norris HT, ed. *Pathology of the Colon, Small Intestine, and Anus.* New York: Churchill Livingstone; 1991:263.
241. Young RH, Gilks CB, Scully RE. Mucinous tumors of the appendix associated with mucinous tumors of the ovary and pseudomyxoma peritonei: A clinicopathologic analysis of 22 cases supporting an origin in the appendix. *Am J Surg Pathol.* 1991;15:415.
242. Moertel CG, Weiland LH, Nagorney DM, et al. Carcinoid tumor of the appendix: Treatment and prognosis. *N Engl J Med.* 1987;317:1699.
243. Thomson WH. The nature of hemorrhoids. *Br J Surg.* 1975;62:542.
244. Hosking SW, Johnson AG. Bleeding anorectal varices: A misunderstood condition. *Surgery.* 1988;104:70.
245. Nothmann BJ, Schuster MM. Internal anal sphincter derangement with anal fissures. *Gastroenterology.* 1974;67:216.
246. Ramanujam PS, Prasad ML, Abcarian H, et al. Perianal abscesses and fistulas: A study of 1023 patients. *Dis Colon Rectum.* 1984;27:593.
247. Bubrick MP, Hitchcock CR. Necrotizing anorectal and perineal infections. *Surgery.* 1979;86:655.
248. Lobert PF, Appelman HD. Inflammatory cloacogenic polyps: A unique inflammatory lesion of the anal transitional zone. *Am J Surg Pathol.* 1981;5:761.
249. Wexner SD, Milsom JW, Dailey TH. The demographics of anal cancers are changing: Identification of a high risk population. *Dis Colon Rectum.* 1987;30:942.
250. Daling JR, Weiss NS, Hislop TG, et al. Sexual practices, sexually transmitted diseases, and the incidence of anal cancer. *N Engl J Med.* 1987;317:973.
251. Wells M, Griffiths S, Lewis F, et al. Demonstration of human papillomavirus types in paraffin processed tissue from human anogenital lesions by in situ DNA hybridization. *J Pathol.* 1987;152:77.
252. Singh R, Nime F, Mittelman A. Malignant epithelial tumors of the anal canal. *Cancer.* 1981;48:411.
253. Slater G, Greenstein A, Aufses AH. Anal carcinoma in patients with Crohn's disease. *Ann Surg.* 1984;199:348.
254. Boman B, Moertel CG, O'Connell MJ, et al. Carcinoma of the anal canal: A clinical and pathologic study of 188 cases. *Cancer.* 1984;54:114.
255. Papillon J, Montbaron JT. Epidermoid carcinoma of the anal canal: A series of 276 cases. *Dis Colon Rectum.* 1987;30:324.
256. Beck DE, Fazio VW. Perianal Paget's disease. *Dis Colon Rectum.* 1987;30:263.
257. Cooper PH, Mills SE, Allen MS. Malignant melanoma of the anus: Report of 12 patients and analysis of 255 additional cases. *Dis Colon Rectum.* 1982;25:693.
258. Ward MWN, Romano G, Nicholls RJ. The surgical treatment of anorectal malignant melanoma. *Br J Surg.* 1986;73:68.

13

The Liver, Biliary Tract, and Pancreas

Jorge Albores-Saavedra and William H. Snyder III

Definition

Although the liver, extrahepatic biliary tree, and pancreas have different histologic structure and function, they derive from the primitive foregut. The histologic similarity between neoplasms of the extrahepatic biliary tree and exocrine pancreas is based upon their common embryologic derivation. Diseases involving the distal biliary-pancreatic ducts may profoundly affect both the liver and the pancreas. Moreover, the evaluation of neoplastic diseases involving the terminal portions of the biliary and pancreatic ducts requires similar diagnostic and therapeutic tools. For these reasons, surgeons and pathologists consider these organs as a single system (the hepato-pancreatic-biliary system). The reported number of hepatic and pancreatic tumors is increasing, due in part to a true increased incidence and in part to improved detection methods. Thus, the hepato-pancreatic-biliary system is of increasing importance to surgeons.

Liver

BIOPSY TECHNIQUES AND PITFALLS

Five types of biopsies are used to evaluate liver diseases: percutaneous core needle biopsy, percutaneous fine needle aspiration (FNA) biopsy, laparoscopic needle biopsy, and open incisional or excisional biopsy. Needle core techniques utilize a cutting needle (Tru-Cut or Menghini needle) to secure a core of tissue. Such specimens are appropriate for diagnosing diffuse diseases of the liver, such as chronic active hepatitis or cirrhosis. In contrast, the FNA is best for space-occupying lesions, especially primary and metastatic neoplasms and hepatic abscesses (see Chap. 3). Computed tomography (CT) or ultrasonography is the best method for guiding aspiration biopsy of hepatic lesions. The sensitivity of this procedure varies from 80 to 90%, with few false-positive diagnoses.[1] However, distinguishing metastatic adenocarcinoma from cholangiocarcinoma may be impossible by the FNA method. Likewise, hepatic adenomas are indistinguishable from focal nodular hyperplasia or well-differentiated hepatocellular carcinoma by FNA. Laparoscopic or open biopsy is used when neither FNA nor core needle biopsy is diagnostic, or when an unsuspected liver mass is found during laparoscopy or laparotomy performed for other diseases.

Both the percutaneous needle core and FNA biopsies are considered safe procedures; however, a variety of complications may result. The most frequent complications are pain, bleeding, and bile leakage. Massive fatal hemorrhage can occur in patients with clotting abnormalities or amyloidosis or with vascular tumors or highly vascularized neoplasms, including hepatocellular carcinoma. Bile leakage is less common than bleeding and usually occurs in patients with biliary obstruction. Perforation of a distended gallbladder with subsequent bile peritonitis is a rare complication.

A frozen section diagnosis of the unsuspected liver mass may be essential for definitive surgical treatment. Such is the case when one or several hepatic nodules are found during resections of gastrointestinal carcinomas. Another clear indication for frozen section diagnosis is the examination of surgical margins in hepatic resections for primary malignant hepatic neoplasms or solitary metastatic lesions. Frozen section diagnosis of liver lesions is usually straightforward; however, three benign tumors can cause problems for the unwary pathologist: liver cell adenoma, bile duct adenoma, and angiomyolipoma. Large hepatic adenomas with cytologic atypia can be virtually impossible to distinguish from well-differentiated hepatocellular carcinomas. Bile duct adenomas are asymptomatic, small, solitary or multiple nodules composed of tubular structures resembling bile ducts, which can be confused with glands of metastatic carcinoma. This is especially true when they are incidental findings during resection of gastrointestinal adenocarcinomas. Angiomyolipomas are hemorrhagic tumors that can reach a large size. Multinucleated giant cells and atypical epithelioid smooth muscle cells are prominent, and fat is inconspicuous. These features may cause confusion with angiosarcoma, malignant fibrous histiocytoma, or hepatocellular carcinoma.

LIVER ABSCESSES

Two types of liver abscess are recognized: pyogenic and amebic. The pyogenic type (bacterial) is more common in the United States, whereas the amebic type is endemic in countries with poor sanitary conditions. Ultrasonography, computed tomography, and FNA have simplified the diagnosis of hepatic abscess. The aspirate from a bacterial abscess reveals sheets of neutrophils. If the purulent material is cultured, the causative microorganism can be identified. In contrast, the aspirate from an amebic abscess shows necrotic hepatic tissue without neutrophils. Trophozoites of *Entamoeba histolytica* can sometimes be identified in the smears with routine stains.

The pathogenic organisms that cause pyogenic abscess may reach the liver via the biliary tree (ascending cholangitis), the portal vein, or the hepatic artery, or by direct extension from subhepatic or subdiaphragmatic infection.[2] The most common source of pyogenic abscess is cholecystitis or biliary obstruction by tumor or stones.[3] Other sources include appendicitis, diverticulitis, pelvic inflammatory disease, generalized sepsis, and portal pyelophlebitis. The origin of the abscess cannot be determined in about 15% of the cases. The most common organisms cultured from liver abscesses are *Escherichia coli, Klebsiella pneumoniae,* and *Streptococcus*, and *Bacteroides* species. Most pyogenic abscesses are multiple and occur more often in the right than in the left hepatic lobe.[4]

Amebic hepatic abscess, the most frequent complication of intestinal amebiasis, is more common in males than in females.[5] The amebas reach the liver through the portal vein. Like pyogenic abscesses, amebic abscesses involve the right hepatic lobe more often than the left. Approximately 30% of patients with hepatic amebic abscesses have symptoms of intestinal amebiasis, although many more eliminate cysts or trophozoites of *E. histolytica*. Complications of amebic hepatic abscess include rupture into the peritoneal, pleural, or pericardial cavities or, less commonly, rupture into abdominal viscera such as stomach, colon, and duodenum or into the retroperitoneum.[6] Abscesses may be solitary or multiple and vary from a few millimeters to 25 cm. In some cases, extensive destruction of the liver parenchyma results.

Microscopic examination reveals abundant necrotic material with few polymorphonuclear leukocytes. Trophozoites of *E. histolytica* may be found at the periphery of the lesion. If secondary infection occurs, histologic features of a pyogenic abscess may supervene.

CYSTS

Congenital, inflammatory, and neoplastic cysts may affect the liver and give rise to diagnostic and therapeutic problems. Congenital cysts are usually small, solitary, and asymptomatic. Only when they enlarge do they become symptomatic (Fig. 13–1). The epithelial lining is low cuboidal and resembles either biliary epithelium or mesothelium. Cytologic examination of the fluid aspirated from the cyst suggests the diagnosis and excludes malignancy. It is clear and may be acellular or contain small groups or sheets of benign cuboidal or flat epithelial cells. Multiple hepatic cysts are associated with polycystic renal disease in approximately 50% of the cases.[7] Inflammatory cysts are caused by parasites and include the hydatid cysts of the larvae of the dog tapeworm *Echinococcus granulosus*. If a hydatid cyst is suspected clinically, FNA biopsy is contraindicated because of the danger of rupture and anaphylactic shock. Histologically, the fibrous wall of the cyst is thick and frequently calcified. Daughter cysts containing several scolices with the characteristic hooks are seen on the inner layer of the cyst wall.

Both *benign* and *malignant* cystic neoplasms originate in the liver and extrahepatic bile ducts and are classified as biliary cystadenoma and cystadenocarcinoma, respectively.[8, 9] These multiloculated cystic tumors are seen almost exclusively among women. Microscopically, the walls of the locules are lined by biliary-type epithelium and contain a characteristic ovarian type of stroma, which usually is estrogen- and progesterone-receptor-positive. Finally, both primary and metastatic carcinomas of the liver may undergo central necrosis and simulate intrinsically cystic neoplasms.

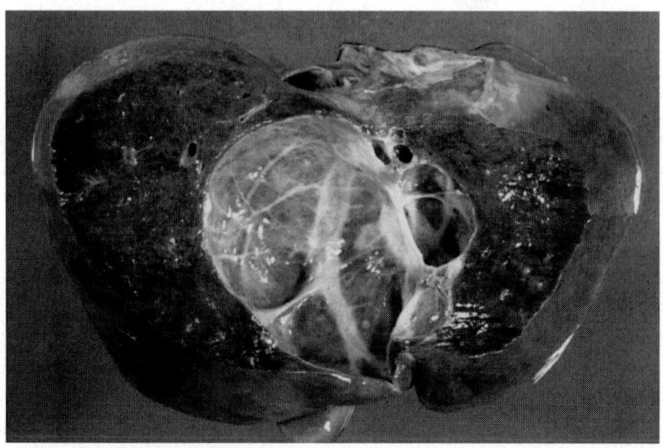

Figure 13–1. Asymptomatic large simple cyst of the liver found incidentally at autopsy.

BENIGN TUMORS

Focal Nodular Hyperplasia

Focal nodular hyperplasia (FNH) is a well-demarcated multinodular hepatic mass in an otherwise normal liver. It is often an incidental finding at autopsy or during a CT scan or a laparotomy for unrelated diseases. Nonoperative diagnosis can also be made by dynamic CT or magnetic resonance imaging (MRI). Focal nodular hyperplasia is most common in females between 25 and 50 years of age.[10, 11] Cases have been described in children and in women using contraceptive steroids, although this association is not as strong as for hepatic adenoma. About one third of patients report mild abdominal pain or a palpable mass. Improved imaging methods now allow better detection and earlier resection of FNH. A core needle biopsy is usually diagnostic, whereas FNA is usually inconclusive.

Focal nodular hyperplasia is a solitary lesion, usually measuring less than 6 cm in diameter. On cross section, it is multinodular, yellow-brown, and with a central or an eccentric depressed scar that radiates toward the periphery and divides the lesion into nodules (Fig. 13–2). Microscopically, it consists of nodules of normal-appearing hepatocytes. The nodules are separated by fibrous septa containing bile ducts, inflammatory cells, and abnormal arteries and veins. Some investigators believe that the vascular malformation is responsible for the hepatocellular hyperplasia.

Hepatocellular Adenoma

Hepatocellular adenomas occur most commonly in women during their reproductive years, usually those with a history of oral contraceptive use.[12, 13] Less frequently, these adenomas are seen in patients receiving androgenic anabolic steroids, patients with type 1a glycogen storage disease, diabetics, or patients with tyrosinemia or iron overload. Rarely hepatocellular adenomas have been described in children,[14] men, or women without a history of oral contraceptive use. Familial cases have also been reported. The most common clinical presentation is a palpable mass associated with right-upper-quadrant discomfort or pain. Rupture of the adenoma leads to intraperitoneal hemorrhage. This is a grave complication and is reported more often in patients taking oral contraceptives.[15] Approximately 10% of hepatocellular adenomas are asymptomatic and are found incidentally. Some adenomas regress following withdrawal of the contraceptive pill, although complete regression may take several years after cessation of estrogenic compounds.[16–18] The tumors are usually single, well-demarcated, and even partially encapsulated. Focal necrosis may be seen in the center but, in contrast to FNH, there is no central scar. They vary in size from 2 to 26 cm. The largest tumors may replace an entire hepatic lobe. Conventional hepatic adenomas cannot be distinguished from focal nodular hyperplasia by aspiration cytology. Microscopically, most hepatocellular adenomas are composed of liver cells arranged in cords with bland cytologic features or without cytologic features of malignancy. There are no portal triads or central veins, so that the normal lobular architecture of the liver is no longer recognizable. Although rare, malignant transformation has been documented in adenomas, usually those associated with anabolic steroid use.

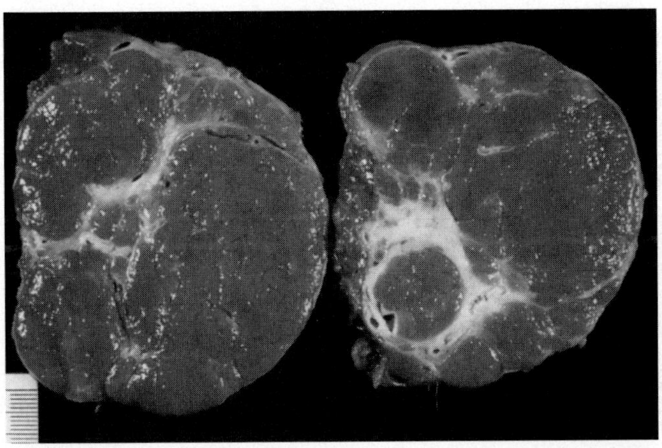

Figure 13–2. Focal nodular hyperplasia. The central scar divides the hepatic tissue into nodules of different sizes.

Adenomas associated with the use of androgenic anabolic steroids predominate in males; they are usually multiple and small. Because of cytologic atypia, these adenomas are often confused with hepatocellular carcinoma by FNA.

Vascular Tumors

Cavernous hemangioma is the most common primary hepatic tumor. It can be differentiated from other mass lesions by isotope scanning or MRI.[19] If hemangioma is suspected due to the risk of hemorrhage, FNA is contraindicated.[20] The majority of hepatic hemangiomas are incidental findings at autopsy. Only large or giant cavernous hemangiomas (10 cm or larger) require surgical treatment because they compress adjacent structures or because of the risk of hemorrhage. Grossly, hemangiomas are usually solitary, less than 5 cm in size, and spongy. On sectioning, they are well-demarcated red-blue nodules.

Infantile hemangioendotheliomas are usually asymptomatic, but they may rupture, producing congestive heart failure or thrombocytopenia (Kasabach-Merritt's syndrome). These vascular tumors are multinodular and have characteristic histologic features. Malignant transformation has rarely been reported.

Epithelioid hemangioendothelioma is a distinctive, low-grade, malignant vascular tumor that is often multicentric and usually involves both hepatic lobes.[21] It is most commonly seen in women. Patients often survive many years after diagnosis regardless of therapy. Until recently, this vascular neoplasm was often confused with cholangiocarcinoma. The neoplastic endothelial cells are large and epithelioid, have vacuolated cytoplasm, and lie in a dense fibrous stroma. Occlusion of sinusoids and veins results in hemorrhage and infarction.

Angiosarcoma is a highly malignant mesenchymal tumor of the liver that can be induced by thorium dioxide or vinyl chloride exposure or by arsenical ingestion. Most patients present with hepatomegaly and die several months after diagnosis. Because it usually appears as a multinodular mass involving both hepatic lobes, angiosarcoma is rarely resectable (Fig. 13–3). Its histologic structure is similar to that of angiosarcoma in other sites.

Bile Duct Adenoma

Bile duct adenoma is a small (less than 1 cm), subcapsular nodule that simulates metastatic disease both grossly and microscopically. The likelihood of such misdiagnosis is increased when these nodules are multiple, found during resection of gastrointestinal adenocarcinomas, and diagnosed with intraoperative frozen sections. These benign tumors are composed of tubular structures resembling normal bile ducts.[22]

MALIGNANT TUMORS

Hepatocellular Carcinoma

Hepatocellular carcinoma is one of the most prevalent and most lethal cancers in the world.[23, 24] It is much more common in sub-Saharan Africa, Southeast Asia, Japan, the Pacific Islands, and Greece than in North America. The incidence of hepatocellular carcinoma is increasing in many parts of the world, including the United States.

The association of hepatitis B virus infection and hepatocellular carcinoma has been established by epidemiologic, virologic, and molecular pathology studies.[10] In the United States, approximately 90% of patients with hepatocellular carcinoma have a history of chronic liver disease, usually posthepatitic cirrhosis.[10] Several studies have shown that a significant proportion of patients with hepatocellular carcinoma are infected with hepatitis C virus, suggesting that this viral infection is a major risk factor for the development of hepatocellular carcinoma.[25, 26] Other etiologic factors related to hepatocellular carcinoma include hemochromatosis; alcoholic cirrhosis; thorium dioxide or vinyl chloride exposure; metabolic diseases such as glycogen storage disease; the Budd-Chiari's syndrome; biliary atresia; aflatoxins; and parasitic infestation, especially schistosomiasis.

The tumor is most commonly reported in men but has also been reported in children. The most common symptoms are weakness, malaise, abdominal pain, hepatic mass, weight loss, jaundice, anorexia, and fever. Although nonspecific, serum alpha-fetoprotein is the best marker for hepatocellular carcinoma and is elevated in 60 to 80% of the patients. In high-risk patients, the combination of periodic serum alpha-fetoprotein measurements, ultrasonography, computed tomography, and FNA have allowed the detection of small tumors (less than 4 cm in diameter). Consequently, the rate of resection has increased.[27, 28]

Fine needle aspiration cytology allows differentiation of well to moderately differentiated hepatocellular carcinoma from metastatic disease.[29, 30] However, poorly differentiated hepatocellular carcinomas are difficult to distinguish from metastatic carcinoma by FNA, and core needle biopsy or open biopsy may be required for definitive diagnosis. Likewise, hepatocellular adenomas with atypia cannot be distinguished from well-differentiated hepatocellular carcinoma by FNA.

The solitary small hepatocellular carcinoma is usually well demarcated, often encapsulated, and located near the hepatic capsule (Fig. 13–4). In contrast, clinically apparent tumors are usually multinodular or diffuse (Fig. 13–5). A massive form is also recognized. Since these tumors are

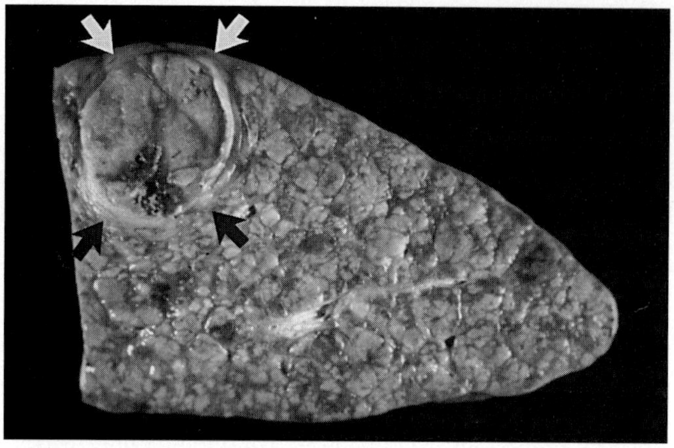

Figure 13–4. Small hepatocellular carcinoma *(arrows)*. The tumor, which was detected by serum alpha-fetoprotein measurements in a patient with posthepatitic cirrhosis, is subcapsular and appears encapsulated.

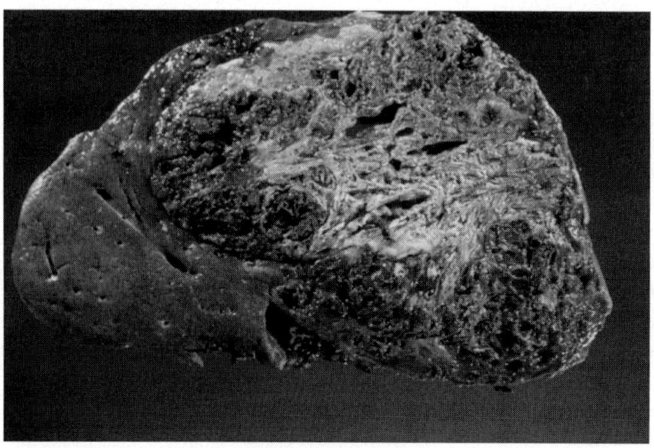

Figure 13–3. Large, hemorrhagic, well-demarcated, and spongy angiosarcoma of liver surgically resected.

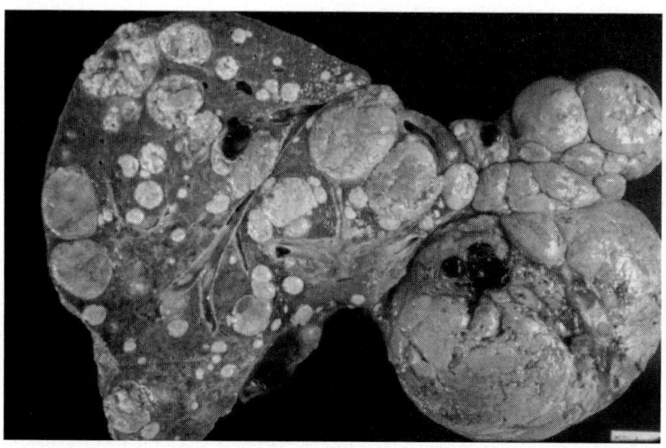

Figure 13–5. Multinodular hepatocellular carcinoma involving both hepatic lobes and resembling metastatic carcinoma.

Table 13–1. TNM Classification and Staging of Liver Tumors

Primary Tumor (T)	
TX	Primary tumor cannot be assessed
T0	No evidence of primary tumor
T1	Solitary tumor 2 cm or less in greatest dimension without vascular invasion
T2	Solitary tumor 2 cm or less in greatest dimension with vascular invasion; or multiple tumors limited to one lobe, none more than 2 cm in greatest dimension without vascular invasion; or a solitary tumor more than 2 cm in greatest dimension without vascular invasion
T3	Solitary tumor more than 2 cm in greatest dimension with vascular invasion; or multiple tumors limited to one lobe, none more than 2 cm in greatest dimension, with vascular invasion; or multiple tumors limited to one lobe, any more than 2 cm in greatest dimension, with or without vascular invasion
T4	Multiple tumors in more than one lobe, or tumor(s) involving a major branch of the portal or hepatic vein(s)
Regional Lymph Nodes (N)	
NX	Regional lymph nodes cannot be assessed
N0	No regional lymph node metastasis
N1	Regional lymph node metastasis
Distant Metastasis (M)	
MX	Presence of distant metastasis cannot be assessed
M0	No distant metastasis
M1	Distant metastasis

Source: From Beahrs OH, Henson DE, Hutter RVP, Kennedy BJ, eds. *Manual for Staging of Cancer,* 4th ed. Philadelphia: Lippincott; 1992:185–186. With permission.

often multicentric and involve both lobes, less than 25% are resectable (Table 13–1).

Microscopically, hepatocellular carcinomas are composed of cells that resemble normal hepatocytes. The commonest pattern is trabecular (Fig. 13–6); however, sheetlike and acinar growth patterns are also relatively common. Although most hepatocellular carcinomas are well to moderately differentiated, poorly differentiated forms exist. These tumors are composed of spindle or giant cells and have a poorer prognosis.

The fibrolamellar variant occurs in adolescents or young adults and has a better prognosis than the conventional hepatocellular carcinoma. It usually arises in noncirrhotic liver.[31–33] Fine needle aspiration cytology does not distinguish this unusual variant from the conventional type of hepatocellular carcinoma. However, the distinction can be made on core needle biopsy or with intraoperative frozen sections. Microscopically, it is characterized by deeply eosinophilic cells separated into cords and trabeculae by lamellar fibrous bands (Fig. 13–7).

Hepatoblastoma

Hepatoblastoma is the most common primary hepatic tumor in childhood and is associated with a high mortality rate. Over 60% of hepatoblastomas are diagnosed in children under 2 years of age.[34] Hypoglycemia, thrombocytosis, sexual precocity, and hemihypertrophy are associated with these tumors. Hepatoblastomas are usually large and multinodular and are composed of fetal hepatocytes. Frequently a mesenchymal component is present, whereas teratoid elements can rarely be recognized.[35]

Cholangiocarcinoma

Cholangiocarcinoma is a malignant tumor composed of ductal structures similar to intrahepatic bile ducts.[36] It is less common than hepatocellular carcinoma and usually arises in a noncirrhotic liver. Elevated serum carcinoembryonic antigen (CEA) and CA19-9 levels are reported in approximately half of the patients. Ultrasonography is the best radiographic method for the detection of cholangiocarcinoma. Core needle or incisional biopsy may be necessary for definitive diagnosis, since aspiration cytology does not distinguish cholangiocarcinoma from metastatic adenocarcinoma. Two clinicopathologic types are described: (1) peripheral cholangiocarcinoma, the most common type, which arises within small bile ducts within the portal space and is usually asymptomatic until it is quite large; and (2) hilar cholangiocarcinoma, which arises in a major bile duct near the hilum and may extend into the left and right hepatic ducts and produce biliary obstruction. Grossly, cholangiocarcinoma may be multifocal and simulate metastatic disease or it may be a single large mass involving most of the liver and mimic hepatocellular carcinoma (Figs. 13–8 and 13–9). Cholangiocarcinomas represent 7 to 8% of all primary hepatic tumors. However, cholangiocarcinomas are relatively common in countries where the parasite *Opisthorchis* is endemic, such as Hong Kong or Thailand. Other predisposing factors for the development of cholangiocarcinoma include cystic lesions of the liver, such as von Meyenberg complexes, Caroli's disease and congenital hepatic fibrosis, inflammatory bowel disease, primary sclerosing cholangitis, intrahepatic calculi, parasitic infestation, thorium dioxide therapy, and many drugs. The tumor is unrelated to hepatitis B virus.

Metastatic Tumors

Metastatic tumors are the most common malignant neoplasms of the liver and are the prime consideration when multiple umbilicated nodules are discovered in the liver of

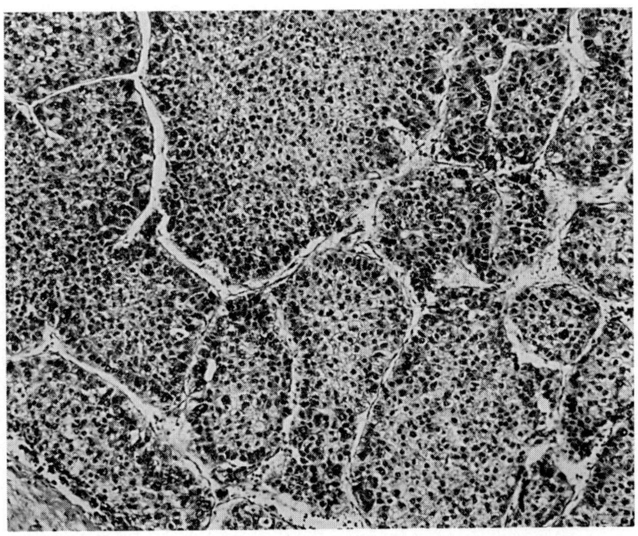

Figure 13–6. The trabecular histologic pattern of hepatocellular carcinoma is illustrated in this photomicrograph.

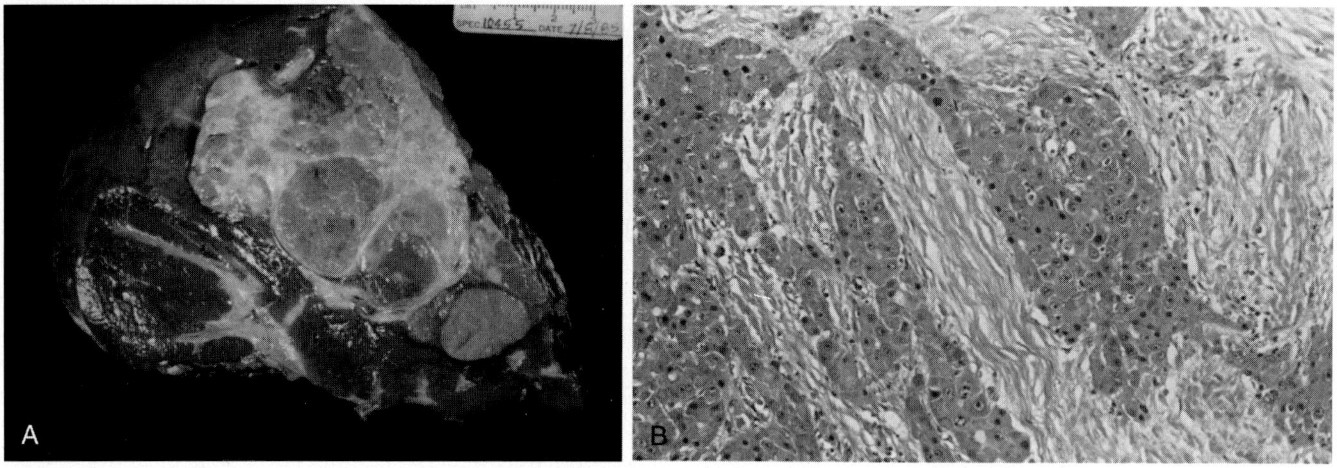

Figure 13–7. *A*, Multinodular fibrolamellar carcinoma that arose in noncirrhotic liver. A scar reminiscent of focal nodular hyperplasia is seen. *B*, Fibrolamellar carcinoma. Cords of neoplastic, deeply eosinophilic cells with prominent nucleoli are separated by dense fibrous bands.

patients over 50 years of age. Although any malignant neoplasms may disseminate and reach the liver through the bloodstream, the most common are lung carcinomas, adenocarcinomas of the gastrointestinal tract, breast carcinomas, prostatic adenocarcinomas, genitourinary carcinomas, and malignant melanomas. Solitary hepatic metastases are usually of colorectal origin and can sometimes be curatively resected. The 5-year survival rate in these patients is between 20 and 30%. Frequently, it is not possible to determine the site of origin of hepatic metastases by microscopic examination of biopsy specimens alone. Even with the aid of immunohistochemistry and electron microscopy, it may be impossible to determine with certainty the origin of the primary tumor.[37]

Gallbladder

INFLAMMATORY PROCESSES

Acute Calculous Cholecystitis

The majority of cases of acute cholecystitis are associated with calculi and are therefore more common in women.[38–40] Obstruction of the neck of the gallbladder or the cystic duct by a stone appears to be the important pathogenetic mechanism. Other contributing factors are mucosal ischemia, formation and release of inflammatory mediators, and mucosal injury by bile acids. Bacterial invasion is probably a secondary event. The inflamed gallbladder is usually enlarged and its wall is thickened by congestion, edema, and fibrinopurulent exudate. The mucosal changes range from moderate edema and congestion to extensive ulceration and necrosis. Microscopically, an acute inflammatory infiltrate is seen in the gallbladder wall. Complications of acute calculous cholecystitis include perforation, abscess, and fistula formation.

Acute emphysematous cholecystitis is a rare variant of acute cholecystitis that usually occurs in diabetic patients and is characterized by the presence of gas in the wall and lumen of the gallbladder.[41] The gas is produced by the infecting bacterial organism, usually *Clostridium welchii* or *perfringens*. Gallstones are found in most cases. Perforation is a relatively common complication.

Acute Acalculous Cholecystitis

Acute cholecystitis in the absence of gallstones is found in approximately 5% of patients undergoing cholecystec-

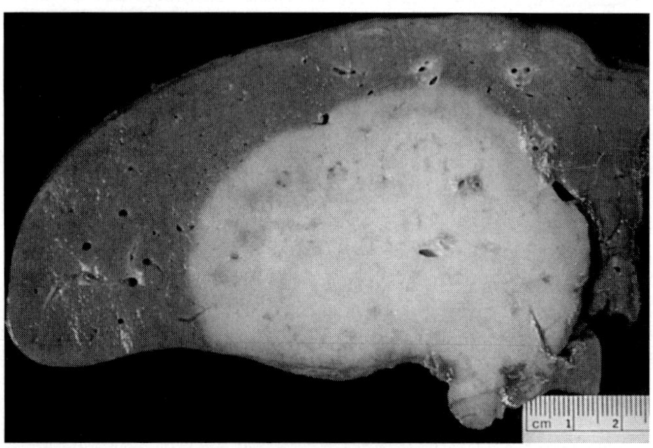

Figure 13–8. Cholangiocarcinoma. A large, well-demarcated, gray-white, firm mass replaces the liver parenchyma.

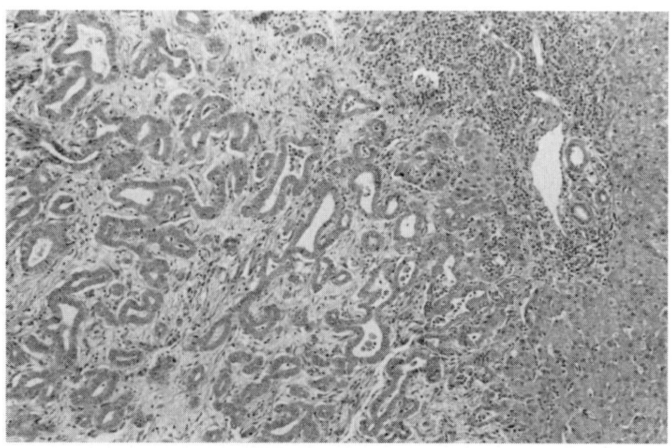

Figure 13–9. Neoplastic tubular structures similar to small bile ducts are lined by cuboidal epithelial cells in this cholangiocarcinoma.

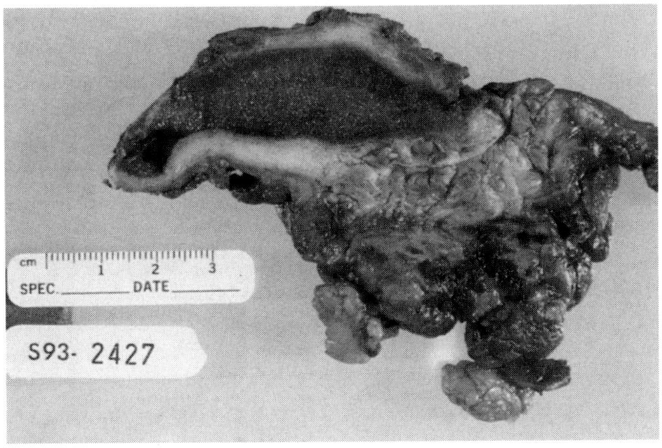

Figure 13–10. Xanthogranulomatous cholecystitis simulating malignancy. The wall of the gallbladder is markedly thickened by a yellow-brown, poorly defined mass that extended to the liver.

tomy. The pathogenesis of acute acalculous cholecystitis is multifactorial.[42] The disease affects individuals with other pathologic conditions including trauma, sepsis, burns, non-biliary surgical procedures, and debilitating systemic diseases such as sarcoidosis, lupus erythematosus, or AIDS.

Patients with AIDS may develop acalculous cholecystitis in which cytomegalovirus and/or *Cryptosporidium* is found.[43–45] Infection with *Mycobacterium avium-intracellulare* has rarely been reported.

Hydrops and Mucocele

Distention of the gallbladder by a clear and watery or mucoid material is known as hydrops and mucocele, respectively. It accounts for 3% of the pathologic gallbladders in adults. The most common cause is an impacted stone in the neck of the gallbladder or cystic duct. Other causes include tumors, fibrosis, or kinking of the cystic duct. The gallbladder is markedly distended by watery fluid or gelatinous mucous material. Its wall is usually thin and contains a few inflammatory cells.

Chronic Cholecystitis

Chronic cholecystitis with cholelithiasis is a common surgical disease.[46] Approximately 500,000 cholecystectomies are done annually in the United States for gallstones. There are two types of gallstones: cholesterol and pigment stones.[38, 39] In Western countries the former are more common than the latter. Pigment stones are either brown or black. Brown stones result from bile infection, while black stones are associated with hemolysis. Most patients with chronic cholecystitis and stones are women of childbearing age. The disease results from an abnormal chemical composition of bile (''lithogenic bile'') that leads to stone formation and injury to the mucosa. The wall of the gallbladder shows chronic inflammation and metaplastic mucosal changes.[47] If the gallbladder wall is markedly thickened, the surgeon should request a frozen section to exclude carcinoma.

Xanthogranulomatous cholecystitis is an uncommon form of chronic cholecystitis that resembles carcinoma both clinically and grossly but can be recognized on frozen sections.[48, 49] The inflammatory response leads to marked thickening of the wall by a poorly demarcated yellow mass measuring up to 7 cm and which may extend into the liver (Fig. 13–10). Microscopically, lipid-laden histiocytes, lymphocytes, plasma cells, and polymorphonuclear leukocytes predominate (Fig. 13–11). Foreign-body giant cells and variable degrees of fibrosis are also found. The inflammatory infiltrate appears to be a reaction to the bile that escapes from ruptured microherniations of the mucosa, so-called Rokitansky-Aschoff sinuses.

Diffuse calcification of the gallbladder gives rise to the ''porcelain gallbladder,'' which carries a 10 to 20% risk for malignant transformation.[50] Because of this, prophylactic cholecystectomy is recommended in patients with porcelain gallbladders.

About 10 to 12% of patients with chronic cholecystitis do not have gallstones. Postinflammatory stenosis or abnormalities of the cystic duct that interfere with the normal emptying of the gallbladder are possible pathogenetic mechanisms.

Biliary Fistulas

Fistulas between the biliary tract and adjacent hollow viscera usually result from stone-associated necrosis and inflammation of the gallbladder and/or bile ducts. A large inflammatory mass forms around the fistula and alters the anatomy of the region. This mass is often confused with a malignant tumor. In the presence of a biliary fistula, cholecystectomy carries a high risk for injury to the bile ducts. The most common fistulas are cholecystoduodenal, followed by cholecystocolic and choledochoduodenal.

Extrahepatic Bile Ducts

CHOLANGITIS

The inflammatory diseases of the bile ducts are classified as simple obstructive cholangitis, recurrent cholangitis syndromes, and primary sclerosing cholangitis.

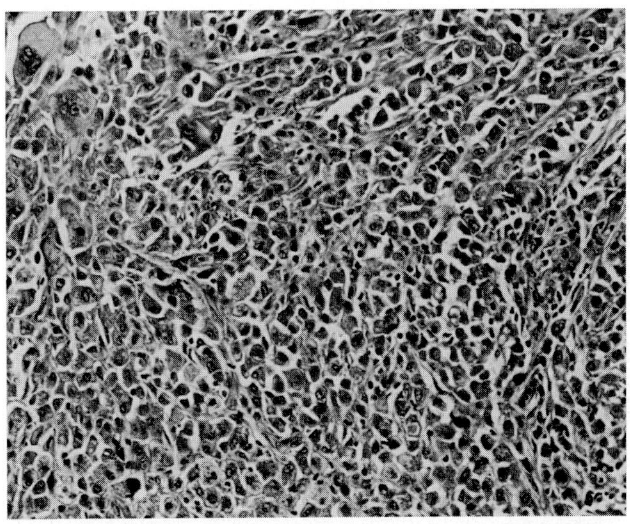

Figure 13–11. Sheets of histiocytes and a few multinucleated giant cells of foreign-body type are present in this example of xanthogranulomatous cholecystitis.

In Western countries, obstructive cholangitis is the most common type and is caused by stones, tumors, or scarring from previous surgical procedures. Most stones originate from the gallbladder and migrate into the bile ducts. The organisms most commonly found in bile are *Escherichia coli, Streptococcus faecalis, Klebsiella, Pseudomonas*, and *Proteus*. In acute obstructive cholangitis, the bile ducts show edema, neutrophilic infiltrate, epithelial erosions, and regenerative changes. In chronic obstructive cholangitis, fibrosis of the wall of the bile ducts ensues. Entrapment of glandlike structures may microscopically simulate carcinoma. However, nonneoplastic glands are arranged in a lobular pattern that is lacking in carcinoma.

Recurrent pyogenic cholangitis (also known as ''oriental cholangiohepatitis,'' ''intrahepatic pigment stone disease,'' and ''biliary obstruction syndrome of the Chinese'') was first described in Hong Kong.[51] In the United States and Canada, the disease is seen predominantly in Asian immigrants and is attributed to chronic infestation of the biliary tree with *Clonorchis sinensis* (now known as *Opisthorchis sinensis*) or *Ascaris lumbricoides*. The adult flukes, worms, or eggs produce biliary obstruction, which leads to bile stasis and bacterial infection with formation of stones. Another theory postulates that recurrent infectious gastroenteritis in malnourished people causes episodes of portal bacteremia and resultant cholangitis. Cholangiocarcinoma develops in 2 to 5% of patients with recurrent pyogenic cholangitis.

Primary sclerosing cholangitis is a rare inflammatory disorder of the intra- and extrahepatic bile ducts.[52, 53] The disease affects mainly young men and carries considerable morbidity and mortality. It is characterized by fatigue, pruritus, jaundice, and slow progression to cirrhosis. Approximately 50 to 70% of cases are associated with inflammatory bowel disease, mainly ulcerative colitis. Some studies suggest immune mechanisms in the pathogenesis of primary sclerosing cholangitis.[54–56] The extrahepatic bile ducts appear as ''fibrous cords.'' Cholangiograms reveal strictures alternating with slightly dilated segments, producing a characteristic ''beaded'' appearance.

Microscopic examination of the extrahepatic bile ducts shows a diffuse inflammatory infiltrate composed predominantly of lymphocytes and plasma cells with epithelial ulceration. Neutrophils are seen within lumens of glandlike structures. Extensive fibrosis of the wall with entrapment of glandlike structures may simulate adenocarcinoma. Primary sclerosing cholangitis is a risk factor for the development of cholangiocarcinoma, particularly when associated with ulcerative colitis.[57, 58]

NEOPLASMS

Benign Tumors of the Gallbladder and Extrahepatic Bile Ducts

Adenomas of the gallbladder are more common in women than men and are found in 0.3 to 0.5% of gallbladders removed for cholelithiasis. According to their growth pattern, these adenomas are classified as tubular, papillary, or tubulopapillary. Cytologically, they are subclassified as pyloric, intestinal, or biliary type.[59]

Adenomas of the gallbladder are small, usually single, and often found incidentally in cholecystectomy specimens.[60, 61] Rarely, they occur in association with Gardner's syndrome or with Peutz-Jegher's syndrome.[60] Their malignant potential is low. Histologically, some resemble intestinal adenomas, whereas others are composed of pyloric-type glands or biliary-type epithelium. Although adenomas of the extrahepatic bile ducts are much less common than those that arise in the gallbladder, they mimic malignant tumors clinically because of resulting biliary obstruction. Histologically, they are similar to neoplasms of the gallbladder.

Granular-cell tumors of the extrahepatic bile ducts are a rare cause of obstruction; they may simulate carcinomas clinically and by imaging techniques.[60] Microscopically, granular-cell tumors can also be confused with malignant tumors because they may extend into the periductal connective tissue, around nerves, and even into adjacent lymph nodes.[61] This is compounded by the fact that these tumors can be multicentric. Carcinoid tumors only rarely originate in the gallbladder and extrahepatic bile ducts.[62]

Carcinoma of the Gallbladder and Extrahepatic Bile Ducts

Although carcinomas of the gallbladder and extrahepatic bile ducts are histologically similar, they differ in their epidemiology, clinical presentation, risk factors, and etiology. They should therefore be considered two separate diseases (Table 13–2). The prevalence of carcinoma of the gallbladder varies in different parts of the world and even in different ethnic groups within the same country. In the United States, for example, this tumor is more common in American Indians and Mexican Americans than in whites or in African Americans.[38] There is no geographic or ethnic variation in the incidence of extrahepatic bile duct carcinoma. The incidence of carcinoma of the gallbladder correlates with the incidence of cholelithiasis. No such correlation exists for extrahepatic bile duct carcinoma, which is seen more often in patients with ulcerative colitis and primary sclerosing cholangitis.[58] Carcinomas of the gallbladder show a strong female predominance, whereas extrahepatic bile duct carcinomas are slightly more common among males. The dominant and initial sign of extrahepatic bile duct cancer is jaundice, which occurs in more than 90% of patients.[63] The symptoms of gallbladder carcinoma are usually those of preexisting cholecystitis with cholelithiasis. Cholangiography is essential for the diagnosis of extrahepatic bile duct carcinoma, whereas ultrasound and CT scan are useful tools for the preoperative detection and staging of gallbladder carcinoma.

Approximately 10 to 15% of invasive gallbladder carcinomas are inconspicuous on gross examination. The macroscopic features in these cases are similar to those of chronic cholecystitis. Surgeons should request frozen sections of gallbladders removed for cholelithiasis but found to have a very thickened wall. Gallbladder carcinomas originate in the fundus in 60% of cases, the body in 30% of cases, and the neck in 10% of cases (Figs. 13–12 and 13–13).

According to their gross features, carcinomas of the extrahepatic bile ducts are classified as nodular, polypoid,

Table 13–2. Comparison of Gallbladder and Extrahepatic Bile Duct Carcinomas

	Gallbladder	Extrahepatic Bile Ducts
Geographic variation in incidence	Yes	No
More common in certain ethnic groups	Yes	No
Female predominance	Yes	No
Associated with stones	Yes	No
Increased incidence with ulcerative colitis and primary sclerosing cholangitis	No	Yes
Biliary obstruction is usually the initial sign	No	Yes
Cholangiography essential to diagnosis	No	Yes
Adenocarcinoma the most common histologic type	Yes	Yes
Elevated serum CEA	Yes	Yes
Poor prognosis	Yes	Yes

or diffusely infiltrating. Not infrequently, however, there is only a focal thickening or an induration of the wall with partial obstruction of the bile duct, showing a roughened or granular mucosa. This type of carcinoma can be easily overlooked by both surgeons and pathologists. It is reported that carcinoma of the bile ducts is missed in up to 20% of patients at the time of initial surgical exploration for obstructive jaundice. This is a problem area for surgeon and pathologist alike. Obtaining intraoperative biopsies of high proximal carcinomas may be extremely difficult. Pathologic interpretation is difficult due to the presence of benign, glandlike structures in the walls of the bile ducts that can simulate carcinoma. Retrograde cholangiography with cytologic brushing sampling can sometimes successfully detect carcinoma in this site preoperatively.

Prognosis of gallbladder and extrahepatic bile duct carcinoma is poor. The two most important prognostic factors are pathologic stage and histologic grade of the tumor (see Tables 13–3 and 13–4).[64–66] Patients with in situ carcinoma of the gallbladder are cured by cholecystectomy. For patients with carcinoma limited to the gallbladder wall, the 5-year survival rate is 32%. Patients with direct extension to adjacent organs or hepatic metastases die soon after the diagnosis is made. Patients with papillary adenocarcinoma have the best survival because these tumors grow into the lumen and infiltrate the gallbladder wall late in their course. Although carcinomas of the extrahepatic bile ducts are better differentiated than carcinomas of the gallbladder, they have a worse prognoses, probably in relation to lack of resectability. The 5-year survival rate for patients with stage I disease was 11% in the largest series recorded so far.[65] Patients with tumors located in the distal third of the common bile duct do better than those with tumors that arise in the proximal ductal system.

Pancreas

BIOPSY TECHNIQUES

Because carcinoma of the pancreas can be confused with chronic pancreatitis, and because both diseases often coexist in the same pancreas, biopsy is imperative to establish the correct diagnosis.[67, 68] Moreover, a great variety of neoplasms (some benign, others of low malignant potential) originate in the pancreas and must be differentiated from the highly lethal ductal carcinomas.

Cytologic examination of pancreatic secretions and brushings obtained during endoscopic retrograde cholangiopancreatography after secretion stimulation has produced limited diagnostic success. Because of its high sensitivity and specificity, CT- or ultrasound-guided FNA is now the

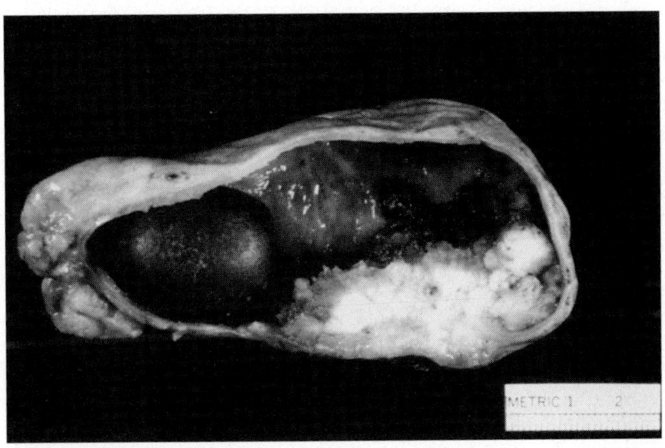

Figure 13–12. Carcinoma of the gallbladder. The polypoid and infiltrating tumor involves the fundus and body of the gallbladder, which contains stones.

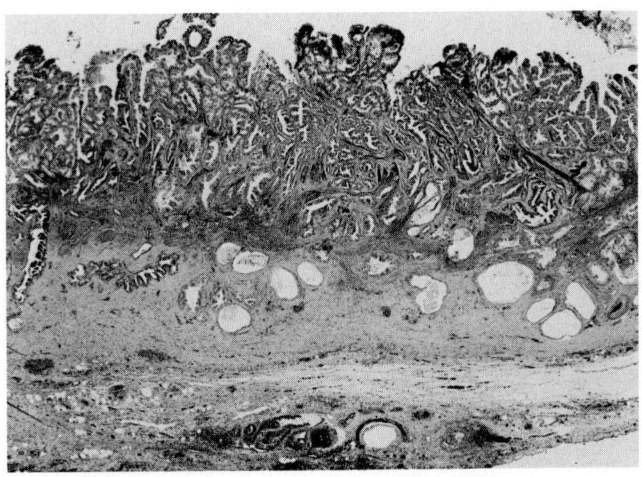

Figure 13–13. Well-differentiated adenocarcinoma of the gallbladder infiltrating the full thickness of the wall.

Table 13–3. TNM Classification and Staging of Gallbladder Tumors

Primary Tumor (T)

TX	Primary tumor cannot be assessed
T0	No evidence of primary tumor
Tis	Carcinoma in situ
TI	Tumor invades mucosa or muscle layer
	T1a Tumor invades the mucosa
	T1b Tumor invades the muscle layer
T2	Tumor invades the perimuscular connective tissue; no extension beyond the serosa or into the liver
T3	Tumor perforates the serosa (visceral peritoneum), directly invades into one adjacent organ, or both (extension 2 cm or less into the liver)
T4	Tumor extends more than 2 cm into the liver and/or into two or more adjacent organs (stomach, duodenum, colon, pancreas, omentum, extrahepatic bile ducts, any involvement of liver)

Regional Lymph Nodes (N)

NX	Regional lymph nodes cannot be assessed
N0	No regional lymph node metastasis
N1	Metastasis in cystic duct, pericholedochal, and/or hilar lymph nodes (i.e., in the hepatoduodenal ligament)
N2	Metastasis in peripancreatic (head only), periduodenal, periportal, celiac, and/or superior mesenteric lymph nodes

Distant Metastasis (M)

MX	Presence of distant metastasis cannot be assessed
M0	No distant metastasis
MI	Distant metastasis

Staging Grouping

Stage 0	Tis	N0	M0
Stage I	T1	N0	M0
Stage II	T2	N0	M0
Stage III	T1	N1	M0
	T2	N1	M0
	T3	N0	M0
	T3	N1	M0
Stage IVA	T4	N0	M0
Stage IVB	Any T	N2	M0
	Any T	Any N	M1

Source: From Beahrs OH, Henson DE, Hutter RVP, Kennedy BJ, eds. *Manual for Staging of Cancer*, 4th ed. Philadelphia: Lippincott; 1992:185–186. With permission.

preoperative method of choice for the diagnosis of pancreatic cancer.[69, 70] Percutaneous transabdominal aspiration provides adequate material in 60 to 90% of the cases, depending upon the skill of the operator. If the tumor appears resectable, aspiration cytology during laparotomy is ideal. This approach allows better localization of the mass by the surgeon and provides diagnostic material in nearly all cases (Fig. 13–14).[69] Both diagnostic techniques have a low complication rate of acute pancreatitis, fistula formation, or implantation of neoplastic cells (see Chap. 3).

Assessment of peritoneal, lymph nodal, and hepatic metastases is done by intraoperative frozen sections if visibly suspect lesions are identified, prior to embarking on a Whipple's procedure or a total pancreatectomy. If metastatic disease is present, biopsy of the pancreatic mass is unnecessary. The presence of hepatic, serosal, or distant nodal metastases indicates unresectable tumor.

The diagnosis of pancreatic carcinoma should be established by cytologic or histologic means prior to a major surgical procedure. However, many surgeons perform a Whipple's procedure or a total pancreatectomy in patients with negative biopsy results, based only upon clinical evidence of carcinoma. Rarely, a Whipple's procedure or a total pancreatectomy is carried out in the patient with metastatic disease or chronic pancreatitis because of failure to secure cytologic or histologic evaluation before resection.

At present, wedge or needle core biopsies are used only infrequently for the intraoperative diagnosis of pancreatic cancer. Such biopsy methods are associated with significant morbidity and multiple samples are often necessary to obtain a definite diagnosis. Common pitfalls with frozen sections include misdiagnosis of malignancy due to hyperplastic ducts in a dense fibrous stroma and that due to perineural endocrine cells as seen in chronic pancreatitis. Both of these features closely simulate carcinoma microscopically.

PANCREATITIS

Most cases of acute pancreatitis are associated with alcoholism, biliary tract disease (stones), or trauma. Rarely, acute pancreatitis is caused by hypercalcemia due to hyperparathyroidism, hyperlipidemia, or drugs. Microscopically, acute pancreatitis may be focal or diffuse and is character-

Table 13–4. TNM Classification and Staging of Extrahepatic Bile Duct Tumors

Primary Tumor (T)

TX	Primary tumor cannot be assessed
T0	No evidence of primary tumor
Tis	Carcinoma in situ
	T1 Tumor invades the mucosa or muscle layer
	T1a Tumor invades the mucosa
	T1b Tumor invades the muscle layer
T2	Tumor invades the perimuscular connective tissue
T3	Tumor invades adjacent structures: liver, pancreas, duodenum, gallbladder, colon, stomach

Regional Lymph Nodes (N)

NX	Regional lymph nodes cannot be assessed
N0	No regional lymph node metastasis
N1	Metastasis in the cystic duct, pericholedochal and/or hilar lymph nodes (i.e., in the hepatoduodenal ligament)
N2	Metastasis in the peripancreatic (head only), periduodenal, periportal, celiac, superior mesenteric, and/or posterior pancreatic or duodenal lymph nodes

Distant Metastasis (M)

MX	Presence of distant metastasis cannot be assessed
M0	No distant metastasis
M1	Distant metastasis

Staging Grouping

Stage 0	Tis	N0	M0
Stage I	T1	N0	M0
Stage II	T2	N0	M0
Stage III	T1	N1	M0
	T1	N2	M0
	T2	N1	M0
	T2	N2	M0
Stage IVA	T3	Any N	M0
Stage IVB	Any T	Any N	M1

Source: From Beahrs OH, Henson DE, Hutter RVP, Kennedy BJ, eds. *Manual for Staging of Cancer*, 4th ed. Philadelphia: Lippincott; 1992:185–186. With permission.

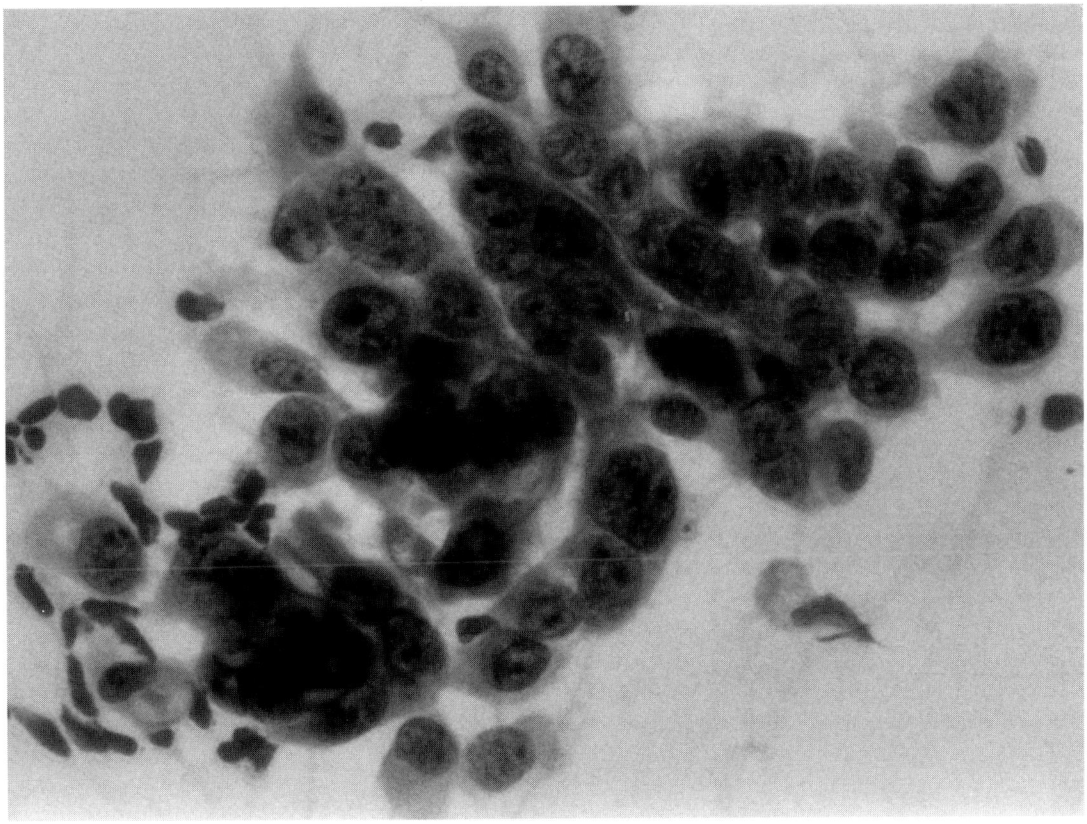

Figure 13–14. Fine needle aspirate from pancreas, obtained intraoperatively, contains clusters of malignant ductal epithelial cells.

ized by necrosis of the acinar tissue, edema, neutrophilic infiltration, and fat necrosis. Pancreatic abscess is reported in up to 5% of patients and is a serious complication of acute pancreatitis.[71] Another complication is pseudocyst formation, which appears in 5 to 10% of patients.[72] Some pseudocysts are quite large (over 15 cm in diameter) and require surgical intervention. They are composed of a fibrous wall devoid of epithelial lining. Pseudocysts can be confused clinically and radiographically with mucinous cystic neoplasms of the pancreas, and vice versa.[73, 74] Because of this, frozen section of the wall of the cyst should be performed to determine the nature of the cyst and avoid drainage procedures, which are inappropriate therapy for cystic neoplasms of the pancreas.

Chronic pancreatitis is most often the result of obstruction of the main pancreatic duct by tumor or fibrosis.[75, 76] Cases of familial chronic pancreatitis have also been documented. Histologically, there is atrophy of the acinar tissue, fibrosis, ductal proliferation, and chronic inflammatory infiltrate. In some cases extensive calcification occurs.[67]

NEOPLASMS

Adenocarcinoma (Pancreatic and Periampullary)

In the United States, ductal carcinoma of the exocrine pancreas is the ninth most common malignancy and the second most common gastrointestinal cancer, being surpassed only by colorectal cancer.[77] Pancreatic carcinoma is responsible for 5% of all cancer deaths. Metastatic disease is often present by the time the diagnosis is made. Of patients with tumors 2 cm or less in size, 61% have lymph node metastasis at surgery (Table 13–5). The frequency of this neoplasm appears to be increasing, especially among black females.[77] Ductal carcinoma of the pancreas is highly lethal.[78, 79] Approximately 95% of patients die within 2 years of diagnosis. With the aid of CT, MRI, and ultrasound, radiologists can detect pancreatic carcinomas of 2 cm or larger; however, even sophisticated imaging techniques fail to detect truly early-stage disease (see Tables 13–5 and 13–6).[80, 81] Differentiating carcinoma from chronic pancreatitis remains a diagnostic problem.

Grossly, these tumors are firm, gray-white masses with poorly defined borders. Extensive necrosis and cystic degeneration are uncommon features of conventional ductal carcinomas but may be seen in giant-cell carcinomas and in some endocrine carcinomas. Ductal carcinomas arise most commonly in the head, followed by the body and tail of the pancreas. Mutations of the K-*ras* oncogene are found in about 90% of cases.[82] A small number of pancreatic carcinomas are familial and inherited as an autosomal dominant trait.[68] Ductal adenocarcinoma is the most common histologic type, accounting for 90% of all malignant tumors of the pancreas (Fig. 13–15). Other types include adenosquamous, mucinous, and giant-cell carcinomas. Carcinomas composed of cells with acinar phenotype are quite rare despite the fact that acinar cells form over 95% of the cell mass of the pancreas.[83]

Of particular interest to the surgeon is the rare intraductal

Table 13–5. TNM Classification and Staging of Tumors of the Pancreas

Primary Tumor (T)
- TX Primary tumor cannot be assessed
- T0 No evidence of primary tumor
- T1 Tumor limited to the pancreas
  - T1a Tumor 2 cm or less in greatest dimension
  - T1b Tumor more than 2 cm in greatest dimension
- T2 Tumor extends directly to any of the following: duodenum, bile duct, or peripancreatic tissues
- T3 Tumor extends directly to any of the following: duodenum, stomach, spleen, colon, or adjacent large vessels

Lymph Node (N)
- NX Regional lymph nodes cannot be assessed
- N0 No regional lymph node metastasis
- N1 Regional lymph node metastasis

Distant Metastasis (M)
- MX Presence of distant metastasis cannot be assessed
- M0 No distant metastasis
- M1 Distant metastasis

Staging Grouping

I	T1	N0	M0
	T2	N0	M0
II	T3	N0	M0
III	Any T	N1	M0
IV	Any T	Any N	M1

Source: From Beahrs OH, Henson DE, Hutter RVP, Kennedy BJ, eds. *Manual for Staging of Cancer,* 4th ed. Philadelphia: Lippincott; 1992:185–186. With permission.

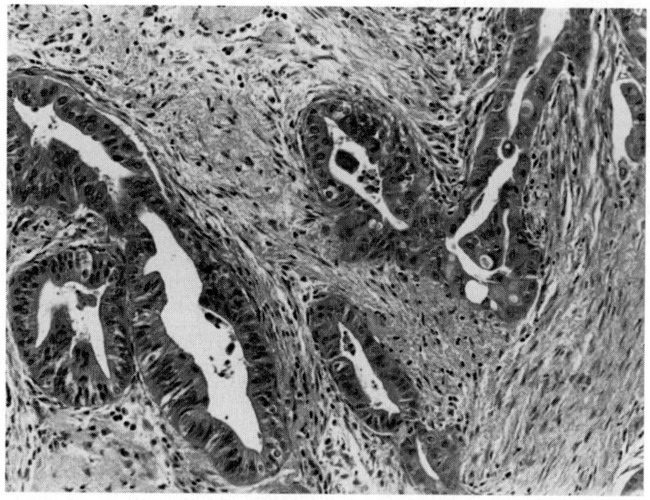

Figure 13–15. Photomicrograph of ductal carcinoma of the pancreas, the most common form of pancreatic cancer. Abnormal ducts featuring dark, atypical epithelium are surrounded by cellular fibrous stroma.

mucin-producing papillary carcinoma. These tumors remain confined to the major pancreatic duct for several years and can therefore be cured by the Whipple's procedure or total pancreatectomy.[84–86] Eventually some of these tumors infiltrate the stroma and behave as conventional ductal carcinomas. Most patients are men older than 50 years with a long history of symptoms suggesting chronic pancreatitis. The tumors usually arise in the cephalic portion of the main pancreatic duct but extend to smaller ducts in a retrograde fashion or by multifocality. K-*ras* mutations have been identified by molecular pathology techniques in some of these intraductal neoplasms. They are composed of cuboidal or columnar cells with minimal, moderate, or marked nuclear atypia. They may produce abundant mucin with marked dilatation of the ducts and may thus be confused with mucinous cystic neoplasms (Table 13–6).

Table 13–6. Comparison Between Intraductal Papillary Carcinoma and Mucinous Cystic Neoplasms of the Pancreas

	IPC	MCN
Origin from ductal epithelium	Yes	Yes
Intestinal differentiation	Yes	Yes
Abundant mucin production	Yes	Yes
Malignant and "benign" cells	Yes	Yes
Ovarianlike stroma	No	Yes
Estrogen and progesterone receptors	No	Yes
More common among females	No	Yes
Often located in the tail	No	Yes
Multiloculated cystic mass	No	Yes
Connected to ducts	Yes	No

Cystic neoplasms of the pancreas are divided into three types according to their microscopic features and biologic behavior: mucinous, microcystic adenoma, and papillary and cystic tumors.[73, 84, 87] Mucinous cystic neoplasms of the pancreas are usually large, multiloculated, and more common in middle-aged females (Fig. 13–16). About 65% of the tumors arise in the tail of the pancreas. Cystadenomas tend to be smaller than cystadenocarcinomas and borderline tumors (Fig. 13–17).

Glycogen-rich microcystic adenomas are almost invariably benign and are more common in the head than the tail of the pancreas. These are seen in females in the sixth decade. Their size varies from 2 to 20 cm, with a mean diameter of 10 cm (Fig. 13–18). They are composed of cuboidal clear periodic acid-Schiff (PAS)-positive cells that line small cystic spaces (Fig. 13–19). Mucinous cystic neoplasms are subdivided into cystadenomas, which follow a benign clinical course; borderline tumors (tumors of low malignant potential), of which only a small proportion recur or metastasize; and cystadenocarcinomas, which recur or metastasize in about 40 to 50% of the cases. Some believe that CT findings are sufficiently distinctive to allow radiologic separation of mucinous cystic tumors from pseudocysts and microcystic adenomas. However, mucinous cystic neoplasms are still confused with pseudocysts, despite claims to the contrary.[73] Fine needle aspiration allows distinction of mucinous tumors from glycogen-rich microcystic adenomas. The aspirates of the former tumor usually contain abundant mucin and high concentration of CEA, whereas the aspirates of glycogen-rich microcystic adenomas show clear fluid that does not contain CEA. Fine needle aspiration biopsy of cystadenomas shows clusters or sheets of benign epithelial cells with vacuolated cytoplasm. In borderline mucinous tumors and cystadenocarcinomas, at least some of the epithelial cells show large, hyperchromatic nuclei and vacuolated cytoplasm. Aspirates of microcystic adenomas contain few cuboidal cells with clear cytoplasm and a small, centrally placed round nu-

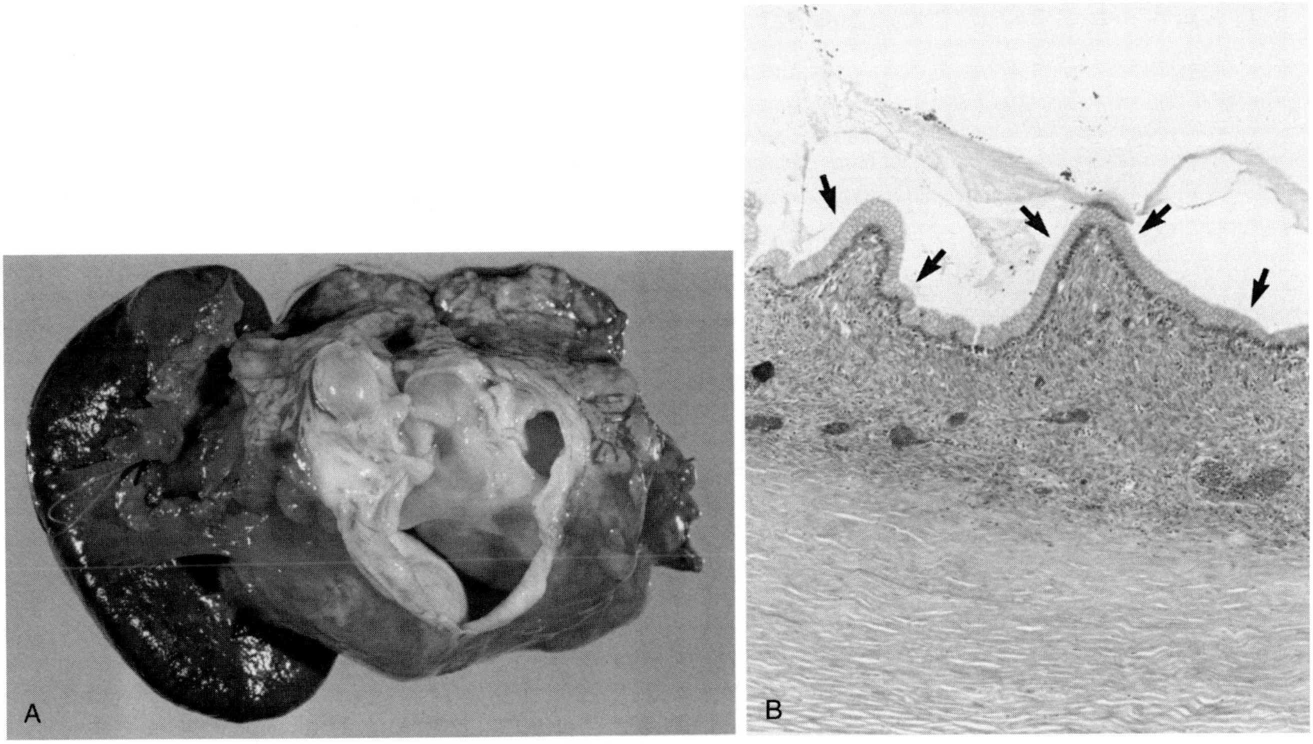

Figure 13–16. *A*, Mucinous cystadenoma of the tail of the pancreas. The tumor is multilocular, has a smooth inner surface, and was resected together with the spleen. *B*, The wall of a mucinous cystadenoma is lined by well-differentiated, tall columnar epithelium *(arrows)* and contains an ovarylike stroma and dense fibrous tissue.

cleus. The cytology of papillary and cystic tumors consists of papillary fronds lined by one or more layers of cuboidal cells with round eccentric nuclei having finely granular chromatin. Small nucleoli may be present. Histologically, mucinous cystadenomas are lined by a benign mucinous epithelium. In borderline tumors the lining epithelium shows focal areas of carcinoma in situ alternating with benign-appearing mucinous epithelium. Cystadenocarcinomas are malignant gland-forming tumors that infiltrate the stroma. Extensive sampling is recommended in cystadenomas and borderline tumors so as to exclude foci of invasive carcinoma.

Papillary cystic tumors occur almost exclusively in adolescent girls or young females.[88] The majority of these tumors are benign and more often affect the body or tail than the head of the pancreas. They may reach a large size (average 10 cm) and may be asymptomatic. Pancreatoblastoma is a rare malignant pancreatic tumor of childhood that may produce an elevation of serum alpha-fetoprotein.

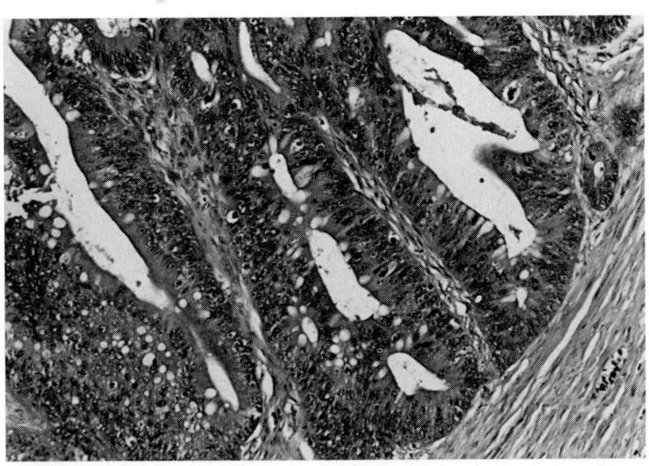

Figure 13–17. Cystadenocarcinoma of the pancreas. Neoplastic glands infiltrate the wall of the cyst. Compare pattern to that of a ductal carcinoma (Fig. 13–15).

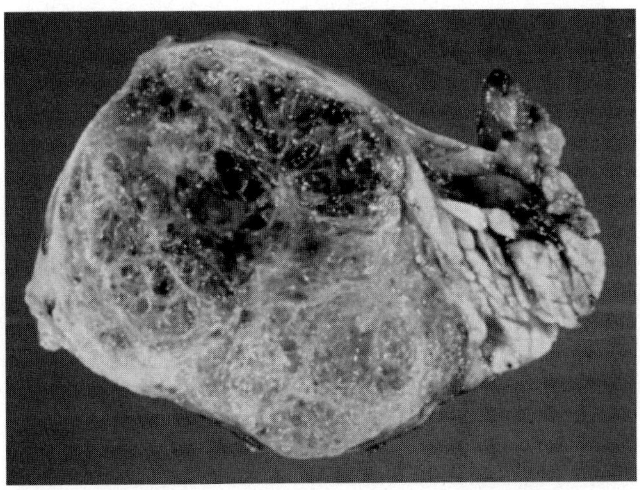

Figure 13–18. Microcystic adenoma of the pancreas. A nodular mass is composed of small cystic structures.

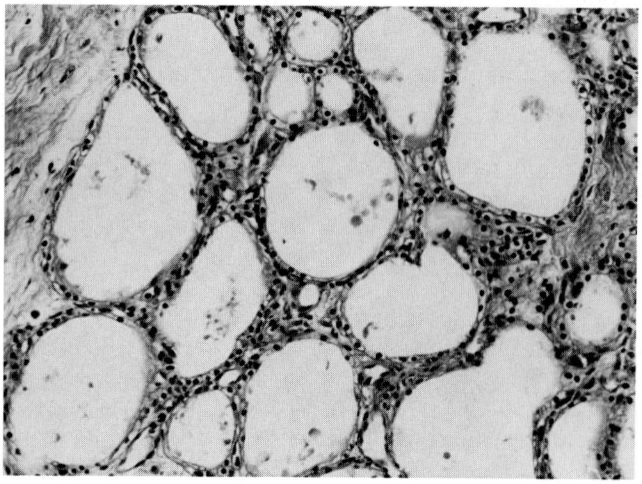

Figure 13–19. Small cystic structures of a microcystic adenoma are lined by cuboidal cells with clear cells containing glycogen.

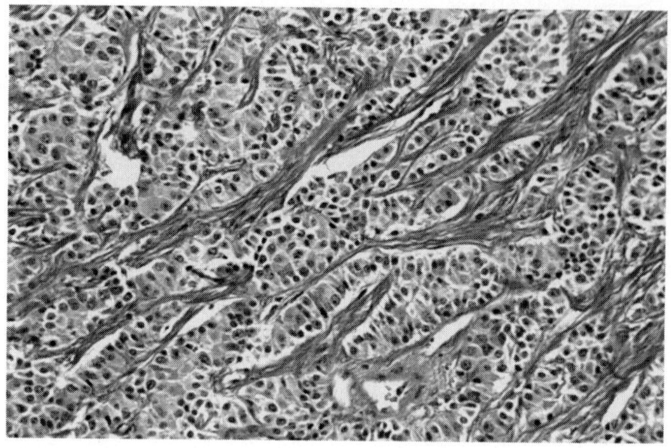

Figure 13–21. Alpha-cell (glucagon-producing) tumor of the pancreas with a prominent trabecular growth pattern.

Endocrine Tumors

Because of their hormonal secretion and the corresponding systemic manifestations, endocrine tumors of the pancreas fascinate both clinicians and pathologists. Clinicopathologic correlation and immunohistochemical assessment are essential to understand the pathobiology of these unusual neoplasms, which are an integral component of multiple endocrine neoplasia type I (MEN I).[89] Malignancy is difficult to evaluate on histologic grounds alone. Extension beyond the pancreas, blood vessel invasion, and metastases are the best indicators of malignant behavior. Even malignant tumors usually pursue long clinical course and are less aggressive than the exocrine carcinomas. Functioning endocrine tumors account for 60 to 80% of all pancreatic endocrine neoplasms. Many of the clinically nonfunctioning tumors contain peptide hormones when studied by immunohistochemical techniques, indicating that they synthesize hormones. However, for a number of reasons, they do not cause a clinical syndrome. Although these tumors are usually associated with a single predominant hormone, immunohistochemical stains show that most endocrine pancreatic tumors actually feature several cell types that produce more than one hormone. Despite this, mixed endocrine syndromes are exceedingly rare. Beta-cell tumors (insulinomas) are the most common functioning tumors of the pancreas (Figs. 13–20 and 13–21). They produce hypoglycemia and hyperinsulinemia. Some tumors also produce excessive amounts of proinsulin and C-peptide. The great majority (90%) of beta-cell tumors are benign, small (usually less than 2 cm), and solitary. Some 1 to 3% are multiple and associated with MEN I. In contrast to beta-cell tumors (insulinomas), alpha-cell tumors (glucagonomas) are usually malignant and produce a characteristic syndrome that includes elevated serum glucagon levels, a necrolytic migratory erythema, diabetes, glossitis, normocytic anemia, and a tendency to develop vein thrombosis. A small proportion of nonfunctioning glucagonomas are associated with MEN I.

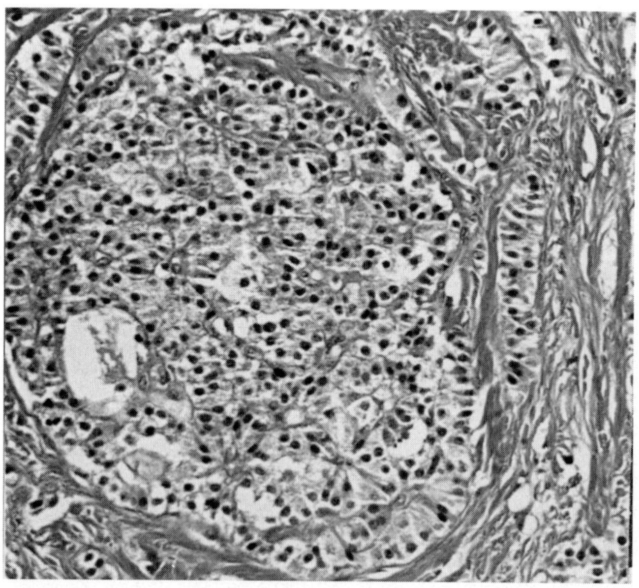

Figure 13–20. Beta-cell (insulin-producing) tumor of the pancreas showing a nodule of neoplastic cells, reminiscent of a pancreatic islet.

G-cell tumors (gastrinomas) are associated with the Zollinger-Ellison's syndrome and are characterized by gastric acid hypersecretion, peptic ulcers in the stomach or small intestine, diarrhea, and elevated serum gastrin levels. Gastrinomas can also occur in the duodenum and stomach, where they are often overlooked because of their small size. The majority of pancreatic gastrinomas are malignant, while gastric and duodenal gastrinomas rarely metastasize. Most patients with pancreatic gastrinomas are adult males in the fourth or fifth decade of life.

Somatostatin-producing tumors (D-cell tumors) are exceedingly rare. They give rise to a clinical syndrome (somatostatinoma) characterized by diabetes mellitus, steatorrhea, diarrhea, cholelithiasis, and elevated serum somatostatin levels. To date, all pancreatic tumors have occurred in adult patients and have followed a malignant clinical course. Extrapancreatic somatostatinomas arise more commonly in the duodenum or ampulla of Vater. In this location they are usually small, nonfunctioning, and clinically less aggressive tumors.

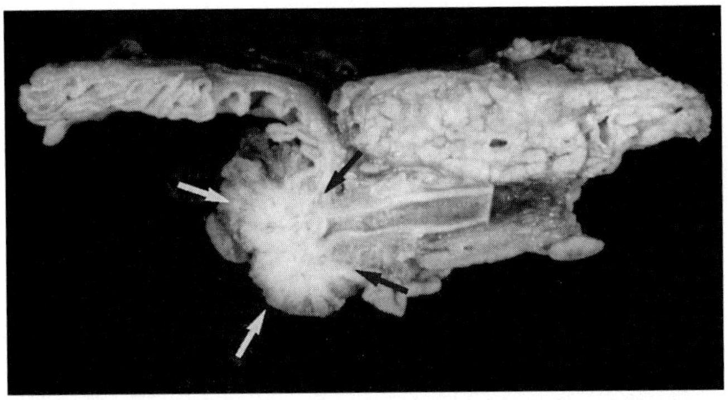

Figure 13–22. Adenocarcinoma of the ampulla of Vater. The tumor *(arrows)* arose in the duodenal mucosa and extended into the common channel.

Tumors that produce excessive amounts of vasoactive intestinal peptide (VIP) give rise to the Verner-Morrison's syndrome, characterized by watery diarrhea, hypokalemia, and achlorhydria. The massive loss of potassium results in muscle weakness, renal tubular changes, and a diabetic glucose tolerance curve. These tumors (VIPOMAS) occur more often in females than in males and are usually large and malignant. The Verner-Morrison's syndrome has also been reported in association with extrapancreatic neoplasms, including ganglioneuromas and ganglioneuroblastomas.

Endocrine tumors of the pancreas that synthesize predominantly pancreatic polypeptide are clinically nonfunctioning tumors. Their importance lies in their common association with MEN I. In this clinical setting, the tumors are usually small and multiple. Pancreatic endocrine tumors have been described in patients with the von Hippel-Lindau's syndrome or with familial pheochromocytoma. Carcinoids and small-cell carcinomas are exceedingly rare endocrine tumors of the pancreas that have been associated with the carcinoid syndrome and Cushing's syndrome, respectively.

Ampullary Tumors

Ampullary neoplasms may arise from the duodenal mucosa, the common channel, the most distal portion of the common bile duct, or the pancreatic duct (Fig. 13–22, Table 13–7). When the site of origin cannot be determined with certainty, the term ''periampullary neoplasm'' or ''periampullary carcinoma'' is employed. Identification of an in situ component suggests the site of origin of the tumor. However, invasive carcinomas arising in the duodenal mucosa may show carcinoma in situ in the common channel, pancreatic or common bile ducts, and vice versa. Tubular and villous adenomas usually arise from the duodenal mucosa and may extend into the common channel. These benign epithelial tumors are either sporadic or represent a component of familial polyposis or Gardner's syndrome. Since adenocarcinomas frequently arise at the base of the adenomas, small endoscopic biopsies often miss the malignant component. The most common malignant tumors are well- to moderately differentiated adenocarcinomas. However, many other histologic types have been reported, including adenosquamous carcinomas, adenocarcinomas with sarcomatoid features, and small-cell carcinomas. Carcinoid tumors, especially nonfunctioning somatostatinomas, are also found in this region and may be associated with MEN I or with neurofibromatosis.[90, 91]

Table 13–7. TNM Classification and Staging of Tumors of the Ampulla

Primary Tumor (T)

TX	Primary tumor cannot be assessed
T0	No evidence of primary tumor
Tis	Carcinoma in situ
T1	Tumor limited to the ampulla of Vater
T2	Tumor invades the duodenal wall
T3	Tumor invades 2 cm or less into the pancreas
T4	Tumor invades more than 2 cm into the pancreas and/or into other adjacent organs

Regional Lymph Nodes (N)

NX	Regional lymph nodes cannot be assessed
N0	No regional lymph node metastasis
N1	Regional lymph node metastasis

Distant Metastasis (M)

MX	Presence of distant metastasis cannot be assessed
M0	No distant metastasis
M1	Distant metastasis

Staging Grouping

Stage 0	Tis	N0	M0
Stage I	T1	N0	M0
Stage II	T2	N0	M0
	T3	N0	M0
Stage III	T1	N1	M0
	T2	N1	M0
	T3	N1	M0
Stage IV	T4	Any N	M0
	Any T	Any N	M1

Source: From Beahrs OH, Henson DE, Hutter RVP, Kennedy BJ, eds. *Manual for Staging of Cancer,* 4th ed. Philadelphia: Lippincott; 1992:185–186. With permission.

The small glands and ducts present within the muscularis of the duodenum may be mistaken for adenocarcinoma in frozen sections, particularly if they are hyperplastic. These structures are usually arranged in lobules and the lining epithelial cells lack nuclear atypia, features that allow distinction from adenocarcinoma. Nevertheless, interpretation of frozen sections from this region is notoriously difficult and requires a thorough understanding of the microscopic anatomy peculiar to this site.

Examination of the Whipple's Specimen

The pathologist should dissect along the common bile duct and the main pancreatic duct and determine whether the latter joins with the distal portion of the common bile duct or empties directly into the duodenum. Sections for histologic examination should include the tumor, duodenal mucosa, common channel, common bile duct, main pancreatic duct, pancreas, and stomach. All peripancreatic and retroduodenal lymph nodes should be examined histologically. The most important margins are usually the proximal common bile duct and the plane of pancreatic transection. The gastric and duodenal margins are nearly always free of tumor in standard Whipple's resections. However, these margins are of great importance in the pylorus-preserving pancreaticoduodenectomy specimens.

PITFALLS FOR THE SURGEON

1. Performance of large needle or incisional biopsy of hemangiomas or other highly vascular lesions with high risk of bleeding. Fine needle aspiration biopsy is infrequently indicated, but it is probably not as dangerous.
2. Proceeding with resection of hepatic lesions without histologic exclusion of focal nodular hyperplasia. For this lesion, resection is indicated only for symptomatic or enlarging lesions.
3. Performance of open drainage of liver abscesses without prior exclusion of hydatid, echinococcal, or amebic lesions. This often includes a therapeutic trial with antiamebic agents.
4. Proceeding with resection of hepatic malignancies in patients with compromised hepatic function, including extensive resections in aged patients. Aged hepatic tissue has little functional margin.
5. Failure to examine the gallbladder at the time of cholecystectomy to detect malignant lesions that may require more extensive local resection.
6. Missing the diagnosis of hydrops of the gallbladder because of mild localized symptoms and findings. Such situations usually progress to acute cholecystitis, with its associated increased morbidity.
7. Failure to institute expeditious drainage by either operative or endoscopic intervention in patients with ascending cholangitis.
8. Failure to pursue the diagnosis of extrahepatic biliary tumors intraoperatively in patients with jaundice unexplained by obvious distal tumors or choledocholithiasis.
9. Performance of a cyst-enteric drainage for the presumed diagnosis of pancreatic pseudocyst without biopsy and frozen section of the cyst wall to confirm the nonneoplastic diagnosis.
10. Failure to differentiate mucinous and glycogen-rich cystic neoplasms of the pancreas in determining the need for resection, especially in those lesions involving the pancreatic head.
11. Proceeding with pancreaticoduodenectomy without thoroughly sampling enlarged lymph nodes outside the field of resection and, in the event that lymph nodes are negative, not attempting cytologic diagnosis of the lesion by FNA. Occasionally, resection is indicated for highly suspicious, possibly curable lesions without prior cytologic or histologic confirmation of malignancy.
12. Failure to thoroughly examine the duodenum for small intraluminal gastrinomas in patients with hypergastrinemia and without evidence of gastrinoma in the pancreas.

PITFALLS FOR THE PATHOLOGIST

1. Attempting to distinguish by FNA biopsy between hepatocellular adenoma with atypia and well-differentiated hepatocellular carcinoma.
2. Inability to distinguish poorly differentiated hepatocellular carcinoma from metastatic carcinoma by FNA or core needle biopsy.
3. Mistaking cholangiocarcinoma for metastatic adenocarcinoma or vice versa by FNA or core needle biopsy.
4. Mistaking xanthogranulomatous cholecystitis for malignant fibrous histiocytoma on the basis of fibrous and histiocytic composition and the presence of a large and poorly defined tumorlike mass.
5. Failing to provide information about depth of invasion in carcinomas of the gallbladder.
6. Mistaking reactive atypia, hyperplastic, and metaplastic lesions of the gallbladder for carcinoma.

Continued

7. Mistaking chronic pancreatitis with marked ductal proliferation for carcinoma of the pancreas.
8. Inadequately sampling large mucinous cystic neoplasms to exclude stromal infiltration (malignancy).
9. Failing to provide information about the surgical margins and lymph node metastases in specimens from the Whipple's procedure for carcinoma.

FURTHER READING

Henson DE, Albores-Saavedra J. *Pathology of Incipient Neoplasia*, 2nd ed. Philadelphia: Saunders; 1993.

Jessurun J, Albores-Saavedra J. *Pathology of the Gallbladder and Extrahepatic Bile Ducts*. In: Damjanov I, Linder J, eds. *Anderson's Pathology*. St. Louis: Mosby-Year Book. In press.

REFERENCES

1. Bell DA, Carr CP, Szyfelbein WM. Fine needle aspiration cytology of focal liver lesions: Results obtained with examination of both cytologic and histologic preparations. *Acta Cytol*. 1986;30:397–402.
2. Frey CF, Zhu Y, Suzuki M, Isaji S. Liver abscess. *Surg Clin North Am*. 1989;69:259–271.
3. Srivastava ED, Mayberry JF. Pyogenic liver abscess: A review of aetiology, diagnosis and intervention. *Dig Dis*. 1990;8:287–293.
4. McDonald MI, Corey GR, Gallis HA, et al. Single and multiple pyogenic liver abscesses: Natural history, diagnosis and treatment with emphasis on percutaneous drainage. *Medicine*. 1984;63:291–302.
5. Adams EB, MacLeod IN. Invasive amebiasis: II. Amebic liver abscess and its complications. *Medicine*. 1977;56:325–334.
6. De Cock KM, Reynolds TB. Amebic and pyogenic liver abscess. In: Schiff L, Schiff ER, eds. *Disease of the Liver*, 6th ed. Philadelphia: Lippincott; 1987;1235–1253.
7. Milutinovic J, Fialkow PJ, Rudd TG, et al. Liver cysts in patients with autosomal dominant polycystic kidney disease. *Am J Med*. 1980;68:741–743.
8. Ishak KG, Willis GW, Cummins SD, Bullock AA. Biliary cystadenoma and cystadenocarcinoma: Report of 14 cases and review of the literature. *Cancer* 1977;38:322–338.
9. Wheeler DA, Edmondson HA. Cystadenoma with mesenchymal stroma (CMS) in the liver and bile ducts: A clinicopathologic study of 17 cases, 4 with malignant change. *Cancer*. 1985;56:1434.
10. Craig JR, Peters RL, Edmondson HA. Tumors of the liver and intrahepatic bile ducts. In: Hartman WH, ed. *Atlas of Tumor Pathology*, 2nd series. Fascicle 26. Washington, DC: Armed Forces Institute of Pathology; 1989.
11. Ishak KG. Benign tumors and pseudotumors of the liver. *Appl Pathol*. 1988;6:82–104.
12. Leese T, Farges O, Bismuth H. Liver cell adenomas: A 12-year experience from a specialist hepato-biliary unit. *Ann Surg*. 1988;208:558–564.
13. Model DG, Fox JA, Jones RW. Multiple hepatic adenomas associated with an oral contraceptive. *Lancet*. 1975;1:865.
14. Wheeler DA, Edmondson HA, Reynold TB. Spontaneous liver cell adenoma in children. *Am J Clin Pathol*. 1986;85:6–12.
15. Flowers BF, McBurney RP, Vera SR. Ruptured hepatic adenoma: A spectrum of presentation and treatment. *Am Surg*. 1990;56:380–383.
16. Buhler H, Pirovino M, Akovbiantz A, et al. Regression of liver cell adenoma: A follow-up study of three consecutive patients after discontinuation of oral contraceptive use. *Gastroenterology*. 1982;82:775–782.
17. Edmondson HA, Reynolds TB, Henderson B, et al. Regression of liver cell adenomas associated with oral contraceptives. *Ann Intern Med*. 1977;86:180.
18. Steinbrecher UP, Lisbona R, Huang SN. Complete regression of hepatocellular adenoma after withdrawal of oral contraceptives. *Dig Dis Sci*. 1981;26:1045–1050.
19. Choi BI, Han MC, Kim CW. Small hepatocellular carcinoma versus small cavernous hemangioma: Differentiation with MR imaging at 2.0 T_1. *Radiology*. 1990;176:103–106.
20. Terriff BA, Gibney RG, Scudamore CH. Fatality from fine needle aspiration biopsy of hepatic hemangioma. *AJR*. 1990;154:203–204.
21. Ishak KG, Sesterhenn IA, Goodman ZD, et al. Epithelioid hemangioendothelioma of the liver: A clinicopathologic and follow-up study of 32 cases. *Hum Pathol*. 1984;165:839–852.
22. Allaire GS, Rabin L, Ishak KG, et al. Bile duct adenoma: A study of 152 cases. *Am J Surg Pathol*. 1988;12:708–715.
23. Edmonson HA, Steiner PE. Primary carcinoma of the liver: A study of 100 cases among 48,900 necropsies. *Cancer*. 1954;7:462.
24. Wands JR, Blum HE. Primary hepatocellular carcinoma. *N Engl J Med*. 1991;325:729–731.
25. Yoshimichi H, Norio H, Kamada T, et al. Expression of hepatitis C virus in hepatocellular carcinoma. *Cancer*. 1994;73:2253–2258.
26. Yuki N, Hayashi N, Kasahara A, et al. Hepatitis B virus markers and antibodies to hepatitis C virus in Japanese patients with hepatocellular carcinoma. *Dig Dis Sci*. 1992;37:65–72.
27. Kanai T, Hiroshashi S, Upton MP, et al. Pathology of small hepatocellular carcinoma. *Cancer*. 1987;60:810–819.
28. Li GH, Li JQ. Localization of small liver tumors. *J Surg Oncol*. 1990;44:115–118.
29. Bottles K, Cohen MB, Holley EA, et al. A stepwise logistic regression analysis of hepatocellular carcinoma: An aspiration biopsy study. *Cancer*. 1988;62:558–563.
30. Sangalli G, Livraghi T, Giordano F. Fine needle biopsy of hepatocellular carcinoma: Improvement in diagnosis by microhistology. *Gastroenterology*. 1989;96:524–526.
31. Brandt DJ, Johnson CD, Stepheans DH, et al. Fibrolamellar hepatocellular carcinoma. *Radiology*. 1985;157:583–587.
32. Craig JR, Peters RL, Edmondson HA, et al. Fibrolamellar carcinoma of the liver: A tumor of adolescents and young adults with distinctive clinico-pathologic features. *Cancer*. 1980;46:372.
33. Saul SH, Titelbaum DS, Gansler TS, et al. The fibrolamellar variant of hepatocellular carcinoma: Its association with focal nodular hyperplasia. *Cancer*. 1987;60:3049–3055.
34. Lack EE, Neave C, Vawter GF. Hepatoblastoma. A clinical and pathologic study of 54 cases. *Am J Surg Pathol*. 1982;6:693–705.
35. Manivel C, Wick MR, Abenoza P, Dehner LP. Teratoid hepatoblastoma: The nosologic dilemma of solid embryonic neoplasms of childhood. *Cancer*. 1986;57:2168–2174.
36. Nakajima T, Kondo Y, Miyazaki M, et al. A histopathologic study of 102 cases of intrahepatic cholangiocarcinoma: Histologic classification and modes of spread. *Hum Pathol*. 1988;19:1228–1234.
37. Ganjei P, Nadji M, Albores-Saavedra J, Morales AR. Histologic markers in primary and metastatic tumors of the liver. *Cancer*. 1988;62:1994–1998.
38. Maurer KR, Everhart JE, Knowler WC, et al. Risk factors for gallstone disease in the Hispanic population of the United States. *Am J Epidemiol*. 1990;131:836.
39. Paumgartner G, Sauerbruch T. Gallstones: Pathogenesis. *Lancet*. 1991;338:1117.
40. Sen M, Williamson RCN. Acute cholecystitis: Surgical management. *Bailliere's Clin Gastroenterol*. 1991;5:817.
41. Mentzer RM, Golden GT, Chandler JG, et al. A comparative appraisal of emphysematous cholecystitis. *Am J Surg*. 1975;129:10.
42. Babb RR. Acute acalculous cholecystitis: A review. *J Clin Gastroenterol*. 1992;15:238.
43. Blumberg RS, Kelsey P, Perrone T, et al. Cytomegalovirus and cryptosporidium-associated acalculous gangrenous cholecystitis. *Am J Med*. 1984;76:1118.

44. Kavin N, Jonas RB, Chowdhury L, et al. Acalculous cholecystitis and cytomegalovirus infection in the acquired immunodeficiency syndrome. *Ann Intern Med.* 1986;104:53.
45. Lebovics E, Dworkin BM, Heir SK, et al. The hepatobiliary manifestations of human immunodeficiency virus infection. *Am J Gastroenterol.* 1988;83:1.
46. Bowen JC, Benner HI, Ferrante WA, et al. Gallstone disease. Pathophysiology, epidemiology, natural history, and treatment options. *Med Clin North Am.* 1992;76:1143.
47. Albores-Saavedra J, Nadji M, Henson DE, et al. Intestinal metaplasia of the gallbladder: A morphologic and immunocytochemical study. *Hum Pathol.* 1986;17:614.
48. Goodman ZD, Ishak KG. Xanthogranulomatous cholecystitis. *Am J Surg Pathol.* 1981;5:653.
49. Howard TJ, Bennion RS, Thompson JE. Xanthogranulomatous cholecystitis: A chronic inflammatory pseudotumor of the gallbladder. *Am Surg.* 1991;57:821.
50. Ashur H, Siegal B, Oland Y, et al. Calcified gallbladder (porcelain gallbladder). *Arch Surg.* 1978;113:594.
51. Lim JH. Oriental cholangiohepatitis: Pathologic, clinical, and radiologic features. *AJR.* 1991;157.
52. LaRusso NF, Wiesner RH, Ludwig J, et al. Primary sclerosing cholangitis. *N Eng J Med.* 1984;310:899.
53. Wiesner RH, Ludwig J, LaRusso NF, et al. Diagnosis and treatment of primary sclerosing cholangitis. *Semin Liver Dis.* 1985;5:241–253.
54. Chapman RW, Varghese Z, Gaul R, et al. Association of primary sclerosing cholangitis with HLA-B8. *Gut.* 1983;24:38.
55. Lo SK, Fleming KA, Chapman RW. Prevalence of anti-neutrophil antibody in primary sclerosing cholangitis and ulcerative colitis using an alkaline phosphatase technique. *Gut.* 1992;33:1570.
56. Snook JA, Chapman RW, Fleming KA, et al. Peripheral blood and portal tract lymphocyte populations in primary sclerosing cholangitis. *J Hepatol.* 1989;9:36.
57. Maarowitz DA, Benbasset RH. Chronic postcolectomy pericholangitis and cholangiocarcinoma. *J Clin Gastroenterol.* 1985;7:323–326.
58. Mir-Madjlessi SH, Farmer RG, Sivak MV. Bile duct carcinoma in patients with ulcerative colitis. *Dig Dis Sci.* 1987;32:145.
59. Albores-Saavedra J, Vardaman C, Vuitch F. Non-neoplastic polypoid lesions and adenomas of the gallbladder. *Pathol Annu.* 1993;28(Part I):145.
60. Albores-Saavedra J, Henson DE. Tumors of the gallbladder and extrahepatic bile ducts. In: Hartman WH, ed. *Atlas of Tumor Pathology*, 2nd series. Fascicle 22. Washington, DC: Armed Forces Institute of Pathology, 1986.
61. Albores-Saavedra J, Henson DE, Sobin LE. *Histological Typing of Tumours of the Gallbladder and Extrahepatic Bile Ducts.* World Health Organization. Berlin: Springer-Verlag; 1991.
62. Goodman ZD, Albores-Saavedra J, Lundblad D. Somatostatinoma of the cystic duct. *Cancer.* 1984;53:498.
63. Rossi RL, Heiss FW, Beckmann CF, et al. Management of cancer of the bile duct. *Surg Clin North Am.* 1985;65:59.
64. Henson DE, Albores-Saavedra J, Corle D. Carcinoma of the extrahepatic bile ducts: Histologic types, stage of disease, grade, and survival rates. *Cancer.* 1992;70:1498.
65. Henson DE, Albores-Saavedra J, Corle D. Carcinoma of the gallbladder: Histologic types, stage of disease, grade and survival rates. *Cancer.* 1992;70:1493.
66. Yamaguchi K, Enjoji M. Carcinoma of the gallbladder: A clinicopathology of 103 patients with a newly proposed stain. *Cancer.* 1988;62:1425.
67. Chari ST, Mohan V, Pitchumoni CS, et al. Risk of pancreatic carcinoma in tropical calcifying pancreatitis: An epidemiologic study. *Pancreas.* 1994;9:62–66.
68. Ekbom A, McLaughlin JK, Karlsson BM, et al. Pancreatitis and pancreatic cancer: A population-based study. *J Natl Cancer Inst.* 1994;86:625–627.
69. Edoute Y, Lemberg S, Malberger E. Preoperative and intraoperative fine needle aspiration cytology of pancreatic lesions. *Am J Gastroenterol.* 1991;86:1015–1019.
70. Nguyen G-K. Percutaneous fine needle aspiration cytology of the pancreas. *Pathol Annu.* 1985;20(Part I):221–238.
71. Camer SJ, Tan EGC, Warren KW, Braasch JW. Pancreatic abscess. A critical analysis of 113 cases. *Am J Surg.* 1975;129:426–431.
72. Klöppel G, Maillet B. Pseudocysts in chronic pancreatitis: A morphological analysis of 57 resection specimens and 9 autopsy pancreata. *Pancreas.* 1991;6:266–274.
73. Albores-Saavedra J, Gould EW, Angeles-Angeles A, et al. Cystic tumors of the pancreas. *Pathol Annu.* 1990;19(Part II):50.
74. Warshaw AL, Rutledge PL. Cystic tumors mistaken for pancreatic pseudocysts. *Ann Surg.* 1987;205:393–398.
75. Sarles H, Bernard JP, Gullo L. Pathogenesis of chronic pancreatitis. *Gut.* 1990;31:629–632.
76. Suda K, Mogaki M, Oyama T, et al. Histopathologic and immunohistochemical studies on alcoholic pancreatitis and chronic obstructive pancreatitis: Special emphasis on ductal obstruction and genesis of pancreatitis. *Am J Gastroenterol.* 1990;85:271–276.
77. Miller BA, Ries LAG, Hankey BF, et al, eds. *SEER Cancer Statistics Review: 1973–1990.* NIH Pub. No. 93–2789. Washington, DC: National Cancer Institute; 1993.
78. Ries LAG, Hankey BF, Miller BA, et al. *Cancer Statistics Review 1973–1988.* NIH Pub. No. 91–2789. Washington, DC: National Cancer Institute; 1991.
79. Warshaw AL, Fernandez del Castillo C. Pancreatic carcinoma. *N Engl J Med.* 1992;326:455–465.
80. Fauconnier J, Faivre J, Quipourt V, et al. Diagnostic modalities and treatment of cancer of the pancreas. *Gastroenterol Clin Biol.* 1993;17:341–346.
81. Thoeni RF, Blankenberg F. Pancreatic imaging. *Radiol Clin North Am.* 1993;31:1081–1113.
82. Urban T, Ricci S, Grange JD, et al. Detection of c-Ki-*ras* mutation by PCR/RFLP analysis and diagnosis of pancreatic adenocarcinomas. *J Natl Cancer Inst.* 1993;85:2008–2012.
83. Klimstra DS, Heffers CS, Oertel JE, et al. Acinar cell carcinoma of the pancreas: A clinicopathologic study of 28 cases. *Am J Surg Pathol.* 1992;16:815–837.
84. Albores-Saavedra J, Vuitch F, Henson DE. The pancreas. In: Henson DE, Albores-Saavedra J, eds. *The Pathology of Incipient Neoplasia*, 2nd ed. Philadelphia: Saunders; 1993.
85. Milchgrub S, Campuzano M, Casillas J, Albores-Saavedra J. Intraductal carcinoma of the pancreas: A report of four cases. *Cancer* 1992;69:651–656.
86. Morohoshi T, Kanda M, Asanuma K, Klöppel G. Intraductal papillary neoplasms of the pancreas: A clinicopathologic study of six patients. *Cancer.* 1989;64:1329–1335.
87. Albores-Saavedra J, Nadji M, Henson DE, et al. Enteroendocrine cell differentiation in carcinomas of the gallbladder and mucinous cystadenocarcinoma of the pancreas. *Pathol Res Pract.* 1988; 183:169–175.
88. Lynch HT, Fitzsimmons ML, McLellan J, et al. Familial pancreatic cancer: Surveillance, diagnostic tests and surgical strategies. *Nebr Med J.* 1990;75:130–133.
89. Klöppel G, Heitz PU. Pancreatic endocrine tumors. *Pathol Res Pract.* 1988;183:155–168.
90. Burke AP, Sobin LH, Federspiel BH, et al. Carcinoid tumors of the duodenum: A clinicopathologic study of 99 cases. *Arch Pathol Lab Med.* 1990;114:700.
91. Burke AP, Sobin LH, Shekitkas KM, et al. Somatostatin-producing duodenal carcinoids in patients with von Recklinghausen's neurofibromatosis: A predilection for black patients. *Cancer.* 1990;65:1591.

14

The Urologic and Male Reproductive Systems

David G. Bostwick and Joseph E. Oesterling

Definition

The urologic and male reproductive systems include the kidneys, ureters, bladder, urethra, testes, paratesticular structures, prostate, seminal vesicles, and external genitalia.

Diseases of the urinary tract and male reproductive system are common. Knowledge of diseases arising at these sites is essential for the surgical management of conditions involving the abdomen, pelvis, retroperitoneum, and inguinal and perineal regions. Women often have bladder infections, and urinary obstructive symptoms are common in older men. Both men and women frequently have calculi and renal parenchymal disease. Tumors are common at all sites of the urinary system; for example, the prostate accounts for the most common benign tumorlike condition (benign prostatic hyperplasia) and malignant tumor (adenocarcinoma) in men. All surgeons should understand the contribution of disorders of the kidney, bladder, prostate, testis, and external genitalia to patient history, physical examination, and clinical evaluation. As with other organ systems, cooperation and communication between the surgeon and pathologist is invaluable. This chapter presents a brief review of diagnostic urologic pathology as it is related to the practice of surgery.

The Kidney

GLOMERULAR DISEASES

Because glomerular diseases have overlapping clinical presentations, percutaneous needle biopsy of the kidney plays a critical role in precise classification. Open biopsy is useful in patients in whom closed biopsy is risky. These patients include those with a solitary kidney, a coagulopathy, or an anatomic kidney abnormality. Open biopsy also decreases the risk of complications of fine needle aspiration biopsy such as hematoma and arteriovenous fistula. The right kidney is preferentially biopsied because of its more caudal location.

Diagnosis and classification of glomerular diseases require correlation of the clinical presentation, physical findings, laboratory studies, and biopsy results.[1-4] Because of the complexity of pathologic interpretation of glomerular diseases, special handling of biopsy material is necessary, with allocation for light microscopy (formalin fixation), immunofluorescence (frozen tissue), and electron microscopy (glutaraldehyde fixation). Biopsy specimens are routinely examined by light microscopy using a variety of stains (hematoxylin and eosin, periodic acid-Schiff, trichrome, and silver methenamine), by immunofluorescence with stains directed against immunoglobulins (IgG, IgM, IgA), C3, C1, C4, fibrinogen, albumin, and others, and by electron microscopy. Immunofluorescent deposits and electron-dense deposits may be continuous along the glomerular and tubular basement membranes, within capillary loops, in the mesangium, or within vascular structures. The combination of biopsy findings and clinical information is used to classify the disease process and to select appropriate management.

TUBULOINTERSTITIAL DISEASES

A wide variety of agents and toxins cause tubulointerstitial nephritis and pyelonephritis, often resulting in acute or chronic renal failure.[1-5] The anatomic pattern of injury is useful for determining etiology. The spectrum of diseases includes acute tubular necrosis, tubulointerstitial nephritis, pyelonephritis, acute interstitial nephritis, analgesic nephropathy, uric acid nephropathy, and myeloma kidney. Needle biopsy is useful for evaluating tubulointerstitial disease. Both the renal cortex and medulla should be sampled. Histologic evaluation determines the severity of the disease and the potential for salvageable kidney function.

VASCULAR DISEASES

Other than benign nephrosclerosis associated with arteriolosclerosis, vascular diseases of the kidney are uncommon.[1–4, 6] These include atheroembolic renal disease, microangiopathic hemolytic anemia, thrombotic thrombocytopenic purpura, sickle-cell nephropathy, malignant nephrosclerosis, and diffuse cortical necrosis. Renal artery stenosis, when detected early with renin serum levels and other studies, is surgically correctable. If uncorrected, hypertension results and eventually damages the other unprotected kidney.

RENAL MASSES

Increased use of abdominal and pelvic imaging studies such as ultrasound, computed tomography (CT), and magnetic resonance imaging (MRI) has improved the accuracy and rate of detection of renal masses. Many renal tumors are now diagnosed at an early stage.[1–4, 7] Sonographically, cystic masses that are simple or are composed of adipose tissue usually require no further workup. In contrast, hyperdense or complex cysts should be investigated, often with cyst aspiration. Solid masses usually require surgery, although fine needle aspiration (FNA) is often employed preoperatively to determine the nature of the tumor (see Chap. 3).

Evaluation

Percutaneous FNA is safe and reasonably accurate and allows evaluation of tumor recurrence in the renal fossa after nephrectomy as well as distinction between renal cysts and neoplasms.

Simple nephrectomy is performed in patients with end-stage kidney disease, calculus disease, obstruction, and trauma, whereas radical nephrectomy is performed in patients with renal cell carcinoma and other malignancies. Regardless of the condition, the pathologist weighs, measures, and slices the specimen carefully at 3-mm intervals to determine multicentricity, anatomic location, and extent of the process. Pathologic staging of renal neoplasms requires evaluation of Gerota's fascia, renal vein and artery, and medulla and pelvis. Multiple sections are obtained through the neoplasm and the adjacent uninvolved kidney for histologic evaluation.

Partial nephrectomy (nephron-sparing nephrectomy) is useful for removal of a variety of benign lesions in the kidney and is employed in select cases with malignant tumors in which preservation of renal function is desired. In such cases, it is important to document the portion of kidney removed. Frozen section evaluation of adequacy of the surgical margins is usually employed in order to spare as much parenchyma as possible without jeopardizing the curative potential of the procedure.

Cysts

Cysts are frequent incidental findings in the kidney and may be confused with tumors.[7] They are often associated with certain forms of chronic renal failure and with cysts in other organs. Cysts arise from partial intratubular obstruction, defective tubular basement membrane production, or abnormal tubular cell growth. Surgical management depends on the clinical setting, including patient age, bilaterality, and association with cysts in other organs.

Childhood polycystic kidney disease is a rare autosomal recessive condition associated with liver and bile duct cysts and congenital hepatic fibrosis. *Adult polycystic kidney disease* is a common autosomal dominant condition associated with liver cysts (40% of cases) and berry aneurysms in the circle of Willis (10 to 30%) (Fig. 14–1).[7, 8] Other cystic diseases include benign simple cysts, cystic renal dysplasia, cystic disease of the renal medulla, and dialysis-associated cystic disease.

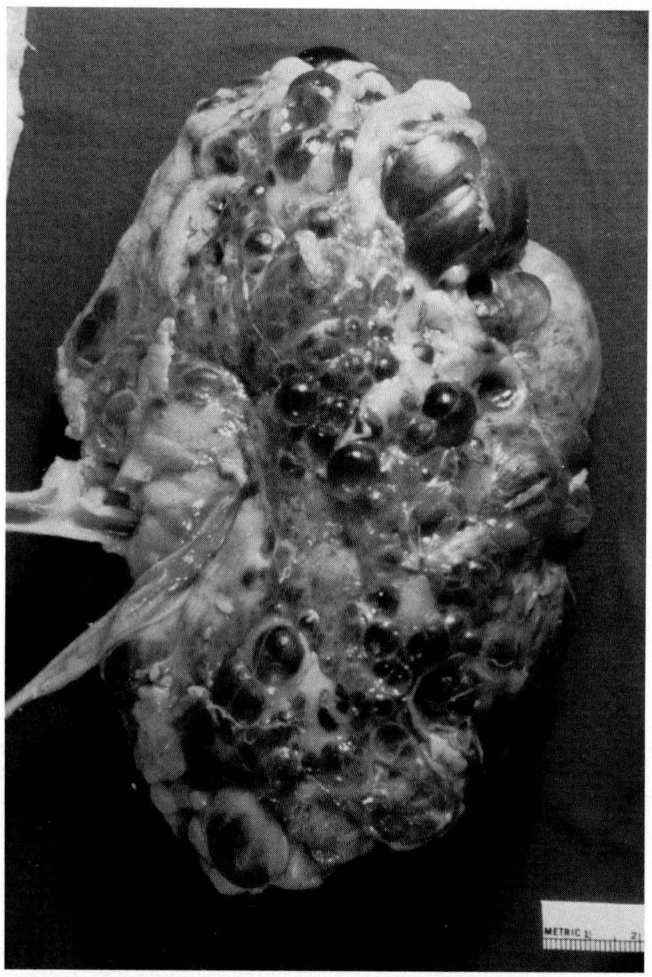

Figure 14–1. Adult polycystic kidney disease. This is a common condition, usually seen in patients over 40 years of age, with bilateral involvement.

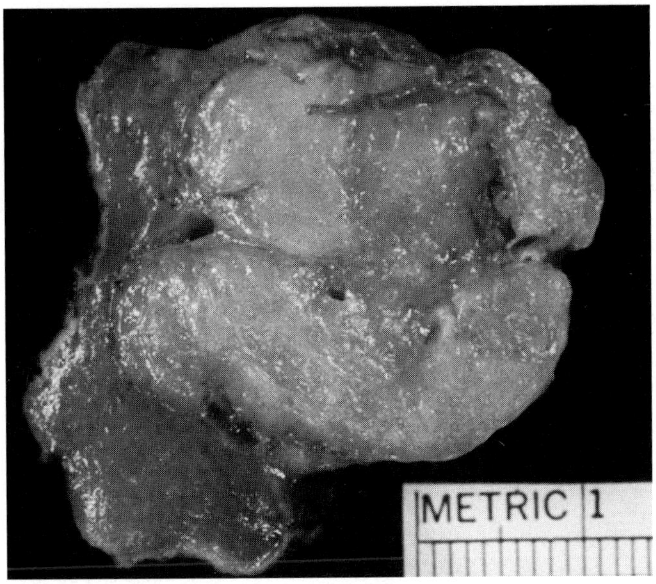

Figure 14–2. Angiomyolipoma of the kidney. This case was unilateral and not associated with tuberous sclerosis.

Benign Tumors

Angiomyolipoma is a hamartoma composed of blood vessels, smooth muscle, and fat and is common in patients with tuberous sclerosis. This syndrome should be considered in all cases, particularly in patients with bilateral angiomyolipoma (Fig. 14–2).[9, 10] *Oncocytoma* is a common benign epithelial tumor of adulthood with large eosinophilic cells containing numerous mitochondria; it may be difficult to distinguish from renal-cell carcinoma (Fig. 14–3). Oncocytoma is large, solitary, encapsulated, and mahogany-brown, with a central stellate scar. Both benign and malignant soft tissue tumors of the kidney are rarities. *Juxtaglomerular cell tumor* is a rare tumor that causes hypertension in young patients. *Fibroma* is a small gray-white nodule within the pyramids composed of fibroblasts and collagen, usually identified incidentally at autopsy.

Malignant Tumors

Renal-cell carcinoma usually occurs in patients over 60 years of age and is more common in men than women.[9, 10] It usually appears as a large, solitary, circumscribed mass, but multifocality is frequently observed in serially sectioned kidneys, a finding that challenges the utility of nephron-sparing surgery (partial nephrectomy) in some cases. As one of the great mimickers in medicine, renal-cell carcinoma can manifest in distant metastatic sites prior to detection of a primary renal tumor; also, it may produce paraneoplastic syndromes such as polycythemia (due to erythropoietin production), hypercalcemia, hypertension (due to renin production), Cushing's syndrome (due to ACTH production), feminization, masculinization, amyloidosis, and others. Microscopically, there are several patterns of renal-cell carcinoma. The most common is a clear-cell pattern (Fig. 14–4). Two histologic patterns—sarcomatoid (Fig. 14–5) and papillary—are associated with the poorest outcomes. Patients with von Hippel–Lindau syndrome, an autosomal dominant disease, often have renal-cell carcinoma, and this syndrome should always be considered in patients with bilateral renal tumors.

Renal-cell carcinoma may invade into the inferior vena cava and propagate upward, causing a right-sided cardiac obstruction due to a solid mass filling the right atrium. Metastases occur following hematogenous spread to the lungs (50% of cases with metastases) and bones (33%). Surgical removal of solitary or even a small number of metastatic nodules is associated with increased survival when compared with alternative treatments. The TNM staging system is presented in Table 14–1.

The most important prognostic variables in renal-cell carcinoma are tumor size, stage, grade, and histologic pattern. Separation of adenoma from carcinoma was originally based on a size threshold of 3 cm, but identification of metastases with occasional smaller tumors has led most investigators to abandon the simple size criterion; a reasonable approach is to refer to small tumors as renal cortical neoplasms without separating "benign" from "malignant." Grading of renal-cell carcinoma is prognostically valuable, and many pathologists use the Fuhrmann classification scheme.[9, 10] DNA ploidy may also provide prognostic information.

Wilms' tumor is an unusual tumor that usually occurs in infancy and childhood, occurring as a large round tumor dwarfing the kidney.[9, 10] Microscopically, Wilms' tumor is composed of a mixture of primitive renal epithelial and stromal elements. Cytogenetic deletion of the short arm of chromosome 3 is characteristic (see Chap. 21). The histologic appearance and grading of urothelial carcinoma of the renal pelvis and ureters are the same as for those corresponding neoplasms arising in the bladder.

The Urinary Tract

COMMON INFLAMMATORY CONDITIONS

Acute inflammation of the urinary tract (collecting system, ureter, bladder, and urethra) results in increased urinary frequency, lower abdominal pain, and dysuria; mucosal biopsy is usually unnecessary. Endoscopic findings include hemorrhage, suppuration, ulceration, and polypoid cystitis.

Chronic cystitis often arises without preceding acute inflammation, usually following ascending infection from the urethra. Special forms of cystitis include *ulcerative*

Table 14–1. TNM Staging System for Kidney Cancer

T1	<2.5 cm, limited to kidney
T2	>2.5 cm, limited to kidney
T3	Into major veins or perinephric invasion
T4	Invades beyond Gerota's fascia
N1	Single <2 cm
N2	Single >2 cm <5 cm, multiple <5 cm
N3	>5 cm
M1	Distant metastases

Source: Simplified from Beahrs OH, Hensen DE, Hutter RVP, Kennedy BJ. *Manual for Staging of Cancer*, 4th ed. American Joint Committee on Cancer (AJCC). Philadelphia: Lippincott; 1992:115–122, 199. With permission.

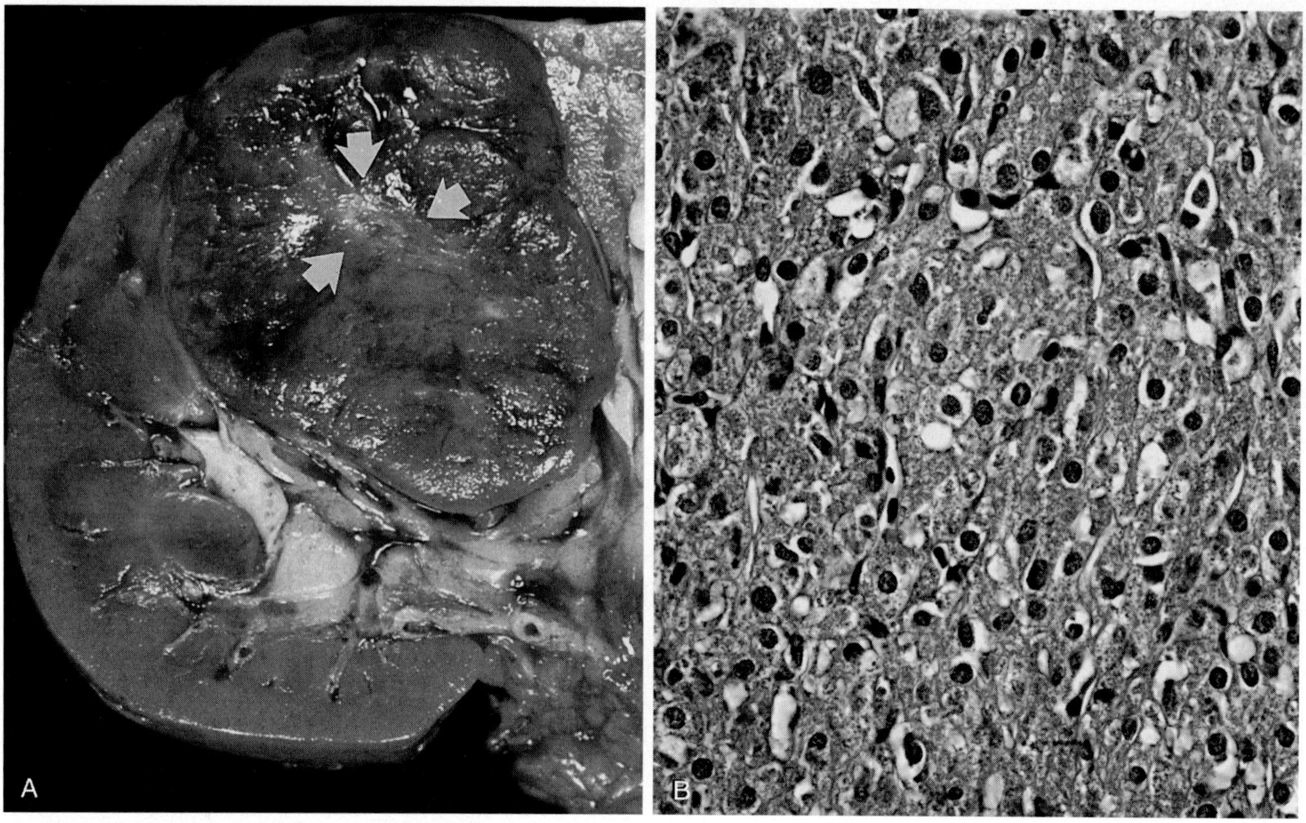

Figure 14–3. Oncocytoma of the kidney. *A.* Grossly, the tumor is solitary, large, and mahogany-brown, with a characteristic central stellate scar (*arrows*). *B.* Microscopically, the cells are uniform, with abundant eosinophilic cytoplasm.

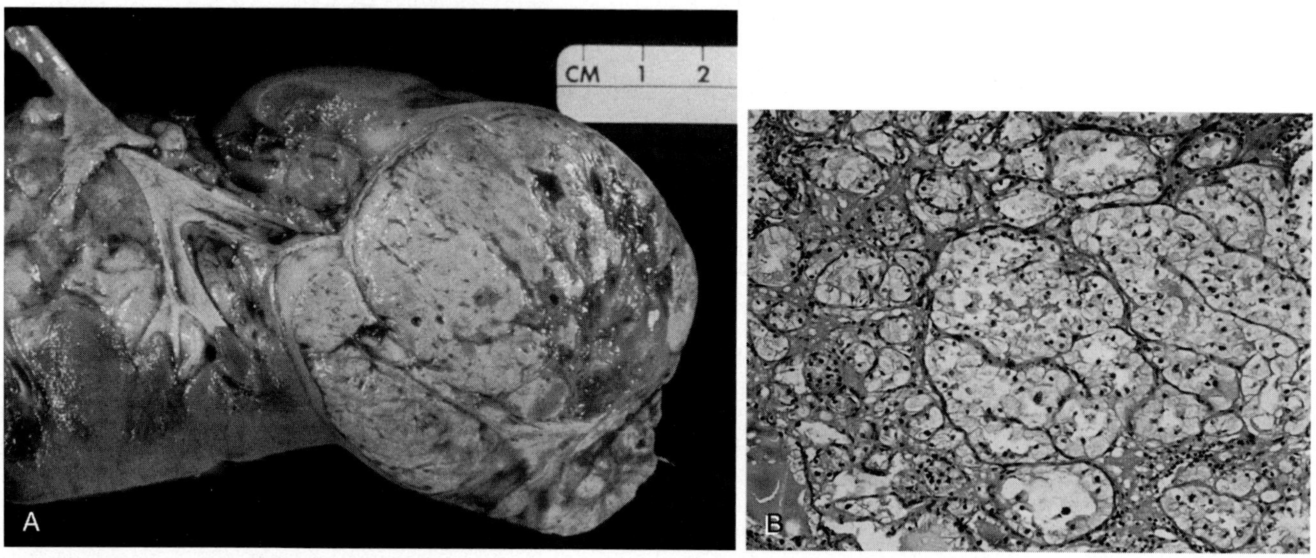

Figure 14–4. Renal-cell carcinoma, clear-cell type. *A.* Grossly, the tumor is large, solitary, and bright yellow. *B.* Microscopically, the tumor cells are uniform, with abundant clear to pale cytoplasm.

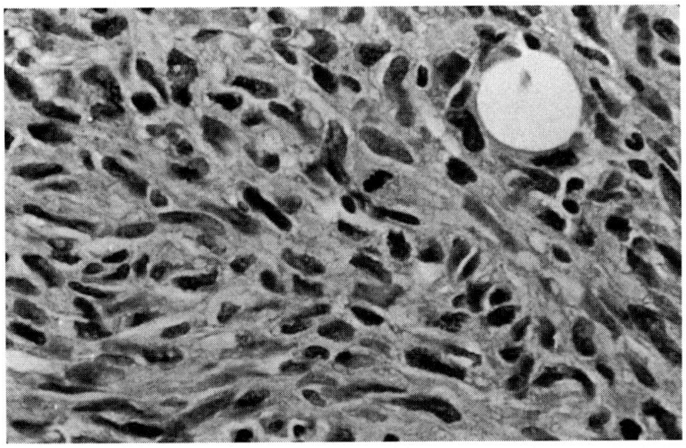

Figure 14–5. Renal-cell carcinoma, sarcomatoid type. This tumor mimics sarcoma histologically, but the cells contain abundant keratin, demonstrated with immunostaining, and show ultrastructural evidence of epithelial differentiation.

interstitial cystitis, a persistent debilitating form of chronic cystitis of unknown etiology, which usually occurs in women; *emphysematous cystitis*, characterized by the presence of gas bubbles in the submucosa and generally limited to diabetics; and *malakoplakia*, a form of chronic cystitis due to defective lysosomal killing of bacteria such as *Escherichia coli*, characterized microscopically by laminated calcospherites (Michaelis-Gutmann bodies) within macrophages. Other causes of cystitis include vesicoureteral reflux and persistent urachus.

Metaplastic changes occur in the urothelium of the bladder or elsewhere in the urinary system as a result of chronic irritation, and the patient may be predisposed to malignancy. Such changes include intestinal metaplasia, nephrogenic metaplasia, and keratinizing and nonkeratinizing squamous metaplasia.

CALCULI

Four main types of calculi occur in the urinary tract:

1. Calcium phosphate and calcium oxalate calculi are the most common, accounting for about 75% of cases; they may arise as a result of hypercalcemia and hypercalciuria, hyperuricuria, and hyperoxaluria, but the cause is often idiopathic; the stones are radiopaque.
2. Struvite calculi (''triple'' stones), composed of magnesium ammonium sulfate, arise following infection by urea-splitting bacteria such as *Proteus* and some staphylococci that convert urea to ammonia; alkaline urine causes precipitation of salt, creating huge stones such as staghorn calculi of the renal pelvis.
3. Uric acid calculi may be seen in patients with gout (hyperuricemia), but more than half of patients do not have hyperuricemia/hyperuricuria; these radiolucent stones form because uric acid is insoluble in acid urine.
4. Cystine calculi.

UROTHELIAL TUMORS

All suspect cystoscopically visible lesions should be sampled to exclude a urothelial tumor. Transurethral resection of the bladder is subject to the same artifacts seen in prostatic curettage, including cautery artifact and tissue shrinkage. Cystoscopic biopsy often shows denudation of the mucosa because of the delicate adherence of the urothelium to the stroma, particularly in inflamed areas. Intraoperative frozen section generally only compounds the problem of interpretation posed by small specimens and is rarely indicated in this clinical setting.

Urine Cytology

Exfoliative urine cytology is an effective method for detecting urothelial carcinoma and for monitoring treatment. For carcinoma of the bladder, cytology has a sensitivity of 50 to 60% for a single specimen and 80 to 90% for multiple specimens, with a specificity of almost 100%; the sensitivity is lower for urothelial neoplasms of the upper urinary tract and for low-grade tumors such as urothelial papilloma.[10, 11] Exfoliative cytology relies on the preferential shedding of malignant rather than benign cells. This phenomenon reflects decreased cell adhesion and greater cell proliferation in cancer. False negative results can occur with advanced cancers, which ulcerate and then reepithelialize with benign urothelium, temporarily losing the capacity for exfoliation of malignant cells into the urine. Catheterized and cystoscopic irrigation specimens often contain mechanically dislodged clumps of benign cells that are difficult to distinguish from low-grade cancer, particularly in the setting of prominent acute and chronic cystitis. Sequential cytology samples at 3- to 6-month intervals are useful for following patients with incipient urothelial carcinoma.

Noninvasive Urothelial Tumors

There are two morphologic patterns of noninvasive (in situ) urothelial neoplasia that differ clinically and pathologically.[10–12] The first, *noninvasive papillary urothelial carcinoma*, is common and usually low-grade and tends to recur multiple times prior to subepithelial invasion (Fig. 14–6). The local recurrence rate is 40 to 70%, usually within 2 years, with progression to higher grade in about 30%. A small (less than 2 cm diameter), solitary, low-grade papillary urothelial tumor in patients less than 50 years of age is considered by most pathologists to be low-grade carcinoma, although such a neoplasm is referred to as transitional-cell papilloma by the World Health Organization. Regardless of nomenclature, the malignant potential is low. The second form of urothelial neoplasia, flat *carcinoma in situ*, is uncommon, is usually high-grade, and tends to progress to invasive carcinoma rapidly (Fig. 14–7). Both forms of noninvasive urothelial neoplasia are initially treated by intravesicular therapy such as bacille Calmette-Guérin (BCG); however, resective surgery is often necessary in cases that progress to invasion (Table 14–2).

Invasive Urothelial Tumors

Urothelial carcinoma (*transitional-cell carcinoma*) accounts for about 90% of bladder cancers in the United States.[10–12] It is rare before 40 years of age and much more

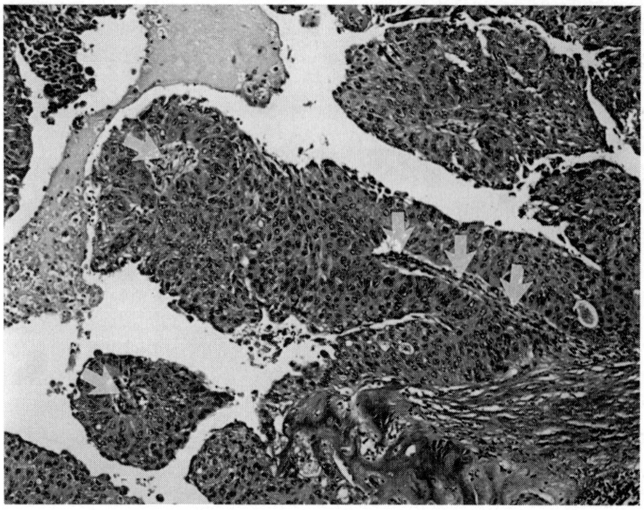

Figure 14–6. Grade 1 noninvasive papillary urothelial carcinoma of the bladder. Papillary projections of well-differentiated epithelium contain stromal cores (*arrows*); stroma without tumor invasion is present in the lower right corner.

common in men than women. The tumors are grossly papillary, sessile, nodular, or infiltrating. Although most common in the bladder, this tumor can arise anywhere in the urinary tract. Microscopically, three grades are recognized: *grade 1* consists of an orderly but thickened growth of urothelial cells with mild nuclear abnormalities such as enlargement, hyperchromasia, and variation in shape; *grade 2* is similar to grade 1 except that there is greater architectural distortion with loss of cell maturation and orderliness as well as moderate to marked nuclear abnormality; and *grade 3* consists of urothelial cells with marked nuclear abnormalities that lack maturation and polarity.

Surgery and radiation therapy are commonly utilized for invasive bladder cancer regardless of histologic features. Prognostic factors of importance include grade, histologic type, growth pattern, stage, lymphatic invasion, nuclear DNA content (ploidy), and blood group antigen expression.

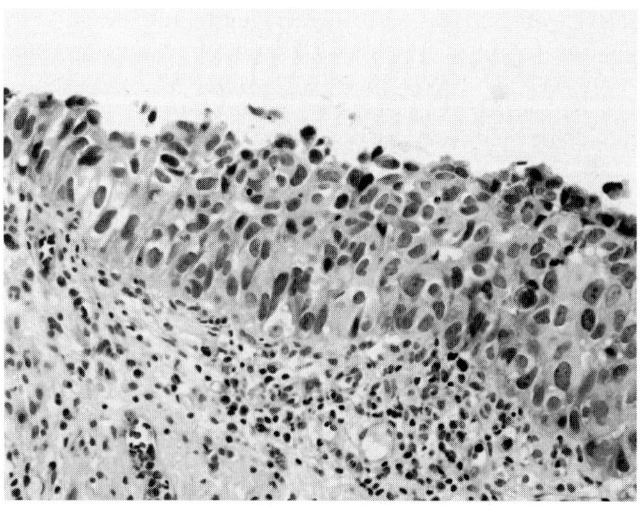

Figure 14–7. Carcinoma in situ (*flat pattern*) of the bladder. Highly atypical, dark, irregular epithelial nuclei remain within the mucosal surface.

Table 14–2. TNM Staging System for Cancer of the Urinary Bladder

Tis	In situ flat tumor
Ta	Papillary noninvasive
T1	Subepithelial connective tissue invasion
T2	Superficial muscle (inner half) invasion
T3	Deep muscle or perivesical fat invasion
T3a	Deep muscle (outer half) invasion
T3b	Perivesical fat invasion
T4	Prostate, uterus, vagina, pelvic wall, abdominal wall invasion
N1	Single <2 cm
N2	Single >2 cm <5 cm, multiple <5 cm
N3	>5 cm
M1	Distant metastasis

Source: Simplified from Beahrs OH, Henson DE, Hutter RVP, Kennedy BJ. *Manual for Staging of Cancer,* 4th ed. AJCC. Philadelphia: Lippincott; 1992:115–122, 203.

Other Tumors

Squamous-cell carcinoma is the most common form of bladder cancer in countries such as Egypt, where *Schistosoma haematobium* is endemic. It is also seen in patients with diverticula and other irritative conditions and in paraplegics with chronic indwelling catheters. Squamous-cell carcinoma tends to be clinically aggressive, manifesting at a high stage. Keratinizing squamous metaplasia is considered to be a precursor lesion in some cases.

Adenocarcinoma is a rare and aggressive form of bladder cancer that often arises in the urachus, in extrophic bladders, and in those infected with schistosomiasis. The tumors can be papillary, glandular, mucin-producing, of the signet ring–cell type, or clear-cell adenocarcinoma. Other rare forms of urothelial carcinoma include small-cell undifferentiated carcinoma and sarcomatoid carcinoma.

Benign soft tissue tumors and tumorlike conditions that occur in the bladder include inflammatory pseudotumor, postoperative spindle-cell nodule, leiomyoma, pheochromocytoma, amyloidosis, and endometriosis. Malignant soft tissue tumors are rare and include sarcoma botryoides (embryonal rhabdomyosarcoma) in infants and leiomyosarcoma in adults. The bladder is rarely involved by metastatic malignancy.

Male Reproductive System

PROSTATE AND SEMINAL VESICLES

Prostatic Inflammation

Patchy acute and chronic inflammation is so common in prostates of adults as to be considered a normal finding. When the inflammation is severe and extensive or clinically apparent, the term ''prostatitis'' is warranted. There is a wide spectrum of prostatitides. Acute bacterial prostatitis is a medical emergency. The patient presents with sudden onset of fever, chills, irritative voiding symptoms, and pain in the lower back, rectum, and perineum. The prostate is swollen, firm, tender, and warm. Microscopically, there are sheets of neutrophils surrounding and invading prostatic glands, often with marked tissue destruction and abundant cellular debris. The stroma is edematous and hemorrhagic, and microabscesses may be present. Diagnosis is based upon culture of urine and expressed prostatic secretions. Biopsy is actually contraindicated due to the potential for sepsis. Most cases of acute prostatitis are caused by the same pathogens that cause other urinary tract infections. Acute prostatitis responds to antibiotics. Abscess is a rare complication, usually occurring in immunocompromised patients such as those with acquired immunodeficiency syndrome.

Chronic bacterial prostatitis is a common cause of relapsing urinary tract infection and is usually due to *E. coli*.[10, 13] Diagnosis is difficult, often requiring multiple urine cultures obtained after prostatic massage. Treatment is also frustrated by the inability of most intravenous antibiotics to enter the prostate and prostatic fluids even when the prostate is overrun with chronic inflammation. Prostatic calculi serve as a nidus of recurring infection, with the bacteria embedded in the mineral matrix. Chronic aseptic prostatitis is more common than bacterial prostatitis and rarely follows infection elsewhere in the urinary tract. Patients often complain of painful ejaculation. Culture findings from urine and expressed prostatic secretions are negative. The etiologic agent is unknown, but *Chlamydia, Ureaplasma*, and *Trichomonas* have all been suggested. This form of prostatitis has an indolent course characterized by relapses and remissions.

Granulomatous prostatitis includes morphologically distinct forms of chronic prostatitis caused by a variety of inciting agents, including infection and biopsy instrumentation (Fig. 14–8).[13–16] The majority of patients have a history of urinary tract infection. The prostate is often hard, fixed, and nodular, and cancer is often suspected clinically. Urinalysis shows pyuria and hematuria, but biopsy is required for definitive diagnosis. The common pathogenetic mechanism of granulomatous prostatitis is blockage of prostatic ducts with stasis of secretions, regardless of the inciting agent. It is important to recognize the various causes of granulomatous prostatitis and the histologic clues that allow its distinction from other entities. Most cases elude a causative explanation and are considered idiopathic.

Benign Prostatic Hyperplasia

Enlargement of the prostate, referred to as benign prostatic hyperplasia (BPH), consists of overgrowth of the glandular and fibromuscular tissues of the transition zone and periurethral area.[17–19] It is extremely common, accounting for up to 400,000 prostatectomies annually, making this the most common surgical procedure in American men. Symptoms are caused by interference with muscular sphincteric function and by obstruction of urine flow through the prostatic urethra. Symptoms include urgency, hesitancy in starting urination, diminished size and force of stream, increased frequency, sensation of incomplete bladder emptying, and nocturia. Androgens are required for development and maintenance of the prostatic epithelium, with morphologic regression of BPH and cancer after orchiectomy and androgen-deprivation therapy. Orchiectomy or pharmacologic hormonal manipulation is useful for treating BPH. Effective drugs include progestational agents, pure antiandrogens, gonadotropin-releasing hormone agonists, and 5-alpha-reductase inhibitors.

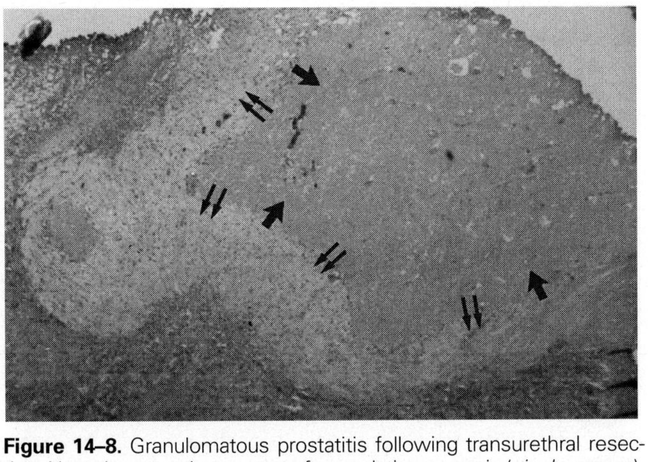

Figure 14–8. Granulomatous prostatitis following transurethral resection. Note the central gray zone of coagulative necrosis (*single arrows*), surrounded by a granulomatous giant-cell reaction (*double arrows*).

Benign prostatic hyperplasia consists of variably sized nodules that are usually firm, rubbery, and yellow-gray; these bulge from the cut surface upon transection. Prominent epithelial hyperplasia, in addition to stromal hyperplasia, creates soft and spongy nodules that ooze a pale-white watery fluid. If the BPH is predominantly fibromuscular, there is diffuse enlargement or numerous trabeculations without prominent nodularity. Degenerative changes include calcification and infarction, often with reactive microscopic changes in the epithelium at the periphery, including squamous metaplasia and transitional-cell metaplasia.

Benign prostatic hyperplasia and its associated benign lesions have numerous histologic variants. Some of these can mimic carcinoma microscopically. Atrophy is a common microscopic finding, consisting of small distorted glands with flattened epithelium, hyperchromatic nuclei, and stromal fibrosis. It is usually idiopathic, and the prevalence increases with age. Postatrophic hyperplasia consists of atrophic glands with benign proliferating luminal cells. Basal-cell hyperplasia is characterized by proliferation of basal cells, forming two or more cells in thickness at the periphery of prostatic glands and acini, usually occurring in the setting of BPH. Adenoid basal-cell tumor consists of basaloid cell nests of varying size infiltrating the stroma without circumscription. Rare cases display perineural invasion and extension into the periprostatic soft tissues, but there have been no reports of metastases or deaths due to these tumors. Cribriform hyperplasia is a histologic variant of BPH that consists of a nodule of glands with a distinctive cribriform pattern with pale to clear cytoplasm and small uniform nuclei with inconspicuous nucleoli.

Atypical adenomatous hyperplasia is a localized proliferation of small glands within the prostate, usually seen in transurethral resection specimens from the transition zone, that may be mistaken for carcinoma. Atypical adenomatous hyperplasia is distinguished from well-differentiated carcinoma by its inconspicuous nucleoli, infrequent crystalloids, lack of basophilic mucin, and fragmented basal-cell layer as seen immunohistochemically with basal-cell–specific antikeratin antibodies. The basal-cell layer is characteristically discontinuous and fragmented in atypical adenomatous hyperplasia, whereas carcinoma has an absent basal-cell layer. This diagnostic feature can be demonstrated immunohistochemically in routine formalin-fixed sections. The identification of atypical adenomatous hyperplasia should not influence or dictate therapeutic decisions, but close surveillance and follow-up are indicated. Caution is warranted in interpretation of scant specimens, cauterized or distorted specimens, and specimens submitted with incomplete patient history.

In contrast to atypical adenomatous hyperplasia, sclerosing adenosis shows striking myoepithelial metaplasia of the basal-cell compartment with prominent stroma composed of fibroblasts and loose ground substance. The basal cells in this condition are positive for S-100 protein and muscle-specific actin and demonstrate thin filament collections and dense bodies on electron microscopy. This immunophenotype is unusual in the prostate, because normal prostatic basal cells do not demonstrate myoepithelial differentiation; consequently, most believe that sclerosing adenosis is a form of metaplasia.

Stromal hyperplasia with atypia consists of stromal nodules in the setting of BPH with increased cellularity and nuclear atypia. Despite the cellular changes, stromal hyperplasia with atypia has no malignant potential, and the atypical cells are considered degenerative.

Most cancers arise in the prostate with concomitant BPH. Cancer is found incidentally in a significant number (10%) of transurethral prostatectomy specimens. It is important to exclude the possibility of underlying cancer in patients presenting with symptoms of urinary obstruction presumed due to BPH.

Transurethral Resection and Adenectomy

Transurethral prostatic resection (TURP) specimens consist of tissue from the transition zone, urethra, periurethral area, bladder neck, and anterior fibromuscular area.[20] Studies of radical prostatectomies performed after TURP reveal that the resection does not usually include tissue from the central or peripheral zone, and some of the transition zone usually remains.

Well-differentiated cancer found incidentally in TURP chips usually represents cancer that has arisen in the transition zone. Such tumors are frequently small and may be completely resected by TURP; however, there is no accurate method to determine the completeness of excision. In contrast, poorly differentiated cancer usually represents part of a larger tumor that has invaded the transition zone from the peripheral zone.

The optimal number of chips to submit for histologic evaluation from a TURP specimen remains controversial, with some experts advocating complete submission even with large specimens that would require many cassettes. The Cancer Committee of the College of American Pathologists (1994)[21] and the Consensus Committee on Staging and Grading of the American Cancer Society (1992)[22] recommend a minimum of 6 cassettes for the first 30 g of tissue and 1 cassette for every 10 g thereafter.

In patients with massive benign prostatic hyperplasia, open suprapubic surgical excision may be preferable to TURP. The specimen usually consists exclusively of transition-zone tissue and periurethral tissue with grossly visible nodules.

Prostatic Intraepithelial Neoplasia

Prostatic intraepithelial neoplasia (PIN) represents the putative precancerous end of the morphologic spectrum of cellular proliferations within prostatic ducts, ductules, and acini.[23] Two grades of PIN, low and high, are identified. Only high-grade PIN is considered a precursor of invasive carcinoma (Fig. 14–9). The continuum of atypia between high-grade PIN and early invasive cancer is characterized by disruption of the basal cell layer, progressive loss of markers of secretory differentiation, increasing nuclear and nucleolar abnormalities, increasing proliferative potential, and increasing variation in DNA content (aneuploidy). The clinical importance of recognizing PIN is based upon its strong association with carcinoma. Its identification in biopsy specimens of the prostate warrants further search for concurrent invasive carcinoma. Some pathologists report only the presence of high-grade PIN, recognizing the difficulty in identifying low-grade PIN and distinguishing it from other histologic mimickers such as atypical basal-cell hyperplasia. Follow-up biopsy is suggested at 3 months and thereafter at 6-month intervals. Identification of PIN alone should not dictate surgical intervention.

Adenocarcinoma

Prostate cancer is the most common cancer among men in the United States and is second only to lung cancer as a cause of cancer death. In 1995, it is estimated that 40,400 men died of prostate cancer and 240,000 new cases were diagnosed.[24] Although most prostatic cancers grow relatively slowly and will not be manifest during the man's lifetime, the clinical course is often unpredictable in its rate of progression. This is perhaps due to the heterogeneity of histologic grade and other factors that influence tumor growth. Despite an autopsy prevalence of up to 80% by age 80 years, the clinical incidence is much lower, indicating that most men die *with* prostate cancer rather than *of* prostate cancer. Little is known about the causes of prostate

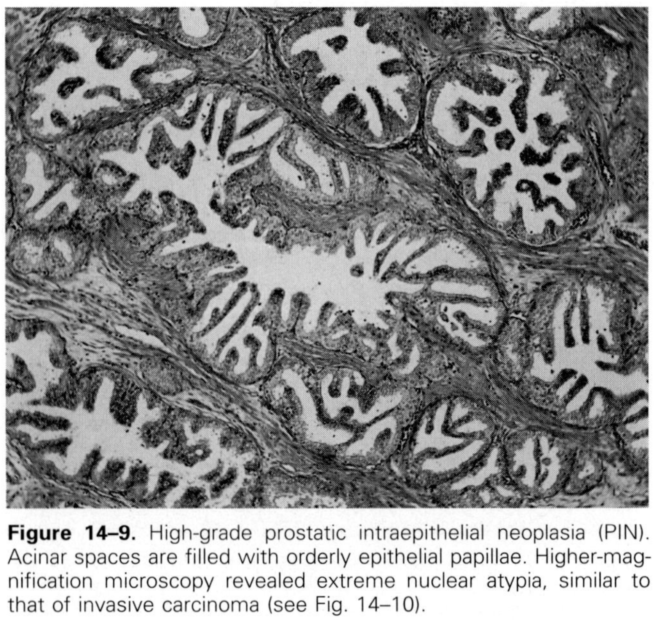

Figure 14–9. High-grade prostatic intraepithelial neoplasia (PIN). Acinar spaces are filled with orderly epithelial papillae. Higher-magnification microscopy revealed extreme nuclear atypia, similar to that of invasive carcinoma (see Fig. 14–10).

cancer despite its high incidence and prevalence. Interestingly, the prevalence of latent cancer is similar in different geographic and ethnic groups despite variation in clinical incidence. The incidence is low in American Indians, Hispanics, and Orientals but high in African Americans and whites.

Definitive diagnosis of prostate cancer requires confirmative microscopy. About 95% of cancers are adenocarcinomas. Evaluation of glandular proliferations in the prostate can be a challenge, particularly when the specimen or suspected focus is small. Diagnosis relies on a combination of architectural and cytologic findings, which may be aided by ancillary studies such as immunohistochemistry. Architectural features include haphazard arrangement of packed glands, irregular glandular contours, and variation in gland size and shape. Comparison with the adjacent uninvolved prostatic gland is helpful. Cytologic features include nuclear and nucleolar enlargement, luminal mucin, and crystalloids. The basal-cell layer is absent in carcinoma, whereas it is present at the periphery of benign glands. Perineural invasion is common in cancer but is seen only rarely with benign glands. Microvascular invasion is also an indicator of malignancy.

Inflammation is important to note when evaluating small glandular proliferations, particularly when the architectural features are equivocal and one is relying on the cytologic findings of large nuclei and nucleoli for the diagnosis of carcinoma. Reactive atypia within glands may result from inflammation, radiation, infarction, and other insults to the prostate. Granulomatous prostatitis is a vexing problem, and caution is warranted in the interpretation of biopsy specimens with this feature.

Biopsy

The combination of an automated spring-loaded 18-gauge needle core biopsy gun with transrectal ultrasound guidance has numerous advantages over the traditional wider 14-gauge needle biopsy performed under digital direction alone. In one study the rate of post-biopsy infection fell from 7.39% to 0.81%, and there was a decline in urinary clot retention from 3.2% to less than 1%. The false-negative rate declined to 11%, and the quality of the tissue sample improved, with little or no compression artifact. The 18-gauge biopsy allows systematic sextant biopsies of the prostate with minimal patient discomfort. The main disadvantage is that it provides less than half the amount of tissue per core for pathologic examination than does the traditional biopsy.

When compared with matched prostatectomy specimens, needle core biopsy underestimates tumor grade in 33 to 45% of cases and overestimates grade in 4 to 32%.[25] Grading errors are greatest in biopsies with small amounts of tumor and low-grade tumors and are probably due to tissue sampling error, tumor heterogeneity, and undergrading of needle biopsy samples. There is no correlation of biopsy grading error and clinical staging error.

Fine needle aspiration remains popular for cytologic examination of the prostate in parts of Europe but is rarely used in the United States, in deference to the ease of the 18-gauge needle core sampling.[26] Both techniques have similar sensitivity in the diagnosis of prostate cancer, and both are limited by small sample size. They are best considered as complementary techniques. Complications of FNA occur in less than 2% of cases and are similar to those with needle core biopsy, including epididymitis, transient hematuria, hemospermia, fever, and septicemia.

Prostate-Specific Antigen

Prostate-specific antigen (PSA) is the most important, accurate, and clinically useful biochemical marker of the prostate because it is, for all intents and purposes, produced by and specific for prostatic tissue.[27–31] This 34-kDa serine protease is normally synthesized by the epithelial cells and secreted into the prostatic ductal system, where it catalyzes the liquefaction of the seminal coagulum after ejaculation. Serum levels are normally below about 4.0 ng/mL but vary according to patient age.[27] Any process that disrupts the normal architecture of the prostate allows diffusion of PSA into the stroma, where it gains access to the blood through the microvasculature. Elevated serum PSA level is seen with prostatitis, with BPH, and transiently following biopsy. The most striking and prolonged elevations are seen with prostatic adenocarcinoma. Although cancer produces less PSA *per cell* than benign epithelium, the greater number of malignant cells and the associated stromal disruption account for elevated *serum* PSA concentration.[28]

Serum PSA evaluation increases the likelihood of detecting early, potentially curable prostate cancer when used in combination with existing detection methods (digital rectal examination and transrectal ultrasound). In some patients, elevated serum PSA may be the only indication of cancer. In comparison, some palpable cancers fail to release detectable serum PSA. Therefore, it is critical that serum PSA alone *not* be used as a substitute for a comprehensive multimodality approach for early detection. Although the benefit of early detection remains controversial, most believe that definitive therapy should be offered to men with a life expectancy of at least 10 years who have organ-confined prostate cancer. Serum PSA concentration is also utilized to detect tumor recurrence after resection, hormonal therapy, or radiation therapy as well as to follow untreated patients (active surveillance). Other clinical measures of PSA include PSA density (serum PSA per volume of prostatic tissue), PSA cancer density (serum PSA per volume of cancer after controlling for gland volume), and PSA velocity (rate of change in serum PSA over time).

The major form of measurable PSA in the serum is a complex between the PSA molecule and alpha-1-antichymotrypsin; there is a higher proportion of complexed PSA in the serum of patients with cancer than in that of other patients; this serum fractionation may be diagnostically useful.[31] New microassays for serum PSA allow detectability at concentrations as low as 0.1 ng/mL.

Immunohistochemical detection of PSA is diagnostically helpful for the pathologist in distinguishing high-grade prostate cancer from urothelial carcinoma, colonic carcinoma, granulomatous prostatitis, and lymphoma.[32] It also allows recognition of prostatic origin in metastatic adenocarcinoma (see Chap. 2). The expression of PSA is generally greater in low-grade tumors than in high-grade tumors, but there is significant variation from case to case and from cell to cell. Up to 1.6% of poorly differentiated cancers will be negative for both PSA and prostatic acid phosphatase.

In addition to PSA, other diagnostic and prognostic markers are used for the evaluation of prostate cancer. Prostatic acid phosphatase (PAP) helps to identify the presence and extent of prostate cancer but has fallen into disfavor because of inherent problems in accuracy of measurement in comparison with PSA. Analysis of DNA content of prostate cancer by flow cytometry and static image analysis may provide independent prognostic information that supplements histopathologic examination. Patients with diploid tumors have a more favorable outcome than those with aneuploid tumors; for example, among patients with lymph node metastases treated with radical prostatectomy and androgen-deprivation therapy, those with diploid tumors may survive 20 years or more, whereas those with aneuploid tumors die within 5 years. However, the ploidy pattern of prostate cancer is often variable regionally, creating potential problems of sampling error.

Grading of Adenocarcinoma

The histologic pattern of prostate cancer correlates significantly with biologic malignancy, and many useful systems of grading are available. The most popular system in the United States, the Gleason grading system, is based upon the degree of glandular differentiation, reflecting tumor heterogeneity by assigning a primary pattern for the dominant grade and a secondary pattern for the nondominant grade; the histologic *score* is derived by adding these two patterns together (Fig. 14–10).[33] The success of the Gleason system is due to four factors: (1) the histologic patterns are identified by their degree of glandular differentiation without relying on morphogenetic or histogenetic models; (2) a simplified and standardized artist's representation of growth patterns in relation to grades was created; (3) the study provided invaluable prospective information that allowed objective development of this self-defining grading system; and (4) unlike any other grading system, the Gleason system provided for tumor heterogeneity by identifying primary and secondary patterns.

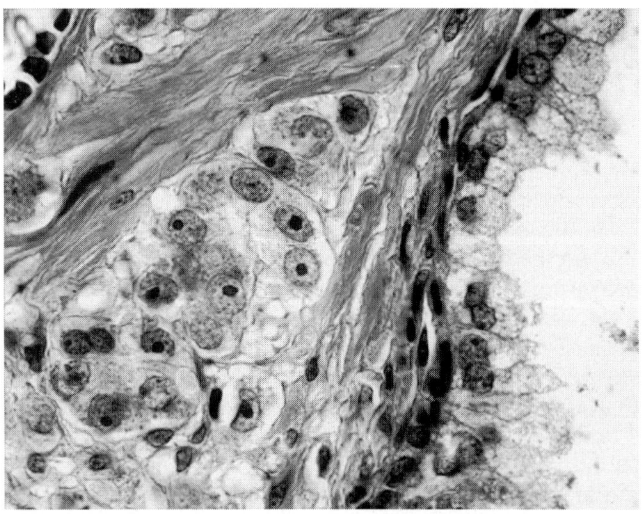

Figure 14–10. Invasive high-grade prostatic acinar carcinoma. Tumor cells (*left side of field*) show large nucleoli in vesicular nuclei, in contrast to delicate features of benign glandular epithelium (*right side*).

Table 14–3. Staging of Prostatic Adenocarcinoma

	American	TNM[b]
Nonpalpable cancer		
≤ 5% of TURP tissue[a]	A1	T1a
> 5% of TURP tissue[a]	A2	T1b
Cancer detected other than by biopsy (e.g., elevated serum PSA)	B0	T1c
Palpable or visible cancer clinically confined		
≤ Half of one lobe	B1	T2a
> Half of one lobe but not both lobes	B1	T2b
Both lobes	B2	T2c
Cancer with local extracapsular extension		
Unilateral	C1	T3a
Bilateral	C1	T3b
Seminal vesicle invasion	C2	T3c
Invasion of bladder neck, rectum,	C2	T4a
levator muscle, or pelvic wall	C2	T4b
Metastatic cancer		
Single regional lymph node ≤2 cm	D1	N1[c]
Single regional lymph node 2–5 cm, or multiple regional lymph nodes ≤ 5 cm	D1	N2
Single regional lymph node >5 cm	D1	N3
Distant metastasis	D2	M1
Nonregional lymph node(s)	D2	M1a
Bone(s)	D2	M1b
Other sites	D2	M1c

Stage groupings for TNM staging systems

Stage 0	T1a	N0	M0	G1[d]
Stage I	T1a	N0	M0	G2,3,4
	T1b	N0	M0	Any G
	T1c	N0	M0	Any G
	T1	N0	M0	Any G
Stage II	T2	N0	M0	Any G
Stage III	T3	N0	M0	Any G
Stage IV	T4	N0	M0	Any G
	Any T	N1,2,3	M0	Any G
	Any T	Any M	M1	Any G

[a]Different definitions exist for substaging A1 and A2 cancers.
[b]N0 or NX, M0 for T1–T4.
[c]NX: regional lymph nodes are not assessable; MX: distant metastasis is not assessable.
[d]G = grade on a scale of 1 to 4.
From Bostwick DG, Myers RP, Oesterling JE. Staging of prostate cancer. *Semin Surg Oncol 1994*; 10:60–73 and Schroder FH, Hermanek P, Denis L, et al: The TNM classification of prostate carcinoma. *Prostate* (Suppl) 1992; 4:129–138. Reprinted by permission of Wiley-Liss, Inc., a subsidiary of John Wiley & Sons, Inc.

Staging of Adenocarcinoma

The stage of a prostate cancer reflects its anatomic extent and burden of tumor, based upon the best available data.[34, 35] Two major systems are currently used: the modified American system and the TNM system [primary tumor (T), regional lymph node (N), and metastases (M)]. The TNM system, revised in 1992, is considered the international standard for prostate cancer staging (Table 14–3). Both systems stratify cases according to the method of tumor detection, distinguishing nonpalpable ''incidental'' prostate cancer detected during transurethral resection for clinically benign prostatic hyperplasia from palpable cancer detected during digital rectal examination. This reliance upon palpability of the tumor is unique among organ staging systems and is hampered by the low sensitivity, low specificity, and low positive predictive value of digital rectal examination. These staging systems also recognize nonpalpable tumors detected by either elevated serum PSA concentration or abnormal transrectal ultrasound image.

Radical Prostatectomy

There are two surgical approaches to radical prostatectomy. The first, retropubic prostatectomy, is the most popular approach in the United States, allowing preliminary regional lymphadenectomy with intraoperative pathologic evaluation prior to removal of the prostate; many urologists will not proceed with prostatectomy if there are lymph node metastases.[36] The second surgical approach, perineal prostatectomy, does not usually allow lymph node removal during the same operation owing to the anatomic approach employed.

The completeness of pathologic sectioning of radical prostatectomies affects the determination of pathologic stage. When the results of limited sectioning (sections of palpable tumor and two random sections of apex and base) are compared with complete sectioning (whole-organ step-sectioning procedure), the latter approach results in a significant increase in positive surgical margins (12% versus 59%, respectively) and higher pathologic stage.[37] The detection of extraprostatic extension in clinical stage T2 (B) cancer (and hence pathologic stage) is related to the amount of the prostate examined.

The capsule of the prostate consists of variable amounts of smooth muscle and collagen.[38] At the apex, bladder base, and anterior aspect of the gland, the capsule is poorly defined, composed of a mixture of fibrous connective tissue, smooth muscle, and striated muscle. As a result, the prostatic capsule should not be considered as a well-defined anatomic structure with constant features.

Complete and careful submission of tissue for histologic evaluation requires the following: (1) unequivocal orientation of specimen and tumor (left, right; transition zone, peripheral zone; anterior, midposterior; apex, base); (2) thorough evaluation of the extent and location of positive surgical margins; (3) thorough assessment and quantitation of the extent and location of capsular perforation and seminal vesicle invasion; (4) quality-control data for the surgeon, particularly in regard to surgical margins in nerve-sparing prostatectomy; (5) postoperative measurement of tumor volume for correlation with imaging studies; and (6) complete evaluation of tumor for grading (e.g., poorly differentiated cancer).

Treatment and Outcome

Treatment of prostate cancer remains controversial, consisting of at least four major options: radical prostatectomy, radiation therapy, androgen-deprivation therapy, and active surveillance (watchful waiting). There is currently no role for cytostatic chemotherapy. The choice of treatment is based upon patient age and health, life expectancy, clinical stage, serum PSA concentration, and tumor grade. Clinical management of prostate cancer is addressed in a number of reviews.[39, 40]

Other Tumors

Several rare benign stromal tumors and tumorlike proliferations arise in the prostate, including postoperative spindle-cell nodule, inflammatory pseudotumor, prostatic melanosis, and blue nevus.[10]

Malignant soft tissue tumors of the prostate are rare and account for less than 0.1% of the primary prostatic neoplasms. One third of these occur in children under 10 years of age and most are rhabdomyosarcoma. Leiomyosarcoma is the most common sarcoma in adults and accounts for 26% of all prostate sarcomas. Other rare sarcomas reported in the prostate include malignant phyllodes tumors, fibrosarcoma, osteosarcoma, malignant fibrous histiocytoma, angiosarcoma, chondrosarcoma, neurofibrosarcoma, and undifferentiated sarcoma. Sarcomatoid carcinoma, carcinosarcoma, and metaplastic carcinoma are not primarily mesenchymal but are included in the differential diagnosis of pleomorphic spindle-cell neoplasms with necrosis and significant mitotic activity. Recognition of the transition of carcinoma to sarcomatous differentiation as well as immunostaining with cytokeratin, PSA, and PAP may be helpful. Malignant lymphoma and leukemia are rare and usually involve the prostate gland following systemic spread.

Neoplasms arising in the seminal vesicle are rare except for contiguous or metastatic involvement by prostatic adenocarcinoma, observed in about 12% of radical prostatectomy specimens from patients with cancer otherwise confined to the prostate.[41] There are three patterns of seminal vesicle invasion: (1) direct spread along the ejaculatory duct complex into the seminal vesicles, (2) prostatic capsular perforation followed by extension into the periprostatic soft tissues with spread into the seminal vesicles, and (3) isolated deposits of cancer in the seminal vesicles. Urothelial carcinoma of the bladder may also invade the seminal vesicle by direct extension or spread along the mucosa of the prostatic urethra, ejaculatory ducts, and seminal vesicles. A variety of rare benign and malignant soft tissue tumors have been described in the seminal vesicles.

TESTIS AND PARATESTICULAR STRUCTURES

Infertility

Testicular biopsy for infertility is usually bilateral, and more than 25% of cases show differences between the paired specimens.[10] The biopsy specimen is taken from the testicular aspect opposite from the rete testis through a 4- to 5-mm incision of the tunica albuginea, allowing herniation of testicular parenchyma that can be sampled. Specimens are usually placed in Bouin's fixative (for optimal nuclear detail), routinely processed, and stained with hematoxylin and eosin. Serial sections are stained with elastic tissue stains to accentuate the tubular profiles. The biopsy sample should contain at least 20 to 30 tubules, and detailed quantitative analysis is often necessary, including tubular diameters and relative number of spermatogonia and other tubular cells (Fig. 14–11). Common abnormalities include maturation arrest, ''Sertoli cell–only'' tubules, tubular hyalinization, hypospermatogenesis or other alterations in spermatogenesis, and mixed tubular atrophy.

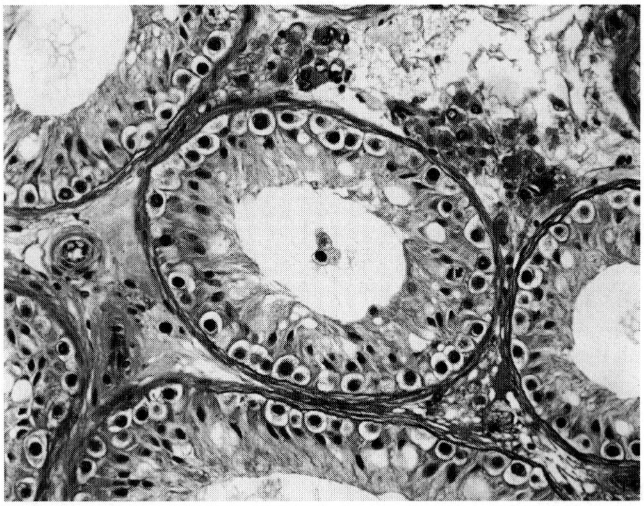

Figure 14–11. Testicular biopsy showing maturation arrest and peritubular fibrosis. Large vesicular nuclei of immature sperm precursor cells are absent.

Inflammation

Testicular inflammation (orchitis) is usually viral or idiopathic. Idiopathic granulomatous orchitis (also known as autoimmune orchitis) usually occurs in patients with azospermia or oligospermia and is typically associated with sperm granulomas in the epididymis. Characteristic pathologic findings include extensive lymphoplasmacytic inflammation, with destruction of progenitor cells within seminiferous tubules; however, the specificity of these findings is uncertain. Most cases of acute and chronic orchitis are infectious, arising as a result of retrograde spread from the vas deferens and epididymis. Clinically, there is swelling and pain, with or without systemic illness. Acute inflammation includes neutrophilic infiltration with destruction of the seminiferous tubules and the interstitium. In chronic orchitis, there is atrophy and peritubular fibrosis.

The most frequent type of viral infection of the testis is mumps orchitis, although other viruses have also been described. Testicular involvement by mumps is rare in children but occurs in 20% of adult cases. Approximately half of these adult cases develop testicular atrophy, usually only unilateral. Less than 10% of adults with mumps develop sterility, with orchitis developing approximately 1 week after the onset of parotid gland swelling. This is due to direct viral infection of the testis. Granulomatous orchitis has also been associated with fungi, tuberculosis, rickettsia, parasites, and malakoplakia. Rarely, systemic vasculitis may be manifest in the testis, including about 85% of cases of polyarteritis nodosa.

Torsion and Varicocele

Testicular torsion usually occurs in children and adolescents, often in association with anatomic abnormalities.[42] Torsion rapidly leads to venous infarction and should be considered a surgical emergency, with testicular viability declining within a few hours if the torsion is not corrected.

Varicocele is caused by congenital absence or insufficiency of the internal spermatic vein valves, with inversion of blood flow and reflux causing varixlike distention of the pampiniform plexus. This is the most common single cause of infertility, accounting for up to 37% of cases, usually associated with hypospermatogenesis.

Cryptorchidism

Cryptorchidism (undescended testis) may be unilateral or bilateral and is more frequent in premature than in term infants; less than 1% of infants have cryptorchidism by age 1 year.[10] It is usually unilateral and not associated with other abnormalities. Orchiopexy during early childhood probably reduces the likelihood of subsequent infertility. About 10% of germ-cell tumors arise in cryptorchid testes.

Intratubular Germ-Cell Neoplasia

Intratubular germ-cell neoplasia (ITGCN) consists of abnormal germ cells within the seminiferous tubules and is considered the precursor of testicular germ-cell tumors (Fig. 14–12).[10] Intratubular germ-cell neoplasia has invasive potential and may occur in the absence of a testicular mass. It is frequently observed in patients with gonadal dysgenesis, in the contralateral testis of patients with invasive germ-cell tumor, in patients with cryptorchidism (2 to 8%), and in patients with androgen receptor disorders. At least 50% of untreated patients with cryptorchidism and ITGCN followed for several years develop invasive germ-cell neoplasms, and bilateral testicular biopsy may be of value. Screening biopsies are recommended for those with cryptorchidism between the ages of 18 and 20 years, because negative findings suggest minimal risk. The neoplastic cells of ITGCN react strongly with antibodies to placental alkaline phosphatase (PLAP), a finding that may be useful in microscopic differential diagnosis.

Germ-Cell Tumors

Testicular germ-cell tumors are the most common cause (13%) of cancer death in 20- to 34-year-old American

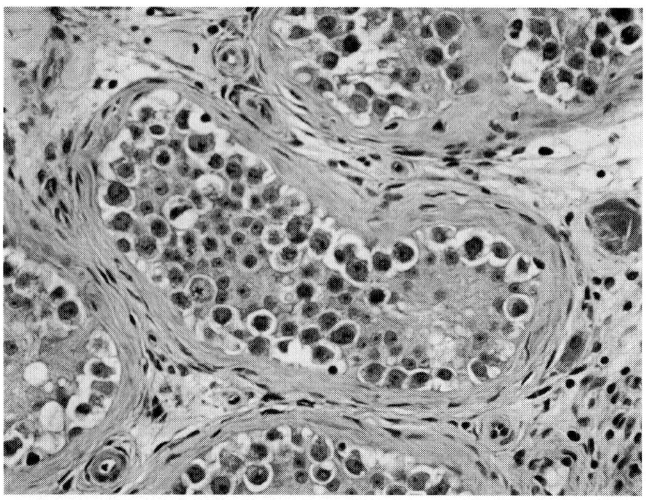

Figure 14–12. Intratubular germ-cell neoplasia of the testis (ITGCN). Immature vesicular nuclei are abundant and unaccompanied by normal maturation.

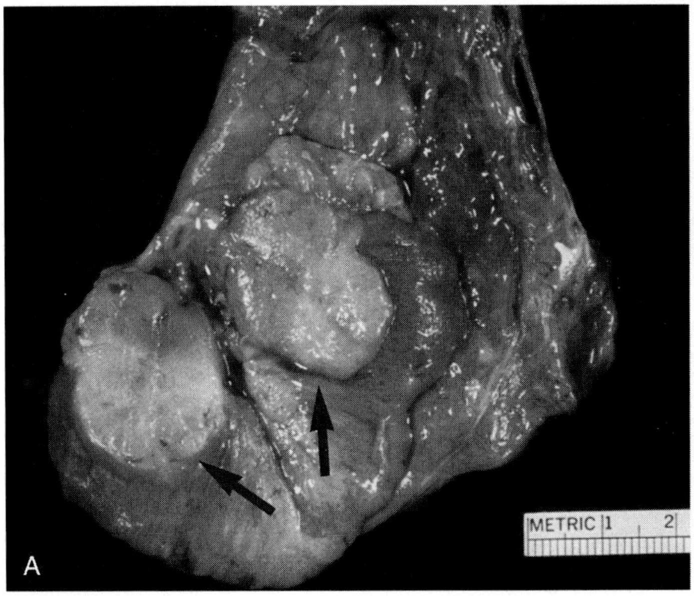

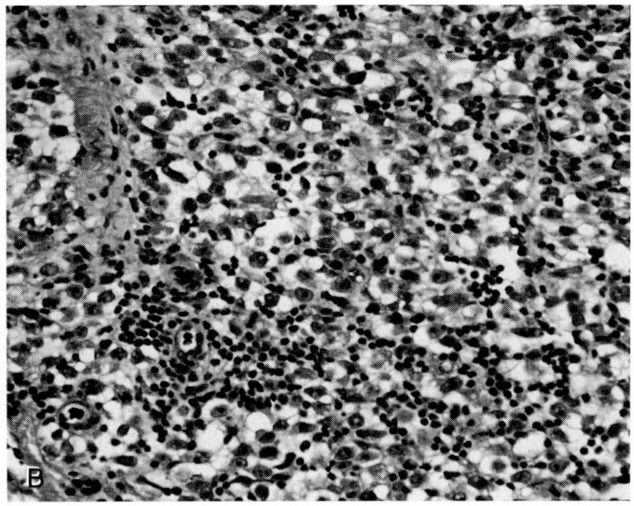

Figure 14–13. Testicular seminoma. *A.* Grossly, a solitary uniform nodule has been bisected (*arrows*). B. Microscopically, the tumor cells are uniform and large, with clear cytoplasm. There is a conspicuous infiltration by small, reactive lymphocytes.

males.[10, 43–45] These tumors are rare among blacks in both the United States and Africa. Risk factors include family history (16% of cases), cryptorchidism (10%), and infection. Germ-cell tumors are frequently asymptomatic. Even with enlargement, there may not be associated pain. Other types of neoplasms can occur in the testicular tunics, rete testis, and other adnexal structures, but these are rare. They include cysts, benign hyperplastic growths, and neoplasms (see following text).

Serum concentration of germ-cell tumor markers should be obtained preoperatively. These markers include beta–human chorionic gonadotropin (HCG), alpha-fetoprotein (AFP), and PLAP. For correct diagnosis and treatment, orchiectomy with removal of the cord is usually indicated. Final treatment depends upon the histology of the primary tumor, the serum concentration of tumor markers after orchiectomy, and the presence and histologic type of metastases.

There are five main types of germ-cell tumor: (1) *seminoma* (Fig. 14–13), (2) *embryonal carcinoma*, (3) *yolk-sac tumor*, (4) *choriocarcinoma*, and (5) *teratoma*. Frequently, mixed tumors are seen, thus dictating the need for adequate histologic sampling and thorough examination. *Seminoma* is the most common, usually occurring in patients 30 to 50 years of age. It contains variable numbers of lymphocytes and is bilateral in 2% of cases. In pure seminoma, AFP and HCG are negative but tumor cells contain abundant glycogen. Cells are aneuploid. Seminoma with numerous mitotic figures (more than three per high-power field) and cellular anaplasia is considered to be the anaplastic variant, but this subtyping has no apparent prognostic value. One variant of seminoma, referred to as spermatocytic seminoma, almost always occurs in older men and has never been associated with other germ-cell tumors. Its occurrence is restricted exclusively to the male gonad, having no histologic counterparts in ovaries or in extragenital sites. Unlike typical seminoma, spermatocytic seminoma tumor cells are diploid, suggesting that they have not undergone reduction division, and do not express PLAP.

Embryonal carcinoma is a primitive germ-cell neoplasm of adolescence and adulthood that rarely occurs in pure form but is seen as a component in about 47% of germ-cell tumors; it is not observed in infants or children. In pure embryonal carcinoma, there may be marginal elevation of AFP concentration, probably due to inapparent yolk-sac tumor elements. Human chorionic gonadotropin is not observed in these cells.

Yolk-sac tumor, also called endodermal sinus tumor, occurs in infants and children and previously has been termed ''adenocarcinoma of the infant testis.'' In pure form, it is rare in adults; but as a component, it is present in about 41% of mixed germ-cell tumors. Typical histologic patterns include anastomosing tubuloacinar structures, papillary structures, and Schiller-Duval bodies. Alpha-fetoprotein is considered a marker of yolk-sac tumor.

Choriocarcinoma is a rare and aggressive testicular tumor, usually detected clinically as manifestations of metastatic tumor. Human chorionic gonadotropin is markedly elevated in the serum and present within tumor cells; AFP is usually negative. Two cell types are observed: syncytiotrophoblastic and cytotrophoblastic. Unlike other testicular germ-cell tumors, choriocarcinoma metastasizes by hematogenous as well as lymphatic routes.

Teratoma composed exclusively of mature tissues is clinically benign and does not require treatment other than orchiectomy. Most teratomas occurring in prepubertal children are mature and, even when immature, are clinically benign. In adults, teratomas that have areas with immature tissues are considered malignant.

Staging of Germ-Cell Tumors

Numerous staging protocols for testicular germ cell tumors have been proposed; the most recent TNM staging system is shown in Table 14–4.

Table 14–4. TNM Staging of Testicular Cancer

Extent of primary tumor (T)			
TX	Primary tumor cannot be assessed (in the absence of radical orchiectomy, TX is used)		
T0	Histologic scar or no evidence of primary tumor		
Tis	Intratubular tumor: preinvasive cancer		
T1	Tumor limited to testis, including rete testis		
T2	Tumor invades beyond tunica albuginea or into epididymis		
T3	Tumor invades spermatic cord		
T4	Tumor invades scrotum		
Regional lymph nodes (N)			
NX	Regional lymph nodes cannot be assessed		
N0	No regional lymph node metastasis		
N1	Metastasis in a single lymph node, 2 cm or less in greatest dimension		
N2	Metastasis in a single lymph node, more than 2 cm but not more than 5 cm in greatest dimension, or multiple lymph nodes, none more than 5 cm in greatest dimension		
N3	Metastasis in a lymph node more than 5 cm in greatest dimension		
Distant metastasis (M)			
MX	Presence of distant metastasis cannot be assessed		
M0	No distant metastasis		
M1	Distant metastasis		
Stage grouping			
Stage 0	Tis	N0	M0
Stage I	T1	N0	M0
	T2	N0	M0
Stage II	T3	N0	M0
	T4	N0	M0
Stage III	Any T	N1	M0
Stage IV	Any T	N2, N3	M0
	Any T	Any N	M1

Source: From Beahrs OH, Henson DE, Hutter RVP, Kennedy BJ. *Manual for Staging of Cancer,* 4th ed. AJCC. Philadelphia: Lippincott; 1992:115–122, 189.

Treatment and Outcome

In determining therapy, testicular germ-cell tumors are commonly divided into two types: seminoma and nonseminoma. Seminoma is radiosensitive. Patients with clinical stage I or nonbulky stage II tumor are managed by orchiectomy and irradiation of paraaortic, paracaval, and ipsilateral pelvic lymph nodes, with a 95% cure rate. Patients with advanced-stage seminoma or bulky retroperitoneal tumor are managed by chemotherapy, with a cure rate of up to 80%. Proposed prognostic factors in seminoma include prominent lymphoid tumor reaction, elevated serum HCG concentration, and advanced stage. The recognition of nonseminomatous elements in otherwise typical seminoma carries a worse prognosis.

The management of low-stage nonseminomatous germ-cell tumor includes orchiectomy with or without nerve-sparing retroperitoneal lymph node dissection. Orchiectomy alone cures 60 to 70% of patients with stage I tumors, and combination chemotherapy in those with nodal involvement or nodal relapse results in greater than 95% survival. Factors indicating poor prognosis include advanced patient age, microvascular invasion, predominant or pure embryonal carcinoma, prominent neovascularization, absence of a yolk-sac component, presence of choriocarcinoma, preorchiectomy AFP value greater than 80 ng/mL, slow decline in AFP concentration after orchiectomy, high S-phase fraction, and aneuploid DNA content. Patients with bulky stage II tumor or advanced stage are treated by orchiectomy, tumor debulking, and chemotherapy, with 70 to 80% survival.

Most germ-cell tumors metastasize by lymphatic channels to the iliac and periaortic lymph nodes and subsequently spread to the lungs, liver, and mediastinal lymph nodes. By contrast, seminoma often spreads to bone, and choriocarcinoma spreads by hematogenous routes, sometimes to the brain. After treatment, germ-cell tumors recur as metastases, usually within 2 years.

Metastatic germ-cell tumor displays differentiation disparate from the primary tumor in up to 44% of cases. Interestingly, the primary tumor may regress histologically, leaving only a scar despite aggressive progression of metastases; in rare instances, a metastasis is the first manifestation of tumor with no palpable abnormality of the testis.

Orchiectomy

The testis and attached tunics and spermatic cord should be weighed, measured, and examined in the fresh state soon after surgical removal. Immersion of the intact specimen in fixative does not allow penetration through the tunics, often resulting in autolysis of the testicular parenchyma. For this reason, rapid processing is essential. If delay in pathologic examination is anticipated, the surgeon should make a single deep incision through the testis to allow penetration of fixative. The cord should be measured and palpated for neoplasm, as should the tunica vaginalis and tunica albuginea. The testis should be bisected, preferably through the hilum, and then serially sliced with parallel cuts. The size, gross appearance, and location of any neoplasms should be recorded, and multiple blocks should be submitted to encompass the entire mass of small tumors or at least 10 blocks of larger tumors. Thorough sectioning is essential to identify heterogeneous elements in many germ-cell tumors, recognizing that the presence of even a microscopic field of any other type of tumor within a seminoma alters therapy. The uninvolved testis should be sectioned, as well as the epididymis, the spermatic cord margin, midcord, and proximal cord, and any grossly suspicious areas.

Other Tumors

A variety of rare tumors are observed in the testis, testicular tunics, and adnexal structures. These include sex cord–stromal tumors (Leydig's cell and Sertoli's cell tumors, both of which are usually benign, and patients may present with symptoms such as gynecomastia due to steroid hormone production by tumor cells); malignant lymphoma (the most common testicular tumor in men over 50 years of age); and a variety of benign and malignant soft tissue tumors.[10]

EXTERNAL GENITALIA AND PERINEUM

Inflammation

A variety of infectious and inflammatory processes can affect the external genitalia. *Fournier's scrotal gangrene* (fusospirochetal infection) is an ulcerative lesion of the glans penis or scrotum occurring in injured or debilitated patients as a result of infection by fusobacteria and anaerobic treponemes. Diagnosis requires smears that demonstrate elongate gram-negative rods and coiled spirochetes.

Plasma cell balanitis is a circumscribed plaquelike lesion of the glans penis of uncircumcised men—its etiology is unknown. Its diagnosis requires biopsy, showing epidermal atrophy without atypia, lichenoid plasma cell dermatitis, and hemosiderin deposition.

Lichen sclerosus et atrophicus is a degenerative condition of the glans penis that appears as white atrophic patches; diagnosis may be made clinically, but biopsy reveals epidermal atrophy, homogenization of the superficial dermis, and patchy, nonspecific inflammation.

Gonorrhea and nongonococcal urethritis are the most common venereal diseases; their diagnoses rely upon clinical impression and culture findings. Reiter's syndrome usually occurs in young men with nongonococcal urethritis, arthritis, and conjunctivitis; there is often a psoriasiform lesion of the glans penis. Syphilitic chancre is a hard but painless plaque, often with erosion, caused by *Treponema pallidum*. Diagnosis can be made by smear, with silver stain revealing numerous spirochetes. Chancroid appears as multiple painful ulcers, usually associated with regional lymphadenitis, caused by *Haemophilus ducreyi*. Culture or smear, with the organisms appearing as parallel chains of gram-negative bacilli, provides the diagnosis. Granuloma inguinale appears as chronic spreading ulcers with scarring, caused by *Calymmatobacterium granulomatis*. Diagnosis can be made by culture or biopsy results revealing ulcer with acanthosis, prominent granulation tissue response with a paucity of lymphocytes, and distinctive Donovan bodies within histiocytes on silver stain. Lymphogranuloma venereum appears as small vesicles (which are often overlooked) associated with bilateral inguinal lymphadenopathy and caused by *Chlamydia trachomatis*. The diagnosis is based upon clinicopathologic correlations. Lymph node biopsy is the most common procedure, revealing follicular hyperplasia with stellate necrosis rimmed by macrophages. Herpes progenitalis infection causes a vesicular eruption that regresses and recurs and is usually caused by herpesvirus type II. Diagnosis is confirmed with clinical features and findings on smear or biopsy with identification of typical intranuclear inclusions. Condyloma acuminatum appears as one or more soft exophytic masses caused by human papillomavirus (usually HPV-6 and HPV-11). Diagnosis is usually reached clinically, but the biopsy specimen reveals typical epidermal papillomatosis and distinctive koilocytotic changes of the epidermis. Pediculosis pubis may cause erythema or vesicles and is caused by pubic louse infection. Scabies appears as multiple pruritic nodules caused by *Sarcoptes scabiei*. Demonstration of the organisms in biopsy specimens is diagnostic, but clinical impression is often sufficient. Molluscum contagiosum appears as multiple small papules caused by a *DNA poxvirus*. Clinical appearance and biopsy identification of pathognomonic intracytoplasmic molluscum bodies within the epidermis support the diagnosis. Superficial mycoses such as tinea cruris may also involve the external genitalia and perineum and are best diagnosed by clinical impression, scrapings stained by silver stain, biopsy, or culture.

Tumors

Noninvasive squamous-cell carcinoma in situ (penile intraepithelial neoplasia; previously referred to as Bowen's disease) usually appears as a poorly circumscribed erythematous change or multiple papules of the penis, sometimes associated with human papillomavirus types 16 and 18. Biopsy reveals epidermal thickening with a disordered maturation sequence, enlarged hyperchromatic nuclei, and increased numbers of mitotic figures.[10, 46, 47] *Extramammary Paget's disease* occurs in patients over 50 years of age as pruritic erythematous macules. Biopsy reveals mucin-producing cells within the epidermis. In some cases, there is an underlying carcinoma.

Squamous-cell carcinoma is the most common malignancy of the external genitalia and perineum and occurs most frequently on the glans penis of uncircumcised men. The tumor may be large, exophytic, and noninvasive (verrucous carcinoma), with an excellent prognosis following treatment, or it may be ulcerative and invasive (typical squamous-cell carcinoma), with the prognosis based upon the grade and extent of invasion. Other neoplasms include basal-cell carcinoma (rare), malignant melanoma (rare but aggressive), and metastases, often from the prostate.

PITFALLS FOR THE SURGEON

Kidney

1. Determining true positive margins in cases of enucleation or partial nephrectomy.
2. When doing a partial nephrectomy, determining if there are other tumors in the remaining kidney.

Bladder and Urothelium

1. Mucosal folds may be mistaken for papillae.
2. Urothelial carcinoma in situ may be cystoscopically difficult or impossible to identify.
3. Superficial biopsies of thickened urothelium may yield insufficient tissue to determine the presence or extent of invasion of cancer.

Continued

Prostate and Seminal Vesicles

1. On digital rectal examination, the seminal vesicles may have a variable anatomic location, mimicking prostatic nodularity.
2. Apical dissection is critical in radical prostatectomy for cancer, balancing the need for uninvolved surgical margins with preservation of the narrow and delicate external striated sphincter that controls continence.
3. Benign enlargement of lymph nodes may be mistaken for metastatic carcinoma.

Testis and Paratesticular Adnexae

1. Embryonic remnants in the paratesticular adnexae may mimic tumor.

External Genitalia and Perineum

1. Squamous-cell carcinoma in situ may be mistaken for genital warts.

PITFALLS FOR THE PATHOLOGIST

Kidney

1. Interpretation of a biopsy for glomerular disease without sufficient number of glomeruli creates potential for misdiagnosis due to sampling error.
2. Oncocytoma is a common adult renal tumor with large eosinophilic cells that may be mistaken for renal-cell carcinoma on frozen section and even on permanent sections.
3. Possibility of bilateral angiomyolipoma should always be considered to avoid missing a case of tuberous sclerosis.

Bladder and Urothelium

1. Normal squamous epithelium, which is often present at the trigone in women, may be mistaken for squamous metaplasia.
2. Falsely negative results occur with advanced cancers that ulcerate and reepithelialize with benign urothelium, thereby temporarily losing the capacity for exfoliation of malignant cells into the urine.

Prostate and Seminal Vesicles

1. Needle biopsy containing tissue from the seminal vesicle, ejaculatory duct, or Cowper's gland may be misinterpreted as prostatic adenocarcinoma.
2. Granulomatous prostatitis, glandular atrophy, xanthoma, and sclerosing adenosis are vexing diagnostic problems and may easily be mistaken for carcinoma.

Testis and Paratesticular Adnexae

1. Interpretation of a biopsy for fertility without sufficient number of tubules[15–20] creates potential for misdiagnosis due to sampling error.
2. Thorough sectioning is essential to identify mixed elements in seminoma, recognizing that a single focus of another type of tumor alters therapy.

FURTHER READING

Bostwick DG, Eble JN, eds. *Urologic Surgical Pathology*. Philadelphia: Mosby-Year Book; 1996. In press.

Holleb AI, Fink DJ, Murphy GP, eds. *American Cancer Society Textbook of Clinical Oncology*. Atlanta: American Cancer Society; 1991.

Petersen RO. *Urologic Pathology*. Philadelphia: Lippincott; 1993.

Walsh PC, Retik AB, Stamey TA, Vaughan ED, eds. *Campbell's Urology*, 6th ed. Philadelphia: Saunders; 1992.

REFERENCES

1. Heptinstall RH. *Pathology of the Kidney*, 4th ed. Boston: Little, Brown; 1992.
2. Tisher C, Brenner BM. *Renal Pathology, with Clinical and Pathological Correlations*, 2nd ed. Philadelphia: Lippincott; 1994.
3. Schrier RW, Gottschalk CW, eds. *Diseases of the Kidney*, 5th ed. Boston: Little, Brown; 1993.
4. Couser WG. Pathogenesis of glomerulonephritis. *Kidney Int*. 1993; 44:S19.
5. Brezis M, Epstein FH. Cellular mechanisms of acute ischemic injury to the kidney. *Annu Rev Med*. 1993; 44:27.
6. Bonventre J. Mechanisms of ischemic renal failure. *Kidney Int*. 1993; 43:1160.
7. Gardner KD Jr, Bernstein J. *The Cystic Kidney*. Dordrecht: Kluwer; 1990.
8. Parfrey PS, Bear JC, Morgan J, et al. The diagnosis and prognosis of autosomal dominant polycystic kidney disease. *N Engl J Med*. 1990; 323:1085.
9. Eble JN, ed. *Tumors and Tumor-like Conditions of the Kidneys and Ureters*. New York: Churchill Livingstone; 1990.
10. Bostwick DG, Eble JN, eds. *Urologic Surgical Pathology*. Philadelphia, Mosby-Year Book; 1996. In press.
11. Young RH, ed. *Pathology of the Urinary Bladder*. New York: Churchill Livingstone; 1989.
12. Murphy WM, Farrow GM, Beckwith B. Tumors of the urinary bladder, urethra, ureters, renal pelvis, and kidneys. Washington, DC: Armed Forces Institute of Pathology; In: *Atlas of Tumor Pathology*, 2nd series. Fascicle 1994.
13. Helpap B. Histological and immunohistochemical study of chronic prostatic inflammation with and without benign prostatic hyperplasia. *J Urol Pathol*. 1994; 2:49–64.
14. Stillwell TJ, Engen DE, Farrow GM: The clinical spectrum of granulomatous prostatitis: A report of 200 cases. *J Urol*. 1987; 138:320–323.
15. Sebo TJ, Bostwick DG, Farrow GM, et al. Prostatic xanthoma: A mimic of prostatic adenocarcinoma. *Hum Pathol* 1994; 25:386–389.
16. Presti B, Weidner N. Granulomatous prostatitis and poorly differentiated adenocarcinoma: Their distinction with the use of immunohistochemical methods. *Am J Clin Pathol*. 1991; 95:330–334.
17. Bostwick DG, Cooner WH, Denis L, et al. The association of benign prostatic hyperplasia and cancer of the prostate. *Cancer*. 1992; 70:291–301.
18. Guess HA. Benign prostatic hyperplasia: Antecedents and natural history. *Epidemiol Rev*. 1992; 14:131–153.
19. McNeal JE. The pathobiology of nodular hyperplasia. In: Bostwick DG, ed. *Pathology of the Prostate*. New York: Churchill Livingstone; 1990:31–36.
20. McNeal JE, Bostwick DG. Anatomy of the prostate: Implications for disease. In: Bostwick DG, ed. *Pathology of the Prostate*. New York: Churchill Livingstone; 1990:1–14.
21. Henson DE, Hutter RVP, Farrow GM. Practice protocol for the examination of specimens removed from patients with carcinoma of the prostate gland: A publication of the cancer committee, College of American Pathologists. *Arch Pathol Lab Med*. 1994; 118:779–783.
22. Graham SD Jr, Bostwick DG, Hoisaeter A, et al. Report of the committee on staging and pathology. *Cancer*. 1992; 70(suppl):359–361.
23. Bostwick DG. High grade prostatic intraepithelial neoplasia: The most likely precursor of prostatic adenocarcinoma. *Cancer*. 1995; 75:1823–1836.
24. Wingo PA, Tong T, Bolden S. Cancer statistics, 1995. *CA*. 1995; 45:8–30.
25. Bostwick DG. Gleason grading of prostatic needle biopsies: Correlation with grade in 316 matched prostatectomies. *Am J Surg Pathol*. 1994; 18:796–803.
26. Maksem JA, Galang CF, Johenning PW, et al. Aspiration biopsy cytology of the prostate. In: Bostwick DG, ed. *Pathology of the Prostate*. New York: Churchill Livingstone; 1990:161–191.
27. Oesterling JE, Jacobsen SJ, Chute CG, et al. Serum prostate-specific antigen in a community-based population of healthy men: Establishment of age-specific reference ranges. *JAMA* 1993; 270:860–866.
28. Blackwell KL, Bostwick DG, Myers RP, et al. Combining prostate specific antigen with cancer and gland volume to more reliably predict pathologic stage: The influence of PSA-cancer density. *J Urol* 1994; 151:1565–1570.
29. Ruckle HC, Klee GG, Oesterling JE. Prostate-specific antigen: Critical issues for the practicing physician. *Mayo Clin Proc*. 1994; 69:59–68.
30. Ruckle HC, Klee GG, Oesterling JE. Prostate-specific antigen: Concepts for staging prostate cancer and monitoring response to therapy. *Mayo Clin Proc*. 1994; 69:69–79.
31. Lilja H. Significance of different molecular forms of serum PSA: The free, noncomplexed form of PSA versus that complexed to alpha-1-antichymotrypsin. *Urol Clin North Am*. 1993; 20:681–686.
32. Bostwick DG. Prostate-specific antigen: Current role in diagnostic pathology of prostate cancer. *Am J Clin Pathol*. 1994; 102(suppl 1):S31–S37.
33. Gleason DF. Histologic grading of prostatic carcinoma. In: Bostwick DG, ed. *Pathology of the Prostate*. New York: Churchill Livingstone; 1990:83–93.
34. Bostwick DG, Myers RP, Oesterling JE. Staging of prostate cancer. *Semin Surg Oncol* 1994; 10:60–73.
35. Shroder FH, Hermanek P, Denis L, et al. The TNM classification of prostate carcinoma. *Prostate*. 1992; 4(suppl):129–138.
36. Walsh PC, Lepor H, Eggleston JC. Radical prostatectomy with preservation of sexual function: Anatomical and pathological considerations. *Prostate*. 1983; 4:473–485.
37. Hall GS, Kramer CE, Epstein JI. Evaluation of radical prostatectomy specimens: A comparative analysis of sampling methods. *Am J Surg Pathol*. 1992; 16:315–324.
38. Ayala AG, Ro JY, Babaian R, et al. The prostatic capsule: Does it exist? Its importance in the staging and treatment of prostatic carcinoma. *Am J Surg Pathol*. 1989; 13:21–30.
39. See WA, Williams RD. Management of prostate cancer: Stage by stage. In: Das S, Crawford ED, eds. *Cancer of the Prostate*. New York: Marcel Dekker, 1993:397–420.
40. Scardino PT. Early detection of prostate cancer. *Urol Clin North Am*. 1989; 16:635–655.
41. Ohori M, Scardino P, Lapin S, et al. The mechanisms and prognostic significance of seminal vesicle involvement by prostate cancer. *Am J Surg Pathol*. 1993; 17:1252–1261.
42. Sheldon CC. Undescended testis and testicular torsion. *Surg Clin North Am*. 1985; 65:1303.
43. Talerman A, ed. *Pathology of the Testis and Its Adnexae*. New York: Churchill Livingstone; 1986.
44. Ilson DH, Bosl GJ, Motzer R, et al. Genetic analysis of germ cell tumors: Current progress and future prospects. *Hematol Oncol Clin North Am*. 1991; 5:1271.
45. Brodsky GL. Pathology of testicular germ cell tumors. *Hematol Oncol Clin North Am* 1991; 5:1095.
46. Kaye V, Zhang G, Dehner LP, Fraley EE. Carcinoma in situ of penis: Is distinction between erythroplasia of Queyrat and Bowen's disease relevant? *Urology*. 1990; 36:479.
47. Sarkar FH, Miles BJ, Plieth DH, Crissman JD. Detection of human papillomavirus in squamous neoplasms of the penis. *J Urol*. 1992; 147:389.
48. Beahrs OH, Henson DE, Hutter RVP, Kennedy BJ. *Manual for Staging of Cancer*, 4th ed. American Joint Committee on Cancer (AJCC). Philadelphia: Lippincott; 1992:115–122, 203.
49. Beahrs OH, Henson DE, Hutter RVP, Kennedy BJ. *Manual for Staging of Cancer*, 4th ed. American Joint Committee on Cancer (AJCC). Philadelphia: Lippincott; 1992:115–122, 199.
50. Beahrs OH, Henson DE, Hutter RVP, Kennedy BJ. *Manual for Staging of Cancer*. 4th ed. American Joint Committee on Cancer (AJCC). Philadelphia: Lippincott; 1992:115–122, 189.

15

Obstetric and Gynecologic Pathology

Steven G. Silverberg and Jeffrey Y. Lin

Definition

Obstetric and gynecologic pathology is a field that has been the subject of several major textbooks. Although most of the diseases encountered in this field are diagnosed and treated by the general obstetrician-gynecologist, others are best managed by subspecialists such as gynecologic oncologists. Conditions encountered by the general surgeon fall into two categories: (1) lesions that are gynecologic in origin but impinge on, invade into, or metastasize to other organs outside the female genital tract and (2) gynecologic conditions that are acute surgical emergencies with a differential diagnosis that includes nongynecologic diseases. In this chapter, we emphasize conditions most likely to be encountered by the general surgeon.

Patients with gynecologic diseases present with a variety of signs and symptoms. Common clinical presentations that bring the patient to an obstetrician-gynecologist include abnormal vaginal bleeding (menometrorrhagia and other forms of irregular bleeding, amenorrhea, and postmenopausal bleeding), vaginal discharge, vulvar masses or dermatologic complaints, an abnormal Papanicolaou smear, and clinical manifestations of an intrauterine pregnancy. Patients with other complaints, such as chronic pelvic pain or virilization, may be seen by either a general surgeon or an obstetrician-gynecologist; however, in these instances, the diagnosis is usually made preoperatively and the patient is operated on by the appropriate specialist. In acute presentations of gynecologic diseases and pelvic mass, the patient is often referred to a general surgeon.

Since the clinical presentations of disease of the female genital tract determine whether the general surgeon will become involved with patient management, we begin this chapter with the most common clinical presentations of gynecologic diseases. We then discuss diseases likely to be encountered by general surgeons. These include diseases of the ovary, the fallopian tubes, the uterine corpus and cervix, and the peritoneum. The latter is included because a number of pathologic lesions are encountered in the peritoneum of women and are rarely if ever seen in men. Several of these conditions can involve the genital tract locally or diffusely and are usually treated by gynecologists; however, if manifestations are primarily extragenital, they may be treated by the general surgeon.

Intrauterine pregnancy and its complications are not discussed in detail in this chapter. Pregnant women can develop any of the diseases that are discussed elsewhere in this text, and pregnancy can complicate the diagnosis and management of many of these diseases. Ectopic pregnancy is discussed in the section on diseases of the fallopian tube, since it can occur as a surgical emergency and thus be treated by the general surgeon. Diseases of the vulva and vagina are discussed only in relation to surgical considerations, since these diseases are managed in large part medically by the obstetrician-gynecologist.

Clinical Manifestations of Gynecologic Disease

Gynecologic conditions should always be considered in the differential diagnosis of women presenting with pelvic or abdominal symptoms. Women undergoing laparotomy or laparoscopic procedures are often diagnosed incidentally with gynecologic pathology. The proximity of the müllerian tract and the urinary and gastrointestinal systems complicates accurate preoperative diagnosis. Furthermore, pregnancy or concern regarding fertility may complicate surgical management.

ABDOMINAL OR PELVIC PAIN

The patient with ectopic pregnancy may present with acute onset of pelvic pain or hypovolemia. Torsion of an adnexal tumor may also cause acute pain with minimal fever and leukocytosis. Even small ovarian tumors and cysts may cause hemorrhage into the peritoneum or within the tumor itself. Salpingitis may cause acute or chronic pain and lead to pelvic abscess formation. Chronic, progressive pelvic pain may be due to endometriosis in reproductive-age women. Degenerating uterine leiomyomata may also produce severe pain, especially during pregnancy.

MENSTRUAL DISTURBANCES

Although the most common cause of secondary amenorrhea is pregnancy, endocrinologic disturbances such as hypothyroidism, pituitary adenoma, or virilizing ovarian neoplasms must also be considered. Oligomenorrhea is most commonly associated with polycystic ovary syndrome and is often accompanied by mild hirsutism and infertility. Menometrorrhagia or postmenopausal bleeding may be related to intrinsic endometrial or myometrial pathology such as endometrial polyps, hyperplasia, carcinoma, or sarcoma. The endometrium may be excessively stimulated by hormonally active ovarian neoplasms or by supplemental estrogen. Postmenopausal bleeding is an alarming clinical finding and lower genital tract malignancy must be excluded, since it is the cause in 15 to 20% of these patients.[1]

INTESTINAL OBSTRUCTION

Small-intestinal obstruction, particularly in postmenopausal women, may be related to metastatic ovarian carcinoma. Generally, the obstruction is in the distal ileum and is secondary to carcinomatosis. Obstruction may also result from radiation enteritis, a late sequel of radiotherapy for cervical or ovarian carcinoma. Low-grade colonic obstruction may occur with extrinsic compression of the rectosigmoid by an ovarian mass. Complete colonic obstruction may develop from deep infiltration of the rectosigmoid by extensive cul-de-sac tumor or from a large omental metastasis extending through the transverse colon.

FEVER AND SEPSIS

Salpingitis with concomitant tuboovarian abscess is the most common serious infectious gynecologic problem. Patients may present with pelvic pain, peritonitis, gastrointestinal disturbances, and signs of sepsis. Broad-spectrum antibiotic therapy is the mainstay of therapy, with surgery reserved for severe cases. Rarely, patients with ovarian carcinomatosis may develop sepsis from spontaneous peritonitis.

ASCITES AND PLEURAL EFFUSION

Ovarian carcinoma often produces ascites or even a pleural effusion. Although cytologic examination of the fluid may suggest a malignant process, exploratory surgery is often necessary to confirm the diagnosis, define extent of disease, and resect tumor. The patient with primary peritoneal serous adenocarcinoma almost always presents with ascites and pleural effusion; occasionally, an ill-defined pelvic or abdominal mass is noted. Rarely, benign ovarian neoplasms cause ascites with pleural effusion (Meigs' syndrome).

Ovary

ANATOMY AND HISTOLOGY

During the reproductive years, ovaries weigh 5 to 8 g and measure 3 to 4 cm in maximum dimension. Ovarian size increases during pregnancy and decreases after the age of 30, progressing to postmenopausal atrophy (2.5 cm maximal dimension). The ovary is located behind and above the fallopian tube, behind the broad ligament, and in front of the rectum. It is attached to the lateral pelvic wall by the infundibulopelvic ligament, to the cornu of the uterus by the uteroovarian ligament, and to the fallopian tube by the tuboovarian ligament. The ovary is supplied by the ovarian artery, a branch of the abdominal aorta that anastomoses with the ovarian branch of the uterine artery. The venous drainage of the ovary forms a plexus at the hilum, which then drains into the right and left uteroovarian and ovarian veins. The lymphatic drainage of the ovaries is to the lower paraaortic and pelvic lymph nodes.

Histologically, the ovary consists of a stromal mass containing the follicles and their derivatives, surrounded by a single layer of coelomic surface epithelium derived from peritoneal mesothelium. Although this epithelial layer is inconspicuous in the normal adult ovary, it is thought to be the tissue from which most malignant ovarian tumors arise.

The external or cortical zone of the ovary consists of a characteristic connective tissue stroma and contains follicles in different stages of maturation, the number of which progressively decreases with age. Most of the approximately 400,000 follicles present at birth degenerate, but those that mature become known as corpora lutea ("yellow bodies," an excellent descriptive term for these corrugated, bright yellow structures) after the oocytes are expelled at ovulation. The mature corpus luteum measures up to 1.5 cm in diameter. A normal corpus luteum of pregnancy is considerably larger, although it begins to regress after the third month of pregnancy. If conception does not occur, the corpus luteum involutes, resulting in a convoluted, hyalinized scar known as a corpus albicans (''white body,'' again describing the gross appearance of this structure).

The normal mature follicle is lined by small, round granulosa cells, which are surrounded by larger thecal cells. Depending upon their location and stage of maturation, thecal cells are either spindled and fibroblastlike or large and polygonal, with voluminous eosinophilic cytoplasm. Each of these elements can also give rise to neoplasms; however, these tumors are not as common as epithelial tumors. The third major type of ovarian neoplasm arises from the germ cells. The ovarian medulla consists predominantly of stroma, blood vessels, lymphatics, and nerves. Few pathologic conditions arise in this region.

NONNEOPLASTIC CYSTS

Although the ovary is occasionally involved by malformations, premature atrophic conditions, and inflammatory diseases, the most common pathologic conditions are nonneoplastic cysts and benign and malignant neoplasms. The cysts can be incidental microscopic findings, or they can be large and/or multiple and occur as palpable masses.

A convenient classification schema divides the ovarian cysts into those of germinal, epithelial inclusion origin and those of follicular origin. The former represent invaginations of the overlying surface epithelium into the ovarian cortex; they accumulate fluid and enlarge to microscopic or clinical size. The latter are derived from one or more layers of the ovarian follicle or corpus luteum. All of these benign cysts tend to be unilocular and filled with clear, colorless or amber-colored fluid. An exception is corpus luteum cysts, which are often hemorrhagic and may occur with rupture and hemoperitoneum. The *corpus luteum cyst* is also recognized grossly by the bright yellow to orange color of its wall, analogous to that of the normal corpus luteum.

Microscopically, *germinal inclusion cysts* are initially lined by a single layer of flattened to cuboidal epithelial cells. These cells may undergo differentiation into various types of müllerian epithelium and then be designated serous, mucinous, or endometrioid (see the discussion of ovarian neoplasms in the following text). *Follicular cysts* are lined by a layer of small round granulosa cells surrounded by larger spindled or polygonal theca cells, as in a normal follicle. Either of these layers may be luteinized, in which case the cells are enlarged and their cytoplasm filled with eosinophilic to foamy to clear material, which represents steroid hormones. Depending upon which layer is luteinized, the cyst is designated a granulosa lutein or theca lutein cyst.

These cysts can have clinical associations. Multiple follicular cysts with varying degrees of thecal luteinization are a prominent feature of the *polycystic ovary syndrome*, also known as the *Stein-Leventhal syndrome*.[2] In this condition, the ovaries are considerably enlarged and have a thick, pearly white capsule overlying multiple cysts. Women with this condition tend to be obese, hirsute, and infertile and tend to display various menstrual irregularities, primarily oligomenorrhea and metrorrhagia. The ovaries in this condition produce increased amounts of androgens, which may be metabolized to estrogens, and insufficient progesterone. The initial amenorrhea in these patients may be followed by profuse and irregular vaginal bleeding due to the precocious development of endometrial hyperplasia or adenocarcinoma.

Other nonneoplastic cysts can also be associated with clinical conditions but are less common than the polycystic ovary syndrome and, rather than infertility, are associated with pregnancy, either normal or abnormal. *Hyperreactio luteinalis*, for example, is characterized by massive bilateral ovarian enlargement secondary to multiple theca lutein cysts and develops in about 25% of women with gestational trophoblastic neoplasia.[3] It is also occasionally seen in women with both normal and abnormal pregnancies and in women undergoing ovulation induction for infertility. The *luteoma of pregnancy* usually also presents as bilateral ovarian enlargement but is unilateral in about one third of the cases. This condition is characterized by multiple nodules, occasionally cystic, of luteinized thecal or stromal cells.[4, 5] Large (up to 30 cm or greater) *solitary follicular cysts* with considerable cytologic atypia are occasionally discovered during pregnancy or in the puerperium.[5]

Other benign cysts are included in the differential diagnosis of some of the lesions discussed. A *simple cyst* results when the pressure of the intraluminal contents erodes the lining cells and they are no longer recognizable. These cysts are lined by fibrous tissue or granulation tissue (Fig. 15–1). Presumably, all simple cysts initially possessed features that would have permitted recognition as a specific cyst type. *Paraovarian* or *paratubal cysts* are lined by müllerian-type epithelium, usually displaying differentiation into epithelium resembling the normal mucosa of the fallopian tube. These cysts may become quite large and may be multiple, but they are almost always thin-walled, unilocular, and contain clear fluid. They are located adjacent to but not within the ovary and fallopian tube. Any of the epithelial neoplasms of the ovary discussed subsequently may rarely develop within one of these cysts, the most common being the serous tumor of low malignant potential.

Endometriosis is another common benign cystic lesion of the ovary. Because this condition is also seen throughout the female genital tract and elsewhere in the peritoneal cavity, it is discussed in more detail with diseases of the female peritoneum.

The major *pitfall for the surgeon* is performing unnecessary surgery on benign, nonneoplastic cysts. Most of the unilateral solitary cysts can be locally excised, sparing the

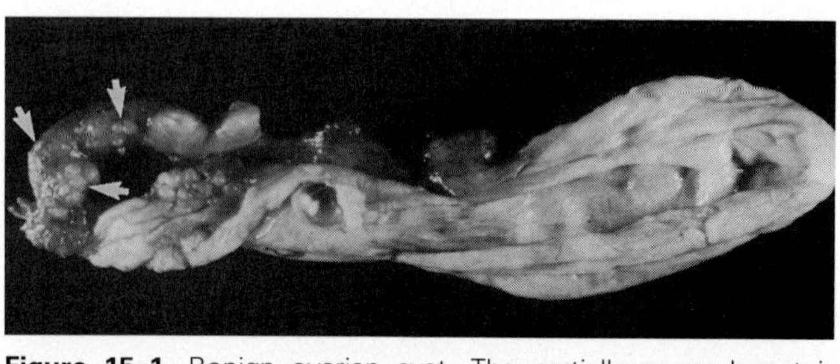

Figure 15–1. Benign ovarian cyst. The partially opened cyst is unilocular and thin-walled, with a smooth inner lining. The attached fallopian tube on the left shows a few serosal nodules of endosalpingiosis (*arrows*).

uninvolved ovarian tissue. Since most of these conditions occur predominantly in young women, this approach is particularly appropriate if the contralateral ovary has been removed or cannot be visualized. Similarly, the bilateral conditions described often regress with appropriate hormonal intervention. This approach means cessation of pregnancy for hyperreactio luteinalis or luteoma of pregnancy, or specific hormonal therapy for the polycystic ovary syndrome. Wedge biopsy or, in some cases, unilateral oophorectomy may be required for diagnosis, but bilateral oophorectomy is contraindicated. Bilateral wedge biopsy of polycystic ovaries may be therapeutic as well as diagnostic, because normal ovulation may resume following this maneuver.

The major *pitfall for the pathologist* is distinguishing between hyperreactio luteinalis, or pregnancy luteoma, and an ovarian steroid (lipid)-cell tumor, luteinized thecoma, or hilar-cell tumor, since the latter, if large and mitotically active, have potential for malignant behavior.[6] The hilar-cell tumor is virtually always unilateral, so that bilateral involvement effectively eliminates this from consideration. Because pregnancy luteomas may be unilateral and steroid-cell tumors may occur in pregnant patients, this situation poses a diagnostic problem. Even so, pregnancy luteomas usually consist of multiple nodules, whereas steroid-cell tumors are usually single nodules.

OVARIAN NEOPLASMS

Ovarian neoplasms are one of the most complex topics in gynecologic pathology and indeed in all of surgical pathology. In addition to the numerous tumors that metastasize to the ovaries, there are over 75 separate primary ovarian neoplasms! This discussion emphasizes the classification of ovarian neoplasms, their recognition as benign or malignant, and some important clinicopathologic correlations associated with specific neoplasms or groups of neoplasms.

Classification

Most primary ovarian neoplasms are derived from one of the following[7]:

1. The coelomic surface epithelium (peritoneal mesothelium) covering the ovary—epithelial tumors
2. The ovarian stroma and/or structures derived from the embryonic sex cords—sex cord–stromal tumors
3. The germ cells—germ-cell tumors

There are also several tumors that are not easily categorized because they contain more than one of the three elements listed (e.g., gonadoblastoma), they contain elements that are not considered in one of the three categories (e.g., the steroid-cell tumors), or they are derived from other cell types (primary malignant lymphomas and some soft tissue sarcomas of the ovary).

Up to 10% of malignant neoplasms of the ovary are metastatic, making this a consideration in the evaluation of any ovarian tumor.[8] Many of these—particularly those derived from the gastrointestinal tract—may clinically mimic primary ovarian neoplasms, with the actual primary sites becoming apparent only after microscopic examination. The surgeon encountering bilateral malignant ovarian tumors should explore the pelvis and abdomen to exclude nonovarian origin, since the majority of metastatic ovarian cancers are bilateral.

Epithelial Tumors

As a group, epithelial tumors of the ovary are the most common primary ovarian neoplasms, particularly in adults. They represent about 60% of all primary ovarian neoplasms and over 90% of malignant primary ovarian neoplasms (Table 15–1).[9] The *single* most common ovarian tumor, benign cystic teratoma (''dermoid cyst''), is not an epithelial tumor but a germ-cell tumor.

Epithelial tumors are classified by their pathway of differentiation and their degree of benignity or malignancy (Table 15–2). Most of these tumors are derived from coelomic surface epithelium, which invaginates beneath the ovarian surface, proliferates, and then differentiates into one or more of the epithelial types, most of which are of müllerian origin.[7] Thus, tumors that resemble the mucosa of the fallopian tube are designated *serous*, whereas *mu-*

Table 15–1. Ovarian Cancer: Compiled Statistics

Type of Tumor	Incidence (%)	Bilaterality (%)	5-Year Survival (%)
Serous borderline tumor	10–15	60[a]	95[b]
Serous carcinoma	25–35	60[a]	20
Mucinous borderline tumor	5–10	20[a]	95[b]
Mucinous carcinoma	5–10	20[a]	45
Endometrioid carcinoma	15–30	30[a]	50
Clear-cell carcinoma	4–6	10–30	40
Undifferentiated carcinoma	5–10	55	10
Yolk-sac tumor	<1	<5	>50[c]
Dysgerminoma	1–2	10–20	90
Immature teratoma	<1	<5	>50[c]
Secondary malignant teratoma	<1	0	15
Granulosa cell tumor	<5	5	90[b]
Androblastoma	<1	5	90

[a]Approximately half in stage I.
[b]Late recurrences common.
[c]With appropriate chemotherapy.
Source: From Gompel C, Silverberg SG: *Pathology in Gynecology and Obstetrics,* 4th ed. Philadelphia: JB Lippincott; 1994.

Table 15–2. Histogenesis and Nomenclature of Differentiated Epithelial Tumors of Coelomic Origin

Pathway of Differentiation	Benign Tumor	Borderline Tumor	Invasive Malignant Tumor
Tubal	Serous Cystadenoma Adenofibroma Surface papilloma	Borderline serous tumor	Serous carcinoma
Endocervical or intestinal	Mucinous Cystadenoma Adenofibroma[a]	Borderline mucinous tumor	Mucinous carcinoma
Endometrial	Endometrioid Adenofibroma[a]	Borderline endometrioid tumor[a]	Endometrioid carcinoma
Clear-cell (? endometrial)	Clear-cell adenofibroma[a]	Borderline clear cell tumor[a]	Clear-cell carcinoma
Urothelial	Brenner tumor	Proliferating Brenner tumor[a]	Malignant Brenner tumor[a]

[a]Rare.
Source: From Gompel C, Silverberg SG: *Pathology in Gynecology and Obstetrics,* 4th ed. Philadelphia: JB Lippincott; 1994.

cinous tumors display either endocervical or intestinal differentiation, *endometrioid* tumors contain elements resembling endometrial glands or stroma or both, and *Brenner tumors* and *transitional-cell carcinomas* contain epithelium resembling urinary bladder mucosa. The *clear-cell neoplasms* do not have an anatomic counterpart but are closely related to neoplasms showing endometrioid differentiation. Many ovarian tumors demonstrate more than one pathway of differentiation (*mixed epithelial tumors*), further complicating classification. Still others are so poorly differentiated that they are unclassifiable or are simply designated as *undifferentiated carcinoma.*

In comparison with the other major types, the epithelial neoplasms are more common, more likely to be bilateral, and more likely to be malignant. Likelihood of malignancy increases with age. Invasive carcinomas are rare before the age of 30 and are more frequent with succeeding decades. Symptoms are variable and include discomfort related to compression of adjacent structures, pain, menstrual abnormalities, and abdominal distention due either to the primary tumor or to ascites. As mentioned, nonneoplastic cysts may occur as ovarian masses, but these are generally seen in premenopausal women and usually regress spontaneously. Ovarian enlargement must be considered potentially malignant if it occurs in an older woman or if it does not resolve within 4 to 6 weeks.

Sonographic evaluation and serum CA-125 antibody levels[10] are useful in initially distinguishing between benign and malignant ovarian masses; nevertheless, exploration is necessary in many cases that ultimately are benign or even nonneoplastic. In most of these instances, the general surgeon will not be involved, since the laparotomy or laparoscopy will be performed by a gynecologist. If, however, the patient with an ovarian tumor presents acutely with rupture, hemorrhage, or torsion or if the pelvic or abdominal mass or ascites is thought to be nongynecologic in origin, the general surgeon may be the first physician to treat this patient. For this reason, the general surgeon must be aware of the gross appearances of these neoplasms as well as their operative management.

The *size* of an ovarian mass does not necessarily indicate likelihood of malignancy. Unlike neoplasms of many other organs, which are often discovered in preclinical states, ovarian tumors attract attention when they become palpable or cause symptoms. This finding applies to both benign and malignant tumors, since there is little tendency for the malignant neoplasms to be significantly larger. Indeed, small ovarian cancers may occur with widespread abdominal carcinomatosis, whereas benign ovarian tumors may become quite large before they cause symptoms. Size correlates best with histopathologic type—with benign teratomas and mucinous tumors being among the largest.[9]

Bilaterality also does not predict malignancy. As previously mentioned, metastases to the ovaries are almost always bilateral. Primary epithelial neoplasms are more frequently bilateral than are sex cord–stromal or germ-cell tumors; but among primary epithelial tumors, bilaterality is more closely related to histologic type than to likelihood of malignancy. The highest rates of bilaterality are for serous carcinomas, serous tumors of low malignant potential, and undifferentiated carcinomas. Benign serous tumors are also frequently bilateral (although less so than their malignant counterparts), whereas bilaterality is generally less common (although not negligible) among the various epithelial tumors of other histologic types. Benign teratomas and all metastases to the ovary are also frequently bilateral.

The *cystic versus solid nature* of ovarian tumors also suggests the diagnosis. In general, unilocular thin-walled cysts are benign. In fact, many of these lesions are nonneoplastic (Fig. 15–1). Multilocular cysts without solid or papillary areas are also likely to be benign, although they are much more likely to be neoplastic. Although papillary and solid regions within a tumor correlate with the likelihood of malignancy (Fig. 15–2), there are exceptions to this rule. For example, the firmest—often rock-hard—solid tumors encountered in the ovary are benign fibromas, thecomas, or Brenner tumors. Papillary growth generally indicates a tumor of serous type; when this feature is extensive, it suggests malignancy, but the correlation is far from absolute. The best indication of malignancy is a heterogeneous gross appearance. Thus, a tumor with cystic, papillary, and solid regions, varying in consistency from soft to hard and showing foci of hemorrhage and necrosis, is usually malignant. Such features, however, may not be apparent until the pathologist examines the ovary, so it behooves the surgeon to obtain intraoperative pathologic consultation before proceeding.

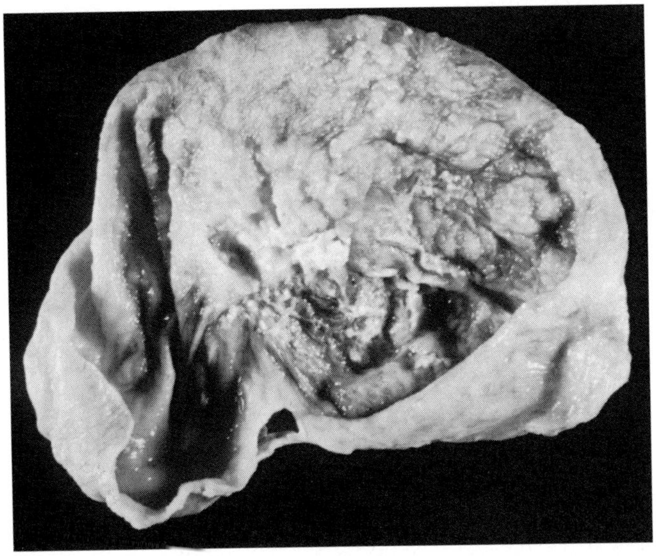

Figure 15–2. Ovarian carcinoma. The largo cyst is filled with a solid and papillary mass with foci of necrosis.

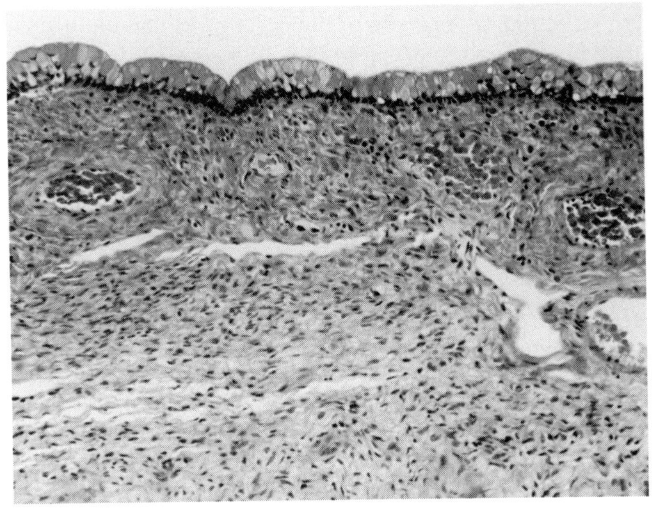

Figure 15–3. Mucinous cystadenoma of ovary. In this benign cystic epithelial tumor, the cyst lining is composed of a single layer of mucinous cells displaying endocervical-type differentiation and no cytologic atypia.

Obviously, the diagnosis of carcinoma gains credibility if there is *local extension* of tumor beyond the ovary, with adhesions to or invasion of adjacent organs, or if there is *metastatic spread.* Even with these findings, however, pelvic inflammatory disease and endometriosis must be ruled out, since these conditions can also be associated with extensive local adhesions or even a ''frozen pelvis.'' Benign conditions such as endometriosis, endosalpingiosis, tuberculosis, and disseminated peritoneal leiomyomatosis can occur with nodules throughout the peritoneal cavity. A careful, directed approach from the pathologist is needed to clarify the diagnosis intraoperatively.

Microscopic Appearance of Epithelial Neoplasms

Because of the variety of ovarian epithelial neoplasms, the microscopic appearances vary considerably. Accordingly, only a few generalities are covered here. In general, *benign epithelial neoplasms* are either cystic or solid. The cysts are generally paucilocular and lined by a single or pseudostratified layer of cells with minimal atypia (Fig. 15–3). In the more solid tumors, a nonreactive stroma is punctuated by glands and cysts lined by epithelium similar to that previously described. Depending upon the pathway of differentiation, this epithelium resembles the mucosa of the fallopian tube (with numerous ciliated cells), the endocervix (with mucinous cells in a ''picket fence'' arrangement), normal proliferative endometrium, or benign urothelium.

Invasive carcinomas, however, are characterized by atypical and mitotically active epithelium invading a reactive stroma. Serous carcinomas have varying amounts of papillary architecture, with papillae more prominent in well-differentiated serous carcinomas than in those that are poorly differentiated (Fig. 15–4). In mucinous carcinomas, small and large glands are lined by cells showing mucin production (goblet cells), which resemble intestinal epithelium. Endometrioid carcinomas mimic endometrial adenocarcinoma and are composed of small round glands of uniform size and shape, frequently associated with sheets of squamous epithelium. Clear-cell carcinomas grow in tubules, papillae, or solid sheets of cells and are characterized by an admixture of clear and hobnail cells. Transitional-cell carcinoma of the ovary resembles its more common counterpart in the urinary bladder. Many malignant epithelial tumors show mixed patterns and should be diagnosed as mixed carcinomas, with the specific types and their relative frequencies specified. Roughly 10% of ovarian carcinomas lack significant differentiation and so are called simply undifferentiated carcinoma.

In most series, undifferentiated and serous carcinomas carry the worst prognosis, and mucinous and endometrioid carcinomas the best.[11] The prognosis is more a function of

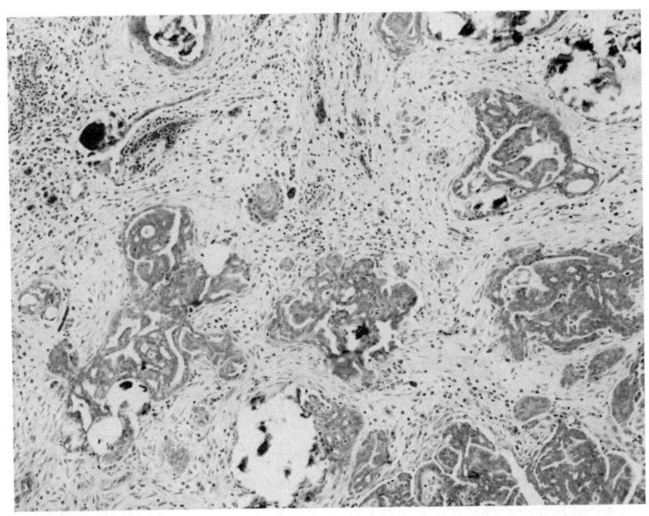

Figure 15–4. Invasive serous carcinoma of ovary. Papillary-glandular tumor nests invade a reactive stroma. The black material in this photomicrograph represents microcalcifications known as psammoma bodies.

extent of tumor than type of tumor—serous and undifferentiated types tend to occur with more advanced disease. The histologic grade of a malignant epithelial tumor may be more important prognostically than its epithelial type, although prognostic differences between grades diminish when patients are treated with chemotherapy.

Between benign epithelial tumors and invasive malignant ones lurk the so-called *borderline tumors or tumors of low malignant potential*.[12, 13] These are primarily serous and mucinous tumors and are defined by malignant cytologic features without stromal invasion (Fig. 15–5). This is often much simpler to describe than to interpret histologically. Stromal invasion in these tumors—particularly the mucinous ones—may be focal. For this reason, extensive sampling (usually defined as one histologic section per 1 to 2 cm of maximal tumor diameter) is essential. A corollary of this statement is that a frozen section diagnosis of a borderline tumor is by definition provisional, since subsequent permanent section may uncover the invasive component that defines malignancy.

As one would expect, *pitfalls for the pathologist* include differentiation of epithelial neoplasms, particularly at frozen section examination. Although pathologists may disagree about the precise epithelial differentiation of a tumor, the more pressing issue is whether a particular tumor is a benign, a borderline, or an invasive cancer. Pathologists who lack experience with borderline tumors are prone to overdiagnose them as invasive carcinomas. This creates a *pitfall for the surgeon*. Reliance on an intraoperative diagnosis of invasive carcinoma may result in unnecessary surgery, particularly in young women. Again, invasive carcinoma of the ovary is rare in women under 30 years of age, whereas borderline tumors are relatively common. It is therefore wise to await permanent section diagnosis before embarking on major operative procedures in women of this age. It is easier to do a subsequent procedure for invasive carcinoma than to explain to a young woman why she has been sterilized for treatment of a tumor that ultimately proved to be borderline or even benign.

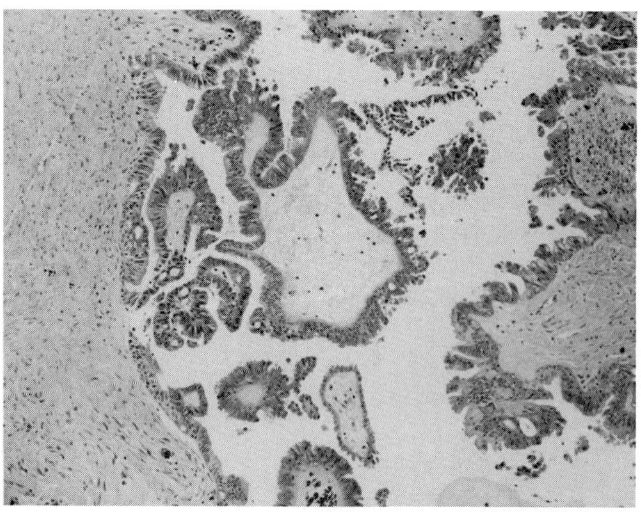

Figure 15–5. Serous tumor of low malignant potential (borderline tumor) of ovary. This tumor is characterized by papillarity, cellular stratification, and atypia (as seen in Fig. 15–4) but lacks invasion into the underlying stroma.

Sex Cord–Stromal Tumors

Like the epithelial tumors, this group of tumors is diverse. Only a few are commonly encountered.[14] The most common stromal tumors are the benign *fibroma* and the *thecoma*, both of which are solid, firm to hard in consistency, and sharply circumscribed. Of the two, the fibroma is more common and represents from 1 to 5% of all ovarian tumors. Although large ones may cause symptoms related to their size or may even be associated with ascites, fibromas are often asymptomatic and discovered incidentally. In comparison, thecomas often display hormonal function, usually estrogenic but occasionally androgenic. Postmenopausal patients typically present with postmenopausal bleeding.[15]

The cut surface of a fibroma is usually white, whereas that of a thecoma is typically yellow, due to its steroid hormone content. Microscopically, both of these tumors are composed of whorled, anastomosing fascicles of uniform cells. In the fibroma, the cells are spindled and separated by variable amounts of collagenous stroma. In thecomas, the cells are ovoid to polygonal with slightly eosinophilic or vacuolated cytoplasm. Fat stains performed on unfixed frozen sections demonstrate cytoplasmic lipid droplets in the cells of thecomas. Malignant thecoma is virtually unknown, and the malignant counterpart of fibroma—fibrosarcoma—is rare.

Less common sex cord–stromal tumors include the *granulosa-cell tumor*[16] and the *Sertoli-Leydig–cell tumor*,[17] which are often characterized clinically by hormonal function, the former generally estrogenic and the latter androgenic. Granulosa-cell tumors are said to make up 1 to 2% of all primary ovarian neoplasms. In our experience, they are frequently overdiagnosed. Many tumors that are called granulosa-cell tumors are actually transitional-cell or undifferentiated carcinomas. Sertoli-Leydig–cell tumors are even less common, representing less than 1% of all primary ovarian neoplasms.

The gross appearance of both of these tumors is variable, with admixture of solid and cystic regions, variation from soft to firm consistency, and color ranging from gray to tan to golden yellow. Their microscopic appearances are correspondingly variable. Granulosa-cell tumors are composed of small, uniform cells with grooved nuclei, which grow in follicular, trabecular, insular, solid, or gyriform patterns or combinations of these. The Sertoli-Leydig–cell tumors often contain tubular elements, but when more poorly differentiated are characterized by cordlike arrangements of the Sertoli cells, among which may be interspersed the large, polygonal, eosinophilic Leydig cells.

Both of these tumors should be considered as tumors of low malignant potential, with 5-year survival rates in the range of 90%. Frequent late recurrences reduce long-term survival. The histologic appearance of the tumor is generally not a reliable predictor of biologic behavior.

Germ-Cell Tumors

Although malignant germ-cell tumors of the ovary are uncommon, they are particularly important in the second and third decades of life. The most common is the *dysgerminoma*, which is analogous to testicular seminoma.[18] This is a fleshy, gray-tan or white tumor that is composed of nests of large, primitive cells separated by a prominent lymphocytic infiltrate within fibrous septa. Like testicular seminoma, dysgerminoma carries a favorable prognosis, with 5-year survival rates well over 90%.

The other malignant germ-cell tumors—*yolk-sac tumor (endodermal sinus tumor), embryonal carcinoma, immature teratoma*, and *choriocarcinoma*—are rare. They occur predominantly in young women and are associated with a poorer prognosis than that of dysgerminoma.[19, 20] Indeed, most of these tumors prove lethal when treated by surgery alone. Triple-agent chemotherapy has achieved frequent cures.[21] Since these tumors are virtually never bilateral and dysgerminoma is bilateral in only 10% of cases or less, the contralateral adnexa and uterus are generally spared in the surgical approach to these tumors. Many patients have subsequently borne healthy children, even after extensive chemotherapy.

In contrast to malignant germ-cell tumors, *benign cystic teratomas* (so-called dermoid cysts) are the most common single primary ovarian neoplasm, accounting for about 25% of all ovarian tumors.[9, 22] They occur in patients of all ages but are commonest between 20 and 50 years of age. Symptoms appear only when the tumor attains a large size, and potentially serious complications—as with other ovarian tumors—include torsion and rupture.

Benign teratomas are grossly recognizable by their unusual cystic contents, which include yellow to white grumous material, oily or clear liquid, tufts of hair, teeth, bone or cartilage, and foci of glial (brain) or thyroid tissue (Fig. 15–6). Accordingly, the microscopic appearance may include a mixture of almost all tissues of the human body, but the predominant—and sometimes the only—component is skin and its adnexae, such as hair follicles, sweat glands, sebaceous glands, and subcutaneous fat. By definition, all of the tissues in a benign teratoma should be histologically benign and mature. Depending upon their size and spatial relationship, these tumors may be treated by oophorectomy or simple tumor excision. The rate of bilaterality is about 10%.

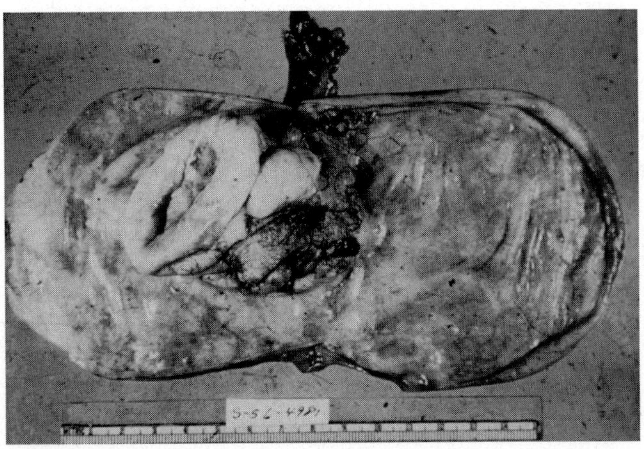

Figure 15–6. Benign cystic teratoma (dermoid cyst) of ovary. This cystic lesion contains sebaceous debris and hair.

Only rarely is malignancy found in ovarian teratomas; it is of two types. First, immature teratoma is seen in children and young adults; it represents a malignant germ-cell tumor in which immature malignant tissues, usually of neuroepithelial type, are superimposed on an otherwise benign teratoma.[23] Like other malignant germ-cell tumors, these neoplasms are sensitive to multiple-agent chemotherapy. Secondly, older women with benign teratomas may secondarily develop malignant tumors of adult type arising in one of the component tissues. These are usually squamous-cell carcinomas, but other carcinomas, sarcomas, melanomas, and other rare tumor types are occasionally encountered.[24] Unfortunately, chemotherapy is generally ineffective for these types of tumors.

Pitfalls for the pathologist involving sex cord–stromal and germ-cell tumors are limited to the malignant variants and stem from the rarity of these lesions. Most pathologists see only a few of these tumors in a lifetime. They are often sent to consultants for confirmatory diagnosis. The main *pitfall for the surgeon* also concerns the malignant germ-cell tumors and is related to inappropriate bilateral oophorectomy for these almost exclusively unilateral tumors occurring in young women. As with epithelial borderline tumors, the temptation to be overly aggressive should be resisted.

Fallopian Tubes

ANATOMY AND HISTOLOGY

The fallopian tubes or oviducts are each situated in the superior wing of the broad ligament and measure from 10 to 12 cm in length and from 0.4 to 0.9 cm in diameter. The interstitial portion of the tube dwells within the uterine wall and progresses externally in sequential order to the isthmus, the ampulla, and the infundibulum or fimbriated portion of the tube. The tubal lumen represents the terminus of a conduit from the external environment to the peritoneal cavity. Histologically, the tubal wall consists of mucosa, submucosa, muscularis, subserosa, and serosa. The serosa consists of peritoneal mesothelium and is subject to the conditions that are discussed further in the section on diseases of the female peritoneum. Tubal mucosa is a mixture of secretory, ciliated, interstitial or "peg," and so-called wandering cells. The latter are mucosa-associated lymphoid tissue (MALT). The ciliated cells are the dominant cell type; indeed, when ciliated cellular differentiation is found in the endometrium or endocervix, this is referred to as "tubal metaplasia."

TORSION

Torsion of the fallopian tube is a fairly common condition that presents in young to middle-aged women as a painful surgical emergency. It is almost always unilateral. Although torsion of an apparently normal tube does occur, most cases are associated with intrinsic abnormalities of the tube or extrinsic causes such as adhesions, tumors, pregnancy, trauma, and pelvic congestion.[25]

At surgery, the twisted tube is usually swollen and usually contains bloody or serous fluid. It is often gangrenous. In about half of the cases, the ovary is involved in the process and must also be removed. Microscopically, the tube shows inflammation, congestion, and edema, occasionally progressing to advanced necrosis. The pathologic features of any underlying disease may be obscured by inflammation or necrosis, and they should be looked for as well.

SALPINGITIS

Inflammation of the tube—salpingitis—is a major gynecologic disease and is frequently treated by the general surgeon because of its clinical presentation as an acute abdominal emergency. Many cases preoperatively diagnosed as acute appendicitis prove instead to be acute right-sided salpingitis, although overall most cases of salpingitis are bilateral.

Gonococcal infection was previously the main cause of acute salpingitis. Common causative organisms today include streptococci, staphylococci, chlamydiae, mycoplasmas, and various anaerobic bacteria.[26] Unilateral salpingitis caused by *Actinomyces* has been seen in association with intrauterine contraceptive devices (IUD).[27] Salpingitis is frequently seen as a postpartum or postabortion complication.

The patient with acute salpingitis presents with pelvic pain, fever, nausea, and vomiting. If not treated in its early stages, acute salpingitis may progress to pelvic and ultimately generalized peritonitis.[28, 29] The involved tube (Fig. 15–7) is swollen, dark red, and edematous, and it is covered by opacified peritoneum, often with adhesions between the tube and neighboring structures. The tube and ovary may be interconnected in a large purulent cavity termed a *tuboovarian abscess*. Identification of the tube or the ovary may require multiple sections through the excised specimen. The normal angularity of the tube is accentuated by the thickening of the tubal wall and the surrounding adhesions. Microscopically, the earliest lesion is endosalpingitis, manifested by neutrophilic infiltration of the tubal mucosa. Postpartum and postabortion infections may begin

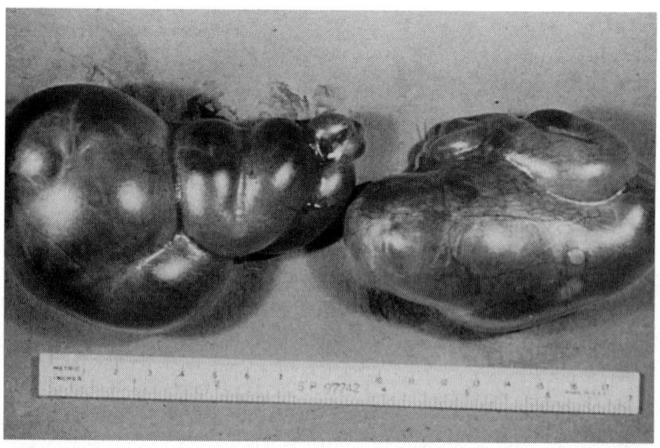

Figure 15–7. Acute salpingitis (pelvic inflammatory disease, or PID). The fallopian tube is kinked, dusky red, and markedly expanded by purulent debris within its lumen (not visualized in unopened specimen here).

as perisalpingitis, with early involvement of the serosa and muscular wall and initial sparing of the mucosa. Vascular congestion and stromal edema usually accompany the inflammation, and either mucosal ulceration or mucosal proliferation may result. Microscopically, mucosal proliferation may be so pronounced as to mimic adenocarcinoma; however, adenocarcinoma of the tube is as rare as salpingitis is common.

Sequelae of acute salpingitis include chronic forms of salpingitis in which the distended tube is filled with pus (pyosalpinx), serous fluid (hydrosalpinx), or blood (hematosalpinx). These conditions, as well as other forms of chronic salpingitis, are common causes of infertility but are rarely treated by the general surgeon, since they do not represent surgical emergencies.

ECTOPIC PREGNANCY

The other major tubal condition encountered by the general surgeon is ectopic pregnancy, which is defined as an implantation anywhere outside the endometrial cavity; 95% of cases occur in the fallopian tubes.[30, 31] Proposed etiologies for ectopic pregnancy include structural disease of the fallopian tube and abnormal fertilization and ovular migration process. Most tubal ectopic pregnancies are preceded by tubal inflammatory disease. Most ectopic pregnancies end after a few weeks by the death of the fetus, which is associated with hemorrhage or rupture of the tubal wall. Fetal development has been known, and delivery of a viable infant has even occurred.

The symptoms of tubal pregnancy, in descending order of frequency, are lower abdominal pain, irregular vaginal bleeding, amenorrhea, nausea, and vomiting. Physical findings include a tender, unilateral adnexal mass, abdominal tenderness, cervical tenderness, and other signs of early pregnancy as well as fluid in the abdominal cavity. The clinical history often includes previous episodes of salpingitis, previous ectopic pregnancy, or the use of an IUD.

The diagnosis of an ectopic pregnancy involves the following steps.[32, 33] After pregnancy is confirmed by an elevated serum beta–human chorionic gonadotropin (beta-HCG), tests are performed to establish whether the pregnancy is intrauterine. These include serial measurements of beta-HCG and transvaginal ultrasonography. A viable intrauterine pregnancy virtually excludes an ectopic pregnancy, since the incidence of a concomitant intrauterine and ectopic pregnancy is about 1:5,000.[32] If, however, a viable intrauterine pregnancy is not confirmed, a dilation and curettage is performed. If no placental tissue is seen, the patient undergoes laparoscopy or laparotomy for removal of the ectopic pregnancy. The triad of a positive pregnancy test, acute abdomen, and hemodynamic shock warrants emergent surgical exploration for a presumed ectopic pregnancy. Ultrasound can often visualize a pregnancy in the adnexa; however, this diagnosis rests on detection of fetal heart motions and not merely the presence of a complex adnexal mass.[33] Normal intrauterine pregnancies have a corpus luteum cyst of the ovary, which may also have a complex appearance on ultrasound.

The involved tube is enlarged, ovoid, and congested. A hemorrhagic mass (Fig. 15–8) is found most frequently in the ampullary portion of the tube, less frequently in the

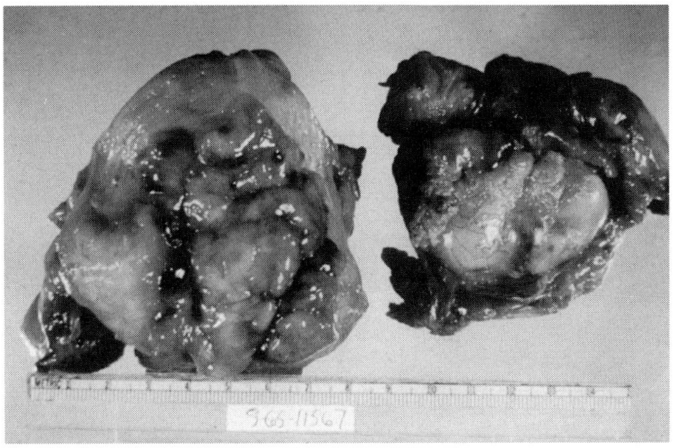

Figure 15–8. Tubal ectopic pregnancy. Edematous, pale, and hemorrhagic chorionic placental tissue has distended and ruptured the tubal wall.

isthmus, and rarely in the interstitial portion. The tubal wall is usually thinned and may be ruptured. Microscopically, the diagnostic finding is the presence of chorionic villi. These are seen in the blood clot within the tubal lumen, within the wall of the tube itself, or, in cases of rupture, outside the tube. These villi are identical to the villi of first-trimester intrauterine pregnancies. Multiple sections of the tube and/or the blood clot may be necessary to demonstrate small numbers of villi. In other cases, a microscopically or even a grossly evident fetus may be present. A stromal decidual response may be observed in the tube, but this is not specific for local implantation. Sections of tube away from the site of implantation usually show evidence of chronic salpingitis or other tubal abnormality.

Therapy involves removal of the gestational products and excision of the ruptured segment of tube, and, in some cases, salpingectomy. Alternative medical therapy with methotrexate is also an option. In cases in which the tube is preserved, subsequent ipsilateral tubal pregnancy may occur; the incidence of subsequent contralateral ectopic pregnancy ranges from 7 to 27%.[34, 35] Infertility is also common because, as previously mentioned, the chronic salpingitis in the affected tube is usually bilateral.

Pitfalls for the pathologist involve misinterpretation of the mucosal proliferative response to an acute or chronic salpingitis as adenocarcinoma. It is also possible to miss a few chorionic villi in a tubal ectopic pregnancy if the specimen is sparsely sectioned. *A pitfall for the surgeon* is leaving behind viable trophoblastic tissue in the remaining portion of the affected tube with a subsequent persistent ectopic pregnancy. Early ectopic pregnancies may be difficult to detect, since there may be minimal tubal distention.

Uterine Corpus and Cervix

ANATOMY AND HISTOLOGY

The uterine corpus and cervix are of mesodermal origin and form a canal continuous with the fallopian tubes above and laterally and with the vagina below. The normal adult corpus measures 4.5 to 5.0 cm in height, 5.0 cm in width, and 2.5 cm in thickness; it weighs 40 to 70 g. Its size is increased in multiparous women, and it undergoes shrinkage after menopause. The cervix forms the inferior third of the uterus; its average length is about 3.0 cm, its diameter at the base is 3.0 cm, and its inferior diameter is 2.5 to 3.0 cm. Its lowest part, which projects into the vagina, is known as the portio vaginalis. This is separated by the external os from the endocervical canal, which communicates with the endometrial cavity of the corpus at the internal os.

Microscopically, the corpus is lined by endometrium, the appearance of which varies with the phase of the menstrual cycle, becoming atrophic after menopause in the absence of exogenous hormone replacement therapy. The underlying myometrium, which forms the bulk of the corpus, is composed of interlacing bands of smooth muscle interspersed with variable numbers of collagen fibers and blood vessels; it is covered by a serosal layer composed of pelvic peritoneum.

The portio vaginalis of the cervix is lined by stratified squamous epithelium and the endocervical canal by mucin-secreting columnar surface mucosa that continues into subjacent glands of similar composition. The junction between the two types of epithelium is known as the transition zone because it is constantly being modified during the reproductive years by successive waves of glandular eversion onto the portio and squamous metaplasia into the endocervical canal. The transition zone is the site of most dysplasias and squamous carcinomas of the cervix.

LEIOMYOMA

Although there are numerous congenital anomalies, inflammatory conditions, and benign and malignant tumors involving the uterine corpus and cervix, few such lesions are likely to be encountered by the general surgeon. The uterine leiomyoma—often called a ''fibroid''—is the most common gynecologic neoplasm. Leiomyomas of the uterus occur in approximately 40% of women after the age of 35 years.[36] Despite their frequency, their pathogenesis is poorly understood, although hormonal factors clearly contribute. The tumor is rarely seen before menarche and generally stabilizes or regresses after menopause. It may increase in size during pregnancy or with oral contraception and usually shrinks when treated with a gonadotropin-releasing hormone agonist such as leuprolide acetate (Lupron).[37]

Many leiomyomas are asymptomatic and are discovered during a routine pelvic examination. Others cause pain, irregular or painful uterine bleeding, urinary disturbances, or constipation. When leiomyomas are large or multiple, they may compress neighboring organs. They are frequently associated with spontaneous abortion and infertility as well as other obstetric complications. Many leiomyomas are clinically undetectable and are only discovered by the pathologist after a hysterectomy has been performed for another reason.

Leiomyomas may be submucous (immediately beneath the endometrium), intramural, or subserous. Subserous myomas are most likely to be encountered by general surgeons, since these may herniate beneath the peritoneal serosa, become pedunculated, or undergo torsion followed by attachment to other pelvic or abdominal organs. In the latter instance, they commandeer a new vascular supply from the host organ and become known as ''parasitic leiomyomas.''

Regardless of location, the leiomyoma is spherical or ovoid, sharply circumscribed, and firm in consistency. Sections demonstrate pearly white tissue with a whorled pattern (Fig. 15–9). Large leiomyomas may undergo degenerative changes with foci of hemorrhage, necrosis, hyalinization, or calcification. Hemorrhage and necrosis, large size, and adhesion to neighboring organs naturally raise the possibility of malignancy (leiomyosarcoma). Leiomyosarcoma is a rare tumor, and even with these grossly worrisome features smooth muscle tumors usually prove to be benign.[38]

Microscopically, the typical leiomyoma consists of interlacing fascicles of uniform spindled cells with bland nuclei, separated by variable amounts of fibrous connective tissue and small blood vessels (Fig. 15–10). Histologic variants include the degenerative patterns mentioned. Less frequently, these tumors may be richly cellular (cellular leiomyoma), contain bizarre giant cells (bizarre, symplastic, or pleomorphic leiomyoma), or contain variable amounts of adipose tissue (lipoleiomyoma). They may be composed predominantly of cells with features resembling those of epithelial cells (epithelioid leiomyoma). These variations represent potential *pitfalls for the pathologist*, since they may be misinterpreted as leiomyosarcoma.[39] Leiomyosarcoma is distinguished from leiomyoma by the presence of hypercellularity, atypia, high levels of mitotic activity, and tumor necrosis. Although grossly typical leiomyomas are generally sampled relatively conservatively,

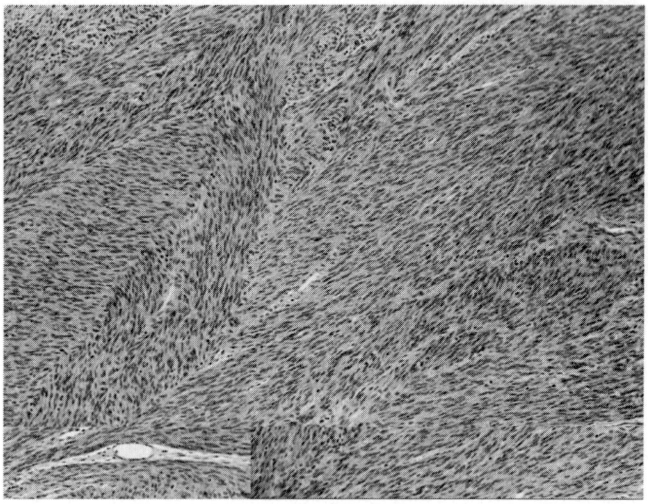

Figure 15–10. Leiomyoma of uterus. Typical microscopic appearance of interlacing fascicles of uniform spindled smooth muscle cells.

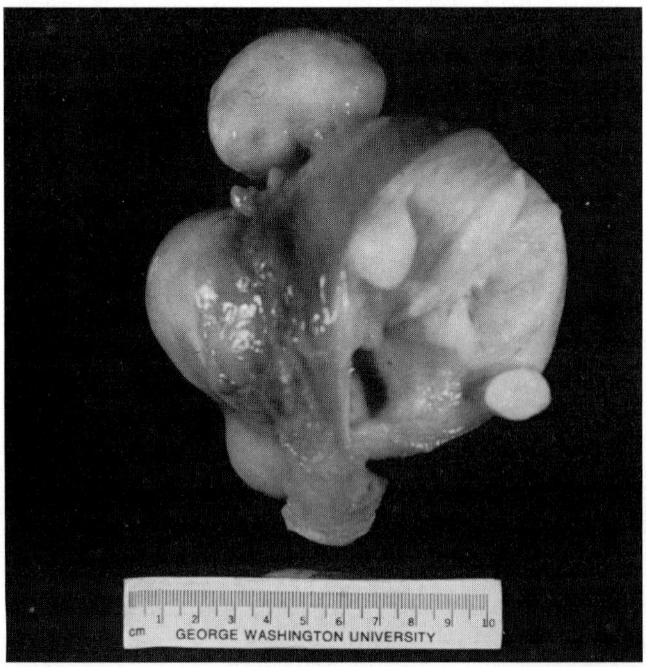

Figure 15–9. Uterine leiomyomas. Multiple, well-circumscribed, firm white tumors are present within the myometrium and fungate out from the serosal surface.

those showing either unusual gross features (softening, necrosis, hemorrhage) or unusual clinical features (for example, rapid enlargement in a postmenopausal woman) should be sampled more extensively, with the general rule being one section per 1 to 2 cm of maximum tumor diameter.[39] Tumors showing unsuspected microscopic findings should also be more thoroughly sectioned.

Cellular or epithelioid leiomyomas may be in the differential diagnosis of endometrial stromal tumors, which may also be found deep in the myometrium. When circumscribed, these leiomyoma variants behave in a benign fashion. In contrast, endometrial stromal tumors that infiltrate the myometrium, even when lacking atypia and mitotic activity, behave as low-grade sarcomas.[40]

The major *pitfalls for the surgeon* are (1) failure to recognize the origin of a tumor that projects from the uterine serosal surface and secondarily involves an adjacent organ and (2) presuming malignancy in a smooth muscle tumor because of its large size, adhesions to adjacent organs, or foci of hemorrhage or necrosis. These errors can be avoided by obtaining intraoperative pathologic consultation, since most pathologists can confirm the smooth muscle nature of the tumor from its gross appearance after sectioning as well as confirm benignity with a frozen section. Simple removal of the leiomyomas (myomectomy) alone with preservation of the uterus is appropriate when childbearing is a consideration; otherwise, hysterectomy is the preferred procedure.

CARCINOMAS OF THE ENDOMETRIUM AND CERVIX

Although these tumors are important topics in gynecologic pathology, they are mentioned only briefly in this chapter because they are likely to be treated by general surgeons in only two situations. First, these tumors may metastasize to a nongynecologic organ such as the bowel serosa, liver, or lung. In the bowel or lung, the distinction from a primary cancer may be difficult, although the serosal rather than mucosal location of metastases is helpful. In the lung, however, a solitary metastatic endometrial or cervical carcinoma may be particularly difficult to distinguish from a primary lung cancer. Second, these tumors are often treated with radiation, with subsequent complications that include radiation enteritis or colitis or a radiation-induced malignant tumor.[41] These processes may be difficult to distinguish preoperatively from recurrent tumor, and the definitive diagnosis may require microscopic examination.

About 95% of malignant tumors of the uterine corpus are adenocarcinomas, whereas a slightly lower but strongly dominant proportion of cervical cancers are squamous-cell carcinomas. The prototype adenocarcinoma of the endometrium is the endometrioid type and is composed of small, round, relatively uniform glands lined by columnar cells with their nuclei oriented perpendicular to the basement membrane. They are often accompanied by a minor or major squamous component. The glandular component may also grow in solid sheets of more anaplastic cells. The histologic grade of the tumor is higher with increasing proportions of this solid growth pattern. Although the majority of endometrial carcinomas are well differentiated, the poorly differentiated forms are more likely to metastasize and come to the attention of the general surgeon.[42] Other less common types of endometrial adenocarcinoma are the serous and clear-cell types that carry a poorer prognosis and a greater likelihood of distant metastases than the usual type of endometrioid adenocarcinoma.[43, 44] Endometrioid carcinomas can also originate in the ovary and, less frequently, in the endocervix, fallopian tube, and foci of endometriosis anywhere in the pelvis or abdomen.

As mentioned, about 85% of invasive cervical cancers are of the squamous-cell type. Most of the remainder are adenocarcinomas. In contrast to endometrial carcinoma, which is a disease of postmenopausal women, many invasive cervical cancers occur in younger women. Unlike ovarian cancer, which may occur with widespread disease and ascites, the majority of endometrial and cervical cancers occur with localized gynecologic symptomatology. Abnormal bleeding from the cervix or corpus is a common presenting symptom. In premenopausal women, this symptom manifests as menometrorrhagia in the case of endometrial cancer and as postcoital bleeding or bloody vaginal discharge in the case of cervical carcinoma. Postmenopausal bleeding is always abnormal and may be a symptom of either cervical or endometrial carcinoma. Moreover, cervical cancer may be detected while still occult or while in a preinvasive state by routine screening with Pap smears. Screening is performed generally on an annual basis beginning when the woman becomes sexually active. Even minor abnormalities, such as repetitively atypical smears or low-grade squamous intraepithelial lesions (LGSIL), may require further evaluation. Often condylomas are detected by Pap smear and certain subtypes of human papillomavirus have been associated more often with both cervical dysplasia and carcinoma. Colposcopy with small directed biopsies can determine whether occult abnormalities are dysplasia or invasive cancer. Occasionally, excisional biopsies such as conization or loop electrosurgical excision are necessary to exclude the presence of invasive cancer. Not all cervical dysplasias require treatment. High-grade dysplasia can be treated in the office with a variety of modalities, such as cryotherapy, CO_2 laser vaporization, and excision.

The treatment of *microinvasive cervical cancer* includes conization, simple hysterectomy, or brachytherapy implant. More advanced disease still confined to the cervix entails radical hysterectomy and lymphadenectomy or external pelvic radiotherapy with subsequent cervical brachytherapy. Disease that extends beyond the cervix is best treated primarily with radiotherapy. Most endometrial cancers are treated by total abdominal hysterectomy with bilateral salpingo-oophorectomy. However, carcinomas that deeply invade the myometrium may require more extensive surgery or postoperative radiotherapy. Chemotherapy is reserved for the uncommon serous type of endometrial carcinoma and for the even rarer primary uterine sarcomas and malignant mixed tumors.

Distant metastases occur relatively late in the course of both endometrial and cervical carcinoma. Metastatic endometrial adenocarcinoma usually demonstrates a characteristic microscopic pattern, and the patient may respond to progestin therapy. In contrast, metastatic cervical squamous carcinoma is nonspecific microscopically, indistinguishable from squamous carcinomas originating in other organs. Thus, a solitary pulmonary metastasis is identical microscopically to a primary squamous carcinoma of the lung. Molecular diagnostic techniques offer hope for resolving such differential diagnosis problems in the future. Analysis of tumor tissue for human papillomavirus (HPV), which is usually present in the cervical cancers, has already been recommended for making the distinction in a series of cases.[45]

More common than distant metastases in lethal cases of cervical carcinoma are extensive pelvic recurrences. These may result in a "frozen pelvis" and cause hydroureter, hydronephrosis, pyelonephritis, and septicemia. Because of this common complication, urologic surgeons may be asked to participate in the management of these unfortunate patients. As the primary treatment of advanced cervical cancer is radiotherapy, it is crucial that the uterine corpus and cervix be preserved to act as a receptacle for afterloading brachytherapy devices. Pelvic disease recurring after irradiation may be treated successfully by pelvic exenteration.

Vagina and Vulva

The vagina and vulva are both lined by squamous epithelium and are therefore susceptible to the same condylomatous, dysplastic, and carcinomatous squamous lesions as is the cervix. With the exception of condyloma acuminatum, these lesions are less frequently encountered in the vagina and vulva than in the cervix. Vulvar skin may be the site of numerous dermatologic diseases, both inflammatory and neoplastic. These, in large part, are similar to those affecting the male external genitalia (see Chap. 14). Structures adjacent to the vagina and vulva, such as the glands of Bartholin and Skene and the female urethra, may also give rise to lesions that occur clinically as vulvovaginal masses.

A variety of benign tumors may arise in the vagina.

Although most are asymptomatic, occasionally dyspareunia may result. These include epidermal inclusion cysts, müllerian (paramesonephric) cysts, and Gartner's duct (mesonephric) cysts. These cysts should be removed only if they are symptomatic. Rarer tumors are fibroepithelial polyps and leiomyomas.

Primary malignant tumors of the vagina are rare; metastatic or locally extensive lesions from the cervix, vulva, uterine corpus, and rectum are more common. Squamous carcinoma of the vagina arises from the mucosal surface and spreads by local invasion and through the lymphatics to the pelvic and inguinal-femoral nodes. Radical surgery may be appropriate treatment; however, most cases are best treated by radiotherapy. Endodermal sinus tumor and embryonal rhabdomyosarcoma are rare primary vaginal tumors of childhood. These are best treated by a combination of radiation, chemotherapy, and surgery. Vaginal adenocarcinomas of clear-cell or endometrioid type are occasionally encountered in women whose mothers received diethylstilbestrol (DES) while pregnant. Far more common are benign microscopic glandular abnormalities (adenosis) and gross anatomic deformities.

Common benign vulvar tumors are condylomas and fibroepithelial polyps. Some 90% of malignant vulvar tumors are squamous-cell carcinomas; 5% are melanomas. The clinical presentation of these tumors includes vulvar pruritus or bleeding accompanied by a visible or palpable lesion. Grossly, these tumors may assume an exophytic, ulcerative, or flat configuration. These cancers generally spread either by direct extension or by embolic metastases to the regional lymph nodes in the groin. Therapy generally involves radical surgical resection of the primary vulvar lesion with dissection of the groin nodes. Radiotherapy may also be utilized as a surgical adjuvant but is poorly tolerated by the moist skin in the groin and vulva. Melanomas are best treated by wide local excision with or without groin dissection. Paget's disease and Bowen's disease are in situ forms of adenocarcinoma and squamous-cell carcinoma, respectively. These are treated by local excision or superficial ("skinning") vulvectomy. Such lesions are frequently multifocal and may involve the perineum and perianal region as well as the vulva.

Female Peritoneum

The same diseases that affect the female genital tract can also affect the peritoneum, giving rise to a spectrum of lesions different from those in the male peritoneum. For example, malignant mesothelioma, a diffuse, highly malignant, and invariably lethal tumor of the peritoneum that is frequently associated with asbestos exposure, is seen 10 times more frequently in men than women, whereas primary peritoneal adenocarcinoma is a disease almost exclusively of women. Benign conditions such as endometriosis and endosalpingiosis are also limited to women.

ENDOMETRIOSIS

Endometriosis is a common and clinically important benign condition defined as the presence of benign endometrial epithelium and stroma in an ectopic site. It is found throughout the peritoneal cavity. In descending order of frequency, sites are the ovary, pelvic peritoneum, rectovaginal septum, fallopian tube, rectum and sigmoid colon, and others. Most of these initially present as serosal disease.[46]

Although debated for many years, the pathogenesis of endometriosis remains unsettled. The theories that best explain the common peritoneal locations are the theory of retrograde menstruation with implantation in the peritoneal cavity and the theory of müllerian metaplasia of coelomic peritoneal mesothelium into endometrial-type tissues.

Endometriosis is predominantly a disease of the postmenarchal and premenopausal years. Some cases are asymptomatic. In the majority, there are symptoms such as dysmenorrhea, menometrorrhagia, dyspareunia, lumbar or rectal pain, and infertility.[47] The pain is usually aggravated during menstruation and is related to bleeding into and around the foci of disease, since the ectopic endometrium cycles in much the same way as intrauterine endometrium. Endometriosis may also cause site-specific clinical manifestations, such as ureteral obstruction, constipation, and symptoms mimicking acute appendicitis, tuboovarian abscess, and rectosigmoid carcinoma.

The gross appearance of endometriosis is protean and varies with the menstrual cycle. The lesions may be small white or yellow nodules, red-brown or blue cysts, or huge hemorrhagic, densely adherent masses (Fig. 15–11). Nonpigmented endometriotic lesions have also been described. Brown and blue nodular or cystic appearances are characteristic of older lesions that have undergone multiple cycles of hemorrhage. Microscopically, endometriosis is composed of endometrial glands, cellular stroma, and occasionally smooth muscle fibers (Fig. 15–12). Following episodes of hemorrhage and resorption, these diagnostic features may be obscured by old and recent hemorrhage; numerous macrophages laden with hemosiderin, lipofuscin, or hemofuscin; granulation tissue; and fibrosis. Multiple sections may be necessary to demonstrate the diagnostic endometrial epithelium and/or stroma. In some cases these are never found and the diagnosis remains a presumptive clinical one. When well-preserved endometrium is present, it varies with the menstrual cycle, so that proliferative, secre-

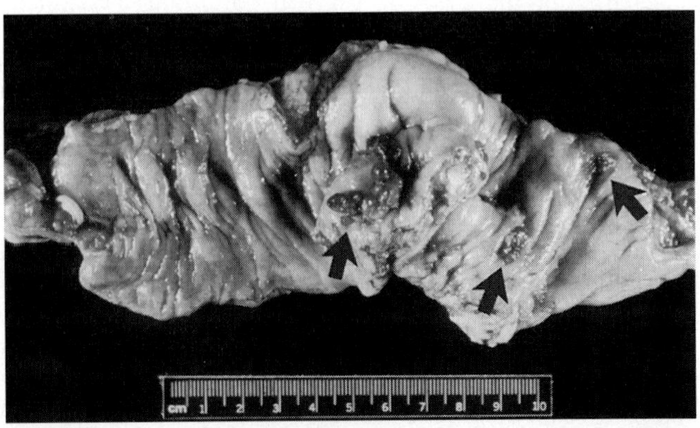

Figure 15–11. Intestinal endometriosis. The initially serosal lesion has extended through the bowel wall and is seen here as a hemorrhagic mass protruding into the lumen (*arrows*).

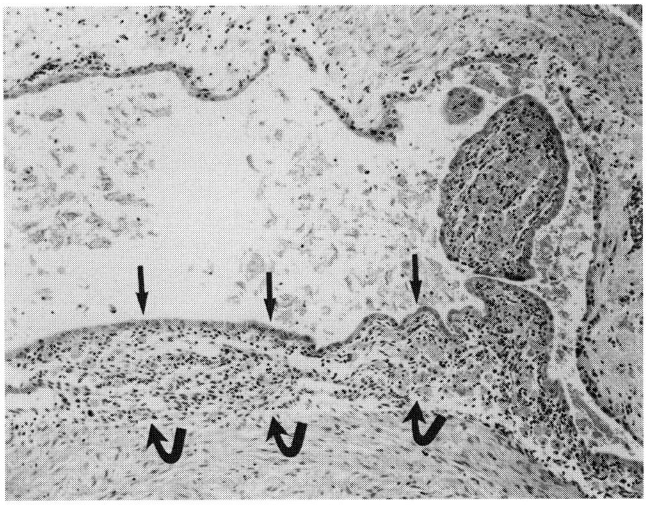

Figure 15–12. Endometriosis. This parovarian cyst is lined by endometrial glandular epithelium (*straight arrows*) and stroma (*curved arrows*).

tory, or even decidual or rare gestational changes may be seen. Marked epithelial atypia may occasionally be observed and probably represents a precarcinomatous change.[48] Endometrioid or clear-cell adenocarcinoma or, rarely, endometrioid sarcoma or carcinosarcoma are complications of endometriosis. These malignant changes must be sought when firm, focally necrotic tissue is encountered within an otherwise typical focus of endometriosis.

Initial treatment of endometriosis is usually medical, including continuous oral contraceptives, other progestational agents, danazol, gonadotropin-releasing hormone alpha (Gn-RH α), and gestrinone.[49] Laparoscopy is used for both diagnosis and treatment, which includes laser vaporization of implants and lysis of adhesions. In women with severe disease who have completed childbearing, hysterectomy and bilateral salpingo-oophorectomy are appropriate. Bowel resection and ureterolysis may be necessary for intestinal or ureteral obstruction. The main *pitfall for the surgeon* lies with the technical expertise required for treatment of severe endometriosis, since the tissue planes are often obscured by inflammation.[50] Clinical recurrence after all forms of therapy is frequent.

Pitfalls for the pathologist are related to the difficulty of demonstrating classic endometrial epithelium and stroma within many of these lesions. They can be confused with hemorrhagic corpus luteum cysts of the ovary, hemorrhagic simple cysts, and, rarely, metastatic adenocarcinomas. This last diagnostic trap is possible when the glandular component overshadows the stromal component.

ENDOSALPINGIOSIS

Endosalpingiosis has only lately been recognized as a common female peritoneal lesion. It is defined as any proliferation of müllerian-type epithelium on a peritoneal surface. As the name suggests, though, these proliferations are most often of tubal epithelial type. Unlike endometriosis, these lesions are rarely symptomatic and are almost always incidental findings. Because they may be encountered during exploratory surgery for female genital or other cancers, their significance lies in their distinction from metastatic adenocarcinoma.[51]

Lesions of endosalpingiosis occur as small, gray or white, firm, and frequently calcified nodules measuring 1 to 2 mm in diameter (see Fig. 15–1). They are most frequently encountered in the omentum, posterior uterine serosa, ovarian surfaces, and rectouterine cul-de-sac. Microscopically, they consist of glands, papillae, or cysts lined by a single layer of cuboidal cells, with transitions to various types of müllerian epithelium, most commonly resembling tubal mucosa with prominent ciliated cells. Foci of calcification (often in the form of psammoma bodies), inflammation, and fibrosis are common. The nuclei, by definition, are small, uniform, and bland. Histologically similar benign glandular inclusions may also be encountered in pelvic and periaortic lymph nodes, again almost exclusively in women.[52]

Because the presence of epithelial glandular or papillary formations in peritoneal or lymph nodal sites is unexpected, the main *pitfall for the pathologist* is misinterpretation of these benign lesions as metastatic adenocarcinoma. Such an error is most likely in cases in which there is a known primary adenocarcinoma elsewhere. Endosalpingiosis is particularly troublesome in patients with borderline serous tumors of the ovary and may cause errors in staging.[52, 53] The differential diagnosis rests upon the benign cytologic appearance of the component cells of endosalpingiosis. The distinction from endometriosis may also prove difficult and rests upon the tubal rather than endometrial appearance of the epithelium as well as the absence of endometrial stroma in endosalpingiosis. The pathologist may create a *pitfall for the surgeon* by confusing endosalpingiosis with metastatic cancer. If the lesions are minute and the patient is young, the possibility of endosalpingiosis should always be entertained even in the presence of a frozen section diagnosis of adenocarcinoma.

ADENOCARCINOMA

Carcinomas in the female peritoneum may be primary or metastatic. Although primary peritoneal adenocarcinoma is the subject of much interest to gynecologic oncologists and pathologists, particularly in the past decade, in most cases carcinoma in the peritoneum is metastatic in nature. Although any malignant tumor can metastasize to the peritoneum, the most common origins are the ovary, endometrium, and large intestine. Metastatic breast cancer, formerly detected at the time of therapeutic oophorectomy or adrenalectomy, is now detected more often in relation to intestinal obstruction. Cervical carcinomas infrequently metastasize to the peritoneum, and those that do are usually adenocarcinomas. When ovarian and endometrial carcinomas metastasize to the peritoneum, they most frequently display serous histology. Such metastases raise the difficult, sometimes virtually impossible problem of distinguishing them diagnostically from primary serous carcinoma of the peritoneum, which is discussed in the following text. Peritoneal fluid washings should always be obtained and sent for cytologic examination in any patient being explored for a primary cancer of any abdominal or pelvic organ.

Two types of cancer metastatic to the female peritoneum that are of particular interest are *pseudomyxoma peritonei*[54] and *gliomatosis peritonei*.[55] The former term refers to mucinous ascites associated with a mucinous tumor of the ovary, appendix, or both. It presents grossly as loculated, yellow-brown, glairy, adhesive mucus on peritoneal surfaces, eventuating in dense mucinous adhesions. Microscopically, relatively small numbers of low-grade mucinous tumor cells are found floating in voluminous pools of extracellular mucin. It is currently controversial whether the ovary, the appendix, or the peritoneum is the source of this lesion.

In peritoneal gliomatosis, the source of the mature glial implants studding the peritoneum is an immature teratoma of the ovary. The implants generally show a higher degree of maturation into benign-appearing tissues than do the primary ovarian tumors, and their behavior is accordingly benign.

The main consideration in the differential diagnosis of metastatic adenocarcinoma—particularly of serous type—in the female peritoneum is *primary serous carcinoma of the peritoneum*.[56, 57] About 10% of disseminated serous carcinomas are peritoneal rather than ovarian in origin, although the distinction between primary peritoneal serous carcinoma and ovarian serous carcinoma with peritoneal dissemination is often subjective. The clinical presentation and gross appearance of these lesions are identical to those of metastatic ovarian serous carcinoma, with the exception that the ovaries are absent (having been removed previously for unrelated disease), present but uninvolved with tumor, or present but minimally involved, with their neoplastic burden limited to a coating of their peritoneal surfaces. It is assumed that the extraovarian peritoneal mesothelium undergoes the same neoplastic transformation that occurs in ovarian epithelial tumors, particularly serous carcinoma. Although this phenomenon has also been reported with other types of cancer, such as endometrioid and clear-cell carcinoma, the majority of the cases are of serous type. Some of these patients may have a synchronous serous carcinoma of the endometrium, often with limited invasiveness in the uterine corpus. The question can again be asked whether there are two or more primary carcinomas (peritoneal and endometrial) or whether the endometrial carcinoma has disseminated into the peritoneal cavity. Regardless of the pathogenesis, the prognosis for long-term tumor-free survival among patients with such tumors is poor. Nevertheless, good and sometimes sustained responses have been achieved with multiple-agent chemotherapy of the sort directed against ovarian cancer. This entity is entirely different from malignant mesothelioma of the peritoneum, emphasizing the importance of this differential diagnosis.

Although the microscopic appearance of peritoneal serous carcinoma is usually characteristic, various histochemical and immunohistochemical stains may be used to distinguish this lesion from either malignant mesothelioma or reactive proliferations of mesothelium. Among the most useful antigens for immunohistochemical studies are the carcinoembryonic antigen (CEA), Leu-M1 (CD15), TAG-72 recognized by monoclonal antibody B72.3, and the antigen recognized by monoclonal antibody BER-EP4. All of these are present in most adenocarcinomas (including metastases to the peritoneum) and absent in all or almost all mesotheliomas.[58]

As indicated, the most important *pitfall for the pathologist* is the distinction of adenocarcinoma from mesothelioma, benign mesothelial proliferations, and such benign lesions as endosalpingiosis and endometriosis. The major *pitfall for the surgeon* is failure to perform an adequate staging laparotomy for definitive diagnosis and to debulk the major masses of intraperitoneal tumor.

Pregnancy

The diagnosis of pregnancy in a woman of reproductive age has obvious important ramifications in the management of surgical diseases. Amenorrhea, weight gain, and nausea should prompt confirmation of pregnancy by beta-HCG testing of urine or serum, a quick and inexpensive study. This is particularly important for patients scheduled for elective surgery or who present with abdominal pain. Ectopic pregnancy has previously been discussed and commonly occurs as an acute surgical abdomen. Normal intrauterine pregnancy may also cause pelvic or abdominal pain by compressing adjacent viscera or causing degeneration of uterine leiomyomas. Premature labor, placental abruption, and intrauterine infection are important obstetric conditions that are associated with abdominal pain and require immediate diagnosis and therapy.

A multitude of maternal physiologic changes accompany pregnancy. There is a progressive increase in plasma volume, glomerular filtration rate, and cardiac output. Because of the normal volume expansion that occurs during pregnancy, a physiologic dilutional anemia is noted frequently, despite an increase in erythrocyte volume. Increased serum levels of progesterone cause relaxation of smooth muscle and resultant cholestasis, decreased lower esophageal sphincter tone, and hydroureter. Compression of the ureters at the pelvic inlet by the gravid uterus also contributes to physiologic ureteral dilation. The enlarging gravid uterus not only reduces operative exposure but may also distort and displace the locations of other organs such as the cecum and appendix. All types of anesthesia are appropriate during pregnancy, and surgical positioning in the supine position is optimal, with a slight degree of lateral rotation to the left to minimize vena caval compression by the uterus. It is critical that teratogenic medications be avoided during the first trimester. Premature labor may be induced by operations performed during the latter half of gestation. Care should be taken to avoid excessive hypotension and manipulation of the uterus. Prophylactic antitoxemic agents such as beta-sympathomimetic agents, magnesium sulfate, and prostaglandin synthetase inhibitors may be indicated to avoid early labor.

The term ''gestational trophoblastic disease'' encompasses a spectrum of aggressive proliferative processes that result from pregnancy. Hydatidiform mole and choriocarcinoma are the most important gestational trophoblastic diseases. Hydatidiform mole may be partial or complete, the distinction being based upon both microscopic examination and flow cytometric ploidy analysis. Both partial and complete moles are characterized by hydropic placental villi with varying degrees of trophoblastic proliferation. The distinction between the two has prognostic implications since complete moles are more likely to persist, invade the uterus, or eventuate in choriocarcinoma. Evacuation of a molar pregnancy must be followed by serial measurements of serum HCG levels. If HCG levels remain elevated, methotrexate chemotherapy is initiated without further tissue examination. Until the chemotherapeutic era, choriocarcinoma was one of the most aggressive and unfavorable human cancers. With modern agents, cure is often achieved, even in the presence of metastatic disease.

PITFALLS FOR THE SURGEON

1. Excessive resection for benign ovarian cysts; excision or, at most, unilateral oophorectomy is adequate in patients still desirous of fertility.
2. Excessive resection for ovarian tumors of low malignant potential; invasive carcinomas are unusual in younger patients, but tumors of low malignant potential are relatively common.
3. Bilateral oophorectomy for malignant germ-cell tumors; these are virtually always unilateral.
4. Missing ectopic tubal pregnancy due to subtle, minimal tubal distention.
5. Failure to remove all trophoblastic tissue from a site of ectopic pregnancy, with resulting persistence of the process.
6. Misjudging uterine leiomyomas to be malignant on the basis of gross findings, such as large size, adhesion to adjacent organs, foci of hemorrhage, or necrosis. For women of childbearing age, myomectomy rather than hysterectomy is usually indicated.
7. Incomplete removal of endometriotic foci on the peritoneum due to obliteration of tissue planes by fibrosis and inflammation. Even worse, however, may be overly aggressive surgery, since small foci of residual disease often respond to medical therapy.
8. Proceeding on an intraoperative diagnosis of metastatic adenocarcinoma when clinical history and gross appearances are consistent with endometriosis or endosalpingiosis.
9. Failure to adequately debulk and sample pelvic, abdominal, and retroperitoneal sites for the staging of peritoneal tumors when intraoperative pathology includes the differential diagnosis of metastatic adenocarcinoma versus primary peritoneal adenocarcinoma.
10. Failure to consider the possibility of primary cervical carcinoma preoperatively, with subsequent simple hysterectomy rather than the radical procedure indicated.

PITFALLS FOR THE PATHOLOGIST

1. Failure to correctly distinguish ovarian steroid-producing stromal-cell processes: *hyperreactio luteinalis* versus pregnancy luteoma versus lipid-cell tumor versus thecoma versus hilar-cell tumor. Bilaterality is a helpful sign of a non-neoplastic nature for this specific differential grouping.
2. Failure to correctly diagnose ovarian epithelial neoplasms—that is, benign versus low malignant potential versus invasive carcinoma. In young patients, the likelihood of malignancy is low, whereas tumors of borderline malignancy are relatively more common. Intraoperative distinction of epithelial type, that is, serous versus mucinous, is of less importance.
3. Difficulty in recognizing sex cord–stromal tumors of the ovary, due to their rarity.
4. Mistaking inflammatory tubal mucosal hyperplasia for adenocarcinoma.
5. Failure to detect intrauterine or ectopic pregnancy by missing rare foci of chorionic villi or trophoblast in scant endometrial or tubal samples.
6. Misinterpreting benign leiomyoma for leiomyosarcoma on the basis of dense cellularity, bizarre symplastic-type giant cells, epithelioid cytologic features, or the presence of mitotic figures within the tumor. These features are recognized to occur in benign smooth muscle tumors.
7. Mistaking endometriosis or endosalpingiosis for other processes, including hemorrhagic corpus luteum cysts, hemorrhagic simple cysts, and adenocarcinoma or borderline tumor.

Continued

8. Failure to inform the surgeon fully that intraoperative differential diagnosis for a sampled peritoneal malignant tumor includes metastatic adenocarcinoma and primary peritoneal adenocarcinoma. A detailed discussion is warranted to emphasize that distribution of tumor may be the decisive criterion and that thorough peritoneal sampling is needed for staging purposes.

FURTHER READING

Fox H, Buckley CH. *Pathology for Gynaecologists*, 2nd ed. London: Edward Arnold; 1991.

Gompel C, Silverberg SG. *Pathology in Gynecology and Obstetrics*, 4th ed. Philadelphia: JB Lippincott; 1994.

Scully RE, Bonfiglio TA, Kurman RJ, et al. *Histological Typing of Female Genital Tract Tumours*, 2nd ed. World Health Organization International Histological Classification of Tumours. Berlin: Springer-Verlag; 1994.

REFERENCES

1. Pacheco JC, Kempers RD. Etiology of postmenopausal bleeding. *Obstet Gynecol.* 1968; 32:40–46.
2. Goldzieher JW, Young RL: Selected aspects of polycystic ovarian disease. *Endocrinol Metab Clin North Am.* 1992; 21:141–171.
3. Wajda KJ, Lucas JG, Marsh WL Jr. Hyperreactio luteinalis: Benign disorder masquerading as an ovarian neoplasm. *Arch Pathol Lab Med.* 1989; 113:921–925.
4. Norris HJ, Taylor HB. Nodular theca-lutein hyperplasia of pregnancy (so-called "pregnancy luteoma"): A clinical and pathologic study of 15 cases. *Am J Clin Pathol.* 1967; 47:557–566.
5. Clement PB, Young RH, Scully RE. Nontrophoblastic pathology of the female genital tract and peritoneum associated with pregnancy. *Semin Diagn Pathol.* 1989; 6:372–406.
6. Hayes MC, Scully RE. Ovarian steroid cell tumors (not otherwise specified): A clinicopathological analysis of 63 cases. *Am J Surg Pathol.* 1987; 11:835–845.
7. Scully RE. Tumors of the ovary and maldeveloped gonads. *Atlas of Tumor Pathology*, 2nd series. Fascicle 16. Washington, DC: Armed Forces Institute of Pathology; 1979.
8. Young RH, Scully RE. Metastatic tumors in the ovary: A problem-oriented approach and review of the recent literature. *Semin Diagn Pathol.* 1991; 8:250–276.
9. Katsube Y, Berg JW, Silverberg SG. Epidemiologic pathology of ovarian tumors: A histopathologic review of primary ovarian neoplasms diagnosed in the Denver Standard Metropolitan Statistical Area, 1 July–31 December 1969 and 1 July–31 December 1979. *Int J Gynecol Pathol.* 1982; 1:3–16.
10. Schutter EMJ, Kenemans P, Sohn C, et al. Diagnostic value of pelvic examination, ultrasound, and serum CA 125 in postmenopausal women with a pelvic mass: An international multicenter study. *Cancer.* 1994; 74:1398–1406.
11. Silverberg SG. Prognostic significance of pathologic features of ovarian carcinoma. *Curr Top Pathol.* 1989; 78:85–109.
12. Bostwick DG, Tazelaar HD, Ballon SC, et al. Ovarian epithelial tumors of borderline malignancy: A clinical and pathologic study of 109 cases. *Cancer.* 1986; 58:2052–2065.
13. Manchul LA, Simm J, Levin W, et al. Borderline epithelial ovarian tumors: A review of 81 cases with an assessment of the impact of treatment. *Int J Radiat Oncol Biol Phys.* 1992; 22:867–874.
14. Gee DC, Russell P. The pathological assessment of ovarian neoplasms: IV. The sex cord-stromal tumours. *Pathology.* 1981; 13:235–255.
15. Sasano H, Sasano N. What's new in the localization of sex steroids in the human ovary and its tumors? *Pathol Res Pract.* 1989; 185:942–948.
16. Young RH, Scully RE. Ovarian sex cord-stromal tumors: Problems in differential diagnosis. *Pathol Annu.* 1988; 23:237–294.
17. Young RH, Scully RE. Ovarian Sertoli-Leydig cell tumors: A clinicopathological analysis of 207 cases. *Am J Surg Pathol.* 1985; 9:543–569.
18. Gordon A, Lipton D, Woodruff JD. Dysgerminoma: A review of 158 cases from the Emil Novak Ovarian Tumor Registry. *Obstet Gynecol.* 1981; 58:497–504.
19. Kurman RJ, Norris HJ. Malignant germ cell tumors of the ovary. *Hum Pathol.* 1977; 8:551–564.
20. Harms D, Janig U. Germ cell tumours of childhood: Report of 170 cases including 59 pure and partial yolk-sac tumours. *Virchows Arch A Pathol Anat Histopathol.* 1986; 409:223–239.
21. Gershenson DM, Morris M, Cangir A, et al. Treatment of malignant germ cell tumors of the ovary with bleomycin, etoposide, and cisplatin. *J Clin Oncol.* 1990; 8:715–720.
22. Dahl N, Gustavson KH, Rune C, et al. Benign ovarian teratomas: An analysis of their cellular origin. *Cancer Genet Cytogenet.* 1990; 46:115–123.
23. Gershenson DM, del Junco G, Silva EG, et al. Immature teratoma of the ovary. *Obstet Gynecol.* 1986; 68:624–629.
24. Stamp GWH, McConnell EM. Malignancy arising in cystic ovarian teratomas: A report of 24 cases. *Br J Obstet Gynaecol.* 1983; 90:671–675.
25. Youssef AF, Fayad MM, Shafeek MA. Torsion of the fallopian tube: A clinico-pathological study. *Acta Obstet Gynecol Scand.* 1962; 41:292–309.
26. Mardh PA. An overview of infectious agents of salpingitis, their biology, and recent advances in methods of detection. *Am J Obstet Gynecol.* 1980; 138:933–951.
27. Vanlancker M, Dierick AM, Thiery M, Claeys G. Histologic and microbiologic findings in the fallopian tubes of IUD users. *Adv Contracept.* 1987; 3:147–157.
28. Hager WD, Eschenbach DA, Spence MR, Sweet RL. Criteria for diagnosis and grading of salpingitis. *Obstet Gynecol.* 1983; 61:113–114.
29. Monif GRG. Clinical staging of acute bacterial salpingitis and its therapeutic ramifications. *Am J Obstet Gynecol.* 1982; 143:489–495.
30. Pauerstein CJ, Croxatto HB, Eddy CA, et al. Anatomy and pathology of tubal pregnancy. *Obstet Gynecol.* 1986; 67:301–308.
31. Stock RJ: Tubal pregnancy: Associated histopathology. *Obstet Gynecol Clin North Am.* 1991; 18:73–94.
32. Weckstein LN. Current perspective on ectopic pregnancy. *Obstet Gynecol Surv.* 1985; 40:259–271.
33. Cacciatore B. Can the status of tubal pregnancy be predicted by transvaginal sonography? A prospective comparison of sonographic, surgical, and serum HCG findings. *Radiology.* 1990; 177:481–484.
34. Stock RJ. Histopathology of fallopian tubes with recurrent tubal pregnancy. *Obstet Gynecol.* 1990; 75:9–14.
35. Langer R, Bukovsky I, Herman A, et al. Conservative surgery for tubal pregnancy. *Fertil Steril.* 1982; 38:427–430.
36. Vollenhoven B, Lawrence A, Healy D. Uterine fibroids: A clinical review. *Br J Obstet Gynaecol.* 1990; 97:285–298.
37. Letterie GS, Coddington CC, Winkel CA, et al. Efficacy of a gonadotropin-releasing hormone agonist in the treatment of uterine leiomyomata: Long-term follow-up. *Fertil Steril.* 1989; 51:951–956.
38. Leibsohn S, d'Ablaing G, Mishell DR Jr, Schlaerth JB. Leiomyosarcoma in a series of hysterectomies performed for presumed uterine leiomyomas. *Am J Obstet Gynecol.* 1990; 162:968–976.
39. Kempson RL, Hendrickson MR. Pure mesenchymal neoplasms of the uterine corpus: Selected problems. *Semin Diagn Pathol.* 1988; 5:172–198.
40. Chang KL, Crabtree GS, Lim-Tan SK, et al. Primary uterine endometrial stromal neoplasms: A clinicopathologic study of 117 cases. *Am J Surg Pathol.* 1990; 14:415–438.
41. Hoffman M, Roberts WS, Cavanagh D. Second pelvic malignancies following radiation therapy for cervical cancer. *Obstet Gynecol Surv.* 1985; 40:611–617.
42. Zaino RJ, Silverberg SG, Norris HJ, et al. The prognostic value of nuclear versus architectural grading in endometrial adenocarcinoma: A Gynecologic Oncology Group study. *Int J Gynecol Pathol.* 1994; 13:29–36.
43. Abeler VM, Kjørstad KE. Clear cell carcinoma of the endometrium:

A histopathological and clinical study of 97 cases. *Gynecol Oncol.* 1991; 40:207–217.
44. Sherman ME, Bitterman P, Rosenshein NB, et al. Uterine serous carcinoma: A morphologically diverse neoplasm with unifying clinicopathologic features. *Am J Surg Pathol.* 1992; 16:600–610.
45. Lancaster WD, Castellano C, Santos C, et al. Human papillomavirus deoxyribonucleic acid in cervical carcinoma from primary and metastatic sites. *Am J Obstet Gynecol.* 1986; 154:115–119.
46. Clement PB. Pathology of endometriosis. *Pathol Annu.* 1990; 25:245–295.
47. Ranney B. Endometriosis: Pathogenesis, symptoms, and findings. *Clin Obstet Gynecol.* 1980; 23:865–874.
48. LaGrenade A, Silverberg SG. Ovarian tumors associated with atypical endometriosis. *Hum Pathol.* 1988; 19:1080–1084.
49. Metzger DA, Luciano AA. Hormonal therapy of endometriosis. *Obstet Gynecol Clin North Am.* 1989; 16:105–122.
50. Candiani GB, Vercellini P, Fedele L, et al. Conservative surgical treatment for severe endometriosis in infertile women: Are we making progress? *Obstet Gynecol Surv.* 1992; 46:490–498.
51. Zinsser KR, Wheeler JE. Endosalpingiosis in the omentum: A study of autopsy and surgical material. *Am J Surg Pathol.* 1982; 6:109–117.
52. Farhi DC, Silverberg SG. Pseudometastases in female genital cancer. *Pathol Annu.* 1982; 17:47–76.
53. Copeland LJ, Silva EG, Gershenson DM, et al. The significance of müllerian inclusions found at second-look laparotomy in patients with epithelial ovarian neoplasms. *Obstet Gynecol.* 1988; 71:763–770.
54. Young RH, Gilks CB, Scully RE. Mucinous tumors of the appendix associated with mucinous tumors of the ovary and pseudomyxoma peritonei: A clinicopathologic analysis of 22 cases supporting an origin in the appendix. *Am J Surg Pathol.* 1991; 15:415–429.
55. Harms D, Janig U, Göbel U. Gliomatosis peritonei in childhood and adolescence: Clinicopathological study of 13 cases including immunohistochemical findings. *Pathol Res Pract.* 1989; 184:422–430.
56. Altaras MM, Aviram R, Cohen I, et al. Primary peritoneal papillary serous adenocarcinoma: Clinical and management aspects. *Gynecol Oncol.* 1991; 40:230–236.
57. Fromm GL, Gershenson DM, Silva EG. Papillary serous carcinoma of the peritoneum. *Obstet Gynecol.* 1990; 75:89–95.
58. Gaffey MJ, Mills SE, Swanson PE, et al. Immunoreactivity for BER-EP4 in adenocarcinomas, adenomatoid tumors, and malignant mesotheliomas. *Am J Surg Pathol.* 1992; 16:593–599.

16

The Cardiovascular System

Jack L. Titus, Demetre M. Nicoloff,
and Jesse E. Edwards

With the possible exception of the emergent evacuation of a life-threatening pericardial effusion by acute care physicians, anything within the pericardium is considered by most physicians to be strictly off limits. This attitude prevails even among most noncardiothoracic surgeons. Nevertheless, a simplified review of the problems that affect the heart and the major vessels, together with the surgical solutions to these problems, is appropriate for all surgeons.

Discussion of some of the anatomic sites requires a review of the normal anatomic features. Accordingly, for acquired abnormalities, presentation is by anatomic location rather than by specific disease. In contrast, the section on congenital anomalies focuses on specific conditions.

Autopsies serve a critical role in cardiovascular surgery—for recognition of successes and failures in diagnostic and therapeutic measures, for development of new knowledge, and for education and training. For these reasons, surgeons must motivate themselves and their colleagues to pursue permission for postmortem studies. Even permits for autopsies limited to the heart have value. In turn, pathologists must provide specialized knowledge of cardiovascular conditions to provide data useful for clinicopathologic correlations. If the necessary expertise is not available on site, intact specimens should be submitted to a consultant. This final examination can thus provide valuable insights into the cause of death, avoiding unfounded and sometimes undesirable speculation.

Cardiac Conduction System

The primary anatomic features of the sinus (sinoatrial) and atrioventricular nodes and His bundle that may be of concern in cardiovascular surgery are reviewed briefly. Some specific conditions in which surgical treatment might affect the structures are mentioned.

SINUS (SINOATRIAL) NODE

The sinus node is situated on the anterior-lateral aspect of the junction of the usual right-sided superior vena cava (SVC) with the right atrium. This small structure (in adults about 5 to 9 mm long, 1 to 5 mm wide, and 1 to 5 mm thick) is both subendocardial and subepicardial, surrounds the sinus node artery, and cannot be identified by gross examination (Fig. 16–1).[1] The node lies on the crista terminalis of the right atrium, near the anterior-superior relation of this muscle bundle to the ostium of the SVC. Surgical procedures in which the sinus node or its artery may be inadvertently injured include (1) cannulation of the right atrium and/or the SVC, especially in small hearts; (2) closure of sinus venosus atrial septal defect; (3) atrial switch procedures (Mustard, Senning operations) for complete transposition of the great arteries; and (4) bidirectional (Glenn operation) procedure when the atrial side of the cava is anastomosed to the right pulmonary artery.

ATRIOVENTRICULAR NODE AND His BUNDLE

The *atrioventricular (AV) node* is situated in the ''floor'' of the right atrium, in the interatrial septum. It lies on the AV fibrous tissue (AV ring), near the base of the septal leaflet of the tricuspid valve, and anterior-superior to the ostium of the coronary sinus (Fig. 16–2). In adults, its size

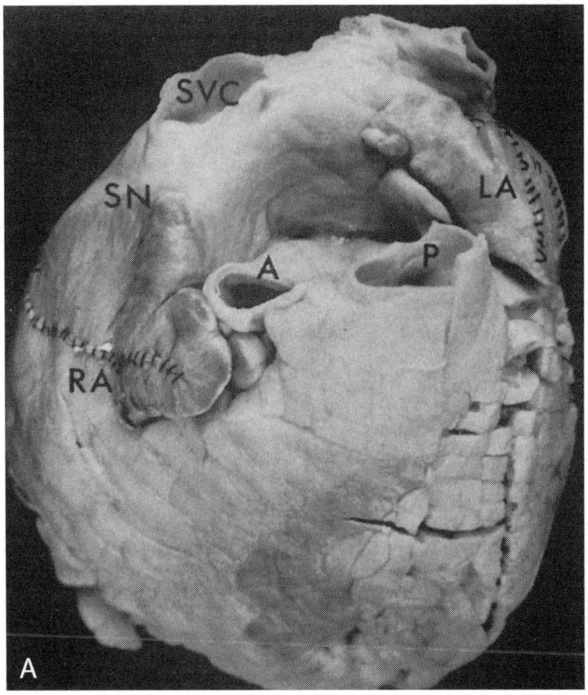

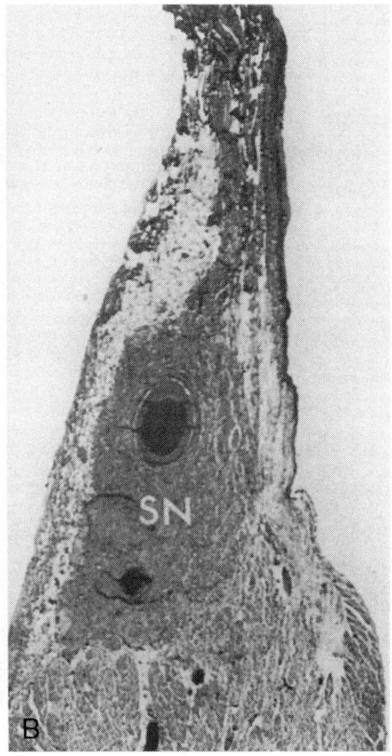

Figure 16–1. *A,* Sinus node. The heart is viewed from an anterior-superior perspective. The position of the sinus node (SN) is at the junction of the superior vena cava (SVC) with the right atrium (RA) near the atrial appendage. A, aorta; LA, left atrium; P, pulmonary artery. (Reprinted with permission from Titus JL. Normal anatomy of the human cardiac conduction system. *Mayo Clin Proc.* 1973; 48:25.) *B,* Histologic sections through the superior vena cava *(upper)* and right atrium *(lower)* demonstrates the sinus node (SN). The nodal tissue surrounds the gelatin-filled sinus node artery. The epicardial surface is leftward, and the endocardium is rightward. (Reprinted with permission from Titus JL. Normal anatomy of the human cardiac conduction system. *Mayo Clin Proc.* 1973; 48:25.)

averages 7.5 × 3.7 × 1 mm.[1] Although the anatomic position often is defined correctly as lying near the apex of the anatomic triangle of Koch, this definition may not be helpful to the surgeon because identification of the boundaries of Koch's triangle usually requires dissection into the atrial musculature. One side of the triangle is formed by the tendon of Todaro, which is a subendocardial and intramyocardial tendonlike cord that passes from the eustachian ridge to the membranous septum. The second side is the annulus of the septal leaflet of the tricuspid valve. The third side, the base of the triangle, is a line drawn between the two sides, just anterior to the coronary sinus ostium and approximately perpendicular to the side formed by the valve annulus. This area is prone to damage in repair of (1) complete AV canal, (2) ostium primum atrial septal defect (ASD), and (3) intraatrial baffle placement with the Mustard, Senning, or Fontan operation.

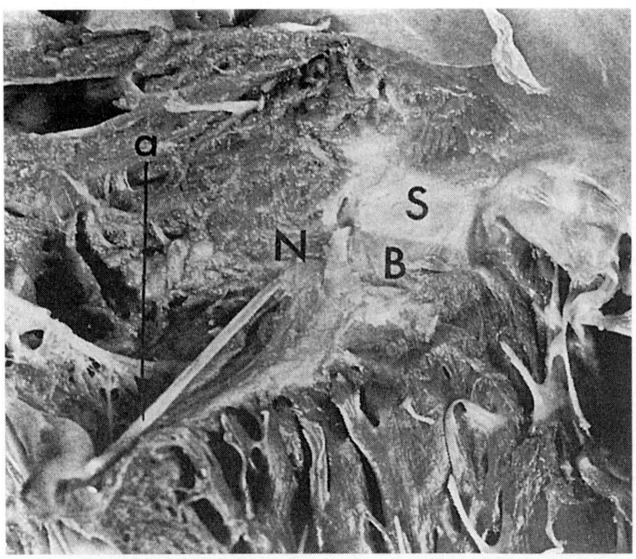

Figure 16–2. The septal region of the junction of the right atrium and ventricle has been dissected to demonstrate atrioventricular node (N) and His bundle (B). The septal leaflet of the tricuspid valve and right atrial endocardium have been removed. S, membranous septum; a, AV nodal artery (it is a branch of the right coronary artery in the posterior atrioventricular sulcus). (Reprinted with permission from Titus JL. Normal anatomy of the human cardiac conduction system. *Mayo Clin Proc.* 1973; 48:26.)

The *bundle of His* usually lies in the inferior part of the membranous septum in its course from the atrial position of the AV node to the crest (base, summit) of the ventricular septum (see Fig. 16–2). The relatively narrow right bundle and the broad left bundle branches originate from the His bundle near the summit of the ventricular septum (Fig. 16–3).

The AV node and His bundle are vulnerable to inadvertent injury in repair of congenital anomalies, such as certain forms of isolated ventricular septal defect (VSD) (e.g., perimembranous VSD) or VSD that is part of another condition, such as tetralogy of Fallot and other conditions. During operations on the left ventricular outflow tract and/or aortic valve, the required dissection may involve the His bundle in the inferior part of the membranous septum (Fig. 16–3).

Mitral Valve Region

Mitral valve dysfunction has many causes and may result in predominant stenosis or predominant insufficiency, or a combination of both. This section focuses on changes in

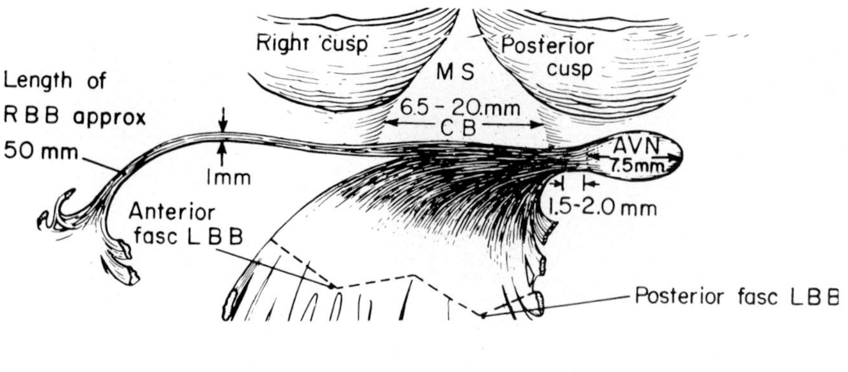

Figure 16–3. The anatomic features of the AV conduction system as viewed in part from the left ventricular septum and aortic valve. This demonstrates the broad origin of the left bundle branch (LBB) from the His bundle (common bundle, CB). In the intact heart, the AV node (AVN) is not visible from this left ventricular outflow prospective. The measurements are average dimensions for adults. Right and posterior aortic cusps and the membranous septum (MS) are labeled. RBB, right bundle branch. The short segment of His bundle between the 1.5 and 2.0 mm is the unbranched portion. (Reproduced with permission from Titus JL. Normal anatomy of the human cardiac conduction system. *Mayo Clin Proc.* 1973; 48:27.)

the mitral apparatus and contiguous structures, related to or resulting from the valvular abnormality (Fig. 16–4). Such changes may complicate the surgical procedure or affect long-term outcome of a procedure. Many of the changes described pertain mainly to valvar replacement, whereas others apply also to reparative (plastic-type) procedures to correct insufficiency or stenosis.

Reparative procedures (e.g., some form of valvuloplasty) or valvar replacement may be influenced by presence and degree of leaflet thickening, commissural fusion, calcification of leaflets or annuli, acquired structural defects from active or healed infective endocarditis (Fig. 16–5), congenital defects (clefts) of the anterior mitral leaflet, and circumference (size) of the valvular annulus. The condition of the chordae tendineae must be evaluated for rupture, presence of tertiary chords attached to the mitral anular area, chords inserting into the muscular ventricular septum, chordal fusion or elongation or shortening, and chordal adherence to posterior or lateral ventricular endocardium in regurgitant myxomatous (floppy) mitral valves (Fig. 16–6). The anatomic integrity and proper positioning in the ventricle of the papillary muscles and the presence of abnormal geometric features of the left ventricle also affect mitral valve function. Valvular regurgitation in particular may be due only to myocardial abnormalities.

Abnormalities of the left atrium can determine the surgical procedure and its outcome. The left atrium may be significantly enlarged secondary to the valvar dysfunction. Thrombotic masses—unorganized, partly organized, or calcified—may be present.[2] Occasionally, surgical retraction of the atrial septal wall leads to postoperative left atrial thrombi. During operation left atrial thrombi should be searched for and removed; some thrombi ''hide'' in the left atrial appendage and continue to be a potential source for embolism after operation.

Most pathologic features listed in the foregoing pertain both to valve replacement with a prosthesis and to repair of the native mitral valve. Even if the initial valve replacement was successful, the need for reoperation or death may be due to prosthesis failure.[3] Conditions that may be encountered by the surgeon include dysfunction due to thrombosis, thromboembolism, active or healed infective endocarditis, and hemodynamic valve dysfunction. Causes of this last problem include structural failure of the prosthe-

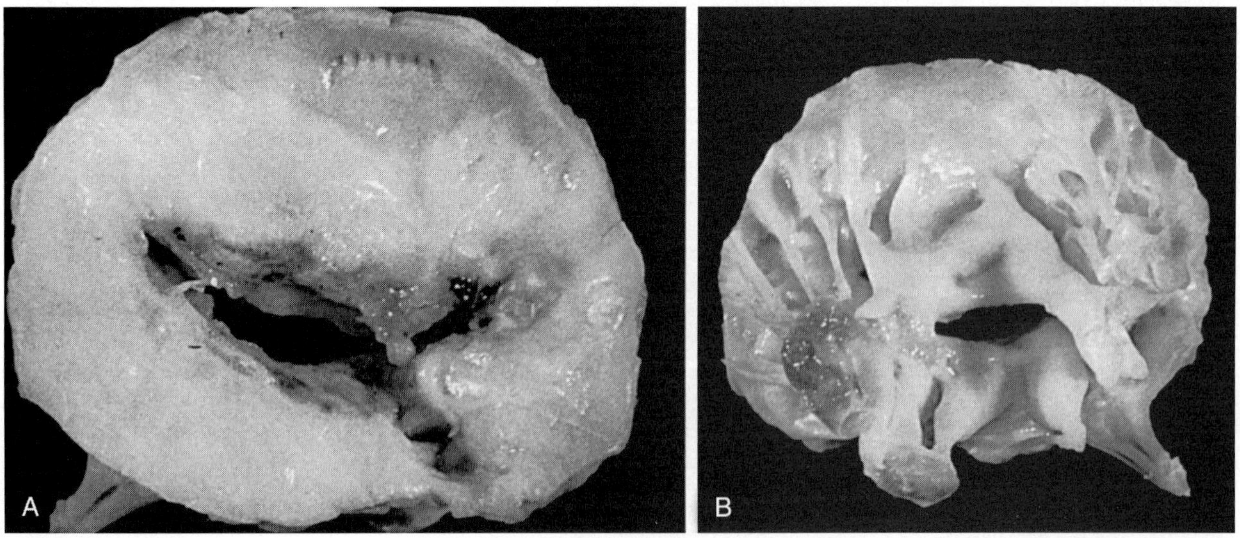

Figure 16–4. The surgically excised mitral valve from a 55-year-old woman has classic morphologic features of postinflammatory (usually postrheumatic) fibrosis. *A*, Small amounts of fibrin (dark material about orifice of valve) are present on atrial aspect of thickened leaflets and fused commissures. *B*, From the ventricular aspect, fibrotic thickening of leaflets and of fused chordae tendineae create more stenosis than is evident in *A*.

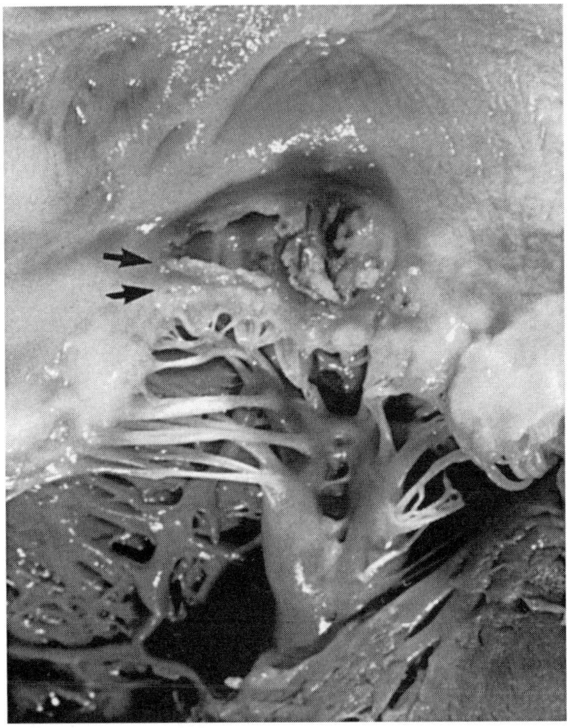

Figure 16–5. The opened left atrium, mitral valve, and left ventricle of this 68-year-old woman display typical features of active infective endocarditis with vegetations *(arrows)*, marked tissue destruction, and invasion of mitral anular region creating abscess (not visible in this view).

sis, obstruction to the left ventricular outflow tract by the prosthesis, dehiscence (sterile periprosthetic leakage), disproportionately large size of the prosthesis to the size of the left ventricular cavity, and excessive endocardial tissue ingrowth into the orifice of the prosthetic valve (Fig. 16–7).

When active infective endocarditis necessitates operation, sometimes on an emergent basis because of a major complication such as significant valvar regurgitation, attempts to extirpate infected annular or other tissue must be made, either as an initial or a secondary procedure. In addition to the threatening effects of septicemia, including myocardial destruction, the process may lead to dehiscence of a prosthetic valve. Eradication of the infection may require removal of the valve and replacement with a new prosthesis.

Sterile periprosthetic valve leaks usually result from separation of sutures from an abnormal annular region; opening of surgical knots; inadequate placement or numbers of sutures for a pathologic annulus; unusual, unpredictable tissue retraction from the valve sewing ring during healing; or inadequate decalcification of the annulus prior to placement of sutures.

Rupture of the left ventricle is a rare complication following operative treatment of mitral valve disease. Most instances have been related to valve replacements. In the past, this was more common in women who had prosthetic valve placement for mitral stenosis.[4] The rupture is usually transmural, resulting in fatal hemopericardium. It most commonly occurs in the lateral or inferolateral aspect of the ventricle in the basilar half. False aneurysm resulting from incomplete (contained) rupture has been reported. The bases for ventricular rupture include operative laceration of the wall due to marked fibrosis and calcification in the region and myocardial infarction due to injury or obstruction of the left circumflex artery, especially when the vessel is deep in the left atrioventricular groove lying close to the endocardium. Major injury or rupture of the left ventricle may also result from overly aggressive excision of papillary

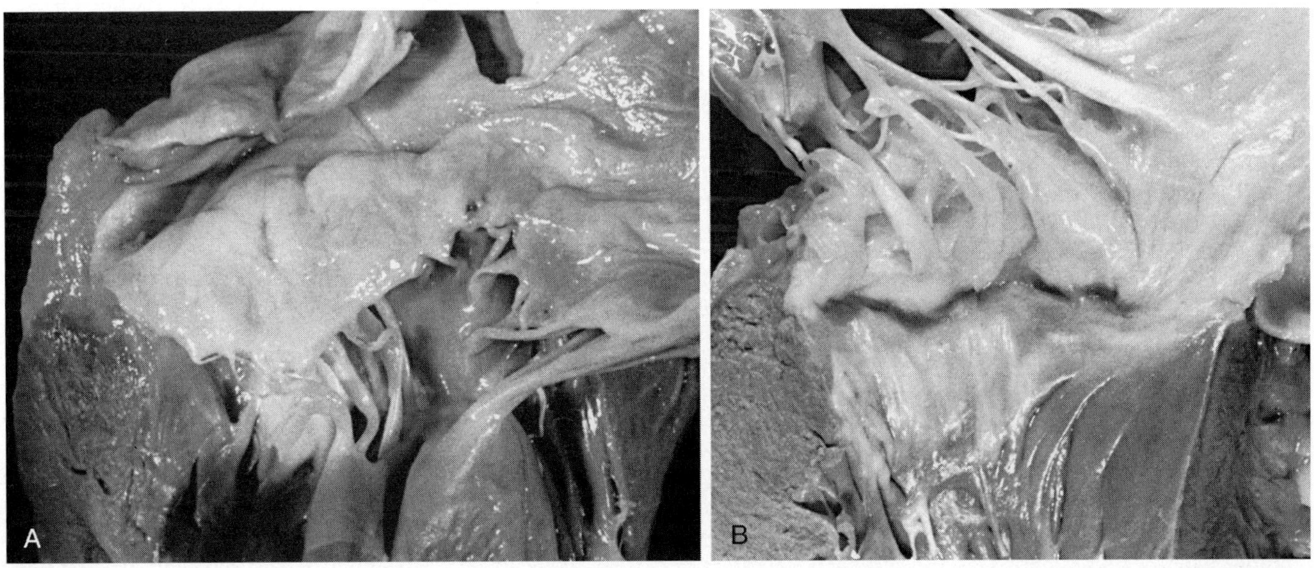

Figure 16–6. A 51-year-old man had known mitral valve prolapse with valvar incompetence. *A*, Part of thickened and enlarged posterior mitral leaflet of the myxomatous valve is shown in leftward half. The anterolateral commissure is central and the anterior leaflet is to the right. The white endocardial thickening of the ventricle beneath the posterior leaflet is an endocardial friction lesion resulting from prolapse. *B*, Ventricular endocardial thickening is better displayed when the posterior leaflet is reflected toward the left atrium *(upward)*; from a 38-year-old male.

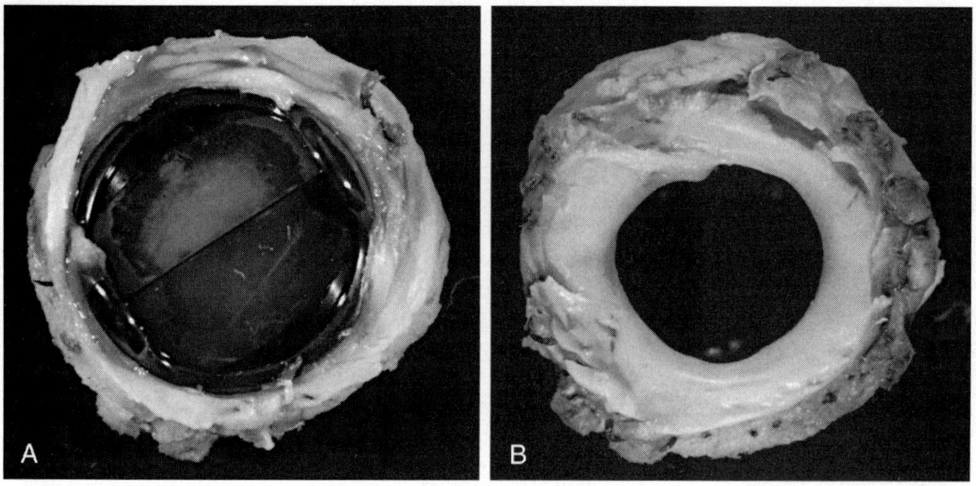

Figure 16–7. This St. Jude mitral prosthesis was surgically excised for severe stenosis. *A,* From the atrial aspect no significant abnormality is apparent; the fibrous tissue growth over the sewing ring is normal for several years postimplantation. *B,* From the ventricular aspect, overgrowth of the fibrous tissue into the valve annulus has created a pannus that obstructs leaflet mobility and narrows the annular orifice.

muscle tissue. Dehiscence of the atrioventricular groove may result from excessive excision of the valve or placement of sutures into the left ventricle muscle.

SURGICAL-PATHOLOGIC CONSULTATIONS

Although intraoperative consultations are uncommon during mitral valve procedures, accurate pathologic evaluation of resected material requires close communication between surgeon and pathologist. The surgeon should expect an evaluation that will contribute to an understanding of the pathogenesis of the valve abnormality. Such information may be necessary for planning immediate or future treatment and for determining prognosis. As indicated in the introductory remarks, in fatal cases every effort should be made to obtain an autopsy.

Aortic Valve Region

In considering the aortic valve it is appropriate to include also the ascending thoracic aorta and the subaortic region of the left ventricular outflow tract.

AORTIC VALVE

Dysfunction of the aortic valve that results in stenosis or insufficiency or both has many causes. In adults in North America stenosis of the aortic valve requiring valvular replacement usually results from one of three processes: (1) acquired fibrocalcific changes in a congenitally bicuspid (rarely unicuspid) aortic valve (Fig. 16–8*A*), (2) senile (degenerative) calcification as an age-related phenomenon (Fig. 16–8*B*), and (3) fibrotic (with or without calcific) changes (scarring) of a postinflammatory, noninfective type, usually related to prior episodes of rheumatic fever with pancarditis. The first and second causes are most common, usually with stenosis as the principal valvar abnormality.

Stenotic aortic valves usually require replacement. Major problems related to or following the surgical procedure are partial obstruction of the ascending aorta,[5] obstruction of coronary arteries (especially the ostia), left ventricular dysfunction, paravalvar leak, and heart block.[3]

Partial *obstruction of the ascending aorta* is uncommon in adult patients. When it occurs it is usually associated with a ''high-profile'' prosthesis, such as a caged ball. This obstruction is due to the relatively narrow channel for blood flow that exists between the ball and the aortic wall.

Coronary arterial obstructions associated with aortic valve replacements have different causes. Most conditions are of historical interest only. In previous years, when cannulation of the coronary arteries often was done for myocardial perfusion, localized stenosing intimal fibrotic thickenings of the ostia sometimes occurred at the site of cannulation. Even more rarely, the cannula passed into the left anterior descending (LAD) coronary artery distal to the origin of the left circumflex (LCX) artery. In this situation, the myocardium in the LCX distribution was ischemic and, with restoration of normal perfusion, hemorrhagic (reperfusion) myocardial lesions resulted. Partial obstruction of coronary ostia may result when a stent of the prosthetic valve lies directly opposite the ostium, especially when the aorta is small. Rarely, a suture may narrow a coronary artery.

Coronary arterial embolism may occur when a calcified valve is manipulated. Such emboli have been identified in essentially all organs, in addition to the heart. Calcific emboli from left heart valves also may occur without manipulation of the valve. This fact needs to be considered when calcific emboli are found in the postoperative period. *Air emboli* are well recognized and discussed in cardiac surgical treatises. They are difficult to demonstrate pathologically; it is likely that some instances of left ventricular hypofunction in the immediate postoperative period are due to unidentified air emboli.

Inadequate left ventricular function after aortic valve replacement is often associated with extreme left ventricular hypertrophy that resulted from preexisting aortic valve disease. In these cases such marked hypertrophy precludes adequate myocardial perfusion during the operation. This may lead to ischemia of sufficient degree and duration to cause subendocardial myocardial infarction. In fatal cases the surgeon should provide detailed information and clari-

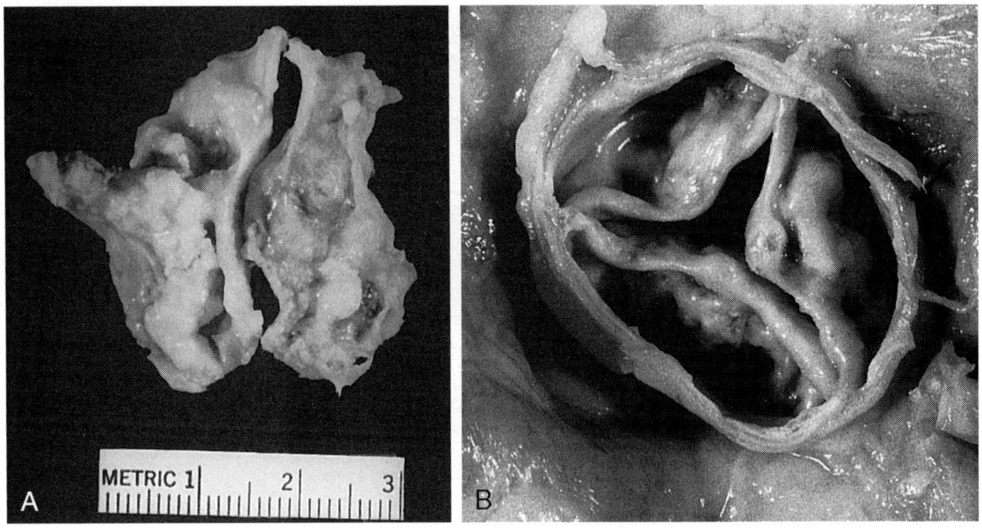

Figure 16–8. *A*, This surgically excised aortic valve demonstrates acquired calcific stenosis of a congenitally bicuspid valve. *B*, This aortic valve has acquired calcific stenosis of a senile (degenerative) type.

fying questions to the pathologist doing the postmortem examination. This problem is less frequent today with the use of retrograde coronary sinus cardioplegia.

Paravalvar leak of bland (sterile) types results from failure of suture knots, atypical degrees of tissue retraction in normal healing processes, abnormal tissues at the annulus, and inadequate decalcification of the aortic annulus.

Active infective endocarditis may be present at the time of valve replacement and may have caused an aortic root abscess (Fig. 16–9). The abscess may be difficult (or impossible) to eradicate completely because of its extent. The abscess may lead to a fistula from the aorta to a cardiac chamber, to the pulmonary trunk, or to the pericardial cavity.[6] The termination of an infected fistulous tract of the aortic root depends upon where the abscess occurs. If the abscess is in the right side of the posterior aortic sinus the fistula may lead to either atrium, more commonly the right. Abscesses involving the rightward half of the left aortic sinus appear near the pulmonary trunk. The region related to the right aortic sinus is the right ventricular infundibulum. Infected tissues of the adjacent part of the left and posterior aortic sinus may lead to perforation of the aortic-mitral intervalvular fibrosa, permitting communication between the left atrium medially and the ascending aorta and pulmonary trunk laterally. This state may be a precursor of bleeding into the pericardial cavity. Because placement of a prosthesis into an infected annulus is prone to infection of the prosthesis, homograft root placement is preferred.

Aortic valve insufficiency can be due to a primary abnormality of the valve (Fig. 16–10) or to dilatation of the aortic root. In contrast to the mitral valve, plastic procedures on the aortic valve to correct insufficiency are less commonly done when the valvular insufficiency is due primarily to cusp abnormality. When the insufficiency is secondary to dilatation of the aortic root the cusps may appear grossly normal with only slight, nonspecific thickenings of their free edges. If minor foci of calcification are present at the base of the cusps the calcification most often is a nonspecific, age-related change without functional significance. Histologically, such cusps may be normal or nearly so. Slight increases in valvar spongiosa may suggest myxomatous change but usually the valvar fibrosa is intact. Accordingly, these minor changes should be viewed as secondary to the insufficiency rather than the cause of it. These pathologic anatomic findings support the concept of possible resuspension of the native cusps after correction of the underlying aortic root problem that originally led to valvar insufficiency.

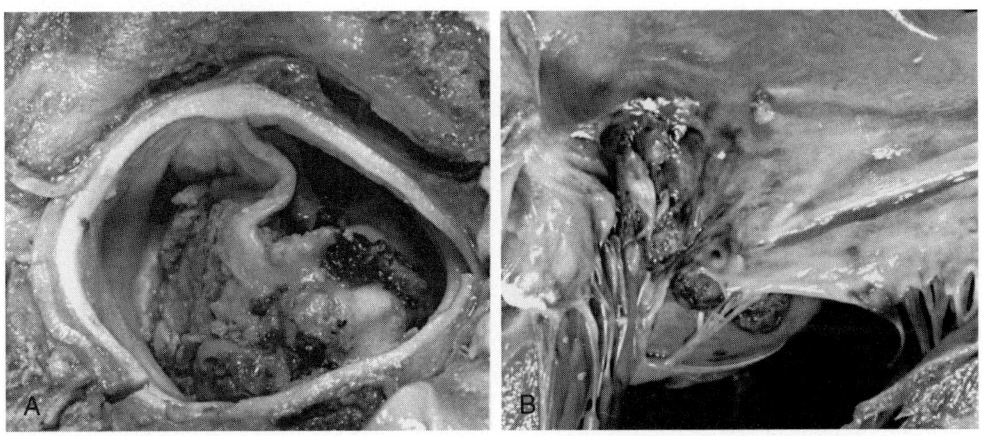

Figure 16–9. Active infective endocarditis of right aortic cusp *(A)* involved right aortic sinus with extension into right atrium *(B)* appearing clinically as abscess in region of septal-anterior commissure of tricuspid valve.

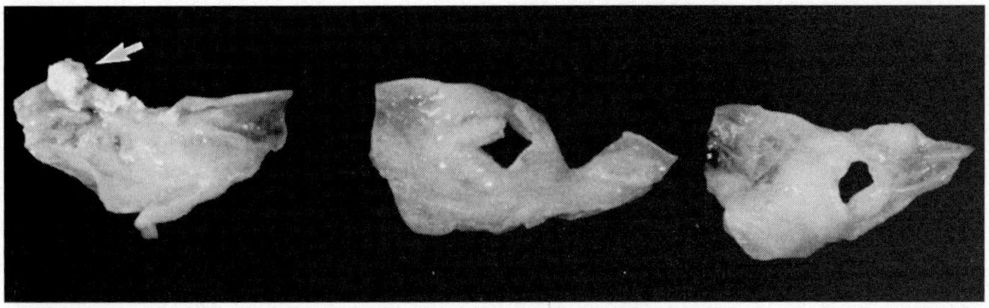

Figure 16–10. These aortic valve cusps were removed for valvular incompetence due to healed infective endocarditis. The two cusps on the right have large central holes with thick fibrotic rims. The leftmost cusp has calcified vegetations on its free edge (top of cusp, *arrow*).

If the abnormal aortic valve is replaced with a prosthesis, the possible complications related to the prosthetic valve are the same as those previously discussed in the section on mitral valve.

ASCENDING THORACIC AORTA

In adults, the most common conditions affecting the ascending aorta are *acquired aneurysms* or *aneurysmal dilatations*. Such enlargement of the aortic root and contiguous ascending aorta may be the primary cause of aortic valve incompetence, as discussed. Aortic dilatation with valvular incompetence may require replacement of both the valve and the aorta with prosthetic materials, often as a composite graft. In addition to the problems discussed in relation to aortic valve replacement, the necessity of an aortic graft adds another dimension of complexities. These include the presence of two circumferential suture lines, reconnection of the coronary arteries to the aortic graft, the nature of the grafts, the graft-host interfaces, and the valve-graft interface.

The pathologic bases for the underlying aortic dilatation merit brief consideration. *Aneurysms of the ascending aorta* result from an abnormality of the aortic media. Medial abnormalities may be developmental, as with hereditofamilial conditions such as the Marfan syndrome, or they may be acquired.[7, 8] Aneurysms of the aortic sinuses of Valsalva are a somewhat special form of medial deficiencies of the aortic root, which may be associated with abnormal runoff from the aorta (Fig. 16–11). Acquired forms are (1) noninflammatory medial degeneration (either an exaggerated aging process or associated with hypertension), (2) noninfective aortitis-Takayasu's disease, giant cell aortitis, and nonspecific aortitis, and (3) infective aortitis of luetic or bacterial cause. Any of these forms of aortitis, except the infective ones, may be associated with aortic dissection. Atherosclerosis is rarely the cause of aneurysm of the ascending aorta, although it may be present as an associated finding.

Histologic examination is necessary for diagnosis of one of these pathologic states. For adequate pathologic evaluation, a full-thickness biopsy of the aortic wall is required. A rather generous strip gives the pathologist a better chance to make the diagnosis because characteristic lesions may be focal in the abnormal wall. Accurate diagnosis will help in planning future treatment, determining prognosis, and perhaps even dictating immediate intervention. Some surgeons believe that anti-inflammatory agents, such as steroids or immunosuppressive agents, should be considered if focal necrosis or active inflammation is present.

SUBAORTIC REGION OF LEFT VENTRICLE OUTFLOW TRACT

Abnormalities of the subaortic region may result in left ventricular outflow obstruction creating *subaortic stenosis*. Among the best known is membranous subaortic stenosis (Fig. 16–12); whether this is a developmental anomaly remains undetermined. Regardless of its pathogenesis, this condition may require surgical excision for two reasons: (1) relief of the subaortic stenosis and (2) prevention of damage to the aortic valve from high-velocity jetflow striking the ventricular side of the cusps. Changes in the cusps resulting from this injury may lead to valve insufficiency. Resected tissue of a subaortic stenotic lesion should be examined histologically to determine its major components. Such knowledge may contribute to understanding of the pathogenesis of the lesion and give an explanation if restenosis occurs.

Muscular subaortic stenosis is usually part of hypertrophic cardiomyopathy. Surgical procedures for relief require

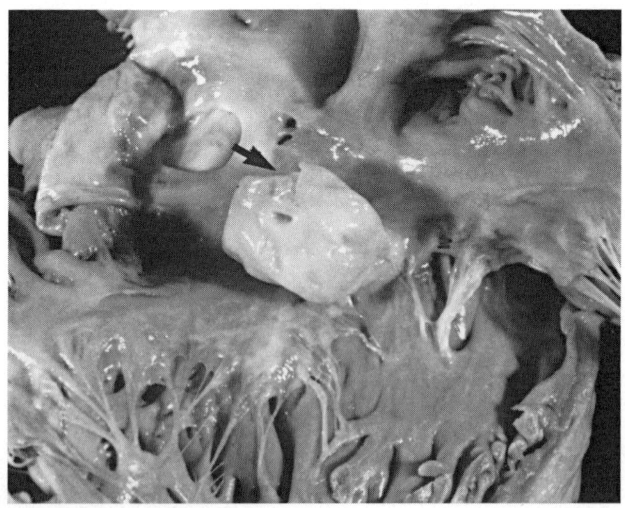

Figure 16–11. Sudden cardiac death occurred in a 20-year-old man. The opened right atrium, tricuspid valve, and right ventricle show a large aneurysm of the right aortic sinus projecting into the right heart. A central small hole in the aneurysmal sac permitted some left-to-right shunting, leading to enlargement of the right atrium and ventricle. An acute tear (uppermost side of aneurysm, *arrow*) resulted in a large and rapidly fatal left-to-right shunt, the functional equivalent of sudden massive aortic incompetence.

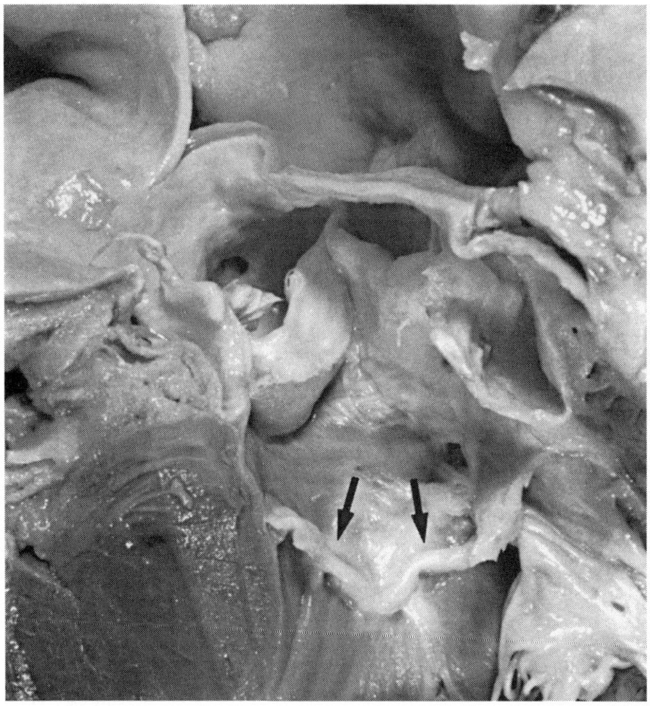

Figure 16–12. An elderly woman had severe aortic stenosis due to a subaortic fibrous membrane, shown *(arrows)* in this view of the opened left ventricular outflow tract and aortic valve. This condition is a rare finding in elderly patients.

excision of subaortic ventricular septal muscle. Because of anatomic location, there is risk for injury to the His bundle (see Fig. 16–2). Histopathologic studies of the resected tissues are needed, partly to confirm clinical diagnosis, but also to help define possible subtypes of the basic condition. Some subtypes have different genetic implications and different prognoses from the classic hypertrophic obstructive cardiomyopathy (asymmetric septal hypertrophy). Pathologic study should assess endocardial thickness and vascularity, myocardial fiber size, myocardial cellular disarray, fiber bundle disorder, and intramyocardial arterial thickness.

Tricuspid and Pulmonic Valve Regions

Abnormalities of the tricuspid valve are relatively infrequent. Acquired conditions of the valve may create stenosis or insufficiency. Postrheumatic scarring is among the more common abnormalities and usually is associated with similar involvement of the mitral and aortic valves.

Tricuspid regurgitation is more often secondary to right ventricular dilatation (from any cause) than to a primary abnormality of the valve. Acquired conditions that cause incompetence include infective endocarditis, carcinoid heart disease (Fig. 16–13), trauma, and floppy (myxomatous) states. Operations for valve insufficiency appropriately first seek to restore competence of the native valve because it may be anatomically normal. When anatomically abnormal, replacement may be required. In general, the same considerations regarding valve prosthesis detailed in the sections on mitral and aortic valves pertain to the tricuspid valve. A major difference for the tricuspid valve is its close relationship to the AV node and His bundle, which are in some danger of injury during operation (see Fig. 16–2).

The *pulmonic valve* only rarely acquires anatomic abnormalities creating dysfunction. In North America the rare conditions of infective endocarditis and carcinoid disease of the pulmonic valve may cause valve regurgitation. As with the tricuspid valve, pulmonic regurgitation most often occurs with an anatomically normal valve, being secondary to pulmonary hypertension.

Aorta and Peripheral Arteries

Discussion of conditions affecting the aorta requires consideration of its different anatomic segments: ascending, arch, descending thoracic, and abdominal. Often the distal part of the thoracic aorta and the proximal part of the abdominal aorta are regarded as a single segment, the thoracoabdominal portion. Based upon pathologic features and pathogenetic factors,[7, 8] conditions affecting the aorta may be classified as developmental (congenital), atherosclerotic, degenerative (noninflammatory medial abnormality), inflammatory infective, inflammatory noninfective (Takayasu's disease, giant cell aortitis, nonspecific aortitis), and traumatic. All of these may cause aneurysms. Some may cause aortic dissection, the exceptions being luetic and bacterial infections and atherosclerosis. Many also lead to narrowing or obstruction of the arch or descending aorta or their major branches. The conditions usually responsible are (1) atherosclerosis with secondary thrombosis and (2) primary inflammatory states with narrowing secondary to reparative fibrotic processes. The healing of any vascular

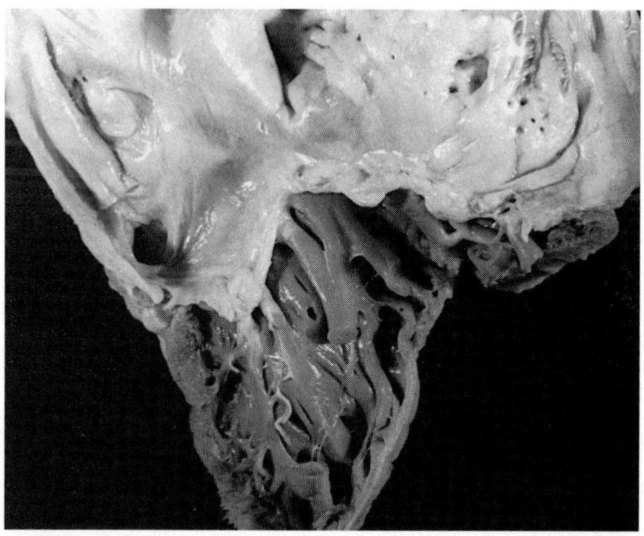

Figure 16–13. Carcinoid heart disease usually is manifested by marked right atrial and modest right ventricular enlargement due to tricuspid insufficiency secondary to fibromuscular proliferations (carcinoid plaques) on the valve and endocardium of the chambers. These findings are shown in the opened right heart of a 71-year-old woman.

injury may result in fibrous tissue narrowing of a channel and does not constitute a specific disease or recurrence of a surgically corrected condition. An example is so-called recoarctation of the aorta after surgical removal of the original congenital coarctation. The recurrent lesion usually is a fibrous tissue proliferation (scar) not redevelopment of the medial abnormality that originally produced the congenital coarctation.

Identification of the underlying disease that produced the condition needing surgical correction may modify or direct current and future management as well as prognosis. Full-thickness biopsy of the vascular wall is needed. If possible, different sites should be sampled including some apparently normal tissue. Intraoperative frozen sections usually are neither needed nor advisable because the freezing process permanently introduces artifacts that obscure subtle diagnostic changes. As always, collaboration between surgeon and pathologist is needed to maximize potential benefits of pathologic studies.

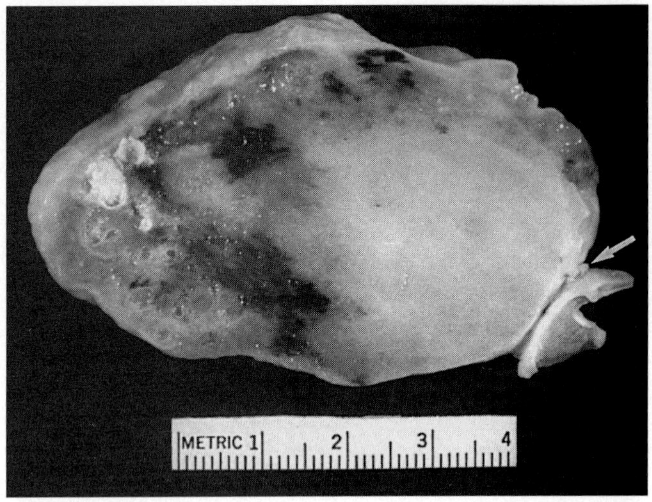

Figure 16–14. A surgically excised left atrial myxoma has been bisected to demonstrate the stalk of the tumor (right side of tumor, *arrow*) attached to the atrial septum; the small portion of atrial septum represents full thickness of this structure. This myxoma has large zones of myxomatous tissue, foci of fibrosis, small cysts, focal hemorrhages, and spotty calcifications (white material near surface of upper left side of tumor).

Endarterectomy, Thrombectomy, and Thromboembolectomy

Although endarterectomy, thrombectomy, and thromboembolectomy are different procedures, from the pathologist's standpoint the tissues obtained are similar. *Endarterectomy* of any artery almost always yields a tissue segment that includes the stenosing lesion with all of the intima as well as some portion of the contiguous media of the vessel. Even though vascular surgeons know well that portions of the elastic lamina and muscular media usually are included, other specialists may need to be advised in this regard. Histopathologic study is needed to confirm the nature of the stenosing lesion, which most often is a complicated atherosclerotic plaque, with or without hemorrhage or thrombosis into the plaque. Occasionally, inflammatory, developmental, neoplastic, or embolic conditions are identified. Such diagnoses may alter treatment indication and prognosis.

Both *thrombectomy* and *thromboembolectomy* are intended to remove occluding luminal lesions. If either type of lesion has been present for even a few days, some organization occurs requiring removal of part of the vascular intima or even the media in older lesions. The importance of histologic study is more than confirmation of the diagnosis. An unsuspected process other than thrombosis (see preceding paragraph) may be first identified in the specimen. Although such unexpected findings are only rarely encountered, failure to do a histopathologic examination may permit a potentially remediable condition to be missed. "Gross only" instructions for the pathologic study of thrombi and emboli are therefore not appropriate. On occasion the thrombus or embolus is secondary to an atrial myxoma, detected only by microscopic examination.

Atrial Conditions

Pathologic consultations in relation to surgical procedures on the atria are infrequent. One condition that may require such interaction is atrial myxoma. Most of these lesions are situated on the atrial septum. Perhaps the most important question answered by pathologic study concerns the stalk of this benign tumor; specifically, is the base of the stalk free of myxoma cells (Fig. 16–14)? To answer this question the surgeon should mark the base of the tumor or its stalk at the line of excision. Of course, when the full thickness of atrial septum has been excised, the question is moot.

Occasionally, the surgeon is asked to close a patent, valve-competent foramen ovale in a patient who has had transient ischemic attacks or stroke. The benefit of this procedure has not been established. Fibrinous thrombotic material encountered in the region should be submitted for histologic study to determine whether the material is thrombus or merely blood coagulum related to the procedure. Aneurysmal dilatation of the fossa ovalis also is associated with thrombi that can embolize.

Coronary Arterial Bypass Surgery

It is uncommon for a surgeon to request an intraoperative pathologic consultation during coronary bypass procedures. However, one of the exceptional situations justifying such an effort is *aortic wall* biopsy, dictated by abnormal anatomic appearances of the aorta. If any of the aortic abnormalities described previously are present, this condition may lead to dissection of the aorta originating at the site of anastomosis of a vein graft to the aorta.

Occasionally, a segment of the harvested *saphenous vein* may appear abnormal and be submitted for histologic study. In such instances nonspecific phlebosclerosis is the most common finding. In rare instances conditions such as venous fibromuscular dysplasia or true phlebitis may be present. If such conditions are diagnosed using frozen section, the involved venous segment should be discarded. Except for an unusually small size, a significant abnormality of an *internal mammary artery* is almost never encountered prior to its anastomosis to a coronary artery.

''Redo'' bypass procedures may yield specimens of previous venous bypass grafts or native coronary arteries. When the internal mammary artery was used as a bypass graft, pathologic changes are limited to slight to moderate intimal thickening at the site of anastomosis. In contrast, changes in venous bypass grafts are universal and well characterized. They are roughly proportional to the amount of time that has elapsed since the bypass operation. The earliest, nearly ubiquitous condition is development of fibromuscular intimal thickening from proliferation of vascular smooth muscle cells. This process is a healing reaction to endothelial cell injury incident to vein harvest. The reaction may create functionally significant luminal stenosis of the vein over time periods that vary greatly among patients or even in different grafts in the same patient. This intimal proliferation reaction is not atherosclerosis. Use of the term ''accelerated atherosclerosis'' is incorrect.

Thrombosis of vein grafts in the early postoperative period may occur, sometimes necessitating reoperation. In past years, some instances were due to technical factors, but today early thrombosis most often is related to poor runoff (blood flow) distal to the venous arterial anastomosis. This is due to atherosclerotic stenosis in the artery distal to the anastomosis. If reoperation is done and if a segment of the thrombosed vessel can be obtained, pathologic study may rarely reveal an underlying venous abnormality.

Atherosclerosis can develop in vein grafts and cause obstruction or aneurysmal dilatation. Major atherosclerotic abnormalities in vein grafts are uncommon earlier than 3 to 4 years after operation. After about 5 years the chances of atherosclerotic disease in vein grafts increase, but significant stenosis does not necessarily proceed, even over long periods. Atherosclerotic plaques in vein grafts tend to be more grumous than those of coronary arteries. They are soft, mushy, and friable with a major component of lipoidal debris admixed with cellular elements and blood proteins. The usual fibrous cap of a classic arterial atheroma is not present in venous specimens; instead their surface is thin and delicate. These features predispose patients with these lesions to experience rupture with extrusion of the materials into the vessels and creation of a thrombogenic surface. At reoperation this same characteristic is responsible for emboli into the distal coronary circulation. One, therefore, should be careful in the handling of old vein grafts.

Myocardial Considerations

Surgical treatment of primary myocardial disease is uncommon as an initial endeavor. Cardiac transplantation for congenital anomalies (e.g., hypoplastic left heart syndromes) or acquired abnormalities (e.g., end-stage cardiomyopathic disease) is not considered in this discussion. The more common situations in which the surgical procedure is directed toward the myocardium are complications of coronary heart disease and, rarely, cardiac tumors.

Surgical treatment of *ischemic heart disease complications* includes operations for true and false ventricular aneurysms, acute rupture of the ventricular septum or free wall or papillary muscle, relief of pericardial tamponade, and mitral insufficiency secondary to abnormal geometry and function of the ischemic ventricle. If tissue for pathologic examination is obtained at operation, the pathologist should estimate the age of infarct, particularly if that is the cause of the condition. If part of a mitral valve is resected, the pathologist should determine whether an underlying abnormality of the valve exists, distinct from the secondary effects of the ischemic ventricle.

During a procedure, biopsy of the myocardium is sometimes appropriate. If possible, the biopsy should be full thickness, i.e., endocardium to epicardium. Prior to biopsy, consultation with the pathologist assures proper fixation, handling, and processing of the specimen. A single negative biopsy finding does *not* exclude the possibility of an inflammatory state, i.e., myocarditis.

Apart from the cardiac myxoma discussed previously, primary cardiac tumors are rare. Some of the benign types are amenable to surgical removal, but the location of the tumor may preclude excision. Metastatic malignant neoplasms are the most common malignant tumors in the heart. The frequency of types encountered essentially parallels that of primary tumor types overall, with the exception of malignant melanoma, which shows a predilection for cardiac metastasis.

Congenital Heart Disease

This section focuses on some of the more common types of congenital heart disease. It should be emphasized that, the more complex the anomalous situation, the more likely it is that iatrogenically induced complications will occur. The following discussion focuses on problems that may arise during surgical intervention for congenital heart disease.

ATRIAL SEPTAL DEFECT

The most common type of atrial septal defect (ASD) is *at the fossa ovalis,* often termed ''secundum type'' ASD. In this condition the posterior aspect of the defect may be the posterior atrial wall. If there is a prominent valve of the inferior vena cava (eustachian valve), the free edge of the valve can be sewn to the anterior edge of the atrial septal defect, thereby directing all inferior venal caval blood to the left atrium (Fig. 16–15). As a result cyanosis that was not present preoperatively will be present postoperatively.

An ASD at the fossa ovalis may be associated with or secondary to mitral stenosis, a combination often termed Lutembacher's syndrome. In some cases mitral regurgitation rather than mitral stenosis is present. Whatever the mitral valvular abnormality, the ASD serves as an ''escape channel'' for the effects of the mitral valvular disease. Thus, closure of the ASD may actually be deleterious. In

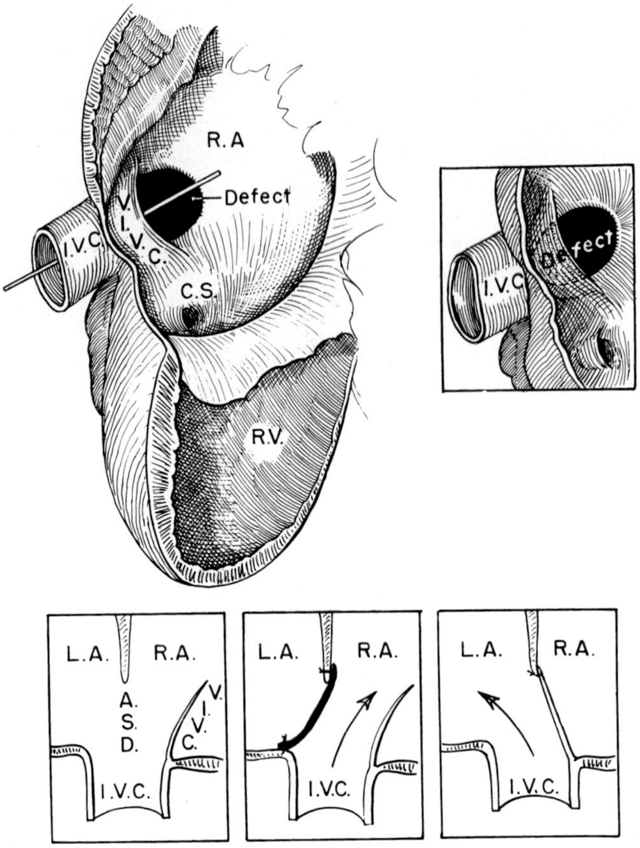

Figure 16–15. In the large drawing at left an ASD (Defect) at the fossa ovalis (secundum defect) is shown from the right atrial (RA) and right ventricular (RV) septal perspective. A probe passes from the inferior vena cava (IVC) and behind the Eustachian valve at the ostium of the inferior vena cava (VIVC) into the defect. The posterior-inferior extent of the defect "behind" the valve is shown in the inset drawing to the right. The lower three panels are views of the same region when hemisected along a base-apex axis. LA and RA are left and right atria, respectively. The ASD is the opening labeled Defect in the upper drawings. VIVC is the valve of the inferior vena cava. In the left panel the basic anatomical relationships are shown. In the center panel the ASD has been closed correctly (heavy black line with "sutures" at ends), so that the IVC is directed entirely to the RA. In the right panel the procedure was incorrect; the valve of the IVC was sutured to the superior rim of the ASD, directing all blood from the IVC to the left atrium.

some cases, the abnormal opening in the atrial septum may be an enlargement of a patent foramen ovale rather than a true ASD, but the functional effects are the same.

The *sinus venosus* type ASD lies posterosuperior to the fossa ovalis partly beneath the superior vena caval junction with the right atrium. Although an uncommon form of ASD, its association with anomalous pulmonary venous connection from the right lung to the right atrium deserves emphasis. Failure to recognize this situation at the time of surgical repair may result in commitment of the superior vena cava to the left atrium and persistence of the anomalous pulmonary venous connection of the right lung to the right atrium.

The rare ASD at the site of the coronary sinus ostium usually is associated with an absence of the coronary sinus and a persistent left superior vena cava joining the left atrium.[9, 10] Closure of the ASD without attention to the left superior vena cava may lead to postoperative cyanosis.

VENTRICULAR SEPTAL DEFECT

Surgical treatment of ventricular septal defect (VSD) consists of either palliative pulmonary arterial banding or closure of the defect. Primary closure of the VSD usually is the treatment of choice. Pulmonary arterial banding may be done as a temporizing palliative procedure, especially when the VSD is part of a more complex condition. Adverse consequences of pulmonary arterial banding occur. The most common is fixed stenosis of the pulmonary trunk, either alone or in combination with stenosis of the origin of the right pulmonary artery. Less commonly, the band may cut through the pulmonary trunk leading to mediastinal hemorrhage or to formation of a false aneurysm. Infection at the band site also occurs. The hemodynamic effects of fixed obstruction of the pulmonary trunk vary with cardiac output. Thus when a band is applied at early age, there may be a balanced state; however, with body growth and increased cardiac output, cyanosis may develop.

Closure of the common types of ventricular septal defect has the potential for mechanical injury to the bundle of His. Better appreciation of the anatomic relationship between different VSDs and the major conduction tissue has reduced the frequency of surgical injury to the conduction tissue.

After apparent surgical closure of a VSD, a residual defect or defects may be present. Some may be so small that the circulation is stable; nevertheless, the danger of infective endocarditis accompanies the presence of a residual small VSD, as with an untreated, congenitally small VSD. Residual VSDs after operation also occur when there are multiple muscular VSDs ("Swiss cheese" ventricular septum). In this condition, intraoperative identification of all the defects in an opened right ventricle may be difficult. This pitfall is avoided by preoperative angiocardiograms or echocardiograms to identify the defects or, if possible, inspection of the septum from the left ventricle.

Among the uncommon complications of closure of VSD is engagement of the anterior mitral leaflet by a suture.

PERSISTENT COMMON ATRIOVENTRICULAR CANAL

The basic anomaly of persistent common atrioventricular canal (AVC) varies considerably from case to case. The anomaly has two principal forms, the partial (incomplete) and the complete types. The partial form has an ASD in the lower part of the atrial septum (primum ASD) and a defect (cleft) in the anterior leaflet of the mitral valve—but does not have interventricular communication. Patients may survive into adulthood without corrective treatment.

The complete range of persistent AVC includes the primum ASD, abnormality of both the septal tricuspid and the anterior mitral leaflets, and major deficiency of the ventricular septum. Surgical repair requires correction of each of these major anomalies. Among problems complicating surgical repair are residual mitral stenosis or insufficiency and subaortic stenosis. The latter results if the narrow left ventricular outflow tract cannot be expanded. Among other cardiac anomalies that may accompany persistent AVC are ASD at the fossa ovalis (secundum ASD) and membranous subaortic stenosis. These conditions must also be corrected at the time of surgical repair of the AVC. Heart block may be a complication of surgical repair, since the complex anomalies present different hazards for surgical injury to the AV node and His bundle.

COMPLETE TRANSPOSITION OF THE GREAT ARTERIES

Complete transposition (d-transposition) of the great arteries (TGA) may be surgically treated by "atrial switch" operations (Senning, Mustard procedures) in which the atrial streams are crossed or by an "arterial switch" procedure. A common palliative procedure in the neonate is the creation of an atrial septal defect by a nonoperative technique (Rashkind procedure). Rare complications include perforation of the left lower pulmonary vein with hemopericardium and puncture of the base of the right atrium with hemopericardium.

Procedures designed to cross the atrial bloodstreams often result in postoperative obstruction of venae cavae, particularly the superior vena cava. Obstruction to pulmonary venous flow may also occur. In the arterial switch operation, a major challenge is transfer of the coronary arteries along with the aorta from the right to the left ventricle.[11] If unsuccessful, acute myocardial infarction may complicate surgical treatment of TGA on the basis of this problem.

TETRALOGY OF FALLOT

The tetralogy of Fallot (TOF) has been treated both palliatively and by total correction. Palliation consists of creation of an aortopulmonary anastomosis. Anastomoses used include the original subclavian-pulmonary arterial shunt (Blalock-Taussig procedure) and direct connections of the aorta to a pulmonary artery (Potts and Waterston procedures). Other palliative procedures include a graft between the ascending aorta and the pulmonary trunk (so-called central shunt). Problems associated with anastomoses include creating too large an acute left-to-right shunt with resulting ventricular failure. Large shunts that are well tolerated may lead to hypertensive pulmonary vascular disease over long periods of time.

Procedures for total correction of TOF are fraught with complications: residual pulmonary stenosis, persisting VSD, heart block, and injury to a coronary artery that has an anomalous course over the anterior wall of the right ventricular infundibulum. To relieve completely the right ventricular outflow obstruction, a patch may be needed to expand the outflow tract. Right ventricular aneurysms may develop.

THORACIC AORTIC AND PULMONARY ARTERIAL ANOMALIES

A few of the many anomalies of the thoracic aorta and the pulmonary arteries that have functional effects are discussed in this section. To fully understand these conditions surgeons and diagnosticians must appreciate the diversity of possibilities.[12]

The following examples serve to illustrate the wide variety of conditions that must be diagnosed accurately to successfully correct them surgically.

1. Vascular rings of aortic origin. Forms that must be distinguished are the angiographically similar right aortic arch and double aortic arch with atresia of the left arch.
2. Pulmonary vascular sling with branches to the left upper lobe of lung.
3. Common sites at which bronchial obstruction may occur owing to pressure of enlarged pulmonary arteries.
4. Compression effect on bronchi by right ductus arteriosus or double ductus arteriosus.
5. Congenital coronary arterial anomalies. Because of difficulty in diagnosis and uncertainty regarding treatment, anomalies of aortic origin of the coronary arteries are of special concern. These can be grouped into ectopic aortic origins or abnormal angles of aortic origin.[13] Pulmonary origin of a coronary artery is well known, both diagnostically and surgically. Coronary arteriovenous and arteriocameral fistulae also require surgical treatment.

Lung Biopsy

The cardiovascular-thoracic surgeon may be asked to perform open-lung biopsy for diagnoses of many conditions. Special considerations apply if the purpose is evaluation of pulmonary vessels as part of the evaluation of cardiac disease and, in particular, a congenital type. Foremost is the need that the biopsy be obtained from somewhere *other than the lingular segment* of the left upper lobe. Findings in this segment are often unrepresentative of other pulmonary vasculature. The pathologist must recognize that interpretation is enhanced by, and indeed often requires, elastic and connective tissue stains in addition to routine hematoxylin-eosin.

The Pericardium

The pericardium presents special challenges to the surgeon and pathologist alike. These include chronic pericardial constriction and problems related to postoperative pericarditis.

CHRONIC PERICARDIAL CONSTRICTION

Chronic pericardial constriction occurs in two forms: (1) fibrocalcific material encasing the heart and (2) chronic pericardial effusion. Treatment of fibrocalcific constriction requires removal of the constricting pericardium, usually consisting of fused parietal and visceral pericardial layers that are thickened and focally calcified, sometimes in large plaques. The fatty layer of the visceral pericardium (epicardial fat) is often preserved and provides a potential plane of dissection to remove the diseased tissue from the heart. However, the potential presence of epicardial coronary arteries in this layer poses a serious risk.

In most cases of chronic pericardial effusion, the major constrictive effect is that of the contained fluid. In some cases of chronic effusion there is also fibrosis of the epicardium. In this circumstance decortication of the thickened epicardium may be necessary after removal of the pericardial fluid.

Of particular importance in instances of long-standing chronic cardiac constriction is atrophy of the myocardial fibers.[14] This process may be the basis for the myocardial insufficiency that commonly appears in the early postoperative period following decortication.

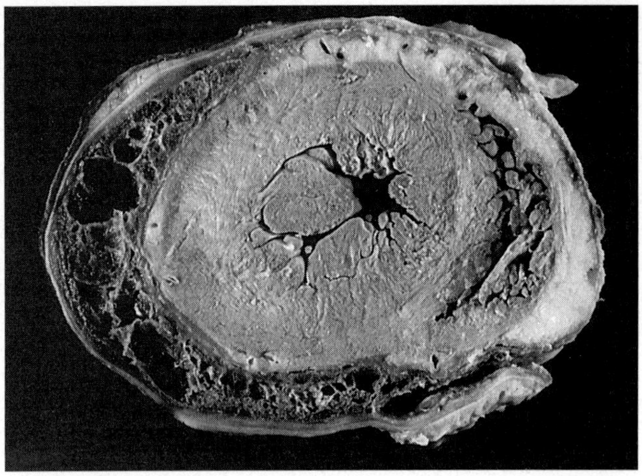

Figure 16–16. Cross section of the ventricles demonstrates an unusual degree of organizing pericarditis related to cardiac surgery 7 weeks prior to death. Acute hemorrhage from the extreme vascularity of the pericarditis caused death. The dark cystlike appearance, best seen about the lateral and posterior (left and inferior in the photograph) aspects of the hypertrophic left ventricle, is organizing pericarditis with hemorrhage.

POSTOPERATIVE PERICARDITIS

Acute fibrinous pericarditis probably occurs following all operations that require opening of the pericardium. In most cases the fibrinous exudate goes through the various stages of organization to form some adhesions between the parietal and visceral layers of the pericardium. Usually the pericardial adhesions are of no functional significance but may present problems to the surgeon if reoperation is necessary. The slightly thickened, adherent pericardial layers may obscure anatomic structures such as epicardial coronary arteries and grafts.

Rarely the organizing postoperative pericarditis may be complicated by hemorrhage (Fig. 16–16). The bleeding occurs from small, newly formed blood vessels within the organizing granulation tissue. The use of anticoagulants may increase the likelihood of hemorrhage. This uncommon cause of bleeding into the pericardium in the early postoperative period (usually 2 to 4 weeks after operation) may be responsible for major complications of hemorrhage, including circulatory failure, and death.

Although some postoperative pericarditis appears to be universal, it is prudent to attempt to avoid drying, mechanical handling, and abrasion by gauze of the exposed pericardium. Often at the conclusion of an operation, the incision in the pericardium is ''left open'' so that a channel for pericardial decompression will be available if needed. Reactive pericarditis may cause the edges of the pericardial incision to adhere to one another or to the chest wall, obliterating this benefit.

PITFALLS FOR THE SURGEON

1. Failing to obtain permission for autopsy on a case posing questions regarding the basis for unsuccessful procedures.
2. Obtaining a less than adequate biopsy sample from aortic aneurysm to allow pathologic assessment.
3. Requesting intraoperative frozen section interpretation of arterial wall biopsy samples, only to satisfy immediate curiosity. Immediate diagnosis is not needed for intraoperative decision making, and freezing artifacts introduced permanently into the samples may compromise final definitive diagnosis.
4. Advising ''gross only'' pathologic evaluation of thrombectomy specimens. Intimal and medial arterial wall elements may reveal microscopic evidence of unsuspected underlying inflammatory or degenerative disease or infectious or neoplastic embolus.
5. Choosing the lingula as a site for pulmonary vascular sampling by lung biopsy. Vessels in this lobe are often unrepresentative of those in the other lobes.
6. Inadequately communicating with the pathologist regarding the clinical presentation and symptoms of the patient.
7. Failing to review the specimen with the pathologist so that there is *direct* communication between the two physicians.

PITFALLS FOR THE PATHOLOGIST

1. Carrying out pathology studies on a surgical or autopsy case without first knowing the issues to be addressed on the part of the surgeon.
2. Proceeding to examine and section a cardiovascular specimen without the understanding and experience necessary to answer the critical questions. When there are doubts, intact specimens should be deferred to a specialist, either within the laboratory or, if necessary, extramurally.
3. Failing to adequately assess myocardium from subaortic outflow tract obstruction procedures.
4. Attempting intraoperative frozen section diagnosis on critical biopsy specimens, when freezing artifact will jeopardize final diagnosis. Before proceeding, the pathologist should communicate directly with the surgeon to be sure that intraoperative decision making depends upon pathology. If it does, the surgeon should be informed that additional samples will be needed, free of freezing artifact, to assure definitive diagnosis.
5. Failing to examine microscopically the arterial wall elements included in thrombectomy specimens for underlying inflammatory or degenerative disorders, or neoplasm.
6. Misinterpreting intimal fibromuscular thickening in a previously implanted venous bypass specimen as "accelerated atherosclerosis."
7. Not utilizing stains for elastic and connective tissues in evaluating vascular biopsy samples.
8. Failing to distinguish normal age-related changes from pathologic conditions.
9. Failing to recognize that diagnosis of different types of acquired valvular abnormalities depends mainly upon *gross examination* and consideration of the *surgical findings*. Histologic sections may obscure the gross diagnostic features.
10. Overdiagnosing some surgically resected valves, e.g., normal-for-age aortic cusps removed in the course of surgery for a dilated aortic root producing aortic valve insufficiency.

FURTHER READING

1. Titus JL, Edwards JE. Pathology of the aging heart. In: Chesler E, ed. *Clinical Cardiology in the Elderly*. Mount Kisco, New York: Futura Publishing Co.; 1994: chap. 1.
2. Titus JL, Edwards JE. Mitral insufficiency other than rheumatic, ischemic, or infective: emphasis on mitral valve prolapse. *Semin Thorac Cardiovasc Surg*. 1989; 1(2):118.
3. Titus JL, Edwards JE. The aortic root and valve. In: Emery RW, Arom KV, eds. *The Aortic Valve*. Philadelphia: Hanley & Belfus; 1991: chap. 1.
4. Titus JL. The heart after surgery for ischemic heart disease. *Am J Cardiovasc Pathol*. 1988; 1(3):339.
5. Titus JL, Edwards JE. Congenital heart disease in the adult: anatomic abnormalities. In: Willerson JT, Cohn JN, eds. *Cardiovascular Medicine*. Edinburgh: Churchill Livingstone; 1995: chap. 1.

REFERENCES

1. Titus JL. Normal anatomy of the human cardiac conduction system. *Mayo Clin Proc*. 1973; 48:24.
2. Ben-Schachar G, Vlodaver Z, Joyce LD, Edwards JE. Mural thrombosis in the left atrium following replacement of the mitral valve. *J Thorac Cardiovasc Surg*. 1981; 82:595.
3. Schoen FJ. Valvular heart disease. In: Schoen FJ, ed. *Interventional and Surgical Cardiovascular Pathology, Clinical Correlations and Basic Principles*. Philadelphia: Saunders; 1989.
4. Kalke B, Korns ME, Goott B, et al. Engagement of ventricular myocardium by open-cage atrioventricular valvular prosthesis. *J Thorac Cardiovasc Surg*. 1969; 58:92.
5. Quaattlebaum FW, Kalke B, Edwards JE, Lillehei CW. Obstruction of the aorta by prosthetic aortic valve. *J Thorac Cardiovasc Surg*. 1968; 55:231.
6. Chesler E, Korns ME, Porter GE, et al. False aneurysm of the left ventricle secondary to bacterial endocarditis with perforation of the mitral-aortic intervalvular fibrosa. *Circulation*. 1968; 37:518.
7. Titus JL, Kim HS, Weilbaecher DG. Surgical pathology of aortic disease. In: Cowgill LD, ed. *Surgery of the Aorta, Cardiac Surgery: State of the Art Reviews*. Vol. 1. Philadelphia: Hanley & Belfus; 1987: 521.
8. Titus JL, Kim HS. Blood vessels and lymphatics. In: Kissane JM, ed. *Anderson's Pathology*. Vol. 1. St. Louis: Mosby; 1990: 766.
9. Raghib G, Ruttenberg HD, Anderson RD, et al. Termination of left superior vena cava in the left atrium, atrial septal defect, and absence of coronary sinus. A developmental complex. *Circulation*. 1965; 31:906.
10. Shrivastava S, Moller JH, Formanek A, et al. Complex of absence of coronary sinus, atrial septal defect, and left superior vena cava joining left atrium associated with ventricular septal defect. *Clin Pathol Conf Am Heart J*. 1977; 94:222.
11. Elliot LP, Neufeld HN, Anderson RC, et al. Complete transposition of the great vessels. I. An anatomic study of sixty cases. *Circulation*. 1963; 27:1105.
12. Edwards JE. Anomalies of the aortic arch system. Birth defects: Original article series, XIII, 3D,47–63. New York: The National Foundation; 1977.
13. Kelly KL, Tetzlaff DR, Titus JL, Edwards JE. Anomalous origin of coronary arteries from the aorta as cause of sudden death. Presented at Am Acad. Forensic Sciences, 46th annual meeting, San Antonio, Tx; February 1994.
14. Dines DE, Edwards JE, Burchell HB. Myocardial atrophy in constrictive pericarditis. *Proc Mayo Clin*. 1958; 33:93.

17

The Hematolymphoid System

Peter M. Banks and Carey P. Page

Definition and Surgical Implications

Unfortunately, the hematolymphoid system is generally perceived by surgeons as remote and more the province of medicine than surgery. Not only are the functions of this system critical for the surgical patient, but the surgeon's role in managing diseases of this system is often pivotal—for diagnosis (biopsy), supportive care (vascular access), and even definitive treatment (splenectomy, tumor resection). The indifference so common among surgeons may stem from the vague anatomy of much of this system; both blood and lymph are fluid, and bone marrow and even lymphoid tissues are normally inconspicuous. Only in disease states do these elements become more apparent on physical examination—for example, in acute lymphangitis or inflammatory or neoplastic enlargement of the tonsils, thymus, lymph nodes, or spleen.

All three functions of the hematolymphoid system are essential for operability and postoperative recovery of surgical patients (Fig. 17–1). Formed elements (platelets) and plasma factors, working in concert, achieve normal hemostasis. Oxygenation depends upon gas exchange within red blood cells as they circulate through tissues. Resistance to infection is conferred by white blood cells. The elements of this diverse and widespread system work together to support tissue viability and wound healing. For example, platelets and coagulation factors are essential to blood vessel regeneration and proliferation. And plasma is the medium through which all nutrients pass to enter peripheral tissues.

The surgeon often acts in a supportive role for patients already diagnosed with hematolymphoid disease—that is, for tissue sampling, tissue harvesting, or providing vascular access (Table 17–1). However, disorders of this system are so common that it may be the surgeon who is the first to suspect or diagnose disorders of this system through history taking, physical examination, and intraoperative evaluation (Table 17–2). For example, is there any history of prolonged bleeding, easy bruising, transfusion requirements, transfusion reactions, recurrent or persisting infections, constitutional symptoms, or slow wound healing? On physical examination are there ecchymoses or petechiae, pallor, persisting open wounds, or enlarged lymph nodes, tonsils, or spleen? During open thoracic, abdominal, or pelvic procedures, is there lymph nodal enlargement, abnormality of serosal surfaces, splenomegaly, or abnormality of consistency or appearance of liver or other viscera? As is the case for other organ systems, basic understanding of the disease processes that affect the hematolymphoid system furnishes the surgeon with insights for patient diagnosis and management.

The Hemic System

PERIPHERAL BLOOD

Blood consists of diverse cellular elements suspended in plasma; these cells derive principally from bone marrow. Survival and health of tissue depends upon its constant perfusion by oxygenated blood. Every patient should undergo a rapid automated complete blood count (CBC) before any major surgical procedure. This test assures that concentrations of red blood cells (erythrocytes), white blood cells (leukocytes), and platelets are within normal limits.[1] Plasma coagulation activity is usually screened as well with both prothrombin time (PT) and partial thromboplastin time (PTT).[2] However, neither of these laboratory panels is completely sensitive. When patient history or physical examination raises the suspicion of an abnormal hemic function, it is advisable to obtain consultation with

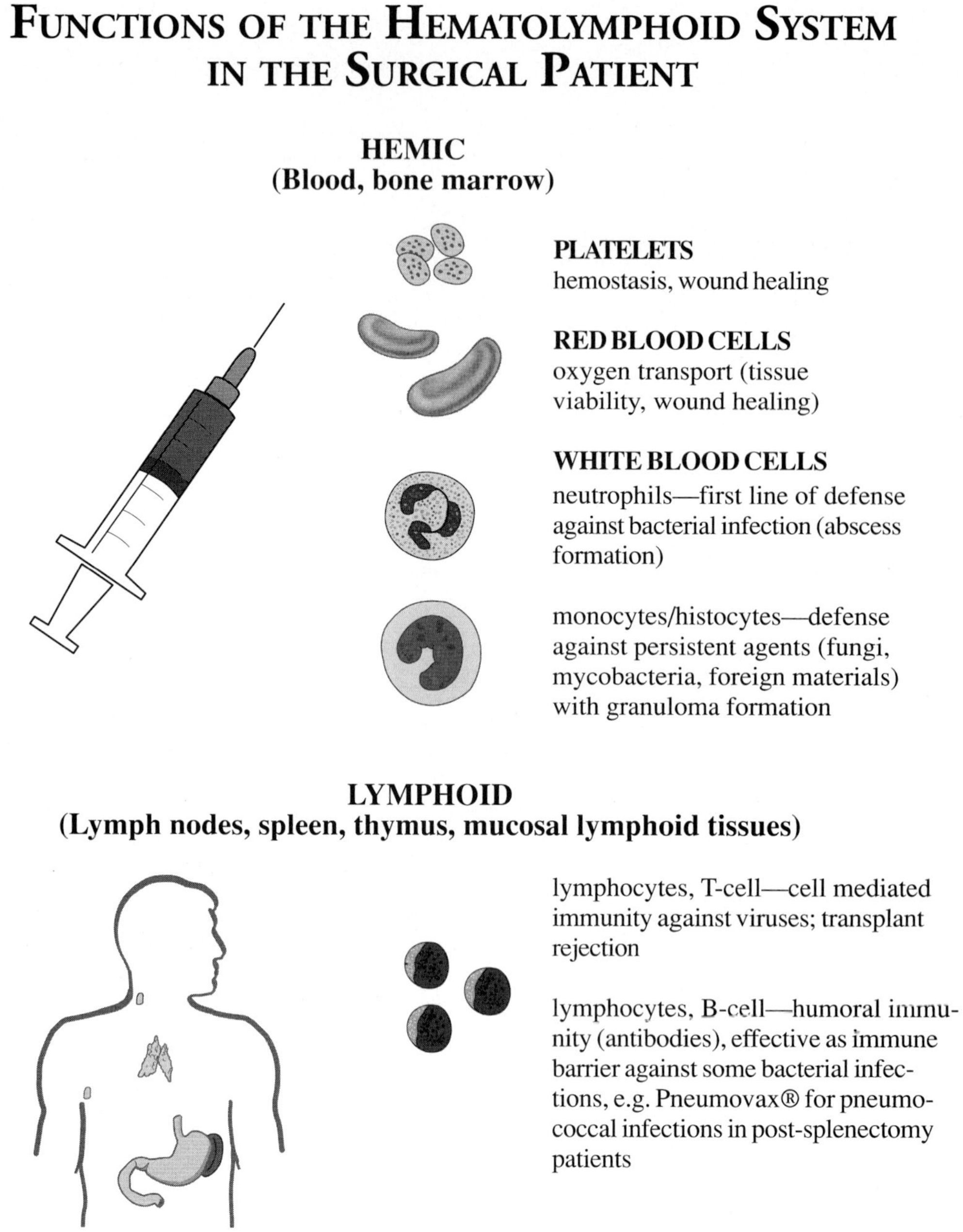

Figure 17–1. The functions of hemic and lymphoid cells in surgical patients are represented in this diagram. Not represented are the nutritional and hydrodynamic functions served by the blood and lymphatic vascular systems.

a hematologic specialist, either a clinical pathologist or a hematologist.

Automated CBCs are performed on EDTA-anticoagulated venous blood specimens (lavender-topped tubes) and PT and PTT on citrated venous specimens (blue-topped tubes). A ''manual differential'' (i.e., a microscopic evaluation of peripheral blood smears) can be performed on such anticoagulated specimens but ideally is performed on nonanticoagulated direct finger-stick samples (Fig. 17–2). Cases in which CBC values are unexpectedly out of normal value range or in which clinical concerns are raised regarding hemic function should always have a ''manual differential'' ordered. This avoids instrument-induced artifacts and permits recognition of subtle diagnoses that can only be detected microscopically. Likewise, a coagulation consultation should be requested when questions arise regarding hemostasis. Though unusual in the absence of a clinical history of excessive bleeding, certain bleeding disorders are not excluded even when PT and PTT are normal. Von Willebrand's disease and drug-induced platelet function abnormalities are examples. In some cases, a bleeding-time procedure may be necessary to establish if the patient can undergo surgery.[3]

An intravenous portal is necessary for most in-hospital patients but is particularly important for those with hematologic disease. This affords constant access both for hematologic evaluation and for intravenous therapy. In cases of chronic disease, peripheral venous access is often difficult, and surgeons are asked to establish central venous lines. A thoughtful approach to this role is essential (Table 17–3*A*

Table 17–1. Signs and Symptoms Possibly Related to Hematolymphoid Disease That May Prompt Surgical Referral

General Category	Specific Observation
Lumps and bumps	Lymphadenopathy (peripheral or Waldeyer's ring)
	Dermal mass or rash
	Subcutaneous mass
	Breast mass
	Thyroid mass
	Salivary gland mass
Abdominal mass	Splenomegaly
	Hepatomegaly
	Retroperitoneal mass
	Intraabdominal mass
Thoracic mass	Mediastinum (thymus, lymphoma)
	Hilar adenopathy

and 17–3*B*). Depending upon the purpose and duration of the venous access required, either a percutaneous or a buried-port type of device is chosen. Insertion and maintenance of both devices should receive the same respect and attention as any major procedure (dedicated environment, professional assistance, barrier precautions, and sterile technique). Prior to installing any device, the central venous system should be assessed. If history, signs, or symptoms suggest occlusion (e.g., swelling of the face, neck, or arm), the patient should be evaluated with duplex Doppler ultrasound examination or with contrast medium injection studies.

Table 17–2. Common History, Physical, and Laboratory Findings Possibly Related to Hematolymphoid Disease

Category	Item or Observation
History	Excessive bleeding
	Brushing teeth
	Dental extraction
	Menstrual flow
	Frequent/difficult nosebleeds
	Hematomas/hemarthroses from minor trauma
	Minor cuts and/or abrasions
	Surgical procedures (reoperation or transfusion)
	Easy bruising
	Recurrent/difficult infections
	Difficult/nonhealing wounds
Physical examination	Lymphadenopathy
	Hepatomegaly
	Splenomegaly
	Anemia
	Petechiae
	Ecchymoses
	Subcutaneous or intradermal mass
Laboratory examination	Complete blood count and differential
	Anemia/abnormal erythrocyte indices
	Leukocytosis or leukopenia
	Thrombocytosis or thrombocytopenia
	Abnormal differential
	Peripheral smear
	Abnormal erythrocyte forms
	Thrombocytopenia or thrombocytosis
	Abnormal/immature/dominant leukocyte differential
	Abnormal prothrombin or partial thromboplastin time

BONE MARROW

The bone marrow is the normal site for production of the cellular blood elements and accordingly is most informative for hematologic evaluation.[4] Whole needle core biopsy specimens, decalcified and sectioned for conventional or special stains, are best for estimation of overall cellularity and detection of metastatic tumors or primary bony neoplasms (Fig. 17–3*A*). For microscopic evaluation of subtle features of hemic cells, air-dried aspirate smear preparations or air-dried imprints from biopsy cores are preferred. Such preparations can be stained with one of the Romanowsky-type stains (Wright, Giemsa, Diff-Quik), which allow evaluation of cellular details such as cytoplasmic granules, Golgi zone, and relative basophilia versus eosinophilia (Fig. 17–3*B*). It is ideal to reserve extra

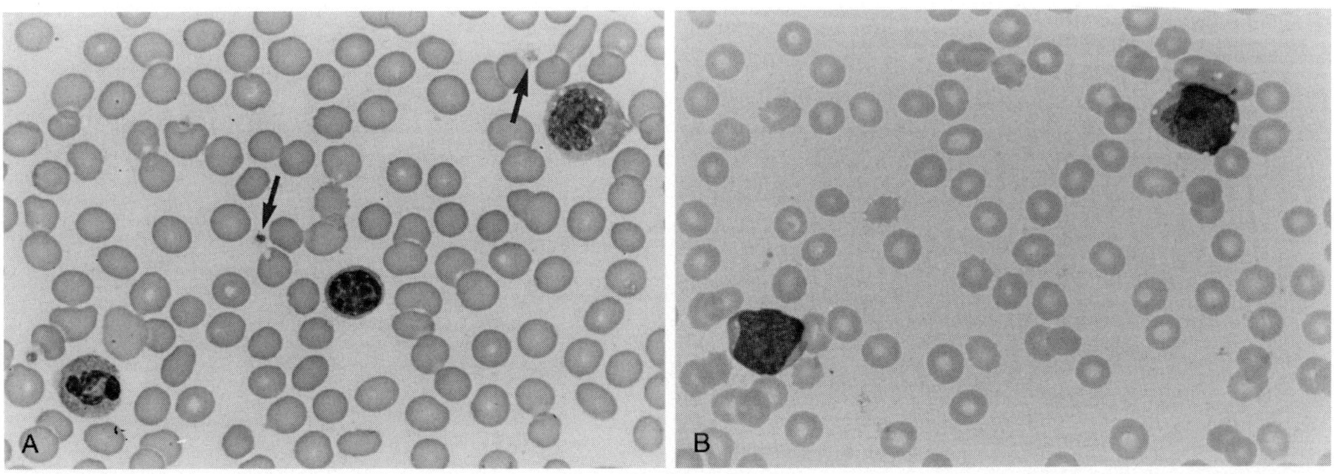

Figure 17–2. *A,* Normal peripheral blood smear shows moderate density of red blood cells in plasma *(throughout field),* platelets *(arrows),* and leukocytes that include a neutrophil *(left lower corner),* a lymphocyte *(center),* and a monocyte *(right upper corner). B,* Peripheral blood smear from a patient with acute leukemia shows relative scarcity of red blood cells in plasma (reflecting anemia), absence of platelets (thrombocytopenia), and abnormal leukocytes. These are blasts, with large nuclei and scant, undifferentiated cytoplasm.

Table 17–3*A*. Central Venous Access (Percutaneous)

Variant	Pattern of Use	Advantages	Comments
Single lumen (subclavian or internal jugular)	Acute care, resuscitation Continuous, long-term infusion One lumen sufficient Venous sampling may be necessary Infusion of blood or blood products may be necessary	Easy to insert and remove "J" wire exchange of catheter for diagnosis and treatment of infection	Outside the operating room procedure to insert Use only chlorhexidine/silver sulfadiazine–bonded catheter with a silver sulfadiazine cuff Sterile technique in site maintenance and access are mandatory Subclavian preferred because of lower incidence of catheter-related infection (vs. internal jugular) Right subclavian rather than left subclavian preferred due to better "lie" in superior vena cava Catheter tip at or above the atriocaval junction (not in the right atrium!) Higher risk of infection than buried ports because of pattern of use and chronic (though protected) breach in skin portal-of-entry barrier Requires more maintenance than buried port (site and hubs)
Multilumen	See above comments for single lumen More than one lumen necessary for multiple medications, blood products, etc.	See above comments for single lumen Multiple lumens for mechanical risk of single catheter	See above comments for single lumen Higher risk of infection than for single lumen (pattern of use and multiple "hubs" to maintain)
"Quinton" (subclavian or internal jugular)	Device of choice for apheresis or dialysis	May be exchanged for and/or replaced by above devices	Situational use is important Insertion and removal (exchange) should ensure shortest duration possible

unstained, unfixed, air-dried slides for the option of subsequent special stains if such are indicated by initial microscopic review.[5]

If hematologic disease is suspected on the basis of preoperative or intraoperative findings, a bone marrow biopsy should be obtained while the patient is still under anesthesia. Sampling the anterior iliac crest with a Jamshidi needle (both core and aspiration) is best for patients in the supine position.[6] The approach can be intraabdominal or percutaneous, depending on the celiotomy incision. For patients with flank or posterior operative approaches and for those not in the operating room, the posterior superior iliac spine is the best biopsy site. Proper techniques include support of the pelvis with a firm roll and strict aseptic procedure. For patients who are awake, intravenous sedation and adequate local anesthesia (including skin, subcutaneous tissue, and periosteum) are needed. If the surgeon is unfamiliar with proper glass slide smear technique,[7] a trained nurse or medical technologist is usually available on short notice for operating room assistance. The pathologist can usually be called upon to coordinate such services.

COMMON DISORDERS

Cellular Deficiency States

Abnormally low numbers of circulating blood cells can be caused by loss or consumption of these elements, by

Table 17–3*B*. Central Venous Access (Buried Port) *Continued*

Variant	Pattern of Use	Advantages	Comments
Peripheral	Chronic, intermittent use Long-term therapy (especially as outpatient) Patient acceptance of needle stick for each access No necessity for blood product administration or sampling	No chronic breach in skin portal-of-entry barrier Requires less frequent maintenance (lumen maintenance) than percutaneous Low-risk insertion for high-risk patients	Operating room procedure Compulsory sterile technique in accessing and maintaining port Use only noncoring needle (Huber needle) for access Needle in port only for duration of infusion New access for each new infusion Removal and insertion more difficult than percutaneous techniques (see Table 17–3*A*) Remove device prior to high-dose chemotherapy/bone marrow transplant (avoids confusion when identifying site of infection)
Central	See above comments for peripheral Peripheral vein not available	See above comments for peripheral (all are applicable except for risk)	See above comments for peripheral

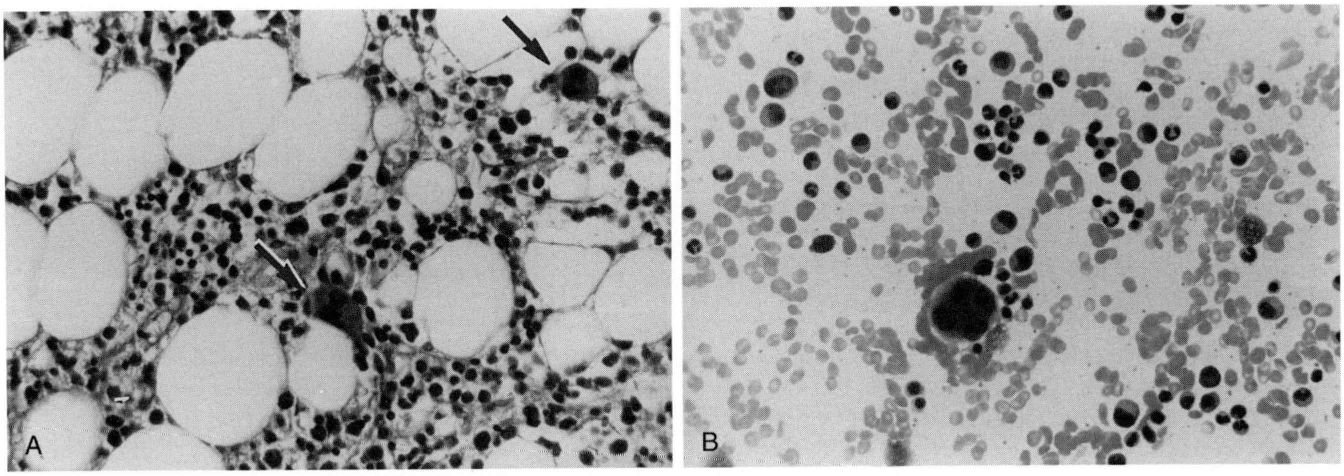

Figure 17–3. *A,* Conventional paraffin section of bone marrow stained with hematoxylin and eosin shows many small precursor hemic cells scattered between large, pale fat cells. Only the very large platelet progenitor cells (megakaryocytes) can be recognized *(arrows). B,* By contrast, marrow aspirate smears or imprints from biopsy cores can be air-dried and stained with a Romanowsky method (Wright's stain or Giemsa stain), allowing recognition of individual cell types by their cytoplasmic and nuclear features: erythroid versus granulocytic versus monocytic versus lymphoid versus megakaryocytic. These two types of sampling and preparation are complementary; biopsy sections are better for cellularity and architectural assessment and for recognition of metastatic tumors; aspirate smears or imprint preparations are better for detailed cellular composition.

defects in their composition, and by inadequate production of these cells in the bone marrow.

The commonest deficiency disorder is anemia resulting from *chronic blood loss* with *iron deficiency.* Such anemia is usual in menstruating women and does not imply any other associated problems. All patients with iron-deficiency anemia, however, should be evaluated for gastrointestinal (GI) tract blood loss from benign or malignant lesions. Minimal evaluation includes stool testing for occult blood. More extensive evaluation is indicated for older patients in whom GI lesions are more prevalent (see Chap. 12). Peripheral blood smears show small hypochromic erythrocytes [low mean corpuscular volume (MCV) and low mean corpuscular hemoglobin content (MCHC) in the CBC]. More specific serum findings include low serum iron, high iron-binding capacity, and low serum ferritin.

Other common causes of chronic anemia are congenital and acquired abnormalities of erythrocyte composition. Peripheral blood smear examination is critical for establishing a differential diagnosis. For example, microspherocytic red blood cells suggest autoimmune hemolytic disease; fragmented forms indicate mechanical damage (cardiac prostheses or intravascular coagulation); target-shaped or sickle-shaped red blood cells point toward hereditary abnormalities of hemoglobin. By narrowing the differential diagnostic considerations, appropriate special studies can then be used to arrive at a definitive diagnosis (e.g., a Coombs test for autoimmune hemolysis, hemoglobin electrophoresis for hemoglobinopathies).

Hypoproliferative states of the bone marrow with deficiency of erythroid, leukocytic, or megakaryocytic cell lines, singly or in combination, can result from a diversity of causes, including nutritional deficiencies, toxins, common pharmaceuticals, and complete or partial aplasia of autoimmune or unknown etiology. In both preoperative and postoperative patients, the bone marrow is second only to the GI tract in its speed of cellular turnover. Therefore, nutritional deficiencies and toxic effects can affect the bone marrow within days or even hours.

Intravascular consumption of hemic cells and platelets can occur rapidly in conditions such as septicemia with disseminated intravascular coagulation, autoimmune cytolysis, and extensive burns. Chronic destruction of cells is associated with vasculitis, heart prostheses, and acquired or congenital abnormalities of erythrocyte composition such as hemoglobinopathies, thalassemias, or sickle-cell disease.

The less common cellular deficiency states may warrant consultation with specialists in hematology because of the bewildering array of disorders, often working in concert, which give rise to these conditions.[8, 9]

For the surgeon, splenic hyperfunction (hypersplenism) is a particularly notable mechanism of blood cell deficiency. Normally, the rate of splenic entrapment of senescent or defective circulating cells equals the rate of marrow production. Hypersplenism is the excessive removal of formed elements of the blood; it may cause anemia, leukopenia, or thrombocytopenia, in isolation or in combination. By contrast, splenomegaly is commonly but not always associated with hypersplenism; the spleen is adept at removing platelets and can do so for long periods without enlargement. In contrast, sequestration and destruction of leukocytes and particularly erythrocytes soon leads to splenic enlargement. In addition, cytopenias can be associated with splenomegaly without being actually *caused* by it—for example, in bone marrow failure from systemic disease that also involves the spleen.

Originally, hypersplenism was divided into ''primary'' and ''secondary'' types. However, these terms are vague and have been supplanted by the terms ''appropriate'' and ''inappropriate,'' which are clearer both in connotation and medical implication.[10] *Appropriate hypersplenism* refers to disorders in which the spleen initially functions normally to remove abnormal formed elements (intrinsically abnormal, antibody-labeled, or altered by a toxin) to produce cytopenia. *Inappropriate hypersplenism* occurs when the spleen is hyperfunctioning and removing essentially normal as well as abnormal cells. This type of hypersplenism results from any process that leads to an enlarged congested spleen. The distinction between these two types of hypersplenism is sometimes unclear, and appropriate hypersplenism, if not corrected quickly enough, can lead to inappropriate hypersplenism.[10] Table 17–4 lists disorders associated with hypersplenism. The decision to perform a splenectomy is often complex and must encompass the potential benefit as well as the immediate and long-term risks of the procedure.

The two major *indications for splenectomy* are trauma and hypersplenism. In some instances it may provide definitive "cure," whereas in others it only reduces the need for cell replacement therapy without significantly altering the disease course. Idiopathic thrombocytopenic purpura (ITP) and many of the congenital hemolytic anemias represent the first category of responses. The latter group, those for which splenectomy provides only palliation, includes most patients with appropriate hypersplenism. Table 17–5 summarizes hematologic disorders for which splenectomy may be useful.

Table 17–4. Disorders That May Be Associated with Hypersplenism

Category	Condition
Appropriate hypersplenism (appropriate removal of abnormal forms)	Congenital hemolytic anemias
	Hereditary spherocytosis
	Hereditary elliptocytosis
	Sickle-cell anemias
	Thalassemias
	Enzyme-deficient anemias (PK, G-6-PD)
	Autoimmune hemolytic anemia (idiopathic, acquired)
	Idiopathic (immune) thrombocytopenic purpura (ITP)
	Thrombotic thrombocytopenic purpura (TTP)
Inappropriate hypersplenism (inappropriate removal of normal forms)	Congestive processes
	Cirrhosis with portal hypertension
	Portal vein thrombosis
	Infiltrative processes
	Infectious mononucleosis
	Lymphoma (Hodgkin's and non-Hodgkin's)
	Leukemia
	Myeloproliferative disorders
	Acute inflammatory processes
	Typhoid fever
	Rubella, chickenpox, and other viral diseases
	Chronic inflammatory processes
	Bacterial (syphilis, tuberculosis)
	Parasitic (malaria, echinococcosis, etc.)
	Autoimmune (rheumatoid arthritis, lupus, etc.)
	Fungal (histoplasmosis, cryptococcosis)
	Reticuloendothelial accumulative disorders
	Gaucher's disease
	Amyloidosis

The risks of splenectomy are divided into the risk of mortality related to the surgical procedure and the long-term risk of overwhelming postsplenectomy infection. Surgical risk is related to the underlying condition (co-morbidity) and the patient's age. Death after staging laparotomy for Hodgkin's disease is rare, but splenectomy for myeloproliferative disorders is associated with an operative mortality rate of roughly 15%.

The rate of overwhelming postsplenectomy infection in patients with some types of hematolymphoid disease is higher than in age-matched patients undergoing splenectomy for trauma (trauma is 0.3% for adults, 0.6% for children). For example, in children with Hodgkin's disease, the rate approaches 4%. In this latter group, however, it is difficult to distinguish the relative contributions of splenectomy, advanced malignant disease, and immunosuppressive therapy. In addition, some hematolymphoid diseases appear to be intrinsically associated with high infection rates (thalassemia, sickle-cell anemia, and autoimmune hemolytic anemia).

All patients undergoing splenectomy should receive vaccines against *Streptococcus pneumoniae* and *Haemophilus influenzae,* two of the encapsulated organisms that can cause overwhelming postsplenectomy infection. Vaccination prior to splenectomy is ideal but is still effective if given postoperatively. Many pediatricians recommend that children undergoing splenectomy be maintained on oral penicillin until they reach adulthood.

Splenectomy is described in many surgical texts and technical manuals. The following description depicts our biases and preferences.

Preparation of the patient for elective splenectomy begins with the immunizations mentioned (10 days to 2 weeks preoperatively). The next step is assuring an adequate supply of blood and platelets. When the blood bank may have difficulty in matching products—autoimmune hemolytic anemia, multiply transfused patients, and so on—this step should begin well in advance of the operation. We prefer single-donor platelets obtained by apheresis. Based upon our own experience, we recommend that patients with hemolytic anemia undergo ultrasound examination for gallstones. Those with gallstones should have their common bile duct "cleared" preoperatively (by endoscopic retrograde cholangiopancreatography, or ERCP, if necessary). Antibiotic and mechanical bowel preparation are generally reserved for patients with splenomegaly. All nonallergic patients receive perioperative antibiotic coverage with cefazolin (1 g before induction of anesthesia, repeated every 2 hours intraoperatively).

Conduct of the operation differs for patients with normal-sized spleens and those with massive splenomegaly. Conceptually, however, both require excellent exposure and a stable operative field. For the former, either a midline incision or a left-upper-quadrant subcostal incision is adequate. The midline approach is used for patients with thrombocytopenia or coagulation abnormalities because it is less bloody. Initial gastric decompression is achieved by an orogastric tube (replaced as a nasogastric tube near the end of case before closing the abdomen), especially in

Table 17–5. Hematolymphoid Disorder for Which Splenectomy May Be Beneficial

Disorder	Comments
Hereditary spherocytosis	Splenectomy is the sole therapy—does not change erythrocytes Good response in correction of anemia and reticulocytosis Leg ulcers heal after splenectomy Gallstones common Splenectomy after age 4 for immune considerations
Hereditary elliptocytosis	Splenectomy only in symptomatic patients Same comments as for spherocytosis
Thalassemia	Splenectomy for hemolysis and high transfusion requirements Splenectomy for symptomatic splenomegaly or infarction High postoperative complication rate
Sickle-cell disease	Splenectomy usually not indicated for hematologic reasons Splenectomy occasionally for acute splenic sequestration Splenectomy for splenic abscess
Autoimmune hemolytic anemia	Splenectomy for steroid failure, complications, or contraindications Favorable response in most patients Difficult to type and crossmatch blood
Idiopathic (immune) thrombocytopenic purpura (ITP)	Occurs in both AIDS and non-AIDS patients; also systemic lupus erythematosus (SLE) Splenectomy for persistence, steroid failure, relapse after steroids Lasting response in about 80% of patients (including those with AIDS and SLE). Accompanying pancytopenia and anemia also improved in most SLE patients Intraoperative platelet transfusion only when necessary and after the spleen is out
Thrombotic thrombocytopenic purpura (TTP)	Fulminant, rapid course and fatal outcome from intracranial hemorrhage is the untreated course Splenectomy for those patients who initially respond to plasmapheresis and later relapse Majority of patients do not benefit from splenectomy
Myeloproliferative disorders	Splenectomy for symptomatic splenomegaly, reduction of transfusion requirements, and to permit chemotherapy in patients with limited marrow reserve Does not alter course of underlying disease Preoperative control of thrombocytosis essential in applicable patients (alkylating agents—e.g., hydroxyurea)
Lymphomas and leukemias	Staging for Hodgkin's disease Palliation for cytopenias and mechanical symptoms for lymphomas Good response in patients with anemia, neutropenia, thrombocytopenia, particularly those with hairy cell leukemia Palliation for mechanical symptoms in patients with chronic myelogenous leukemia Does not alter outcome of disease (except for rare patients with non-Hodgkin's lymphoma confined to spleen—curative)
Secondary hypersplenism	Indicated only for symptomatic cytopenias Add splenorenal shunt at time of splenectomy for patients with cirrhosis and portal hypertension Generally does not alter outcome of underlying disease Curative for patients with isolated splenic vein thrombosis

patients with thrombocytopenia. Mechanical retractors (Upper Hand, Omni Tract, and so on) are essential to a stable operative field and excellent exposure—they do not slip, fatigue, or "fall asleep"! Slight reverse Trendelenburg position brings the spleen into better view. Omental attachments to the spleen are divided. Similarly, the splenocolic ligament is divided between ligatures, permitting inferior displacement of the splenic flexure of the colon by a damp laparotomy pack. The short gastric vessels are identified, doubly ligated, and divided, taking care not to injure the wall of the stomach. Next, the spleen is retracted medially, the splenorenal ligament is incised under direct vision, and the spleen and tail of the pancreas are mobilized into the field by gentle blunt dissection. Splenectomy is completed by separate identification and suture ligation of the splenic artery and vein at the hilum, freeing the tail of the pancreas. Surgical hemostasis is assured by inspecting the operative field and the previously placed ligatures. Platelet transfusions for thrombocytopenic patients are withheld until the spleen is out and all surgical bleeding is controlled. The operation is continued by a thorough search for accessory spleens. Cholecystectomy (for patients with gallstones from hemolytic anemia, and so on) is performed only after all else has been completed and hemostasis assured in the splenic bed.

Though the concepts of a stable, well-exposed operative field are similar, splenectomy for patients with massive splenomegaly is somewhat different. A midline incision is always used. Asymmetric enlargement of the spleen may displace the splenic hilum, the short gastric vessels, and the splenocolic ligament unpredictably, so that the important anatomic markings are no longer in their usual position in the left upper quadrant. In addition, virtually all patients with massive splenomegaly have numerous splenic omental adhesions and dense adhesions to the diaphragm, all of which may be quite vascular. Initial separation of omental adhesions is followed by identification and division of the splenocolic ligament. Next, the lesser sac is entered through the gastrocolic omentum. The splenic artery is identified on the dorsal surface of the pancreas, the overlying peritoneal reflection is incised, and the artery is ligated in continuity until the pulsation in the splenic hilum ceases. This process may necessitate ligation at more than one point because of the hyperdynamic, high-flow nature of the splenic artery in patients with massive splenomegaly and the rich collateral network through the pancreas. This process makes subsequent mobilization of the spleen less bloody, but, because of the fine sinus structure of the splenic circulation, it rarely "decompresses" the spleen or reduces its size significantly.

If they can be visualized, the short gastric arteries are ligated and divided as previously indicated. Once the splenic flexure is packed out of the way, the spleen is mobilized into the wound by separating it from the diaphragm bluntly (to avoid a hole in the diaphragm by sharp dissection). The bed of the spleen is packed with a number of laparotomy pads, and splenectomy is completed by management of the hilar vessels as indicated. Surgical hemostasis is also assured as discussed. The argon laser is particularly useful for controlling "oozing" from the raw surface of the diaphragm and retroperitoneum. Such oozing is a particular problem in patients with massive spleens due to chronic myeloproliferative disorders. The left upper quadrant is not drained unless the tail of the pancreas has been injured.

Postoperatively, nasogastric suction is continued until bowel function returns and gastric emptying is signaled by a reduction in nasogastric output.

Cellular Excess States

Some disorders involving excessive circulating formed elements are distinct from the overtly neoplastic leukemias. These include responses of normal bone marrow to conditions such as chronic hypoxemia (reactive polycythemia), persisting infections or other inflammatory stimuli (reactive leukocytosis or "leukemoid reaction"), and underlying visceral malignancies (reactive thrombocytosis). By contrast, some patients manifest persistent elevation of one or more hemic cell lines without explanation.

Some of these disorders, such as polycythemia rubra vera, are believed to represent autonomous clonal stem-cell abnormalities that are premalignant—i.e., most patients eventually develop acute leukemia. These processes are best classified as chronic myeloproliferative disorders (see subsequent discussion).[11] In some cases of long-standing "essential" thrombocytosis, hypereosinophilic syndrome, and so on, no stem-cell clonal abnormality can be demonstrated. They never progress to overt leukemia.[12] These cases may represent abnormalities of cytokine-mediated regulatory control mechanisms that normally act to control marrow cellular proliferation and differentiation (e.g., involving erythropoietin, thrombopoietin, or granulocyte colony stimulating factor).

Malignant or Autonomous States

Leukemias are malignancies of circulating hematolymphoid cell populations. For management purposes, the major distinctions are between *acute* and *chronic* leukemias and between lymphoid ("lymphocytic") and myeloid ("myelogenous" or "nonlymphocytic") types.

Acute leukemia is an emergent clinical situation. Patients' signs and symptoms usually reflect deficiency of normal hemic cells rather than the presence of high numbers of malignant cells—anemia, thrombocytopenia, and neutropenia (Fig. 17–2*B*). Surgical consultation is usually requested for establishment of indwelling venous catheters (see Table 17–3) or for drainage of perirectal abscess, and so forth.

Acute lymphoid leukemia is a malignancy of lymphoblasts, cells that normally proliferate during fetal development in the thymus, bone marrow, and gut mucosa to generate diverse clones for the immune system's response to antigens. Acute lymphoid leukemias occur mostly in childhood and adolescence.[12] Fortunately, they are responsive to intensive chemotherapy. A high percentage of these young patients are cured. In some patients, the lymphoblastic malignancy develops as a solid neoplasm in thymus or lymph nodes without involvement of blood or even bone marrow. In these cases, the malignancy is designated as lymphoblastic lymphoma rather than leukemia—the distinction is merely distributional.

Acute myeloid leukemia is a malignancy of myeloblasts, the immature precursor elements of the bone marrow cell lines. Although microscopic and enzyme cytochemical and immunologic phenotypic criteria can be used to subclassify acute myeloid leukemias,[4] there is little difference in clinical behavior and prognosis among the types. This group of malignancies occurs in patients of all ages, with a peak incidence in middle-aged adults.[13] Patients who can tolerate rigorous chemotherapy, possibly with allogeneic bone marrow transplantation, have about a 50% chance of cure. Evidence from chromosomal and genetic probe studies suggests that patients with leukemias either from preexisting myelodysplastic disorders or in the setting of previous chemotherapy for another malignancy have a poor prognosis.[14] Older patients typically experience a particularly unfavorable course. They tolerate therapy poorly and often have underlying myelodysplasia (see subsequent discussion).

Chronic lymphoid leukemia is usually an indolent neoplasm of mature-appearing, small lymphocytes. Its solid-tumor counterpart is a low-grade lymphoma, small lymphocytic or "well-differentiated lymphocytic" type. Surgeons may be involved in the management of this disorder in its late phases when complications of chronic cytopenias occur or when the process transforms into high-grade malignant lymphoma (Richter's syndrome). Patients with chronic lymphoid leukemia are usually middle-aged or elderly; occasionally splenomegaly and hypersplenism require splenectomy (see Table 17–5; see Fig. 17–9).

Chronic myeloid leukemia affects predominantly middle-aged adults and is based on a well-defined chromosomal translocation, the "Philadelphia chromosome," which results in an abnormal clonal replacement of the marrow's stem cells. Although clearly neoplastic, the process exhibits deceptively normal-appearing maturation into erythrocytes, granulocytes, and platelets. The chronic phase of this disease is managed with little or no chemotherapeutic intervention for a period of 1 to 5 years; however, splenomegaly may be pronounced and require splenectomy for directly related symptoms. Eventually the neoplastic clone becomes more aggressive, with either gradual "progression'' or sudden ''blastic transformation'' into acute leukemia.

Chronic myeloproliferative disease is a loosely defined group of disorders that includes chronic myeloid leukemia, polycythemia rubra vera, essential thrombocytosis, and agnogenic myeloid metaplasia (chronic myelofibrosis).[11] As mentioned, these disorders are considered chronic stem-cell clonal abnormalities with long-term risk for acute leukemic transformation. Massive splenomegaly often develops in these conditions because of the chronicity of their course, the intrinsic abnormalities in the formed elements in the blood, and the tendency to colonize sites outside the bone marrow for myeloid cell proliferation. This situation may require splenectomy, particularly in the late or ''spent'' phase of disease when cytopenia rather than cellular excess is the problem (Fig. 17–4).[15] When patients have a depleted bone marrow reserve, due to either myelofibrosis or cytotoxic therapy, intraoperative platelet transfusions following splenic artery ligation may be indicated to avoid prolonged oozing following splenectomy.

Myelodysplastic states may be secondary to known toxic exposures or drugs, or they may be ''primary,'' i.e., of unknown etiology. Chromosomal studies of bone marrow are useful for predicting outcome; patients with clonal abnormalities have a poor prognosis.[14] Even if acute leukemia does not supervene, prolonged myelodysplastic disease requires expert clinical management of problems associated with pancytopenia.

The Lymphoid System

LYMPH NODES

Lymph nodes develop at the crossroads of lymphatics as vascular expansions filled with lymphocytes. Early in fetal differentiation, lymphocytes deriving from thymus (T cells) and from bone marrow (B cells) home to these structures, which are strategically positioned as immune barriers to foreign or infectious elements traveling into lymphatics from tissue interstitial space. Surgical oncologists must learn the distribution of lymph nodes draining a particular anatomic region, since these serve as the first barrier to the spread of malignancies.[16]

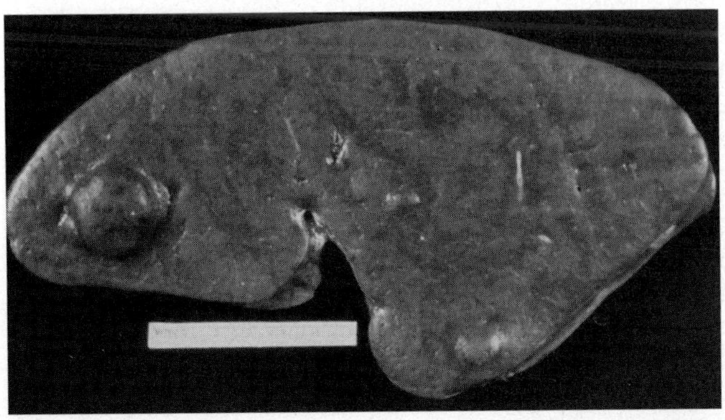

Figure 17–4. Massive splenomegaly in a patient with chronic myeloproliferative disorder (agnogenic myeloid metaplasia or so-called myelofibrosis). This spleen weighed nearly 3,000 g and was removed for worsening pancytopenia caused by a combination of fibrotic replacement of normal marrow elements and secondary (inappropriate) hypersplenism due to enlargement and congestion from extramedullary hematopoiesis. The nodules at extreme left and bottom right represent concentrations of platelet-producing cell clusters, or ''megakaryocytic plums.''

Lymph Node Biopsy

Biopsy of lymph nodes is a common reason for surgical consultation in patients with persistent inflammatory disorders of uncertain nature or with suspected hematolymphoid malignancy (Table 17–6). The surgeon must know the indication for lymph node sampling in order to select the appropriate technique. Fine needle aspiration (FNA) biopsy is a rapid, effective method for sampling superficial nodes. It is particularly useful for the detection of metastatic carcinoma and some types of infectious processes with stainable organisms—e.g., *Mycobacterium avium-intracellulare.* It is also useful for diagnosing or at least raising the suspicion of Hodgkin's disease and high-grade non-Hodgkin's lymphomas. The microscopic distinction of immune reaction from low-grade lymphoma is usually difficult or impossible by FNA (see Chap. 3). However, even small FNA samples are sometimes sufficient for automated flow immunophenotypic analysis. This procedure permits recognition of processes that are qualitatively abnormal or restricted in immunoglobulin light chain expression and thereby neoplastic. In patient settings in which intensive therapeutic intervention cannot be tolerated—as in lymphoma related to acquired immunodeficiency syndrome (AIDS)—precise classification of lymphoma is not as critical as distinguishing between immune hyperplasia and lymphoma.

An excised lymph node is usually needed for definitive diagnosis and classification of malignant lymphoma. Table 17–6 contains useful guidelines for nodal biopsy. The pathologist must assess not only cellular detail but architectural growth patterns (see Figs. 17–7, 17–10, 17–12, and 17–16). Therefore, it is critical that an intact, representative node be submitted, free of crush artifact, fresh, and unfixed. A common misconception is that intraoperative evaluation of lymph node biopsy specimens should be avoided. While it is true that the diagnosis and classification of lymphoma cannot and usually need not be made on this basis, intraoperative evaluation is often critical both to assess the adequacy of sampling (Fig. 17–5) and to limit the differential diagnosis for prioritizing the allocation of tissue for special studies.

The pathologist can use imprint or scrape-smear cytology preparations without consuming tissue and without the infectious disease risks inherent in performing frozen sections. In many cases, particularly when sample size is not a limiting factor, intraoperative frozen sections are indicated as a guide to specimen adequacy (see Fig. 17–5). Furthermore, the frozen tissue block can be transferred still frozen to −70°C storage as a potentially valuable tissue allocation for methods such as frozen section immunohistochemistry, genetic probe analysis, or even microbial culture. When an infectious process is included in the preoperative differential diagnosis, microbial cultures should be requested. It is best for the surgeon to divide the fresh

Table 17–6. Considerations Pertaining to Lymph Node Biopsy

Item	General Rule	Caveat/Rationale
Sampling technique	Needle aspiration to distinguish lymphoid from epithelial (especially for head and neck) "Open" biopsy to define and categorize lymphoid malignancies	High-grade lymphomas may appear cytologically similar to carcinomas; may not be separable by fine needle technique Adequate sampling and specimen management are critical; maximum tissue (within reason)
Selection of node for biopsy	Dominant node Anatomic site preferred Neck Axilla Groin	Smaller adjacent nodes may be uninvolved "reactive" nodes Biopsy of groin nodes associated with higher complication rate (infection, lymphatic fistula, and so on); groin nodes more likely to be histopathologically scarred because of prevalence of injury/inflammation in lower extremity
Surgical technique	Maximum adherence to sterile technique, minimum foreign material in wound Anesthetic and incision adequate for easy exposure Excisional biopsy preferred when practical Incisional biopsy of large nodes with portion of capsule Titanium or absorbable clips on lymphatic channels	Patients with hematolymphoid disease have higher incidence of infection Atraumatic handling of node important to pathologist's interpretation. Hemorrhage may obfuscate architecture. No "keyhole" node biopsies around important structures (axilla, neck, groin) Architecture of entire node may be important in diagnosis Avoid damage to surrounding structures. Subcapsular portion for architecture Avoid lymphocele/lymphatic fistula. Avoid interference with subsequent imaging evaluations (CT, MRI)
Tissue allocation and management	Fresh specimen management Pathologist examination and touch-prep/scrape-prep; tissue allocation; sterile technique	Representative tissue Adequate tissue for histopathology, surface markers, culture, and so on

specimen within the sterile region of the operating room rather than to ask the pathologist to attempt this in the frozen section laboratory where there is a universal presence of microorganisms!

In the lamentable situation in which a lymph node is biopsied without a pathologist for intraoperative evaluation and allocation of tissue, the surgeon should divide the specimen in half, putting one part in a sterile container with sterile saline. This portion is then stored in a conventional 4°C refrigerator, where it will remain useful for up to 24 hours. The other half should be divided into sections no thicker than 3 to 4 mm and placed in standard buffered (3.7%) formaldehyde solution.

Infectious Precautions

Although it is appropriate to "flag" cases of known infectious disease risk—individuals infected with human immunodeficiency virus (HIV) and hepatitis B and C—it is critical to remember that *all* patients, particularly those with hematolymphoid disorders, should be handled with universal precautions. Although most universal precautions are intrinsic to disciplined operating room conduct, their application is often less than ideal. Increased emphasis on minimizing the risk of exposure to HIV is necessary. Most exposures occur during the recapping of used needles or from the improper disposal of needles and scalpel blades. Most are the result of carelessness and have obvious remedies. Operative techniques aimed at minimizing the use of the scalpel, eliminating the conventional transfer of scalpel to the surgeon by the scrub technician or nurse, and maximizing the use of stapling devices rather than sutures are all worthwhile. In addition to conventional barrier precautions, surgeons should double-glove, wear protective eyewear in the operating room, and wash with an iodophor solution after each operation. The issues of appropriate airway protection and the risk of electrocautery smoke are unresolved and remain the subject of heated discussion.

EXTRANODAL LYMPHOID TISSUES

The immune apparatus is concentrated not only in lymph nodes but also in the spleen, thymus, and bone marrow, and in the mucosa of the upper respiratory and digestive tracts, which represent barriers to microorganisms. Even tissues normally endowed with relatively sparse immune cellularity—such as the central nervous system, gonads, and mucosa of the urinary tract—can accumulate dense collections of lymphoid tissue in response to infection. Not surprisingly, the surgeon encounters cases for biopsy or resection in which such extranodal tissues may be involved by inflammatory or neoplastic proliferations of the hematolymphoid system. Again, intraoperative pathology evaluation is needed so that such samplings can be allocated in a manner analogous to that previously described for lymph node biopsy.

All types of pathologic processes elicit a fibrous proliferation in locations such as the mediastinum and retroperitoneum (see Chap. 10). Because of concern about entering vascular structures within these areas of fibrosis, surgeons are tempted to submit only superficial wedge biopsy specimens from these sites. Although understandable, such caution can cause disappointment when, the day after a large open procedure, the pathology report reads "nondiagnostic." To avoid this setback, intraoperative pathology

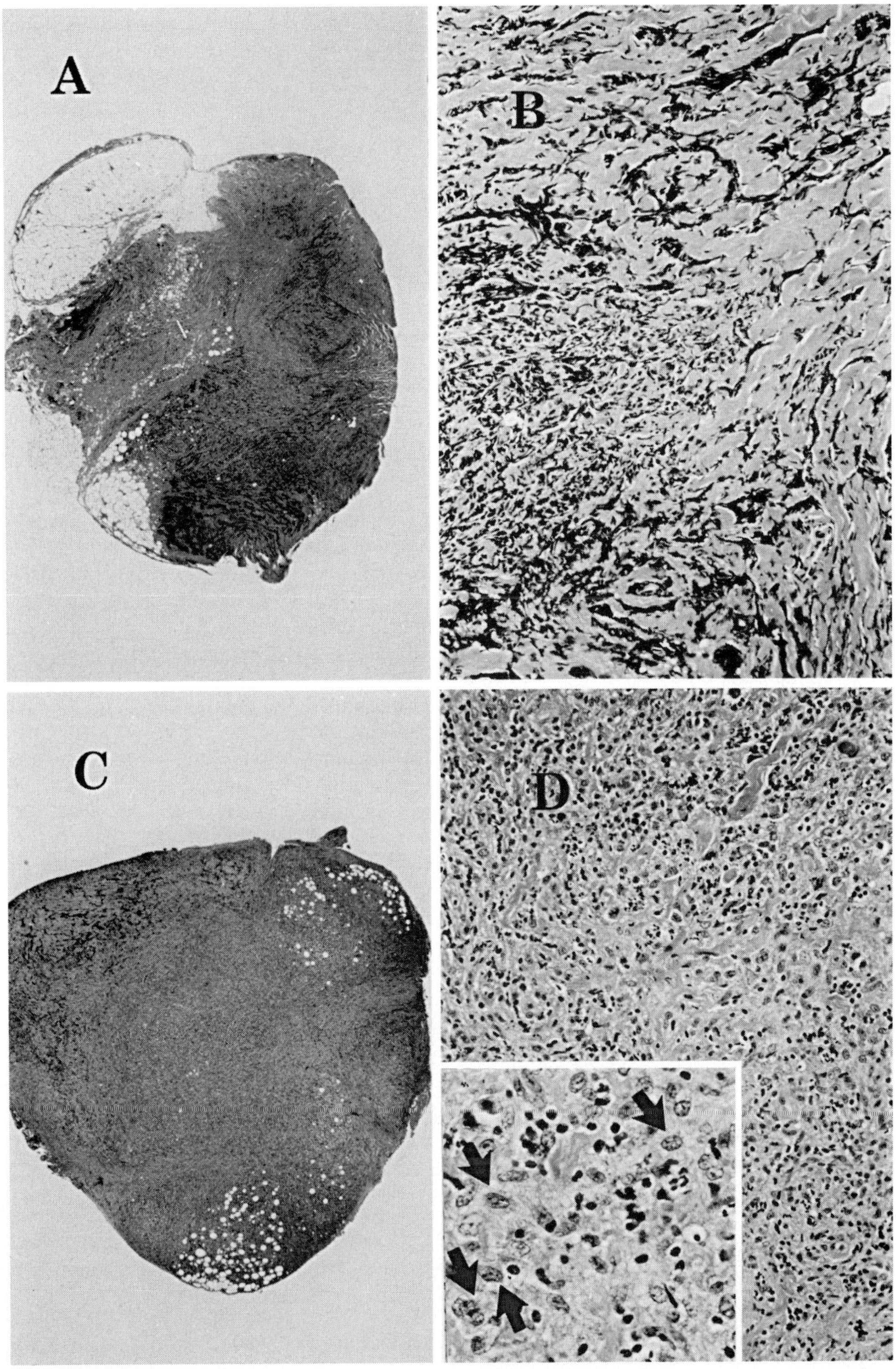

Figure 17–5. Variation in adequacy of mediastinoscopic forceps biopsies of identical size. *A,* One sample consists predominantly of collagenous matrix. *B,* At higher magnification, there is total obscuration of cellular detail by crush artifact, due to fragility of individual cells surrounded by collagen. *C,* Another sample includes greater cellularity. *D,* At higher magnification, intact cellularity is recognizable, including large atypical cells *(arrows, inset)* diagnostic for large-cell lymphoma. Intraoperative frozen sections can be used to monitor such sampling adequacy.

evaluation is crucial to assess adequacy of the specimen in this situation.

COMMON DISORDERS

Lymphoid Hyperplasia

Because the immune system must rapidly respond to challenges with cellular proliferation, benign nodal hyperplasia may be dramatic and alarming (Fig. 17–6). Clinical features favoring benign hyperplasia include sudden onset, pain and tenderness, sharp demarcation without infiltration of surrounding tissues, and associated signs and symptoms of inflammation, either localized or systemic. Inflammatory processes should be considered for lymphoid tissues that drain commonly infected sites. Classic examples include tonsillar enlargement with acute infectious mononucleosis

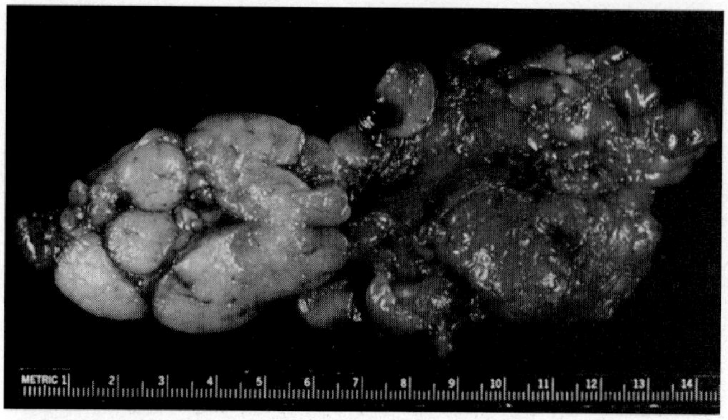

Figure 17–6. Massive enlargement of periparotid lymph node due to benign hyperplasia. Pain and tenderness were reported, which are clinical features favoring benign rather than malignant adenopathy.

or recurrent streptococcal infection, mesenteric lymphadenitis with *Yersinia enterocolitica* infection of the ileum, and inguinal nodal enlargement due to either venereal disease or chronic skin conditions of the lower extremities (dermatopathic lymphadenitis—Fig. 17–7). The experienced pathologist can often suggest a particular etiology for lymphadenitis based upon subtle histologic findings.[17]

For the pathologist, the microscopic hallmark of lymphoid hyperplasia (as opposed to malignancy) is the preservation of functional compartments of the immune system: germinal centers within follicles, paracortical T-cell zones, sinuses with their phagocytic histiocytes, and medullary cords with accumulated plasma cells (see Fig. 17–7).

Castleman's disease or *angiofollicular lymph node hyperplasia* (AFLH) is a peculiar form of nodal hyperplasia for which the surgeon's role is paramount. Patients with this disorder present with massive adenopathy of the mediastinum, celiac axis, or mesentery, often with accompanying features of a chronic inflammatory state. These include hypergammaglobulinemia, anemia, lassitude, and growth retardation.[17] Surgical excision of the nodal mass is curative in cases of true Castleman's disease—i.e., the localized variant of AFLH (Fig. 17–8).

Malignant Lymphomas and Lymphoid Leukemias

Early diagnosis and accurate classification of lymphoid neoplasms are important, because effective and specific therapy is available for most types.[18, 19] By definition, lymphomas are solid neoplasms of the lymphoid system; leukemias are neoplasms with a circulating component. There is considerable overlap between particular types of lymphoma and lymphoid leukemia.

Thanks to the application of high-resolution methods of immunology and chromosomal and molecular genetics analysis, our understanding of these disorders and their classification has greatly improved.[20] For surgical management, only a few broad concepts are important. Most of these are incorporated within the Working Formulation for Clinical Usage published in 1982.[21] Malignant lymphomas, other than Hodgkin's disease, can be grouped into three clinical categories: low-, intermediate-, and high-grade (Table 17–7).

Low-grade lymphomas generally occur in elderly patients and are usually systemic (advanced-stage) at presentation (Fig. 17–9). In fact, one type of low-grade lymphoma—diffuse small-lymphocytic type—is interchangeable with chronic lymphoid leukemia, depending on whether the process involves peripheral blood. The other types of low-grade lymphoma are recognized microscopically by their follicular growth pattern (Fig. 17–10). This reflects their origin from and resemblance to normal follicles of the immune system. Although low-grade lymphomas are incurable in most cases, they are indolent.

By contrast, high-grade lymphomas occur in patients of all ages. They may be localized (early-stage) when first detected, particularly in extranodal sites. High-grade

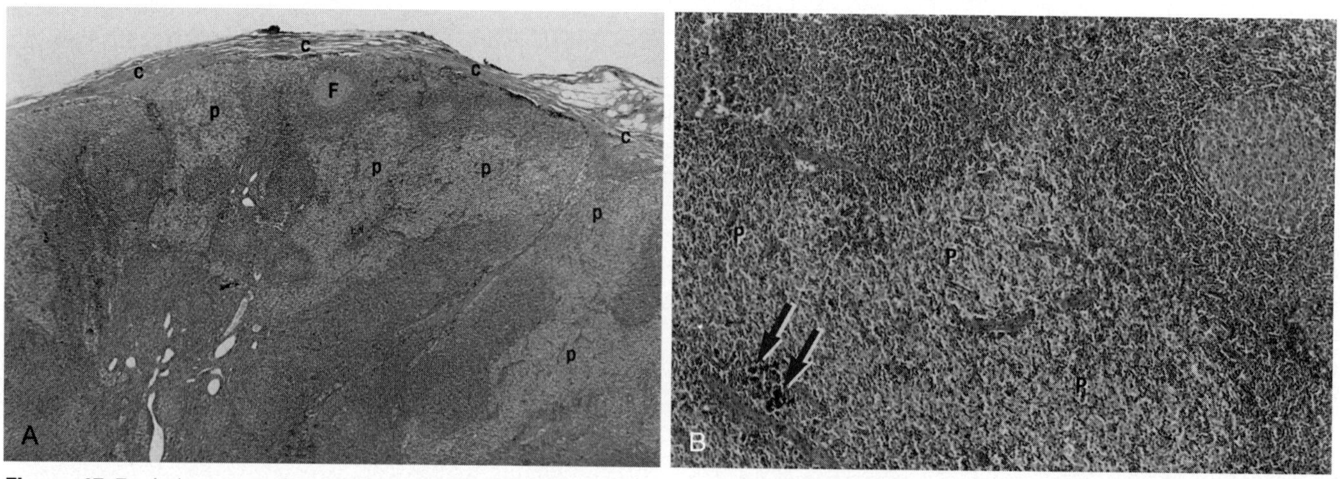

Figure 17–7. *A,* Low-magnification microscopic appearance of a hyperplastic inguinal lymph node. There are recognizable functional compartments of the immune system: follicles (F), paracortex (p), and a retained, intact capsule (c). Compare to pattern of lymphomas, Figures 17–10, 17–12, and 17–16. *B,* Intermediate magnification reveals a pale, mottled appearance of the paracortex (p) due to interspersed histiocytes, some of which contain dark pigment *(arrows).* These features are specific for "dermatopathic lymphadenitis," secondary to inflammatory skin conditions, in this case involving the lower extremities.

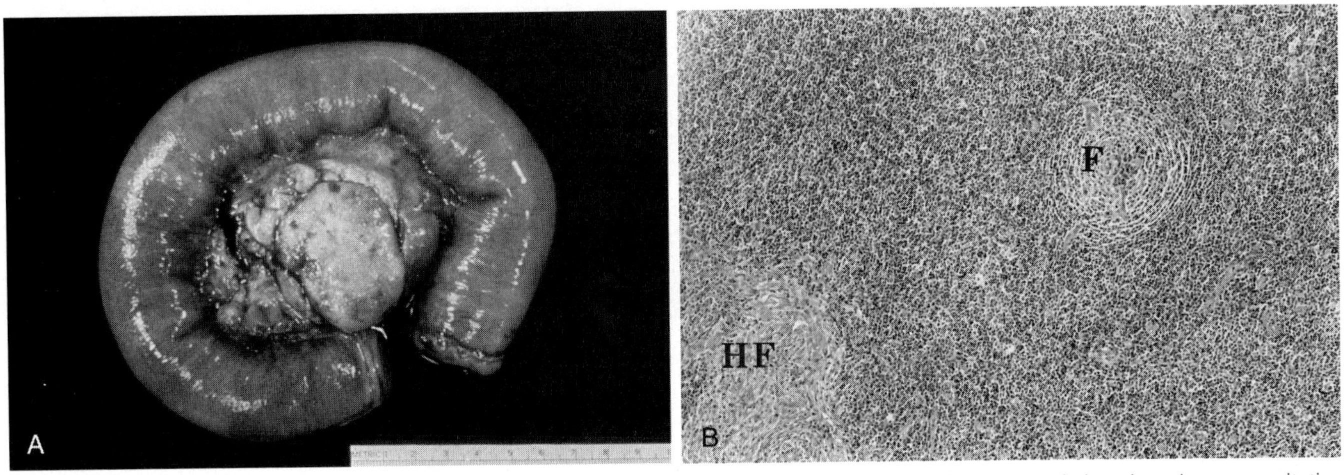

Figure 17–8. *A,* Localized angiofollicular lymph node hyperplasia (Castleman's disease) arose within mesenteric lymph nodes, necessitating a segmental small-bowel resection. *B,* Characteristic microscopic findings included sharply defined, involuted follicles (F) surrounded by expanses of lymphocytes and plasma cells with focal hyaline fibrosis (HF). Although this process produced anemia and hypergammaglobulinemia, the patient was cured by this surgical procedure.

lymphomas are often associated with constitutional symptoms. Because of the high proliferative rate, these tumors are often sensitive to cytotoxic chemotherapy and radiation. As many as 40% of patients with high-grade lymphoma are cured with intensive therapy.[18]

Lymph nodes involved by lymphoma are relatively nontender, firm, and usually fixed to surrounding soft tissues. High-grade lymphomas resemble carcinomas and sarcomas by surgical inspection. Unlike low-grade lymphomas, they do not home to normal lymphoid tissue sites but rather displace and compress adjacent normal structures (Fig. 17–11). Microscopically, high-grade lymphomas have a diffuse growth pattern and are composed of large, rapidly dividing cells (Fig. 17–12). One high-grade type, lymphoblastic lymphoma, is prone to leukemic progression. Thus, the two aggressive lymphoid malignancies are interrelated: lymphoblastic lymphoma and acute lymphoid (lymphoblastic) leukemia.

Intermediate-grade lymphomas show features, both clinical and pathologic, that are between high- and low-grade tumors. This can be a problem for the managing clinician who must choose between a conservative and an aggressive therapeutic strategy.

Although about 85% of non-Hodgkin's lymphomas match one of the histologic types of the Working formulation, new entities with distinct clinical features have also been characterized.[20, 22] One such entity is the low-grade B-cell lymphoma of mucosa-associated lymphoid tissue (MALT). For many years these tumors were thought to be ''pseudolymphomas'' arising in the GI tract (see Chap. 12), lung (see Chap. 11), orbit (see Chap. 7), salivary gland, and so on. Modern immunologic methods prove that these are monoclonal proliferations. If confined to their primary extranodal sites, these MALT-type lymphomas can

Table 17–7. Categorization of Malignant Lymphomas Other Than Hodgkin's Disease

Low-Grade Lymphoma
A. Small lymphocytic (may correspond to chronic lymphoid leukemia)
B. Follicular, small-cleaved-cell
C. Follicular, mixed (small-cleaved-cell and large-cell)

Intermediate-Grade Lymphoma
D. Follicular, large-cell
E. Diffuse, small-cleaved-cell
F. Diffuse, mixed (small-cleaved-cell and large-cell)
G. Diffuse, large-cell*

High-Grade Lymphoma
H. Diffuse, immunoblastic
I. Lymphoblastic (may correspond to acute lymphoid leukemia)
J. Small non-cleaved-cell (Burkitt's and Burkitt's-like variants)

*Although originally included within the intermediate-grade grouping, the diffuse large-cell type has been shown to be difficult to distinguish consistently from the diffuse immunoblastic type, and the survival difference between these two types is not significant.[20]

Source: From The Non-Hodgkin's Lymphoma Pathology Classification Project. National Cancer Institute–sponsored study of classification of non-Hodgkin's lymphomas: Summary and Description of a Working Formulation for Clinical Usage. *Cancer.* 1982; 49: 2112–2135. With permission.

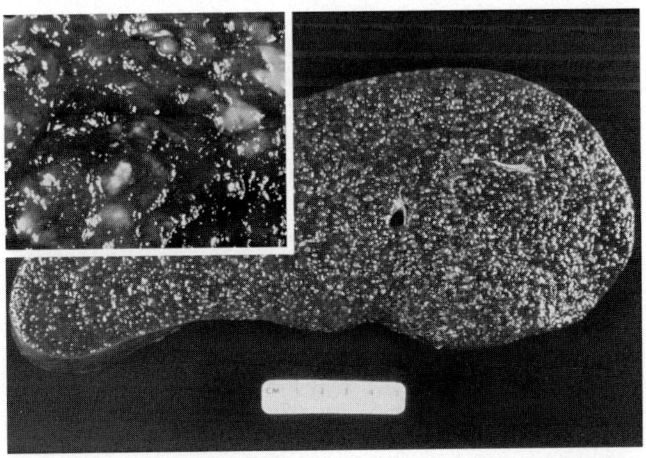

Figure 17–9. Spleen showing gross pathologic features typical of a low-grade lymphoma. Massive enlargement is due to universal expansion of lymphoid pulp component *(inset at small distance).* This appearance reflects homing of well-differentiated lymphomas along normal areas of lymphoid tissues and early systemic spread.

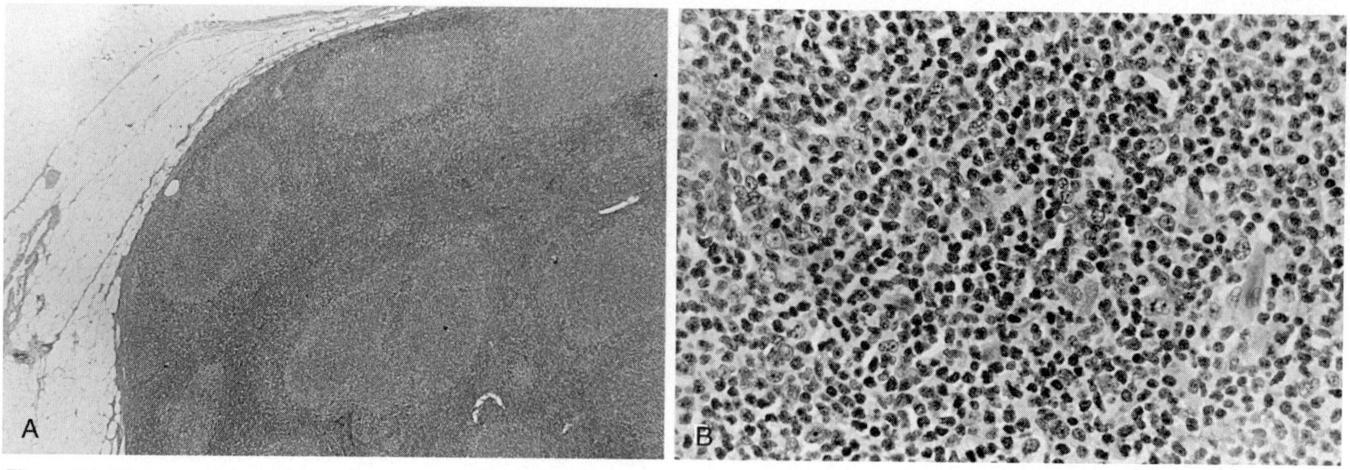

Figure 17–10. Low-grade malignant lymphoma, follicular small cleaved-cell type. *A,* Low magnification reveals a follicular ("nodular") growth pattern closely resembling follicular hyperplasia (compare to Fig. 17–7). *B,* High magnification of follicular cellular composition reveals an abnormally monotonous population of small lymphoid cells with irregular, cleaved nuclei and almost no mitotic figures. Benign follicles contain germinal centers, which feature a mixture of small and large cells.

be resected, often with curative outcome (Figs. 17–13 and 17–14). In the case of MALT-type lymphoma of the stomach, there is strong association with *Helicobacter pylori* infection. In fact, early in the disease course, antimicrobial therapy can actually result in complete regression![23] In other sites of involvement by MALT-type lymphoma, no analogous instigating stimulus has been identified. These lesions must be surgically resected or treated with radiation or chemotherapy. Since many of these tumors arise in parenchyma that is the target of autoimmune disease (e.g., salivary gland in Sjögren's syndrome or thyroid in Hashimoto's thyroiditis), it is likely that the prolonged localized behavior of these tumors reflects their antigen-dependence (i.e., the lymphoma clone is autoimmune-reactive against some local host tissue antigen).

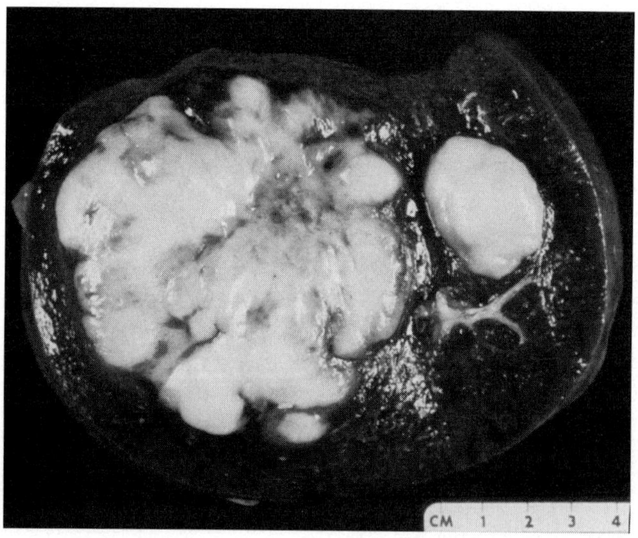

Figure 17–11. Gross appearance characteristic of high-grade lymphomas. In this spleen, the rapidly growing tumors have displaced normal tissues rather than selectively involving lymphoid pulp (compare to Fig. 17–9). High-grade lymphomas are more often localized (early stage) than low-grade lymphomas.

Another newly recognized type is mantle-cell lymphoma. This tumor occurs predominantly in middle-aged and elderly males. It is intermediate in grade and composed of uniform neoplastic small cleaved lymphocytes that correspond to the B-cell follicular mantle zone.[20] This tumor sometimes occurs clinically as the so-called lymphomatous polyposis of the GI tract (Fig. 17–15), initially simulating familial adenomatous polyposis or inflammatory bowel disease.

Hodgkin's disease is a distinct clinical-pathologic group of lymphomas with peak incidence in young adults. It almost always arises in lymph nodes, spreads slowly and predictably along contiguous lymph node-bearing regions, and is frequently associated with constitutional symptoms.[19] Microscopically, Hodgkin's is characterized by a mixture of bizarre tumor giant cells, so-called Reed-Sternberg cells, and benign background host inflammatory cellularity (Fig. 17–16). The pathologist classifies Hodgkin's disease as one of four types, based upon the relative proportion of tumor cells to reactive cellularity and the presence or absence of a nodular sclerosing stromal reaction (Table 17–8).[24]

Staging evaluation is extremely important in managing patients with Hodgkin's disease. The so-called Ann Arbor system[19] is used: stage I disease is confined to a single group of lymph nodes; stage II disease involves two or more lymph node groups all above or below the diaphragm; stage III disease involves lymph nodes and spleen above and below the diaphragm; stage IV disease involves organs other than lymph nodes or spleen (e.g., bone marrow, liver, lungs, skin, and so on). A clinical staging criterion is then appended: A—absence of constitutional symptoms, and B—presence of constitutional symptoms. In general, chemotherapy is advised for patients with advanced stage (III or IV) disease.

Staging laparotomy is indicated when the information provided by celiotomy, splenectomy, liver biopsy, and histopathologic examination of retroperitoneal and mesenteric nodes has the potential for altering therapy: chemotherapy versus radiotherapy or selection of a specific investigational

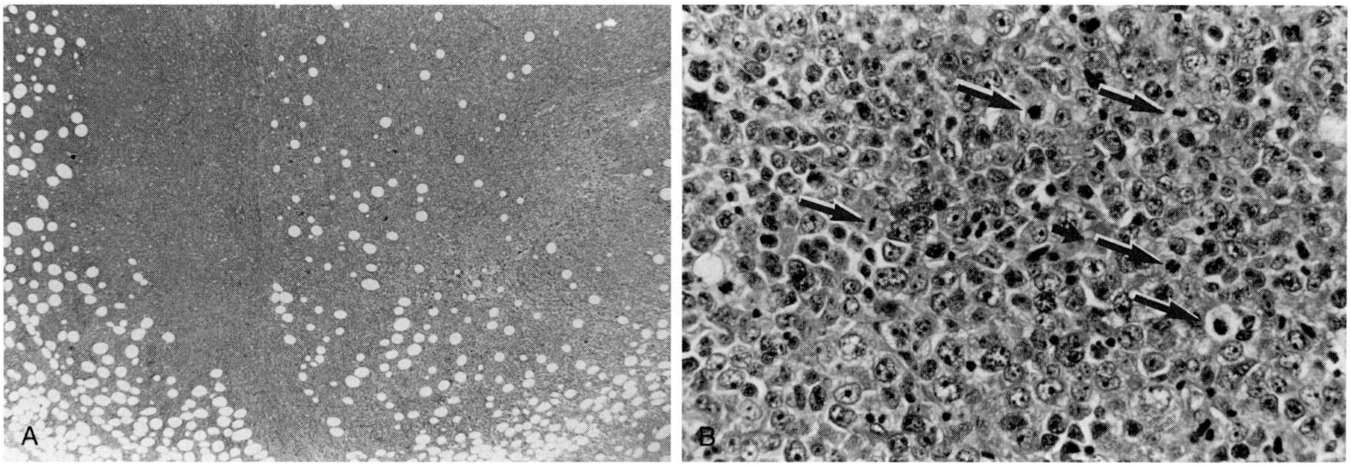

Figure 17–12. *A,* Low-magnification microscopic appearance of a lymph node involved by high-grade lymphoma, showing diffuse growth pattern with effacement of normal functional immune compartments and capsule with invasion of surrounding fat (compare to Fig. 17–7). *B,* High magnification reveals anaplastic cells with vesicular nuclei containing prominent nucleoli. There are many mitotic figures *(arrows),* reflecting a highly proliferative tumor.

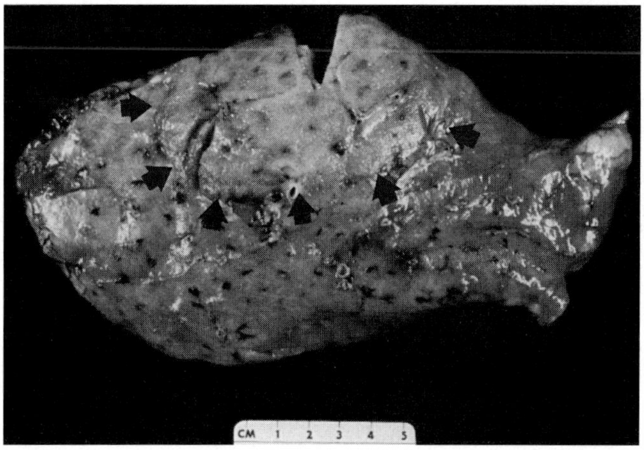

Figure 17–13. A low-grade B-cell lymphoma of mucosa-associated lymphoid tissue (MALT) type. It involves this lobe of lung as a sharply demarcated tumor *(arrows).* Regional lymph nodes were sampled for staging purposes and showed no involvement by lymphoma. Because of their prolonged localized behavior, such extranodal lymphomas are potentially surgically curable (see Chaps. 11 and 12).

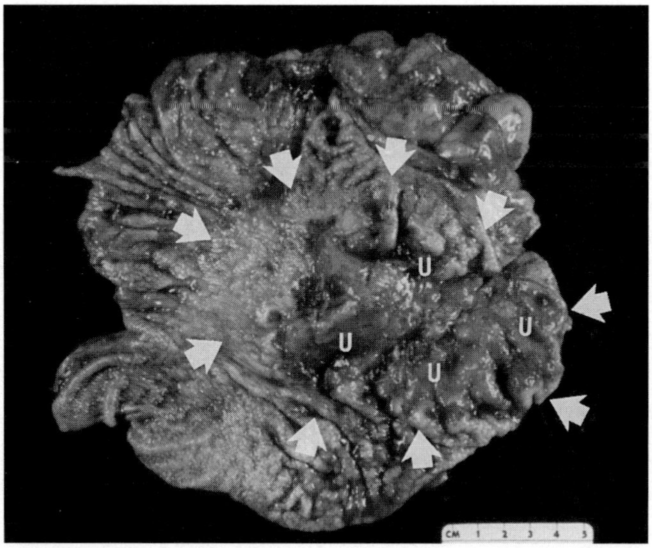

Figure 17–14. Low-grade B-cell lymphoma of MALT type arising in a stomach in association with long-standing follicular gastritis due to *Helicobacter pylori* infection (see Chap. 12). The lymphoma is not clearly demarcated *(arrows)* due to mucosal changes of gastritis, and there is extensive ulceration (U).

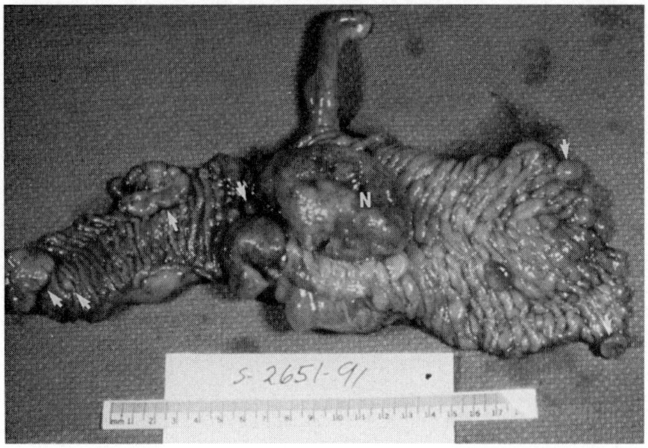

Figure 17–15. Mantle-cell lymphoma has involved the ileocecal region of this middle-aged male patient as lymphomatous polyposis. A large lymphomatous nodule (N) has necessitated surgery for obstruction of the valve; however, innumerable smaller "polyps" represent expansion of the normal mucosal lymphoid tissue by lymphoma *(arrows)*.

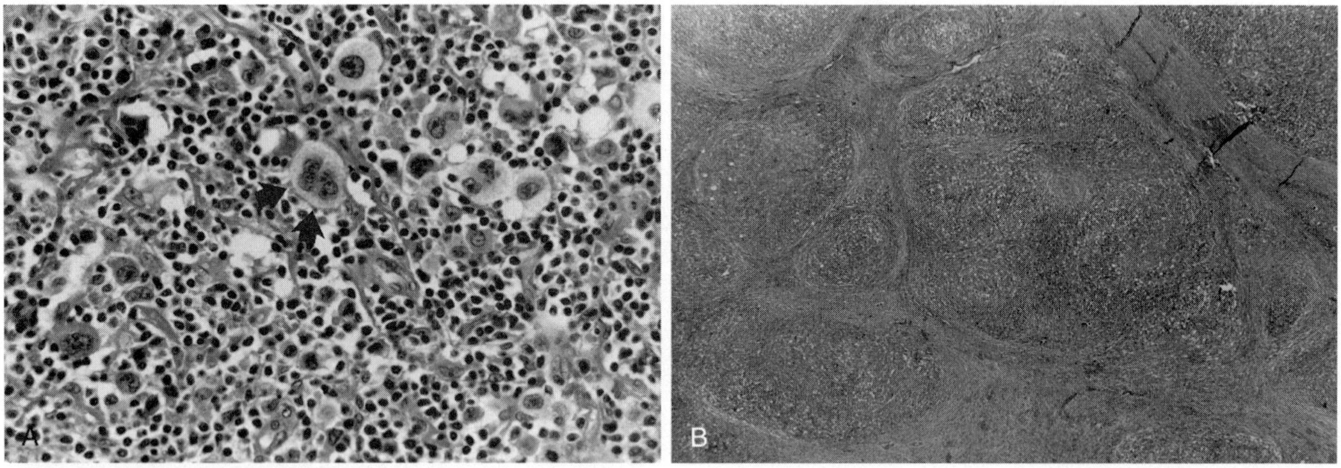

Figure 17–16. *A,* Hodgkin's disease is diagnosed at high magnification on the basis of bizarre tumor giant cells, so-called Reed-Sternberg cells *(arrows)*, featuring two or more nuclei or nuclear lobes, prominent nucleoli, and abundant pale cytoplasm dispersed within a background of benign-appearing inflammatory cells including many small lymphocytes. *B,* Low-magnification features allow classification of this case as nodular sclerosis type, as cellular nodules are surrounded by bands of proliferative fibrosis.

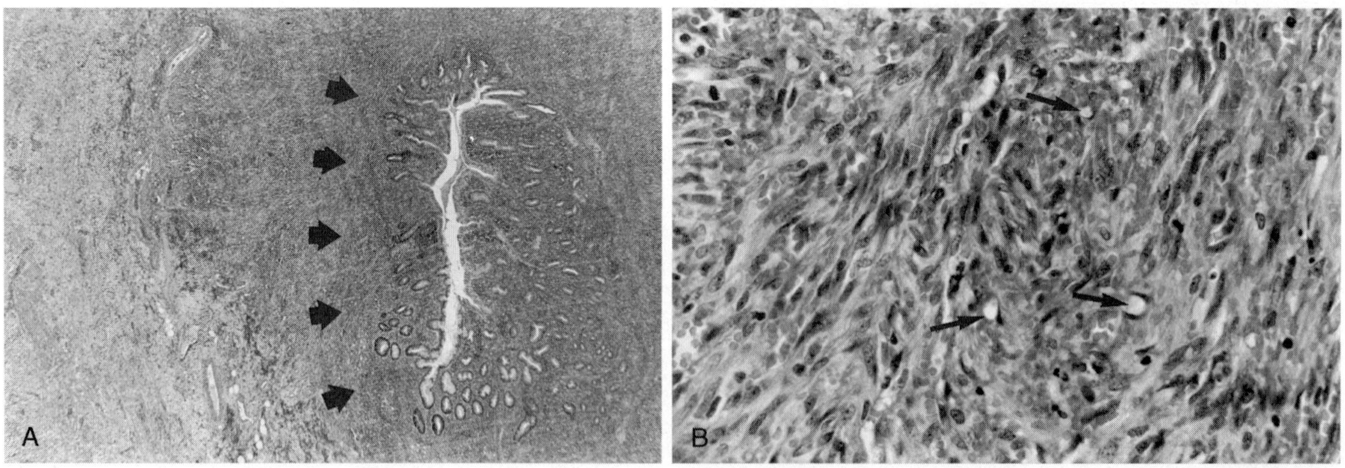

Figure 17–17. Kaposi's sarcoma involving the appendix was identified incidentally in an AIDS patient. Celiotomy was performed for resection of obstructing tumors of the small bowel. *A,* Low-magnification microscopy reveals replacement of mucosal lymphoid tissues (normally dark cellularity) in area adjacent to epithelium *(arrows)* by *B,* pleomorphic spindle-cell process with abortive endothelial lumens *(clear spaces—arrows; high magnification)*.

protocol. Staging laparotomy is not indicated for patients with stage IV disease (involvement of bone marrow, skin, lung, other extranodal sites) or for patients with clinical stage I lymphocyte-predominant Hodgkin's disease (involvement of upper cervical nodes). Revision in stage (by staging laparotomy) is largely a feature of nodular sclerosing-type Hodgkin's disease, the most common histologic type, and occurs in about 40% of patients. Staging laparotomy is performed less often now than in the past because of the ever-increasing sensitivity of radiologic imaging methods. Furthermore, more patients are treated initially with systemic chemotherapy rather than involved field or total nodal radiotherapy, rendering staging less significant.

Staging laparotomy in sequence of performance includes wedge biopsy of the liver; bilateral hepatic lobe needle biopsy; splenectomy; and sampling of periaortic, mesenteric, and periportal nodes. Palpably abnormal tissue is the first choice for sampling. Periaortic node biopsy focuses on the upper aortic chain near the ligament of Treitz and may be facilitated by preliminary lymphangiography and intraoperative radiologic guidance in order to sample the most ''suspicious'' nodes. Accessory spleens should also be removed.

IMMUNODEFICIENCY STATES

Patients who are therapeutically immunosuppressed or intrinsically immunodeficient represent a challenge to both the surgeon and the pathologist. Opportunistic infections must be suspected and pursued in all samples received by the pathologist. Explosive lymphoproliferative disorders driven by the Epstein-Barr virus can mimic high-grade lymphomas, both clinically and microscopically.[25] In immunosuppressed patients, recognition of such ''posttransplantation lymphoproliferative disorders,'' as distinct from true lymphomas, is critical because they remit with reduced immune suppression. The patient will often die if cytotoxic therapy is used (see Chap. 20).

In HIV-infected patients, high-grade lymphomas or Kaposi's sarcoma may initiate the definitional phase of AIDS. In this particular immunocompromised setting, neoplasms often arise in unusual sites, such as the tonsils, adenoids, tongue, and GI tract, particularly the anorectal region (Fig. 17–17). Even though frozen section evaluation is generally not offered for known HIV-positive tissues because of the risk to personnel and the obligatory inactivation of cryotomes for decontamination, intraoperative cytology preparations, imprints or scrape-smears, are useful.[26] For lymph node biopsy, FNA is practical and effective for identifying stainable infectious agents, Kaposi's sarcoma, and carcinomas. It is not useful for distinguishing between AIDS-related lymphadenopathy and lymphoma unless high-resolution methods such as molecular probes or automated flow immunophenotyping can be applied.

Table 17–8. Microscopic Classification of Hodgkin's Disease into Prognostically Relevant Types

Lymphocyte predominance	Most favorable
Nodular sclerosis	Moderately favorable, most common
Mixed cellularity	Unfavorable
Lymphocyte depletion	Unfavorable

Source: Modified from the system of Lukes RJ, Craven LF, Hall TC, et al. Report of the Nomenclature Committee. *Cancer Res.* 1966; 26: 1311.

PITFALLS FOR THE SURGEON

1. *Inadequate sampling.* Biopsies from mediastinum or retroperitoneum and from areas previously treated with radiation or surgery are subject to obscuring fibrosis. Intraoperative evaluation of specimens by the pathologist is crucial to ensure a diagnostic biopsy, as is careful preoperative strategizing, often including detailed imaging studies.
2. *Incorrect submission of tissue.* Only when both surgeon and pathologist are fully informed of the patient's clinical situation can the two function as a team to assure optimal use of biopsied tissue. Tissue suitable for conventional microscopy must always be the top priority; however, in many cases, fresh tissue allocation for automated flow phenotyping, cytogenetics, or microbial culture is also critical. Submission of tissue from locations or at times not conducive to this style of tissue stewardship is not acting in the patient's best interests. If biopsy must be performed in such circumstances, the tissue should be sectioned, a portion refrigerated in sterile saline, and the remainder placed in formalin.
3. *Inappropriate choice of procedure.* Chemotherapy and radiotherapy are the mainstays of lymphoma treatment in most cases. In some instances treating a localized lymphoma as an adenocarcinoma with surgical resection (e.g., primary lymphoma of the stomach) is not inappropriate. However, in many situations only a biopsy and some staging samplings of regional lymph nodes (and possibly liver) are needed if the process is known to be lymphoma. Similarly, mistaking carcinoma or melanoma for lymphoma can lead to undertreatment (e.g., axillary node biopsy rather than a complete axillary dissection). Close intraoperative pathology consultation should be used to avoid this problem.

Continued

4. *Failure to adhere to universal infectious disease precautions.* Patients with known or suspected hematolymphoid disease are at relatively high risk for infection with hepatitis viruses, HIV, and other agents. Lymphadenopathy or blood abnormalities may be the presenting finding for a patient not yet diagnosed with the infection. Only through careful attention to consistently applied universal precaution procedures can the surgeon avoid the risk of infection.

PITFALLS FOR THE PATHOLOGIST

1. Failure to advise the surgeon intraoperatively that the tissue biopsy is inadequate for diagnosis.
2. Failure to appropriately allocate tissue for necessary ancillary studies—e.g., frozen tissue for gene probe analysis to prove whether a microscopically atypical proliferation is benign or malignant.
3. Incorrect intraoperative diagnosis of carcinoma due to residual organ parenchyma, simulating malignant epithelium, associated with an infiltrating lymphoma.
4. Failure to adhere to universal infectious disease precautions (see item 4 in "Pitfalls for the Surgeon," preceding).

FURTHER READING

Kjeldsberg C, Beutler E, Bell C, et al. Hematopoiesis: Peripheral blood and bone marrow examination. In: Kjeldsberg C, ed. *Practical Diagnosis of Hematologic Disorders,* Chicago: ASCP Press; 1991:1–16.

REFERENCES

1. Kjeldsberg C, Beutler E, Bell C, et al. Hematopoiesis: Peripheral blood and bone marrow examination. In: Kjeldsberg C, ed. *Practical Diagnosis of Hematologic Disorders.* Chicago: ASCP Press; 1991:1–16.
2. Harmening DM. Introduction to hemostasis: An overview of hemostatic mechanism, platelet structure and function, and extrinsic and intrinsic systems. In: Harmening DM, ed. *Clinical Hematology and Fundamentals of Hemostasis.* Philadelphia: F.A. Davis; 1992:415–439.
3. Kjeldsberg C, Beutler E, Bell C, et al. Diagnosis of bleeding disorders. In: Kjeldsberg C, ed. *Practical Diagnosis of Hematologic Disorders.* Chicago: ASCP Press; 1991:526–543.
4. Cheson BD, Cassileth PA, Head DR, et al. Report of the National Cancer Institute-sponsored workshop on definitions of diagnosis and response in acute myeloid leukemia. *J Clin Oncol.* 1990;8:813–819.
5. Sun T, Li C-Y, Yam LT. *Atlas of Cytochemistry and Immunochemistry of Hematologic Neoplasms.* Chicago: ASCP Press; 1985.
6. Aycock S, Powers L. Bone marrow aspiration and biopsy. In: Powers LW, ed. *Diagnostic Hematology.* St. Louis: Mosby; 1989.
7. Kass L. Procedures for performing aspiration and biopsy of bone marrow. In: Kass L, ed. *Bone Marrow Interpretation,* 2nd ed. Philadelphia: Lippincott; 1985.
8. Baker WF. Clinical evaluation of the patient with anemia. In: Bick RL, ed. *Hematology: Clinical and Laboratory Practice.* St. Louis: Mosby; 1993:203–230.
9. Peterson L, Foucar K. Granulocytosis and granulocytopenia. In: Bick RL, ed. *Hematology: Clinical and Laboratory Practice.* St. Louis: Mosby; 1993:1137–1154.
10. Erslev AJ. Hypersplenism and hyposplenism. In: Beutler E, Lichtman MA, Coller BJ, Kipps TJ, eds. *Williams Hematology,* 5th ed. New York: McGraw-Hill; 1994:709–714.
11. Silverstein MN. The myeloproliferative diseases. In: Bick RL, ed. *Hematology: Clinical and Laboratory Practice.* St. Louis: Mosby; 1993:1239–1245.
12. Mauer AM. Acute lymphocytic leukemia. In: Beutler E, Lichtman MA, Coller BJ, Kipps TJ, eds. *Williams Hematology,* 5th ed. New York: McGraw-Hill; 1994:1004–1016.
13. Lichtman MA. Acute myelogenous leukemia. In: Beutler E, Lichtman MA, Coller BJ, Kipps TJ, eds. *Williams Hematology,* 5th ed. New York: McGraw-Hill; 1994:272–298.
14. Keating MJ, Freireich EJ. Acute myelogenous leukemia. In: Bick RL, ed. *Hematology: Clinical and Laboratory Practice.* St. Louis: Mosby; 1993:1161–1194.
15. Sheldon GF, Groom RD, Meyer AA. The spleen. In: Sabiston DC Jr, ed. *Textbook of Surgery: The Biological Basis of Modern Surgical Practice,* 14th ed. Philadelphia: Saunders; 1991:1118–1119.
16. Haagensen CD, Feind CR, Herter FP, et al. *The Lymphatics In Cancer.* Philadelphia: Saunders; 1972.
17. Schnitzer B. Reactive lymphadenopathies. In: Knowles DM, ed. *Neoplastic Hematopathology.* Baltimore: Williams & Wilkins; 1992:427–457.
18. Lester EP, Ultmann JE. Lymphomas. In: Beutler E, Lichtman MA, Coller BJ, Kipps TJ, eds. *Williams Hematology,* 5th ed. New York: McGraw-Hill; 1994:1076–1096.
19. Horning SJ. Hodgkin disease. In: Beutler E, Lichtman MA, Coller BJ, Kipps TJ, eds. *Williams Hematology,* 5th ed. New York: McGraw-Hill; 1994:1057–1075.
20. Harris NL, Jaffe ES, Stein H, et al. A revised European-American classification of lymphoid neoplasms: A proposal from the International Lymphoma Study Group. *Blood.* 1994;84:1361–1392.
21. The Non-Hodgkin's Lymphoma Pathology Classification Project. National Cancer Institute–sponsored study of classifications of non-Hodgkin's lymphomas: Summary and Description of a Working Formulation for Clinical Usage. *Cancer.* 1982;49:2112–2135.
22. Banks PM. Pathology of malignant lymphomas. In: Beutler E, Lichtman MA, Coller BJ, Kipps TJ, eds. *Williams Hematology,* 5th ed. New York: McGraw-Hill; 1994:1049–1057.
23. Wotherspoon AC, Doglioni C, Diss TC, et al. Regression of primary low-grade B-cell gastric lymphoma of mucosa-associated lymphoid tissue type after eradication of *Helicobacter pylori. Lancet.* 1993;342:575–577.
24. Lukes RJ, Craver LF, Hall TC, et al. Report of the Nomenclature Committee. *Cancer Res.* 1966;26:1311.
25. Craig FE, Gulley ML, Banks PM. Posttransplantation lymphoproliferative disorders. *Am J Clin Pathol.* 1993;99:265–276.
26. Nochomovitz L, Sidawy M, Jannotta F, et al. *Intraoperative Consultation. A Guide to Smears, Imprints, and Frozen Sections.* Chicago: ASCP Press; 1989.

18

Soft Tissue Tumors

Elizabeth A. Montgomery, Sharon W. Weiss,
and William G. Kraybill

Definition

Soft tissues are defined as nonepithelial extraskeletal tissues exclusive of the reticuloendothelial system and glia. They include muscle, adipose tissue, and supporting vasculature and nerves.[1]

PATHOGENESIS OF SOFT TISSUE TUMORS

The etiology of most soft tissue tumors (STT) is unknown. Benign lesions have been associated with trauma and foreign materials; soft tissue sarcomas (STS) have been associated with several chemical toxins and prior irradiation. The incidence of reported sarcomas following therapeutic irradiation is low, ranging from 0.03 to 0.3%. The latency period is about 10 years, and the most common subtype is malignant fibrous histiocytoma.[2, 3]

Benign and malignant soft tissue tumors are a component of several familial disorders, including neurofibromatosis, Gardner's syndrome, familial retinoblastoma, and the newly described Li-Fraumeni cancer family syndrome.[4] In this syndrome, children and young adults present with a constellation of sarcomas (usually rhabdomyosarcomas), adrenal cortical carcinomas, brain tumors, leukemias, breast carcinomas, and other early-onset malignancies. Germline mutations of the p53 tumor-suppressor gene on chromosome 17 have been demonstrated in these families.[5] Chemical agents that have been implicated in the development of sarcomas include vinyl chloride (used industrially), thorium dioxide, and possibly the phenoxy herbicides.

PATHOBIOLOGY OF SOFT TISSUE TUMORS

The biologic potential of both benign and malignant STT is varied, and at times unpredictable. For example, among benign fibrous proliferations, some lesions, such as nodular fasciitis, proliferate rapidly, whereas others grow insidiously. Still other lesions, such as the fibromatoses, can be locally aggressive but lack metastatic potential.

Similarly, sarcomas show considerable variation in behavior. Even so, a few generalizations can be made. Sarcomas tend to ''respect'' fascial borders unless altered by surgical intervention or advanced growth. Subcutaneous lesions typically expand radially, whereas intramuscular or osseous sarcomas spread longitudinally. Pseudocapsules—consisting primarily of collagen, fibroblasts, newly formed vessels, and inflammatory elements—are a frequent tumor-induced host response. Microscopic extensions of neoplasm are always present within or outside the pseudocapsule. For this reason, local recurrence invariably follows enucleation of what appear to be circumscribed lesions.

Like other malignant neoplasms, STS progress by local extension and by metastasis either hematogenously or, less commonly, to regional lymph nodes. The behavior of STS varies with the histologic type of the tumor, tumor size, and tumor grade (see following text). Low-grade STS rarely metastasize hematogenously, although they may recur locally. Hence, the management of these tumors emphasizes local surgical treatment. High-grade sarcomas may also recur, extending locally and along fascial borders, but they often metastasize hematogenously, most commonly to the lung. The likelihood that a high-grade tumor will metastasize hematogenously is directly related to its size.[6] Although tumor grading is a good general construct, some histologic subtypes independently define the anticipated biologic potential.

Lymph node metastases occur infrequently in sarcomas and are associated with poor prognoses. The regional lymph nodes, therefore, are not usually considered in the management plan of patients with STS. Exceptions to this rule are rhabdomyosarcomas, synovial sarcomas, epithelioid sarcomas, and clear-cell sarcomas, which metastasize to lymph nodes in between 10 and 45% of cases.

Evaluation and Diagnosis of Patients with Soft Tissue Tumors

Benign tumors of the soft tissues are far more common than their malignant counterparts and are usually small and asymptomatic. Most measure less than 3 cm in diameter. Rarely, benign STT may be symptomatic because of their size or location. Patients with these tumors are often referred to a surgeon based upon the concern that they harbor a malignancy.

The management of most benign STT consists of biopsy and excision to exclude malignancy, although occasionally benign lesions require excision because of associated symptoms.

Sarcomas are rare and account for about 1.5% of all malignant neoplasms and about 5% of childhood cancers.[7] The management of STS is increasingly multidisciplinary. Because of this, patients with STS are frequently referred to tertiary care centers. Appropriate management of these patients requires the coordinated efforts of surgeons, pathologists, diagnostic radiologists, radiation therapists, medical oncologists, and rehabilitation staff. Although a minority of surgeons specialize in the care of these complex patients, all surgeons should be familiar with the principles of diagnosis and management of STS.[8]

PATIENT ASSESSMENT AND BIOPSY TECHNIQUES

The assessment of patients with soft tissue masses begins with a careful history and physical examination,[9, 10] including history of exposure to chemical agents suspected of causing these tumors and family history of STT. Duration and growth characteristics of the mass are also important. Although STS are frequently large, they are usually asymptomatic. When symptoms do occur, they are generally attributable to pressure. Large tumor size is more typical of sarcomas; however, benign tumors, especially lipomas, may also be quite large. If the clinician suspects that the lesion is an STS, diagnostic imaging is indicated prior to biopsy. Prebiopsy imaging provides the surgeon with information about positioning for the biopsy by identifying the muscle group involved. Magnetic resonance imaging (MRI) is superior to computed tomography (CT) in the assessment of primary STT of the extremities,[11] whereas CT scans are more effective in the evaluation of tumors of the abdomen and chest. Biopsy prior to imaging may distort the radiographic assessment of the primary tumor.

The three types of biopsy are (1) fine needle aspiration (FNA), (2) core needle biopsy, and (3) open biopsy, either incisional or excisional. The advantages of fine needle aspiration biopsy are minimal trauma, low cost, and avoidance of anesthesia. The puncture site should be amenable to subsequent en bloc excision. An optimal specimen—i.e., one that is quantitatively adequate and free of artifacts—is required. If the Papanicolaou stain is to be used, smeared slides must be fixed immediately to avoid drying artifact. If a satisfactory specimen is obtained, it can also be utilized for immunohistochemical studies (see Chap. 3).

Of the three biopsy types, FNA is most subject to sampling error. The diagnostic information provided by the pathologist is often also of a general nature—malignant or benign. Alternatively, the pathologist may be able to classify the tumor only as "mesenchymal" and unable to state whether it is clearly benign or malignant. Despite its limitations, FNA may be very helpful in situations where the clinical differential diagnosis is limited to lesions having vastly variable histologic features (such as childhood blastic sarcomas versus fibromatosis). FNA is less reliable when the histologic differences are subtle (e.g., in the distinction of nodular fasciitis from sarcoma). Special experience is necessary to perform and interpret FNA biopsy samples. For these reasons, we do not advocate FNA for primary diagnosis of soft tissue tumors but believe it is useful to document recurrent or metastatic disease.

Core needle biopsy offers low cost and minimal tissue damage. Core needle biopsy may be used with relatively little concern about wound healing in patients who will subsequently undergo radiation. The needle puncture wound can be readily removed en bloc. The accuracy of core needle biopsy is about 80%, and this method is being used increasingly as the initial biopsy method in patients with STT. However, in tumors having abundant fibrosis, extracellular matrix, necrosis, or heterogeneous composition, needle biopsy is hampered by sampling error. An example of this is the distinction of a low-grade liposarcoma from a lipoma; the former has diagnostic areas localized to focal areas of the lesion. If the specimen is inadequate or if there is concern that the diagnosis is not consistent with the clinical findings, an open biopsy should be performed (see Chap. 1).

All biopsies, particularly open biopsies, are performed with the ultimate surgical resection in mind. Thus, it is best if the same surgeon plans for both biopsy and potential resection. In the extremities, most incisions are radial. Ill-placed biopsy incisions may preclude limb salvage in some patients (see Case 1–3 in Chap. 1). At the time of biopsy, the tumor is directly visualized and ample tissue is obtained. It may be appropriate to obtain an intraoperative frozen section to confirm adequate sampling, particularly during large open procedures (e.g., abdominal, thoracic, or retroperitoneal explorations). After hemostasis is assured, the wound is closed in layers. If adequate hemostasis cannot be assured or the wound is large, a drain may be used to prevent formation of hematoma or seroma, which could result in extension of the tumor. If a drain is placed, it should be placed so that the tract can easily be excised at the time of definitive surgery.

To summarize, FNA is generally not recommended for initial diagnosis and treatment planning, although it may be recommended for identifying recurrence. Core needle biopsies may be done for definitive diagnosis; however, as in FNA, sampling error may preclude accurate diagnosis. For tumors with fine histologic distinctions, larger specimens are more appropriate, providing the pathologist with more material to study. When an interpretation rendered by FNA or core needle biopsy does not support the clinical impression, it is the surgeon's responsibility to provide appropriate material for complete pathologic evaluation of the tumor. For the most part, we prefer to have a careful and complete staging and pathologic diagnosis prior to proceeding with treatment of STS. Again, it is the surgeon's responsibility to acquire sufficient clinical and pathologic information prior to embarking on a clinical course with irrevocable consequences. This responsibility requires a fundamental awareness of the problems associated with these tumors and good communication between the surgeon and pathologist.

USES OF FROZEN SECTION

The principal uses for intraoperative frozen sections are (1) establishing quantitative and qualitative specimen adequacy, (2) excluding infectious etiology, (3) assessing surgical margins, and (4) in selected instances, assessing benign versus malignant processes.

The adequacy of the material for pathologic diagnosis must be established at this time (see Chap. 2). We rarely utilize frozen section diagnoses to make major therapeutic decisions, although it is appropriate in selected instances. The pathologist should reserve the option to defer diagnosis until permanent sections are available for review. Even on permanent sections, mesenchymal proliferations are among the most difficult challenges for pathologists. Pitfalls include pseudosarcomatous lesions, which may be difficult to distinguish from sarcomas, and spindle-cell areas in metastatic carcinomas, lymphomas, and melanomas that can mimic sarcomas. In these and other instances, frozen section diagnosis for definitive surgery invites error. These difficulties can best be avoided by waiting for permanent sections and special studies. Careful clinical staging can also prevent errors by identifying inapparent primary disease sites.

Whereas frozen sections can assist in the evaluation of selected surgical margins, the size of STS frequently precludes assessment of all margins. Under these circumstances, gross inspection of the mass and surrounding tissue by the pathologist may allow selection of the margin that appears closest to the tumor for frozen section analysis. If frozen section diagnosis is chosen for distinguishing margins, careful communication between the surgeon and pathologist is particularly important. In general, the ideal margin consists of intact tissue, uncomplicated by cautery or clamp crush artifacts. If the pathologist is aware of the diagnostic and therapeutic problems confronting the surgeon, appropriate and useful interpretation of the specimen results.

Treatment and Processing of Specimens

In general, specimens should be reviewed with the pathologist for orientation and surgical margins; anatomic landmarks that are obvious in situ are less so following excision. To avoid spurious contamination by tumor, resection surfaces can be painted with India ink, blotted to avoid smearing, and sampled prior to sectioning through the tumor. Soft tissue and neurovascular margins are sampled. When it is unclear whether the lesion is of skeletal or soft tissue origin, specimen radiographs may identify the epicenter of the tumor. The tumor is measured for staging. One histologic section for each centimeter of tumor should be sampled. Remaining tissue is then examined for satellite nodules. Finally, all lymph nodes are submitted for microscopic examination.

If special studies are contemplated, fresh tissue, either frozen or suspended in media, should be procured. Tiny shave samples placed in glutaraldehyde fixative are of potential use for electron microscopy. If lymphoma is in the differential diagnosis, tissue should be submitted for appropriate studies (see Chaps. 2 and 17). In the case of large sarcoma resections, sufficient material is usually available for tumor banking for research. Photography of the macroscopic specimen is helpful for both documentation and educational purposes. Cytogenetic,[12] molecular, and immunoperoxidase studies are employed increasingly for evaluation of these tumors, especially in pediatric patients. For example, all neuroblastomas should have fresh sterile tissue set aside for karyotyping and fresh frozen tissue allocated for molecular studies for N-*myc* amplification. When sampling allows, fresh frozen tissue from rhabdomyosarcomas should be submitted to the Intergroup Rhabdomyosarcoma Study. The reader is referred to Chapter 2 for additional information on special studies.

Staging of Soft Tissue Sarcomas

Several staging systems are used for STS. The most common system is that of the American Joint Committee on Cancer (AJCC) and the International Union Against Cancer (UICC; see Table 18–1). This system emphasizes the importance of tumor grade but employs the tumor size and the presence of metastases to define prognosis. It correlates well with survival. Another system is based on the anatomic classification of these tumors, which, in addition to tumor grade, utilizes the location of the primary as intracompartmental or extracompartmental (Table 18–2).

Table 18–1. American Joint Committee Staging Protocol for Soft Tissue Sarcoma

Stage	Grade	Tumor	Nodes	Metastases
IA	1	1	0	0
IB	1	2	0	0
IIA	2	1	0	0
IIB	2	2	0	0
IIIA	3–4	1	0	0
IIIB	3–4	2	0	0
IVA	1–4	1–2	1	0
IVB	1–4	1–2	0–1	1

Characteristics
Histologic grade (G)
G1 Well differentiated
G2 Moderately differentiated
G3 Poorly differentiated
Primary tumor (T)
T1 ≤5 cm
T2 >5 cm
Regional lymph nodes (N)
N0 No regional lymph node metastases
N1 Regional lymph node metastases
Distant metastases (M)
M0 No distant metastases
M1 Distant metastases

Source: From Beahrs OH, et al., eds. *American Joint Committee on Cancer: Manual for Staging of Cancer,* 4th ed. Philadelphia: Lippincott; 1992. With permission.

Both systems may be useful, although the AJCC/UICC is more widely known. Separate staging systems have been developed for pediatric sarcomas, particularly rhabdomyosarcomas and neuroblastomas.[13]

Grading of Soft Tissue Sarcomas

One of the most accurate criteria to assess prognosis in these uncommon tumors is tumor grade. Many grading schemes have been developed that attempt to apply uniform grading criteria to all histologic types. This simplistic approach is analogous to using identical criteria to grade carcinomas of all anatomic sites. As previously discussed, low-grade sarcomas virtually never metastasize but may be locally aggressive, whereas high-grade sarcomas threaten not only locally and regionally but also with distant metastasis.

Grading schemes may be two-tiered (low and high) or have up to four grades. By emphasizing various parameters, each of the major grading systems has proven clinical validity. In the United States, use of three grades is the most prevalent approach.[15–17] The histologic features used in grading schemes include (1) degree of tumor differentiation, (2) cellularity, (3) nuclear atypia, (4) cellular pleomorphism (presence of tumor giant cells and bizarre nuclei), (5) mitotic rate, (6) amount of fibrous stroma and myxoid stroma, (7) presence/amount of inflammation, and (8) percent necrosis. This last feature is particularly important. Following preoperative chemotherapy and radiation, however, the foregoing parameters may be profoundly altered, making accurate grading impossible. For example, preoperative radiation may produce geographic necrosis within a tumor, but clearly that feature is a reflection of a therapeutic effect and not an intrinsic tumor characteristic. In such schemes, grading seems useful in fibrosarcoma; leiomyosarcoma; malignant peripheral nerve sheath tumor; and, to a lesser extent, liposarcoma and synovial sarcoma. However, as a result of the inherent heterogeneity of biologic potential based upon histologic type, the National Cancer Institute (NCI)[15] has developed a grading scheme that automatically assigns a low grade to myxoid and well-differentiated liposarcoma and dermatofibrosarcoma protuberans and a high grade to all examples of rhabdomyosarcoma, osteosarcoma, synovial sarcoma, and alveolar soft part sarcoma. Other lesions are assigned a range of grades utilizing histologic criteria.

Some sarcomas are not readily gradable. For example, alveolar soft part sarcoma and epithelioid sarcoma may display deceptively bland features and yet produce metastases in a significant number of cases. Likewise, a grade I lesion does not always equate with an absence of metastatic potential. For example, grade I myxoid liposarcoma may metastasize after a long latency. Surgeons managing patients with STS must be aware of these nuances and apply them to the treatment strategies of these challenging cases.

Grading, of course, is applied only to sarcomas. Application of grading to benign processes is meaningless and misleading. For example, pseudosarcomatous lesions (e.g., nodular fasciitis) may have high mitotic rates and increased cellularity, which would lead to classification as high-grade sarcoma if not recognized as benign.

Standardized Reporting of Soft Tissue Tumors

The pathology report from a resection specimen should include information concerning the following items:

1. Residual tumor

Table 18–2. Enneking Staging System for Soft Tissue Sarcoma

Stage	Grade	Site	Metastases
IA	G1	T1	M0
IB	G1	T2	M0
IIA	G2	T1	M0
IIB	G2	T2	M0
IIIA/IIIB	G1–G2	T1–T2	M1

Characteristics
Grade (G)
G1 Low
G2 High
Site (T)
T1 Intracompartmental
T2 Extracompartmental
Metastases (M)
M0 No regional or distant metastases
M1 Regional or distant metastases

Source: From Enneking WF, et al. *Clin Orthop.* 1980; 153:106–120. With permission.

2. Tumor location (specify anatomic compartment, muscle group, body cavity, or general site, as appropriate)
3. Histologic subtype (e.g., liposarcoma)
4. Histologic grade
5. Surgical margin status (actual distance if margin is close)
6. Presence of tumor deposits in vessels/in lymph nodes/ outside main mass/in joint space/in bone
7. Estimated percent necrosis
8. Tumor size measured from the specimen
9. Results of any special stains used to support the diagnosis
10. Comment: Unusual features of the case should be mentioned as well as expected biologic behavior, if recurrence or metastasis, whether tumor differs in appearance from that of original lesion.

The listed information concerning the primary tumor is the responsibility of the pathologist. Physical findings and pertinent radiographic studies can be used for staging, and a treatment plan with input from the surgeon, medical oncologist, and radiation therapist can then be formulated based upon the expected biologic potential of the lesion.

Histologic Classification of Soft Tissue Tumors

The World Health Organization currently recognizes 165 histologic types of STT.[18] The classification is based upon the light microscopic characteristics of the lesions. Tumors are likened to the adult tissue type that they resemble. For example, a liposarcoma is so classified because its cells to some extent *resemble* normal fat. It does not necessarily imply that the tumor *arose* from fat cells. Described in the following text are those most commonly encountered in clinical practice.

FIBROUS LESIONS

Nodular Fasciitis

Nodular fasciitis is the prototype of the pseudosarcomatous fibroblastic proliferations. It usually occurs as a rapidly growing mass in young adults, most typically in the forearm, attaining a size of 2 to 3 cm. Although the cytologic features are bland, the presence of high cellularity and brisk mitotic activity simulates high-grade malignancy (Fig. 18–1). An alarming proportion of these have been mistaken for sarcomas,[19] with untoward results from unnecessary treatment. Local excision is usually curative.

Fibromatoses

The fibromatoses are classified among benign fibrous proliferations (Fig. 18–2).[18] The identification of clonality[20] suggests that they may be true neoplasms, and their capacity for aggressive local disease has led some observers to regard them as ''fibrosarcomas, grade one-half'' despite their lack of metastatic potential. This term should be

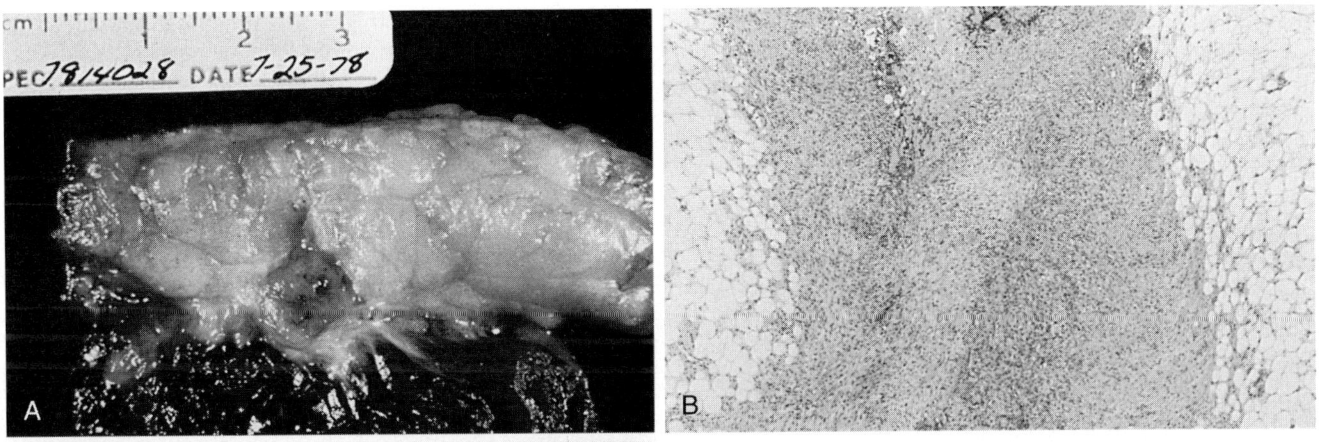

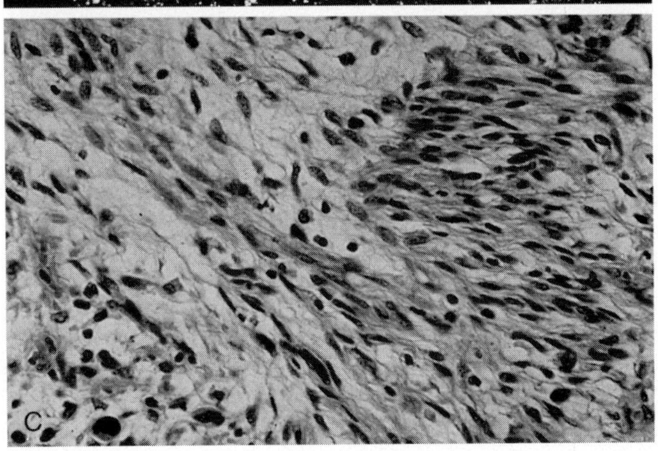

Figure 18–1. Nodular fasciitis typically presents as a relatively superficial, small (2- to 3-cm) tumefaction that attains its maximum dimension in a matter of weeks. *A,* Gross specimen shows a nodule at the interface of subcutaneous fat and fascia. It is cured by local excision or may even regress spontaneously. Nodular fasciitis is characterized by a proliferation of myofibroblasts arranged in a loose storiform pattern punctuated by myxoid stroma, chronic inflammatory elements, and extravasated erythrocytes. Although mitoses may be present, the cytologic features are benign *(B, low magnification; C, high magnification).*

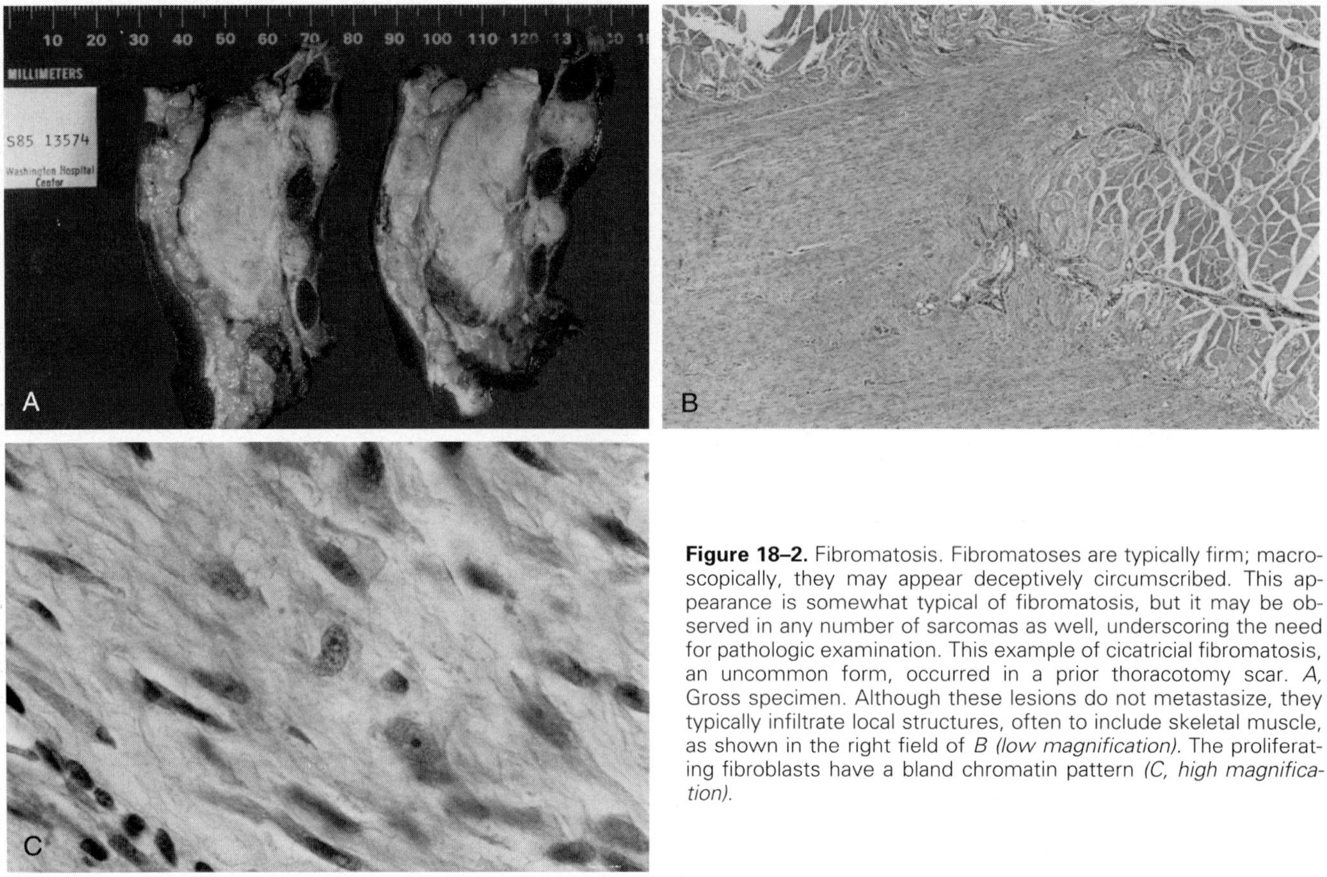

Figure 18–2. Fibromatosis. Fibromatoses are typically firm; macroscopically, they may appear deceptively circumscribed. This appearance is somewhat typical of fibromatosis, but it may be observed in any number of sarcomas as well, underscoring the need for pathologic examination. This example of cicatricial fibromatosis, an uncommon form, occurred in a prior thoracotomy scar. *A,* Gross specimen. Although these lesions do not metastasize, they typically infiltrate local structures, often to include skeletal muscle, as shown in the right field of *B (low magnification).* The proliferating fibroblasts have a bland chromatin pattern *(C, high magnification).*

discouraged, since it potentially confuses fibromatoses with well-differentiated fibrosarcomas, which have a low but definite risk of metastasis. Despite some reports to the contrary, in the absence of radiation, fibromatoses do not transform to fibrosarcomas. Examples purported to represent malignant transformations are probably differentiated fibrosarcomas that were misinterpreted as fibromatoses. Whereas palmar and plantar fibromatoses are readily treated by local excision, fibromatoses in other sites recur in 25 to 50% of cases, and mesenteric lesions may be fatal.

Abdominal fibromatosis usually occurs in women of childbearing age and arises in the rectus or internal oblique muscles. Extraabdominal fibromatosis (musculoaponeurotic fibromatosis, extraabdominal desmoid) most commonly occurs in the shoulder region. Patients with mesenteric fibromatoses present in the fifth decade. These fibromatoses commonly occur in the small-bowel mesentery.[21] Cases associated with Gardner's syndrome (autosomal dominant intestinal polyposis, osteomata, and cutaneous cysts) are more aggressive than de novo cases.

Treatment of fibromatoses should balance the need for complete extirpation of the lesion against the morbidity of the procedure. Radiation therapy may play a role. Efforts to tailor therapy to the presence of hormone receptors identified in some cases appear to be of limited value.

Fibrosarcoma

Fibrosarcomas are rare tumors that typically occur in the deep tissues of the lower extremities of adults in the fifth decade. For the pathologist, this diagnosis should be rendered with caution, as both malignant peripheral nerve sheath tumors and synovial sarcomas can exhibit similar histologic appearances. Distinction between these histologic look-alikes often requires immunohistochemical stains (Fig. 18–3). The infantile form is noteworthy; its microscopic features are indistinguishable from the adult form, but its prognosis is more favorable (see Chap. 21).

FIBROHISTIOCYTIC LESIONS

Dermatofibrosarcoma Protuberans

Dermatofibrosarcoma protuberans (DFSP) is regarded as a tumor of borderline malignancy, as metastases occur in only about 5% of reported cases (4% hematogenous and 1% to lymph nodes). These tumors have a slight male predominance and appear between the third and fourth decades with a predilection for the trunk.[22] The lesions begin as firm plaques but, over several years, become tense, bulging nodules. On microscopic examination, an uninvolved zone underlies atrophic epidermis and the tumor diffusely infiltrates the subcutis.

The reported rates of recurrence for DFSP range from 12 to 50% and are related primarily to adequacy of excision.[23] These locally aggressive tumors require aggressive surgical resection.[24] The Mohs' technique for dermatologic surgery (see Chap. 4) has been successful in some patients with this disease.[25, 26] Regional lymph node excision is not indicated. In cases in which anatomic location (e.g., head

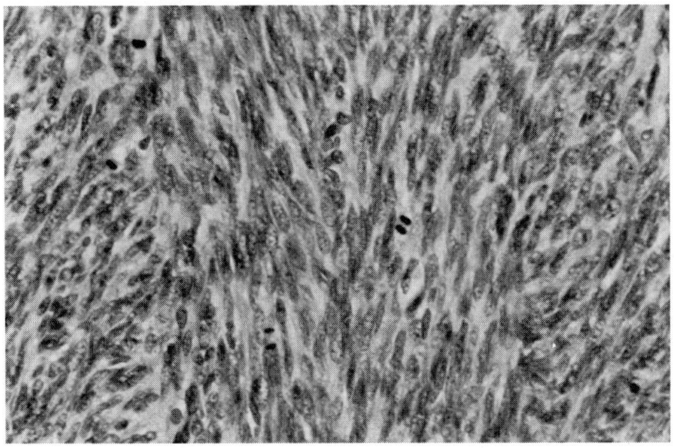

Figure 18–3. Fibrosarcoma. This example of a high-grade fibrosarcoma shows the typical herringbone pattern composed of cytologically malignant spindle cells. This example has a brisk mitotic rate *(high magnification).*

and neck) or operative status precludes resection, radiation may offer an alternative.[27]

Malignant Fibrous Histiocytomas

These are the most common adult sarcomas and typically occur in the sixth and seventh decades, with a modest male predominance.[1, 28] The thigh is the most common location. Variants that have been described include the storiform-pleomorphic or classic form (Fig. 18–4) and the myxoid, giant-cell, and inflammatory types.

Other sarcomas, such as leiomyosarcomas and liposarcomas, may be pleomorphic and can be misinterpreted as malignant fibrous histiocytoma (MFH). Currently, such errors are of no therapeutic consequence. By contrast, melanomas, lymphomas, and carcinomas can simulate MFH by virtue of pleomorphic spindle morphology. It is critical that these masqueraders be unmasked. Immunohistochemical stains can prevent misadventure, and they should be performed in doubtful cases (see Chap. 2). Anti-S100 protein and HMB-45 usually react with melanomas, and antibodies against cytokeratin and epithelial membrane antigen mark most spindled carcinomas.

The overall 5-year survival of all patients with MFH is about 60%. Site and histologic grade are important prognostic determinants. Retroperitoneal tumors are particularly unfavorable. Aggressive surgery with tumor-free margins and radiation are the mainstays of therapy.

LIPOMATOUS TUMORS

Lipoma and Its Variants

Lipomas are the most common mesenchymal neoplasms, typically appearing in the fifth and sixth decades without gender predilection. Many solitary lipomas are associated with rearrangements of the long arm of chromosome 12.[29] Most are superficial, arising in cutaneous fat, although intramuscular, skeletal, mediastinal, retroperitoneal, and articular lipomas are well known. The latter types are frequently less circumscribed than cutaneous examples and may mimic sarcomas clinically. Important variants of lipomas include spindle-cell lipomas[30] and pleomorphic lipomas,[31] which usually affect males in their sixties. They are important to pathologists because they can be mistaken microscopically for sarcomas. Angiolipomas are painful tumors, often multiple, usually arising on the forearms of young adults. Like all benign neoplasms, a small percentage of lipomas may recur locally following incomplete excision.

Lipoblastoma

Lipoblastomas are tumors of infancy that affect boys more frequently than girls.[32] Most examples are solitary, although a diffuse form exists (lipoblastomatosis). Solitary lipoblastomas usually occur on the extremities as well-delineated masses. Patients with these tumors have excellent prognoses and require only conservative excision.

Liposarcoma

Well-Differentiated/Dedifferentiated

Well-differentiated liposarcomas generally occur in the deep soft tissues of the extremities, trunk, retroperitoneum, and spermatic cord. Microscopic patterns include lipoma-like (Fig. 18–5*A*), sclerosing, and inflammatory types. The pathologist must be aware that any large lipomatous neoplasm of the retroperitoneum, mediastinum, or spermatic cord is liposarcoma until proved otherwise (Fig. 18–5*B*). Although most well-differentiated liposarcomas remain histologically bland, a small percentage (10%) may undergo histologic progression (dedifferentiation) to a higher-grade lesion. The so-called dedifferentiated liposarcoma consists of low-grade liposarcoma juxtaposed to high-grade sarcoma indistinguishable from malignant fibrous histiocytoma.[33] This phenomenon is most likely to occur in large retroperitoneal tumors but has also been reported in extremity lesions.[34] Treatment of retroperitoneal lesions is en bloc removal, including adjacent organs and major vessels

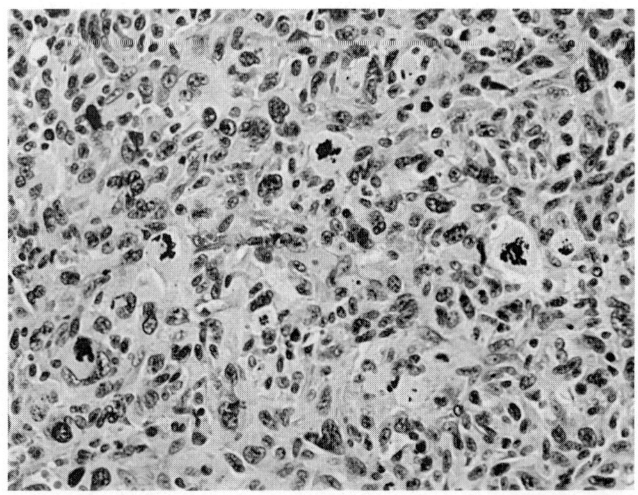

Figure 18–4. Malignant fibrous histiocytoma. This is a typical example of the common pleomorphic form, although several variants have been described. Note haphazardly arranged cells with marked pleomorphism *(high magnification).*

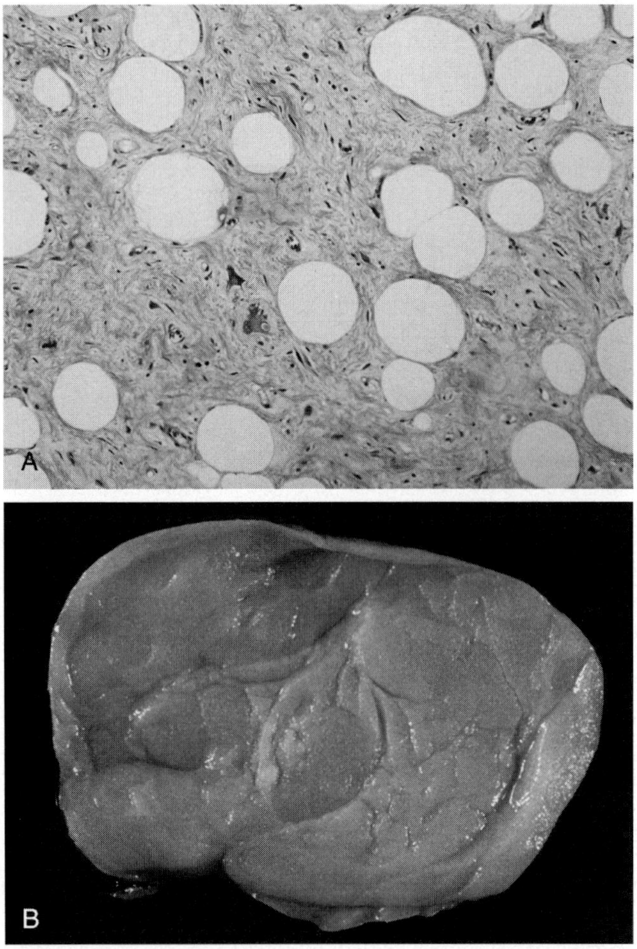

Figure 18–5. Well-differentiated liposarcoma often shows mature-appearing fat and enlarged hyperchromatic cells in a background of fibrosis (sclerosis). Lipoblasts may be infrequent. *(A, intermediate magnification.) B,* Well-differentiated liposarcoma of retroperitoneum, gross specimen. Note that while these tumors appear similar to mature adipose tissue, any fatty tumor of the retroperitoneum should be regarded as liposarcoma until proven otherwise.

(retroperitoneal exenteration). In the absence of dedifferentiation and metastases, death occurs by gastrointestinal/urinary obstruction. Treatment of extremity lesions usually involves complete excision in a function-preserving fashion, as these sites are readily monitored and amenable to reexcision. This approach is reasonable, since liposarcomas of the extremities rarely metastasize.[35]

Myxoid/Round-Cell

Myxoid/round-cell liposarcoma differs from the other subtypes of liposarcoma in several ways. First, these tumors range from hypocellular, myxoid tumors of low malignant potential (myxoid liposarcoma—see Fig. 18–6) to hypercellular, high-grade lesions (round-cell liposarcoma). Grading of these lesions depends upon the percentage of round-cell component. Second, myxoid/round-cell liposarcoma occurs at a younger age than the other types and usually involves the limbs and limb girdles, typically sparing the retroperitoneum. Third, metastases are frequently to the soft tissues rather than to the lungs. Last, a chromosomal translocation is present in over 90% of myxoid/round-cell liposarcoma [(t12;16) (q13;p11)]. Treatment usually consists of surgical resection with or without radiation therapy, depending on tumor grade, size, and location.

Pleomorphic Liposarcoma

Like dedifferentiated liposarcoma, pleomorphic liposarcoma is a highly aggressive neoplasm that occurs in the sixth and seventh decades. The limbs and limb girdles are affected, as well as the retroperitoneum. Histologically, pleomorphic liposarcomas offer the most bizarre malignant cells in human tumors. Unlike other subtypes of liposarcoma, which often require a laborious search for lipoblasts, these tumors have sheets of pleomorphic lipoblasts (Fig. 18–7). As with other high-grade sarcomas, the prognosis is correlated with tumor size, location, and other staging parameters. Treatment is that of high-grade sarcomas.

NEURAL TUMORS

Schwannoma (Neurilemoma)

Schwannomas arise from the Schwann cells ensheathing peripheral nerves and consequently compress the residual peripheral nerve to one side. Microscopically, they exhibit a distinctive pattern of spindled nerve sheath cells (Fig. 18–8). They may occur at any age but predominate between 20 and 50 years without a sex predilection. They involve all sites, including the central nervous system, peripheral soft tissues, or retroperitoneum and mediastinum. In these latter sites, they may achieve impressive dimensions and clinically mimic sarcomas. Despite confusing terminology, schwannomas *virtually never* undergo malignant degeneration into malignant peripheral nerve sheath tumors (malignant schwannomas). This behavior is in contrast to benign neurofibromas, which may undergo malignant transformation. Similarly, a plexiform variety of schwannoma has been reported,[36] which is not associated with neurofibro-

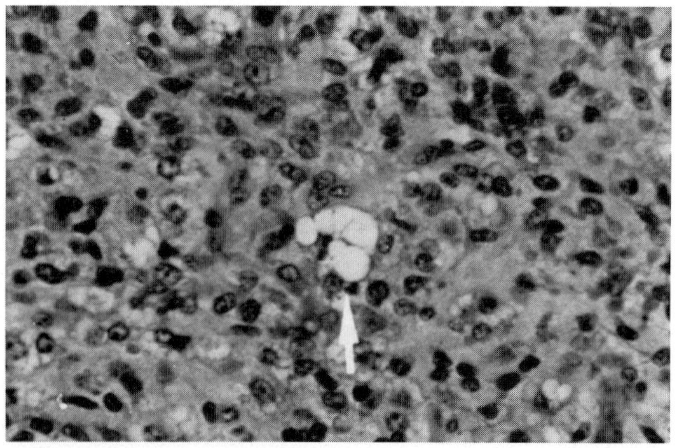

Figure 18–6. Myxoid liposarcoma typically presents a constellation of cystic spaces containing bluish mucopolysaccharide matrix, a prominent vascular pattern, relatively uniform rounded nuclei, and scattered lipoblasts *(arrow)*. Especially cellular examples are referred to as round-cell liposarcoma and behave in a more aggressive fashion than their more paucicellular counterparts *(high magnification)*.

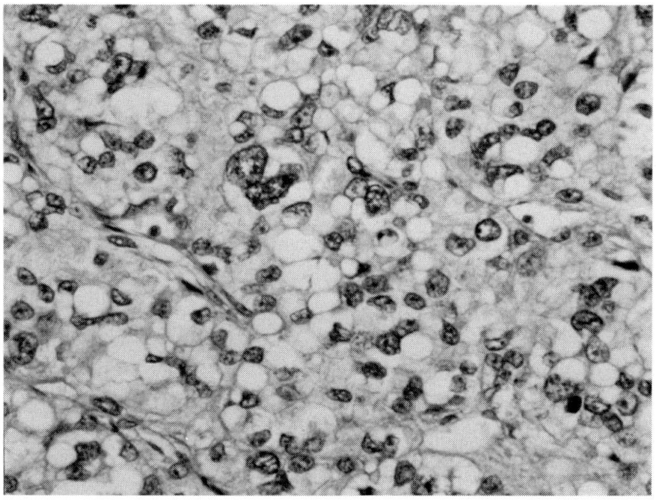

Figure 18–7. Pleomorphic liposarcoma. These high-grade liposarcomas are characterized by sheets of pleomorphic lipoblasts. Whereas the identification of diagnostic lipoblasts is at times challenging in the other variants of liposarcoma, they are readily apparent here *(high magnification).*

matosis, whereas plexiform *neurofibromas* are pathognomonic of neurofibromatosis. Treatment for schwannomas is local excision. In large lesions, where complete resection is not feasible, incomplete excision to relieve compression carries little risk of subsequent malignant degeneration in unexcised tissue.

Neurofibroma and Neurofibromatosis

Solitary neurofibromas represent about 90% of lesions and occur in young adults (20 to 30 years). When they arise in large nerves, they expand within the confines of the perineurium, imparting a fusiform shape to the nerve. Lesions arising in diminutive nerve twigs produce a less well demarcated tumor. Cases associated with neurofibromatosis (NF) are more likely to arise in large nerve trunks (Table 18–3 and see reference 37). The plexiform variant of neurofibroma is a neurofibroma that distorts or contorts a nerve trunk; these lesions are considered pathognomonic for type I neurofibromatosis (NF1) (Fig. 18–9 and Table 18–3). Treatment consists of excision. Large lesions can be difficult to eradicate, since surgical margins may be difficult to establish.

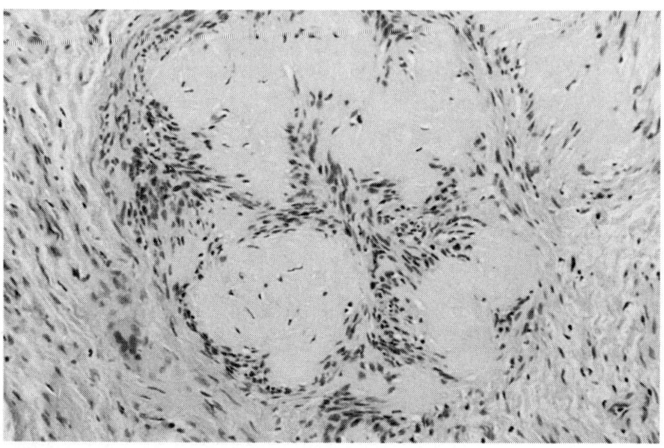

Figure 18–8. Neurilemoma (schwannoma). Neurilemomas are sharply circumscribed, consisting of Schwann cells with slender, serpentine nuclei that align themselves around acellular collagenized zones *(high magnification).*

Malignant Peripheral Nerve Sheath Tumors

Although other terms (malignant schwannoma and neurofibrosarcoma) have been used synonymously for sarcomas arising from nerves, the preferred term is malignant peripheral nerve sheath tumor (MPNST) (Fig. 18–10). It does not specify the exact cell from which these tumors arise (e.g., Schwann cells, perineurium, or fibroblasts), since in most cases this issue remains unresolved.[38]

An MPNST may arise in the setting of NF. Cases not associated with NF occur in 20- to 50-year-olds. NF-associated lesions occur at a younger age. Pediatric cases have been described that behave in an aggressive fashion. The reported incidence of MPNST in NF ranges from 2 to 30%. Among patients with MPNST, those with NF have a total close to 50%. On occasion, heterologous elements—including bone, glandular elements, cartilage and rhabdomyoblasts—may be a component of MPNST. Lesions having the latter heterologous component are referred to as "triton tumors."[39] It has been assumed that MPNST arising in NF1 carries a worse prognosis than that arising de novo; however, this belief may be wrong. When matched for size, location, and grade, there seems to be little difference.[40] For most MPNST, therapy should include aggressive surgery and adjuvant radiation.

SMOOTH MUSCLE TUMORS

Leiomyoma

Almost all leiomyomas occur in the female genital tract and in the GI tract of both sexes. Subcutaneous leiomyomas

Table 18–3. Criteria for Diagnosis of Neurofibromatosis

NF1 (estimated incidence 1:4,000; autosomal dominant)
Previously called von Recklinghausen's disease
Two or more of the following:
- Six or more café-au-lait macules
- Two or more neurofibromas of any type or one plexiform neurofibroma
- Freckling in the axillary or inguinal regions
- Optic glioma
- Two or more Lisch nodules (iris hamartomas)
- A distinctive osseous lesion such as sphenoid dysplasia or thinning of the long bone cortex with or without pseudarthrosis
- A first-degree relative with NF1 by the above criteria

NF2 (estimated incidence 1:50,000; autosomal dominant)
Previously called central neurofibromatosis
One of the following:
- Bilateral eighth nerve masses by CT or MRI
- First-degree relative with NF2 and either unilteral eighth nerve mass

or

Two of the following:
- Neurofibroma
- Meningioma
- Glioma
- Schwannoma
- Juvenile posterior subcapsular lenticular opacities

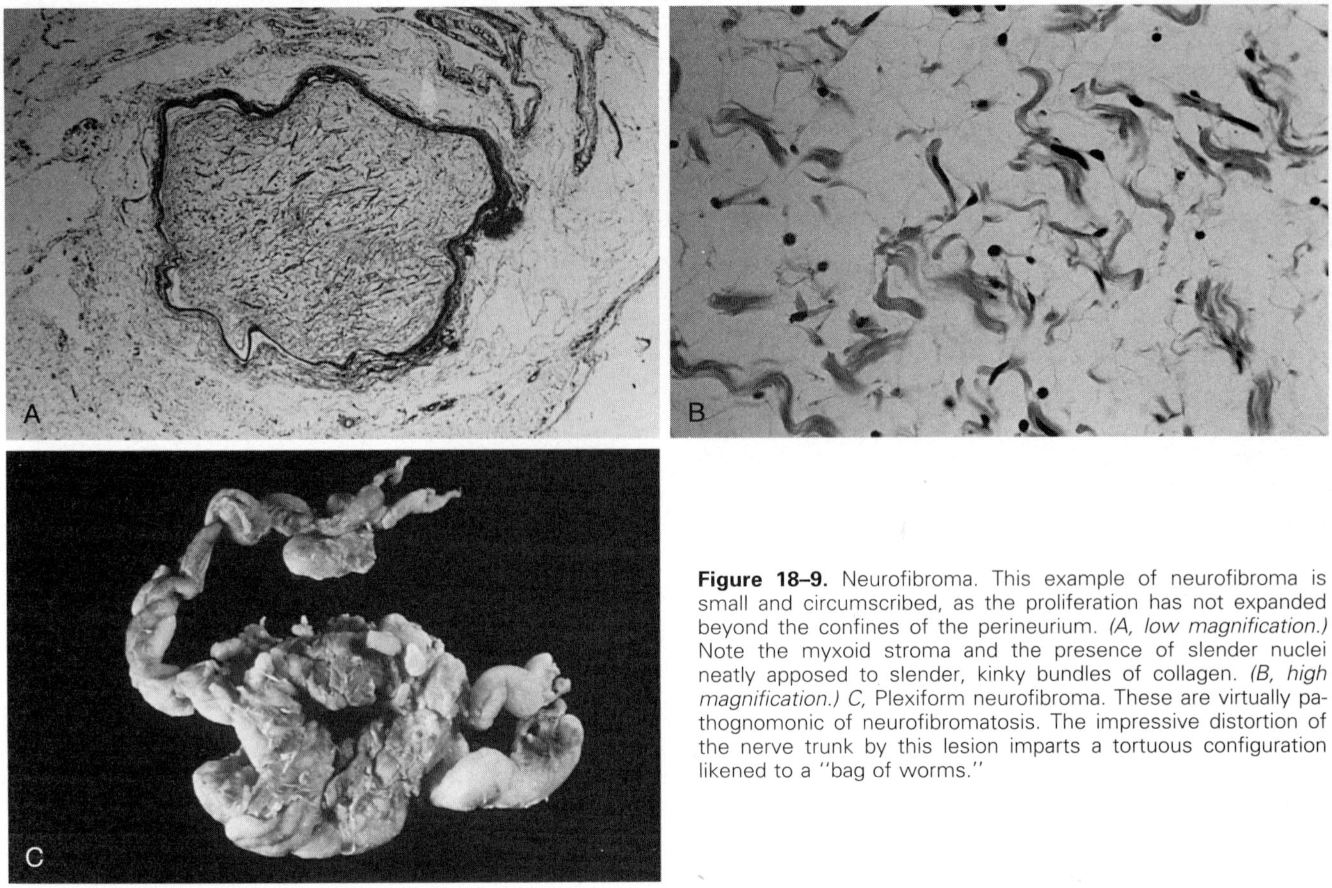

Figure 18–9. Neurofibroma. This example of neurofibroma is small and circumscribed, as the proliferation has not expanded beyond the confines of the perineurium. *(A, low magnification.)* Note the myxoid stroma and the presence of slender nuclei neatly apposed to slender, kinky bundles of collagen. *(B, high magnification.) C,* Plexiform neurofibroma. These are virtually pathognomonic of neurofibromatosis. The impressive distortion of the nerve trunk by this lesion imparts a tortuous configuration likened to a "bag of worms."

are uncommon. Leiomyomas of the deep tissues are rare and must be distinguished from leiomyosarcomas.

Leiomyosarcoma

Leiomyosarcomas of soft tissue predominate in the sixth decade. Although there is a slight male predominance overall, retroperitoneal lesions are substantially more common in women. Leiomyosarcomas may arise from the arrector pili muscles of the skin, vascular walls, and smooth muscle of the female genital tract and GI tract, but the criteria for diagnosis in the latter two sites differ considerably from those for soft tissue lesions.[41]

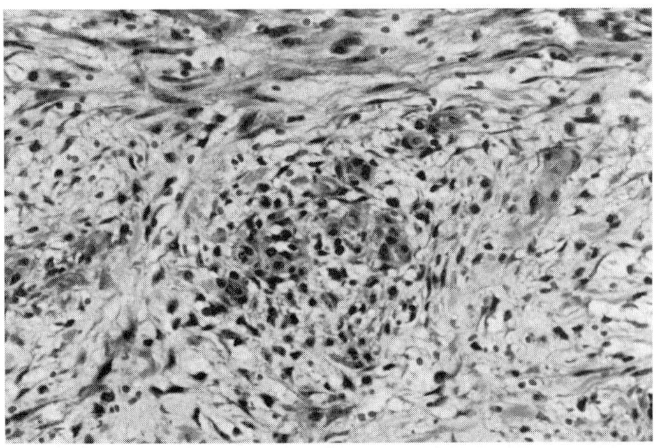

Figure 18–10. Malignant peripheral nerve sheath tumor (malignant schwannoma, neurofibrosarcoma). These tumors consist of cytologically malignant spindle cells that arrange themselves in fascicles, similar to a fibrosarcoma *(high magnification)*. Better-differentiated examples have irregular buckled nuclei, reminiscent of normal Schwann cells.

Microscopically, these neoplasms are composed of plump spindle cells having a fascicular arrangement reminiscent of normal smooth muscle (Fig. 18–11). Whereas occasional mitoses are of no consequence in tumors of the female genital tract smooth muscle, metastases have been observed in retroperitoneal tumors having as few as 1 mitosis per 10 high-power fields. Smooth muscle tumors arising in the retroperitoneum, like fatty tumors, should be considered malignant until proved otherwise. The prognosis for small, superficial (restricted to the dermis) cutaneous tumors is excellent following complete excision, in contrast to the prognosis for deeper, larger lesions. About 40% of subcutaneous and 75% of retroperitoneal tumors metastasize. Wide excision is sufficient therapy for small, superficial tumors, whereas adjuvant radiation should be given to larger tumors.

ROUND-CELL SARCOMAS ("SMALL-CELL," "BLUE-CELL," OR "BLASTIC" SARCOMAS)

Neuroblastoma

Neuroblastomas are tumors of the autonomic nervous system that arise predominantly in the pelvis and account

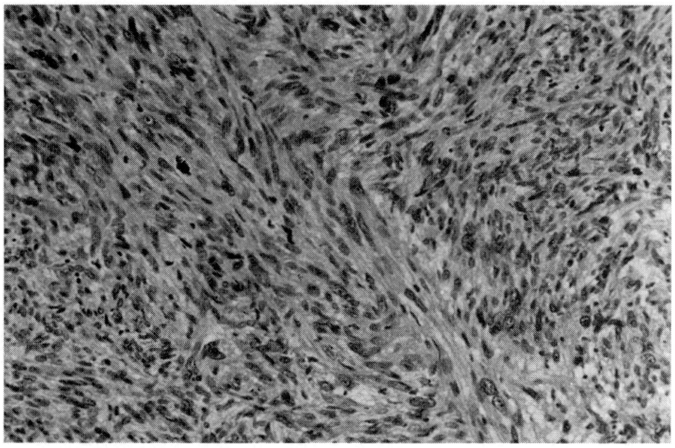

Figure 18–11. Leiomyosarcoma is characterized by perpendicularly oriented fascicles of tumor cells possessing cytoplasmic eosinophilic longitudinal striations and paranuclear glycogen vacuoles, which may indent the nucleus *(high magnification).*

for about 8% of pediatric cancer. They are the most common intraabdominal malignancy of newborns. Like their normal counterparts, neuroblastomas may elaborate various compounds such as neuron specific enolase (NSE), vanillylmandelic acid (VMA), homovanillic acid (HVA), and other catecholamines. High serum NSE and low VMA/HVA ratios have been associated with aggressive tumors. Since the overall survival rate of patients with advanced disease has not improved significantly in the last several decades, there have been numerous attempts to elucidate superior prognostic markers. Prognosis in this disease has been related to stage, patient age, histologic grade, and N-*myc* amplification.[42, 43] A direct relation between amplification of the oncogene N-*myc* and advanced disease has been demonstrated.[44] Moreover, a specific tumor karyotype (del 1p) may be the best overall marker of poor-prognosis lesions (see Chap. 21).[45]

The differential diagnosis includes other sarcomas, lymphomas, and Wilms' tumors, most of which can be excluded by attention to the clinical details and selected immunohistochemical stains. Age and clinical stage are important prognosticators in neuroblastoma; in fact, age is a component in one of the commonly utilized grading schemes.[46] Children under 2 years and those with low-stage disease do well and can be treated with total body irradiation, chemotherapy, and subsequent marrow transplantation. Patients with stage IVS (special) disease are an exception to these general principles; for reasons that are unclear, they generally do well despite the presence of metastases. Patients with stage IVS disease are invariably quite young. These individuals are treated by tumor excision and adjuvant therapy.

Rhabdomyosarcoma

Rhabdomyosarcoma is by far the most common sarcoma in children and young adults; its frequency is similar to all other types combined. Most available data are culled from the Intergroup Rhabdomyosarcoma Study (IRS).[47–49] In adults, rhabdomyosarcomas are vanishingly rare and should be diagnosed with extreme caution (see Chap. 1). In infants, the most common anatomic location is the genitourinary region, followed by the upper airway area. In children and young adults, the extremities are the most common sites, followed by the upper airway region (Fig. 18–12). Rhabdomyosarcomas, unlike most sarcomas, have a tendency to metastasize to lymph nodes.

Rhabdomyosarcoma is one type of sarcoma for which chemotherapy has a well-defined role. The IRS results indicate that initial radical resection of tumors of the trunk and extremities has so favorable an effect on outcome as to justify considerable morbidity.[49]

Ewing's Sarcoma

Ewing's sarcoma of soft tissue is best described as a "small round-cell tumor" in its most primitive form (Fig. 18–13). This tumor occurs in adolescents and young adults with a predilection for the paravertebral region.[50] The microscopic features overlap those of peripheral neuroepithelioma and the so-called Askin tumor,[51, 52] making this a lesion of controversy for surgical pathologists. In addition to many morphologic features, these entities share cytogenetic abnormalities [t(11;22) (q24;q24) or (q24;q12)] and probably represent ends of a common histologic spectrum. Therapy for these aggressive tumors includes a radical excision and an intensive chemotherapy regimen and radiation therapy for unresectable lesions.

MISCELLANEOUS LESIONS—BENIGN

Tenosynovial Giant-Cell Tumor (Giant-Cell Tumor of Tendon Sheath)

Localized tenosynovial giant-cell tumors (giant-cell tumors of tendon sheath) occur most commonly in the hands of women (ages 30 to 50) (Fig. 18–14). The localized form is generally cured by local excision, but up to 20% of lesions may recur. The diffuse form is often locally aggressive but should be regarded as a benign tumor. Therapy should be directed at maintaining function with removal of as much of the lesion as possible.

Focal Myositis

Focal myositis is a benign inflammatory pseudotumor of skeletal muscle of children and adults that typically occurs in the lower extremity, evolving as a painful localized swelling over a period of weeks.[53, 54] At operation, the lesion appears as a pale mass poorly demarcated from the surrounding skeletal muscle. The etiology of this lesion remains obscure. These tumors are unrelated to polymyositis, and a history of trauma is typically lacking. Recurrences have not been reported following local excision.

MISCELLANEOUS LESIONS—MALIGNANT

Synovial Sarcoma

Synovial sarcomas represent about 10% of all sarcomas and arise most commonly in the deep soft tissues of the lower extremities of young adults (Fig. 18–15). There is a

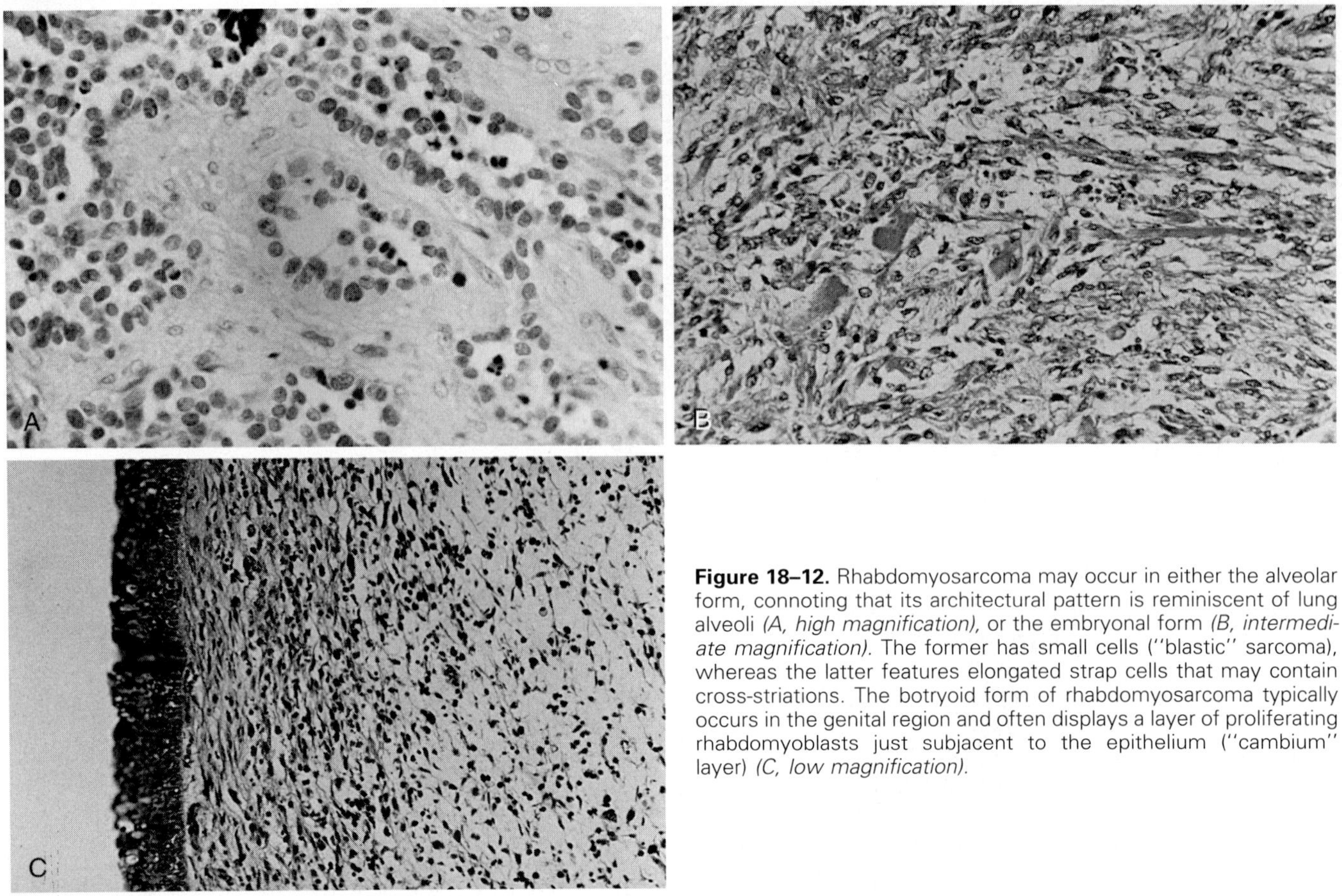

Figure 18–12. Rhabdomyosarcoma may occur in either the alveolar form, connoting that its architectural pattern is reminiscent of lung alveoli *(A, high magnification)*, or the embryonal form *(B, intermediate magnification)*. The former has small cells ("blastic" sarcoma), whereas the latter features elongated strap cells that may contain cross-striations. The botryoid form of rhabdomyosarcoma typically occurs in the genital region and often displays a layer of proliferating rhabdomyoblasts just subjacent to the epithelium ("cambium" layer) *(C, low magnification)*.

slight male predominance. The name is a misnomer; neither does the tumor arise from synovium nor do its cells share features with normal synovial cells. The name synovial sarcoma was chosen decades ago to highlight the superficial microscopic similarities between this tumor and developing synovium.

Synovial sarcoma consists of a biphasic tumor with sharply contrasting gland-forming (epithelial) areas and spindle-cell areas reminiscent of fibrosarcoma (Fig. 18–16). Some tumors lack the epithelial component and are designated as the monophasic fibrous type.[55] A characteristic translocation is seen in synovial sarcoma [t(x;18) (q11;q11)].

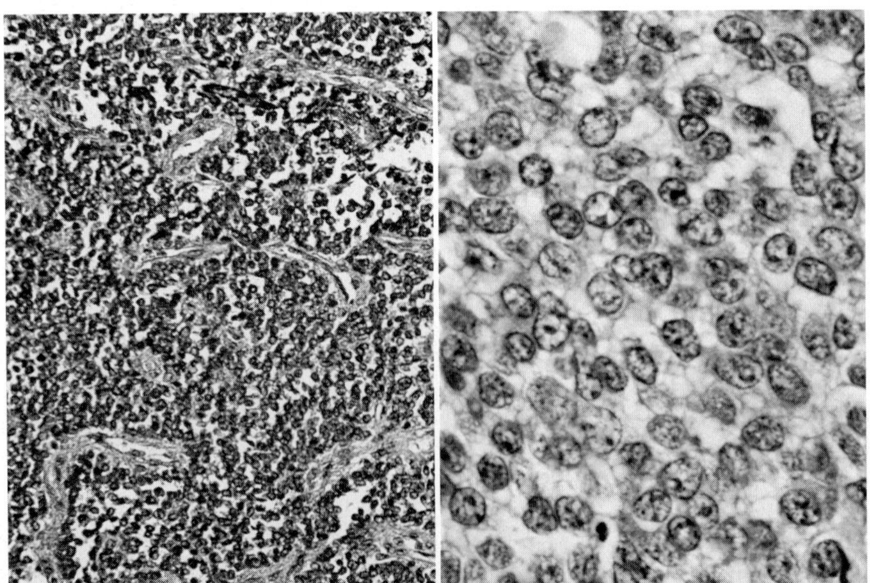

Figure 18–13. Ewing's sarcoma is the prototype of "small round-cell tumors" featuring nests of uniform cells *(left side, low magnification)* with scant cytoplasm, inconspicuous nucleoli, and a brisk mitotic rate *(right side, high magnification)*. These cells frequently contain abundant glycogen.

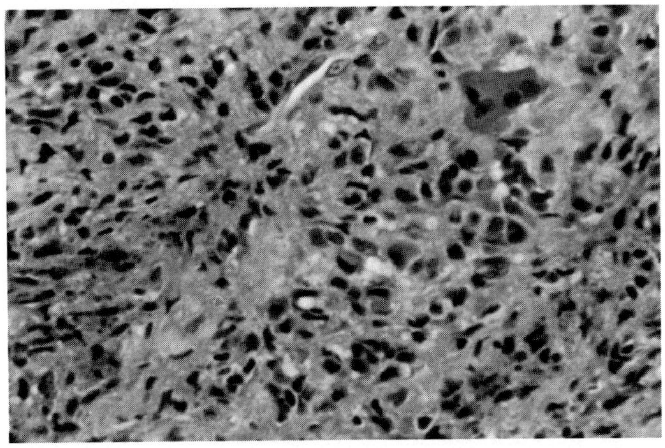

Figure 18–14. Giant-cell tumor of tendon sheath (tenosynovial giant-cell tumor). Although these are most common on the hands of women, they may occur in a variety of anatomic sites and are characterized by uniform rounded cells with eosinophilic cytoplasm with abundant hemosiderin deposition and varying numbers of cytologically bland multinucleated (giant) cells *(intermediate magnification).*

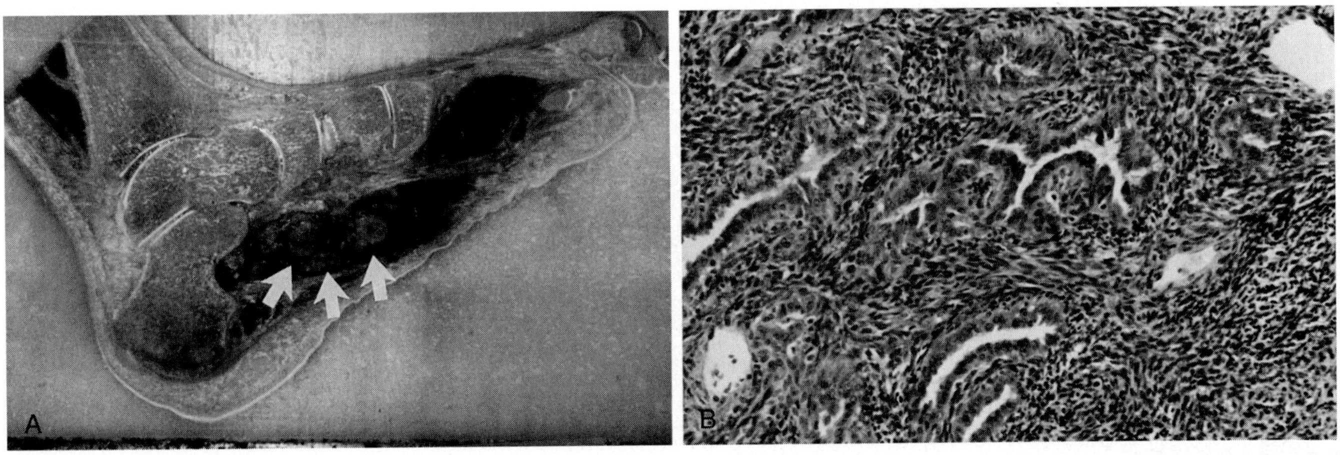

Figure 18–15. Synovial sarcoma. Although synovial sarcoma typically occurs in the extremities, as seen here, examples have been reported in the head and neck, retroperitoneum, mediastinum, and abdominal wall. *A,* Gross specimen. Note the apparent circumscription of the nodules in this example *(arrows).* Contrary to implications of its name, this tumor type does not arise from normal synovial sites. Synovial sarcoma may occur as a monophasic fibrous type, which lacks the epithelial elements, or in its classic biphasic form, which contains both glandular elements and malignant spindle cells *(B, intermediate magnification).*

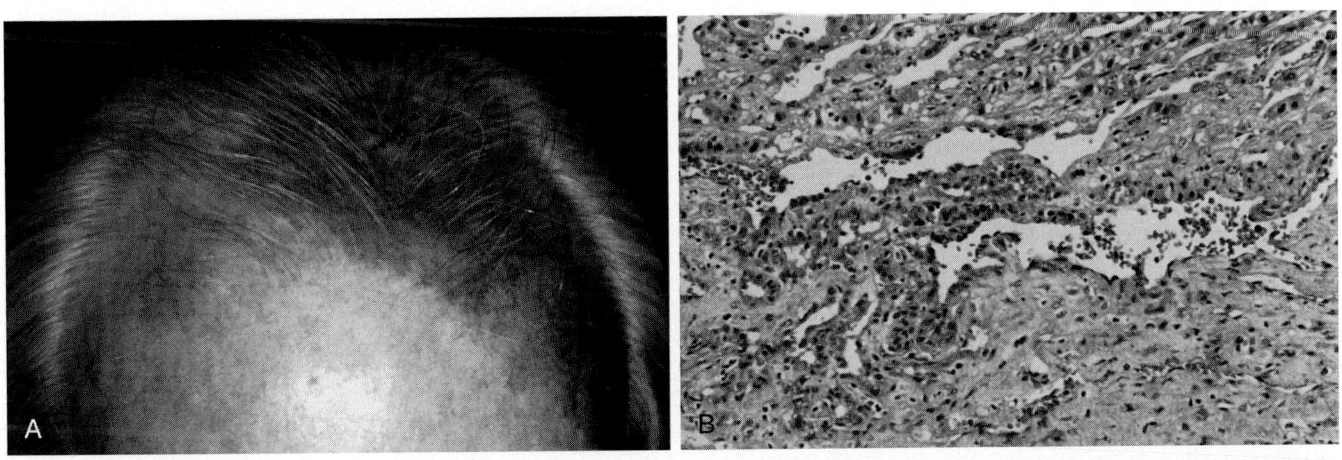

Figure 18–16. Angiosarcoma of scalp; *A,* clinical appearance. Angiosarcomas arise most commonly in the head and neck region of elderly individuals and typically appear as ill-defined purplish mottling. A number of well-documented possible etiologic associations are known. These include a variety of chemical compounds (vinyl chloride, thorium dioxide, arsenic), chronic lymphedema, prior therapeutic irradiation, foreign bodies, neurofibromatosis, and certain dermatologic conditions. (Photograph courtesy of Dr. Yernon Sondak.) Angiosarcoma—*B,* microscopic appearance *(intermediate magnification)* shows poorly formed, dilated neoplastic vascular spaces lined by atypically large, pleomorphic endothelium.

In most cases, both the epithelial elements and the spindle cells are reactive with antibodies directed against several epithelial antigens,[56] although staining is typically focal in the spindled areas. Most grading schemes categorize all synovial sarcomas as high-grade lesions, but certain histologic features—such as low mitotic rates, prominent calcification and/or ossification, and prominent glandular component—have been associated with improved outcome.[57] For therapeutic purposes, these tumors still behave as high-grade soft tissue sarcomas and can metastasize to regional lymph nodes. Treatment should include wide excision or amputation and en bloc removal of regional lymph nodes where feasible. Radiation therapy has a role either preoperatively or postoperatively.

Clear-Cell Sarcoma

Also known as malignant melanomas of soft parts,[58] clear-cell sarcomas of tendons and aponeuroses typically occur in the distal lower extremities. Peak incidence is in the third decade. There is considerable histogenetic and morphologic overlap with malignant melanoma. Despite the overlap, every effort should be made to distinguish the two, since prognosis is vastly different. For example, an excellent prognosis would be anticipated for a 1-cm clear-cell sarcoma, whereas a melanoma the same size would be an ominous lesion.[59] A chromosomal translocation has been demonstrated that distinguishes clear-cell sarcomas from melanoma. More than three quarters of clear-cell sarcomas have a translocation of chromosomes 12 and 22 [t(12;22)(q13-14;q12)].[60] Like synovial sarcoma, rhabdomyosarcoma, and epithelioid sarcoma, clear-cell sarcoma often metastasizes to lymph nodes. Surgical resection with adjuvant radiation is the most effective treatment.

Epithelioid Sarcoma

Epithelioid sarcomas most commonly occur in the hands and forearms of young adults (third decade). They frequently involve aponeuroses and tendon sheaths, producing multinodular masses that may ulcerate.[61, 62] The histology of epithelioid sarcoma may be deceptively bland. Epithelioid sarcomas have recurred in over two thirds of reported cases and have been lethal in about one third. Lymph node metastases are common. Early, aggressive surgical intervention with radiation therapy offers the best chance for cure.[63]

Conclusion

The treatment of STT is a multidisciplinary exercise that presupposes close cooperation between surgery, pathology, medical oncology, and other disciplines. It is the responsibility of the pathologist to be as accurate as possible regarding the histologic type, tumor grade, and adequacy of excision. It is the responsibility of the surgeon to provide adequate biopsy material and pertinent clinical information to the pathologist and to assure that staging studies are carried out in a systematic and thorough fashion. Any surgeon who chooses to participate in the care of patients with STT must have an appreciation for the nuances of proper biopsy techniques and the vagaries of the lesions that may be encountered.

PITFALLS FOR THE SURGEON

1. Poor biopsy site planning.
2. Inadequate prebiopsy or preoperative evaluation and staging.
3. Sampling only necrotic or sclerotic tissues on biopsy.
4. Failure to provide appropriate clinical information to the pathologist.

PITFALLS FOR THE PATHOLOGIST

1. Mistaking pseudosarcomas for sarcomas and vice versa.
2. Mistaking fibromatoses for low-grade sarcomas and vice versa.
3. Interpreting spindle-cell carcinomas/melanomas/lymphomas as sarcomas.
4. Misinterpreting immunohistochemical stains (e.g., aberrant expression of antigens, unusual patterns of cross-reactivity, technical complications).

FURTHER READING

Brennan MF. The James Ewing lecture. *Arch Surg* 1992;127:1290–1293.

Enzinger FM, Weiss SW. *Soft Tissue Tumors,* 2nd ed. St. Louis: Mosby; 1988.

Kraybill WG, Emami B, Lyss AP. Management of soft tissue tumors of the extremities. *Surgery.* 1991;109:233–235.

REFERENCES

1. Enzinger FM, Weiss SW. *Soft Tissue Tumors,* 2nd ed. St. Louis: Mosby; 1988.
2. Robinson E, Neugut AI, Wylie P. Clinical aspects of postirradiation sarcomas. *J Natl Cancer Inst.* 1988;80:233–240.
3. Laskin WB, Silverman TA, Enzinger FM. Postradiation soft tissue sarcomas: An analysis of 53 cases. *Cancer.* 1988;62:2330–2340.
4. Li FP, Fraumeni JF, Mulvhill JJ, et al. A cancer family syndrome in 24 kindreds. *Cancer Res.* 1988;48:5358–5362.
5. Malkin D, Li FP, Strong LC, et al. Germ line p53 mutations in a familial syndrome of breast cancer, sarcomas, and other neoplasms. Science 1990;250:1233–1238.
6. Suit HD, Mankin HJ, Wood WC, et al. Treatment of the patients with stage M_0 soft tissue sarcoma. *J Clin Oncol*: 1988;6:854–862.
7. Ross JA, Severson RK, Davis S, Brooks JJ. Trends in the incidence of soft tissue sarcomas in the United States from 1973 through 1987. *Cancer.* 1993;72:486–490.
8. Mankin HJ, Lange TA, Spanier SS. The hazards of the biopsy in patients with malignant primary bone and soft tissue tumors. *J Bone Joint Surg.* 1982;64A:1121–1127.
9. Kraybill WG, Emami B, Lyss AP. Management of soft tissue tumors of the extremities. *Surgery.* 1991;109:233–235.
10. Brennan MF. The James Ewing lecture. *Arch Surg.* 1992;127:1290–1293.
11. Bland KI, McCoy DM, Kinard RE, Copeland EM III. Application of magnetic resonance imaging and computerized tomography as an adjunct to the surgical management of soft tissue sarcomas. *Ann Surg.* 1987;205:473–481.
12. Fletcher JA, Kozakewich HP, Hoffer FA, et al. Diagnostic relevance of clonal cytogenetic aberrations in malignant soft tissue tumors. *N Engl J Med.* 1991;323:436–443.
13. Beahrs OH, Henson DE, Hutter RVP, Myers MH, eds. *American Joint Committee on Cancer: Manual for Staging of Cancer,* 3rd ed. Philadelphia: Lippincott; 1988.
14. Enneking WF, Spanier SS, Goodman MA. A system for the surgical staging of musculoskeletal sarcoma. *Clin Orthop.* 1980;153:106–120.
15. Costa J, Wesley RA, Glatstein E, Rosenberg SA. The grading of soft tissue sarcomas: Results of a clinicopathologic correlation in a series of 163 cases. *Cancer.* 1984;53:530–541.
16. Hashimoto H, Daimaru Y, Takeshita S, et al. Prognostic significance of histologic parameters of soft tissue sarcomas. *Cancer.* 1992;70:2816–2822.
17. Suit HD, Mankin JH, Schiller AL, et al. Staging system for sarcoma of soft tissue and bone. *Cancer Treat Symp.* 1985;3:29–36.
18. Weiss SW. *Histological Typing of Soft Tissue Tumors,* 2nd ed. *In* Sobin LH (ed): World Health Organization Series of International Histological Classification of Tumours. Berlin: Springer-Verlag; 1994.
19. Montgomery EA, Meis JM. Nodular fasciitis: Its morphologic spectrum and immunohistochemical profile. *Am J Surg Pathol.* 1991;15:942–948.
20. Bridge JA, Sreekantaiah C, Mouron B, et al. Clonal chromosomal abnormalities in desmoid tumors: Implications for histopathogenesis. *Cancer.* 1992;69:430–436.
21. Burke AP, Sobin LH, Shekitka KM. Mesenteric fibromatosis: A follow-up study. *Arch Pathol Lab Med* 1990;114:832–835.
22. McPeak CJ, Cruz T, Nicastri AD. Dermatofibrosarcoma protuberans: An analysis of 86 cases—Five with metastases. *Ann Surg.* 1967;166:803–816.
23. Connelly JH, Evans HL. Dermatofibrosarcoma protuberans: A clinicopathological review with emphasis on fibrosarcomatous areas. *Am J Surg Pathol.* 1992;16:921–925.
24. Brabant B, Revol M, Vergote T, et al. Dermatofibrosarcoma protuberans of the chest and shoulder: Wide and deep excisions with immediate reconstruction. *Plast Reconstr Surg.* 1993;92:459–462.
25. Hruza JG. Mohs micrographic surgery. *Otolaryngol Clin North Am.* 1990;23:854–864.
26. Kraybill W, Emami B, Lyss AP. Use of Mohs' micrographic surgery in management of soft tissue sarcomas (letter). *Surgery.* 1992;111:718–719.
27. Mark RJ, Bailet JW, Tran LM, et al. Dermatofibrosarcoma protuberans of the head and neck: A report of 16 cases. *Arch Otolaryngol Head Neck Surg.* 1993;119:891–896.
28. Pritchard DJ, Reiman HM, Turcotte RE, Ilstrup DM. Malignant fibrous histiocytoma of the soft tissues of the trunk and extremities. *Clin Orthop Rel Res.* 1993;289:58–65.
29. Mandahl N, Hoglund M, Mertens F, et al. Cytogenetic aberrations in 188 benign and borderline adipose tissue tumors. *Genes Chromosom Cancer.* 1994;9:207–215.
30. Enzinger FM, Harvey DA. Spindle cell lipoma. *Cancer.* 1975;36:1852–1859.
31. Shmookler BM, Enzinger FM. Pleomorphic lipoma: A benign tumor simulating liposarcoma: A clinicopathologic analysis of 48 cases. *Cancer.* 198;47:126–133.
32. Chung EB, Enzinger FM. Benign lipoblastomatosis: An analysis of 35 cases. *Cancer.* 1973;32:482–492.
33. Evans HL. Liposarcoma: A study of 55 cases with a reassessment of its classification. *Am J Surg Pathol.* 1979;3:507–523.
34. Weiss SW, Rao V. Well-differentiated liposarcoma (atypical lipoma) of deep soft tissue of the extremities, retroperitoneum, and miscellaneous sites: A follow-up study of 92 cases with analysis of the incidence of "dedifferentiation." *Am J Surg Pathol.* 1992;16:1051–1058.
35. Azumi N, Curtis J, Kempson RL, et al. Atypical and malignant neoplasms showing lipomatous differentiation. *Am J Surg Pathol.* 1987;11:161–183.
36. Woodruff JM, Marshall ML, Godwin TA, et al. Plexiform (multinodular) schwannoma: A tumor simulating the plexiform neurofibroma. *Am J Surg Pathol.* 1983;7:691.
37. National Institutes of Health Consensus Development Conference. Neurofibromatosis: Conference statement. *Arch Neurol.* 1988;45:575–578.
38. Erlandson RA, Woodruff JM. Peripheral nerve sheath tumors: An electron microscopic study of 43 cases. *Cancer.* 1982;49:273–287.
39. Woodruff JM, Chernik NL, Smith MC, et al. Peripheral nerve sheath tumors with rhabdomyosarcomatous differentiation (malignant "triton" tumors). *Cancer.* 1973;32:426–439.
40. Hruban RH, Shiu MH, Senic RT, Woodruff JM. Malignant peripheral nerve sheath tumors of the buttock and lower extremity. *Cancer.* 1990;66:1253–1265.
41. Wile AG, Evans HL, Romsdahl MM. Leiomyosarcoma of soft tissue: A clinicopathologic study. *Cancer.* 1981;48:1022–1032.
42. Joshi VV, Cantor AB, Altshuler G, et al. Age-linked prognostic categorization based on a new histologic grading system of neuroblastoma. *Cancer.* 1992;69:2197–2211.
43. Brodeur GM, Azar C, Brother M, et al. Neuroblastoma: Effect of genetic factors on prognosis and treatment. *Cancer.* 1992;70:1685–1694.
44. Brodeur GM, Seeger RC, Schwab M, et al. Amplification of N-*myc* in untreated human neuroblastoma correlates with advanced disease stage. *Science.* 1984;224:1121–1124.
45. Phillips WS, Stafford PW, Duvol-Arnold B. Neuroblastoma and the clinical significance of N-*myc* oncogene amplification. *Surg Obstet Gynecol.* 1991;172:73–80.
46. Shimada H, Chatten J, Newton WA, et al. Histopathologic prognostic factors in neuroblastic tumors: Definition of subtypes of ganglioneuroblastoma and an age linked classification. *J Natl Cancer Inst.* 1984;73:405–416.
47. Newton WA, Soule EH, Hamoundi AB, et al. Histopathology of childhood sarcomas: Intergroup rhabdomyosarcoma studies I and II: clinicopathologic correlation. *J Clin Oncol.* 1988;6:67–75.
48. Rodary C, Gehan EA, Flamant F, et al. Prognostic factors in 951 nonmetastatic rhabdomyosarcomas in children: A report from the intergroup rhabdomyosarcoma workshop. *Med Pediatr Oncol.* 1991;19:89–95.
49. Hays DM. Rhabdomyosarcoma. *Clin Orthop Rel Res.* 1993;289:36–49.
50. Angervall L, Enzinger FM. Extraskeletal neoplasm resembling Ewing's sarcoma. *Cancer.* 1975;36:240–251.
51. Askin FB, Rosai J, Sibley RK, et al. Malignant small cell tumor of

the thoracopulmonary region in childhood: A distinctive clinicopathologic entity of uncertain histogenesis. *Cancer.* 1979;43:2438–2451.
52. Dehner LP. Primitive neuroectodermal tumor and Ewing's sarcoma. *Am J Surg Pathol.* 1993;17:1–13.
53. Heffner RR, Armbrustmacher VW, Earle KM. Focal myositis. *Cancer.* 1977;40:301–306.
54. Heffner RR, Barron SA. Denervating changes in focal myositis, a benign inflammatory pseudotumor. *Arch Pathol Lab Med.* 1980;104:261–264.
55. Evans HL. Synovial sarcoma: A study of 23 biphasic and 17 probable monophasic examples. *Pathol Annu.* 1980;15:309–331.
56. Ordonez NG, Mahfouz SM, Mackay B. Synovial sarcoma: An immunohistochemical and ultrastructural study. *Hum Pathol.* 1990;21:733–749.
57. Cagle LA, Mirra JM, Storm K, et al. Histologic features relating to prognosis in synovial sarcoma. *Cancer.* 1987;59:1810–1814.
58. Enzinger FM. Clear cell sarcoma of tendons and aponeuroses: An analysis of 21 cases. *Cancer.* 1965;18:1163–1174.
59. Montgomery EA, Meis JM, Ramos AG, et al. Clear cell sarcoma of tendons and aponeuroses: A clinicopathologic study of 58 cases with analysis of prognostic factors. *Int J Surg Pathol.* 1993;1:89–100.
60. Fletcher JA. Translocation (12;22) (q13-14;q12) is a nonrandom aberration in soft tissue clear cell sarcoma. *Genes Chromosom Cancer.* 1992;5:184.
61. Chase DR, Enzinger FM. Epithelioid sarcoma: Diagnosis, prognostic indicators, and treatment. *Am J Surg Pathol.* 1985;9:241 263.
62. Chase DR, Enzinger FM, Weiss SW, Langloss JM. Keratin in epithelioid sarcoma: An immunohistochemical study. *Am J Surg Pathol.* 1984;8:435–441.
63. Evans HL, Baer SC. Epithelioid sarcoma: A clinicopathologic and prognostic study of 26 cases. *Semin Diagn Pathol.* 1993;10:286–291.

19

Tumors and Tumorlike Conditions of Bones and Joints

Michael G. Rock and Krishnan K. Unni

Definition

Bone lesions cause anxiety among surgeons for two reasons. First, there is minimal experience with such conditions during residency. Second, bone lesions are relatively infrequent even in specialized orthopedic practice and rare in general surgical practice. Most tumors occurring in patients less than 20 years old will prove to be benign conditions of cartilage (osteochondromas and enchondromas), fibrous tissue (metaphyseal fibrous defects), or benign cysts (solitary or unicameral bone cysts).[1] In contrast, most bone lesions in patients older than 40 years are due to metastatic tumors.[2–4]

It is estimated that cancer will be diagnosed in 1 million Americans this year.[5] Approximately 50% of these patients will manifest metastatic disease at some point in their clinical course. After lung and liver, bone is the third most common site for metastasis.[6] About half of newly diagnosed cancers in the United States are tumors that commonly metastasize to bone. These include tumors of breast, lung, prostate, kidney, and thyroid.[7] Of the expected 150,000 patients who develop bony metastases, approximately 5 to 8% will experience pathologic fracture requiring fixation. This translates as 8,000 to 12,000 pathologic fractures that will require surgical intervention for stabilization or replacement—and this number does not include the patients in whom biopsy is performed only to confirm metastatic disease.

When these figures are compared with the annual national incidence of primary malignant bone tumors—3,000—it is clear that surgeons are far more likely to encounter metastatic disease of bone than a primary malignancy. On the average, a practicing orthopedic surgeon sees a case of osteosarcoma once every 10 years, a chondrosarcoma once every 15 years, and Ewing's sarcoma once every 25 years. Inappropriate management of these rare primary tumors can be both limb- and life-threatening.

Unlike patients with metastatic bone disease, who have limited life expectancy, patients with primary tumors (if treated appropriately) may be cured of underlying disease. It is therefore critical to recognize the patient with a primary bone tumor. This is accomplished by a careful, logical, and cost-conscious diagnostic strategy that minimizes inappropriate management of patients with primary bone malignancy and affords optimal care of patients with metastatic disease.

Clinical Assessment

HISTORY

Pertinent patient historical information includes age, date of onset and duration of symptoms, severity of pain, and presence of concomitant constitutional symptoms. Since primary malignant bone tumors occur over a finite age distribution, the patient's age is an important diagnostic feature. Most primary malignant conditions of bone occur before the age of 20 years (Table 19–1). Therefore, an aggressive and a progressive lesion of bone in this age

Table 19–1. Age as a Diagnostic Factor in Bone Tumors

Age 20 or Below	Age 20–60	Age 60 or Above
Osteochondroma	Giant-cell tumor	Lymphoma
Aneurysmal bone cyst	Hemangioma	Myeloma
Simple cyst	Hemangioendothelioma	Metastases
Chondroblastoma	Infection	Paget's disease
Histiocytosis X	Hyperparathyroidism	
Infection	Lymphoma	
Osteosarcoma	Fibrosarcoma	
Ewing's sarcoma	Chondrosarcoma	
Leukemia		

group should be presumed to be a primary malignancy. A similar lesion in an older patient is much more likely to be metastatic disease, particularly if there is a history of prior malignancy. In the latter case additional bone involvement and underlying primary malignancy should be sought.[8, 9] Symptoms that suggest malignancy include severe, often nocturnal pain and the relatively short duration of symptoms—in weeks, rarely in months. Constitutional symptoms—including malaise, weight loss, and fever without known cause—point to an aggressive lesion. Furthermore, patients experiencing primary bone malignancy, particularly malignancy involving the appendicular skeleton, complain of rapid swelling and warmth, along with decreased function. This finding is due to pain, weakness, and decreased motion of the contiguous joints.[10]

PHYSICAL EXAMINATION

Physical examination reveals localized discomfort; warmth overlying the area of involvement; decreased motion of contiguous joints; pain with movement; and decreased function caused by pain, weakness, or even neurologic involvement. Because of the rapid evolution of primary bone tumors, extraosseous soft tissue extension with distortion of surrounding soft tissue architecture is common. The presence of a hard, fixed mass that is attached to the underlying bone, generally associated with greater warmth and superficial venous dilatation, suggests an aggressive process that is probably malignant. Lesions in the appendicular skeleton are detected earlier than those in the pelvis or trunk. This is due to the extra volume within the pelvis and to the retroperitoneal regions that are available to accommodate the expanding tumor. An example is Ewing's sarcoma, which can reach huge dimensions in such sites before becoming clinically evident to the patient and the physician.

Radiating pain with a burning quality suggests primary malignancy.[11] Because other symptoms bring the patient to medical attention before tumor progression occurs, arterial supply is usually spared.

In contrast, patients with metastatic disease have a boring, dull, unrelenting discomfort in the involved area but rarely manifest the additional local symptoms as mentioned. Of the five organs from which tumors commonly metastasize to bone, three are accessible to palpation; these are the thyroid, breast, and prostate.

LABORATORY ANALYSIS

A few laboratory tests provide useful diagnostic information. These include serum protein electrophoresis in patients suspected of having multiple myeloma; prostate-specific antigen determination in patients suspected or known to have disseminated prostate cancer; and serum parathyroid hormone level in patients in whom the radiographic features and serum calcium levels suggest hyperparathyroidism. Alkaline phosphatase level is also elevated in many of these lesions, although dramatic elevations are associated only with osteosarcoma and Paget's disease.

Imaging

The most useful diagnostic test may be plain radiography.[12] The advances made in diagnostic imaging during the past 10 to 15 years allow the clinician and surgeon to investigate the lesion thoroughly, permitting accurate diagnosis in 85 to 90% of cases; however, cost-containment considerations place the responsibility on the surgeon to limit investigations to those needed for identification of the lesion's nature. The selection of radiographic imaging techniques performed is dictated by the clinical history, physical findings, and laboratory results. Plain radiographs, when obtained in two planes at right angles to each other, define the anatomic localization, intraosseous extent, distortion of surrounding soft tissue planes, margination of the tumor with the host, and periosteal reaction. Tumors of bone have a very distinct predilection to involve certain anatomic sites of long bones (Table 19–2).

One of the more discriminating features on plain radiography is margination with the host bone. Sharp delineations, sclerotic borders, and lack of periosteal reactions suggest a benign process. Conversely, permeative appearance suggests rapid tumor progression that has left islands of entrapped viable bone. This feature is more consistent with a malignant process. Scalloping of the endosteal surface of cortical bone suggests eccentric growth in a lobular fashion, a common feature in tumors of cartilage, fat, and vascular origin. Slow evolution of a tumor results in deposition of a homogeneous mass of new bone, as that seen with osteomyelitis or osteoid osteoma (Fig. 19–1). Rapid evolution of tumor growth and expansion causes lamination or "onionskinning" of the periosteum, with formation of Codman's triangle at its juncture with the soft tissue (Fig. 19–2). This finding is common in osteosarcoma and Ewing's sarcoma.

Further imaging is indicated to determine extent of dis-

Table 19–2. Site as a Diagnostic Factor in Bone Tumors

Epiphysis	Metaphysis	Diaphysis
Giant-cell tumor	Chondromyxoid fibroma	Hemangioma
Chondroblastoma	Aneurysmal bone cyst	Adamantinoma
Clear-cell chondrosarcoma	Unicameral bone cyst	Ewing's sarcoma
	Infection	Paget's disease
Hyperparathyroidism	Osteosarcoma	Lymphoma
	Lymphoma	Myeloma
	Metastases	Metastases

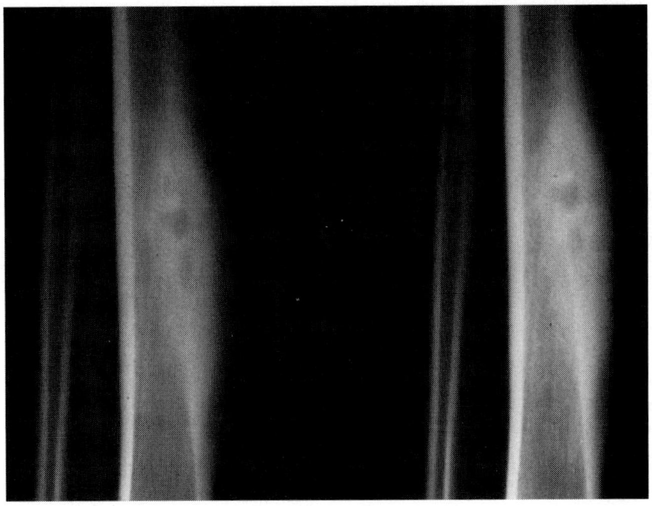

Figure 19–1. Typical mature cortical hypertrophy surrounding intracortical nidus of osteoid osteoma in an 18-year-old man.

ease and additional areas of involvement when evaluating metastatic disease, hyperparathyroidism, Paget's disease, eosinophilic granuloma, or fibrous dysplasia. Bone scintigraphy identifies other areas of involvement and facilitates biopsy site selection.[13–18] Although bone scintigraphy is a highly sensitive test, it has low specificity. In rare cases, activity is decreased at the anticipated site of bone involvement. This pattern is observed in patients who have multiple myeloma and patients who are cachectic and thereby incapable of concentrating tracer.

Computed tomography (CT) and magnetic resonance imaging (MRI) have virtually replaced plain tomography, ultrasonography, and arteriography. Arteriography still is used for therapeutic embolization of highly vascular tumors such as myeloma and metastatic hypernephroma before biopsy or fixation.[19, 20] Conventional tomography confirms the benign nature of cystic lesions. In some cartilaginous lesions, it also assesses endosteal surface scalloping.[21]

The advantage of CT is its better resolution of mineralized or ossified tissue (Fig. 19–3),[22, 23] particularly of mineralization within cartilage lesions such as enchondromas or chondrosarcomas. Computed tomography also better defines lesions that produce ossification, such as osteoblastomas, osteoid osteomas, osteomyelitis, and osteosarcomas. Furthermore, it accurately determines the integrity of the cortex, which even in benign aggressive lesions, such as giant-cell tumor and aneurysmal bone cyst, may be disrupted by the underlying intramedullary process. Aneurysmal bone cysts have thin cortical shells that are often diagnostic of the underlying process and are easily detected on CT. With careful review of axial cuts, intraosseous extent of tumor and its association with adjacent structures can be determined. Undoubtedly, CT is the imaging method of choice to determine chest metastases in patients with primary malignant tumors of bone[24, 25] and in those with a unifocal metastatic deposit of unknown origin.[26, 27] The resolution of CT is superior to that of conventional tomography for identifying suspected nodules within the lungs.

Magnetic resonance imaging has revolutionized the management of patients with bone tumors. The ability to image in multiple planes—including sagittal, coronal, axial, and even oblique—allows accurate determination of local disease. This is accomplished by weighting the image to contrast the tumor and the adjacent tissue. This practice allows greater appreciation of the tumor's margination with the host, its proximity to important vital structures, the intramedullary extent of the tumor, and the presence of skip lesions in areas of the same bone remote from the principal site of involvement (Fig. 19–2*D* and *E*).[28–30] Furthermore, joint involvement and epiphyseal extension can be more accurately determined by MRI than CT. Finally, the beam-hardening artifacts seen on CT around metallic devices are less apparent with MRI. As a consequence, MRI is the method of choice for follow-up of the patient who has had local resection or management for primary disease with metallic implant.

Magnetic resonance imaging has the unique ability to distinguish scar tissue, blood, and seroma. For this reason, it is the imaging tool of choice to follow patients in whom major resections and reconstructions have occurred and in whom these lesions might mimic recurrence on CT. General criteria suggesting malignancy on MRI include a large lesion (more than 5 cm), an absence of capsule, an invasion of contiguous structures, a nonhomogeneous signal, necrosis (with or without calcification), and a marked signal enhancement on T_2-weighted images.[28]

The obvious disadvantages of MRI include the inability to image patients with pacemakers and those with other forms of ferromagnetic substances. Approximately 10% of patients are claustrophobic and cannot tolerate the time needed, enclosure, and noise accompanying MRI techniques. These techniques may also exaggerate the intramedullary extent of tumor because of tumor-induced edema.

In summary, MRI is superior for demonstrating intraosseous and extraosseous tumor extension, tumor necrosis, and interface between tumor and normal tissue, and for detecting local recurrence. Computed tomography is superior for identifying cortical destruction, calcification, and ossification and for determining the presence or absence of chest metastases.[29] Neither CT nor MRI can predict the histogenesis or the aggressiveness of the process imaged.[31] For such information, pathology is needed.

Biopsy

Besides clinically and radiographically benign tumors and diffuse metastatic disease in patients with known primary lesions at no risk of fracture, most bone lesions require biopsy for histologic confirmation. Biopsies are often assumed to be innocuous procedures[32]; however, a review of patients who had poorly designed biopsies prior to referral to tertiary oncologic centers found results to the contrary.[33] The frequency of significant problems caused by inappropriate biopsy was 20%. At least 8% of biopsies done elsewhere produced a significant adverse effect on prognosis; 5% of biopsies precluded limb-sparing techniques. These figures underscore the need for cooperation and communication among surgeon, radiologist, and pa-

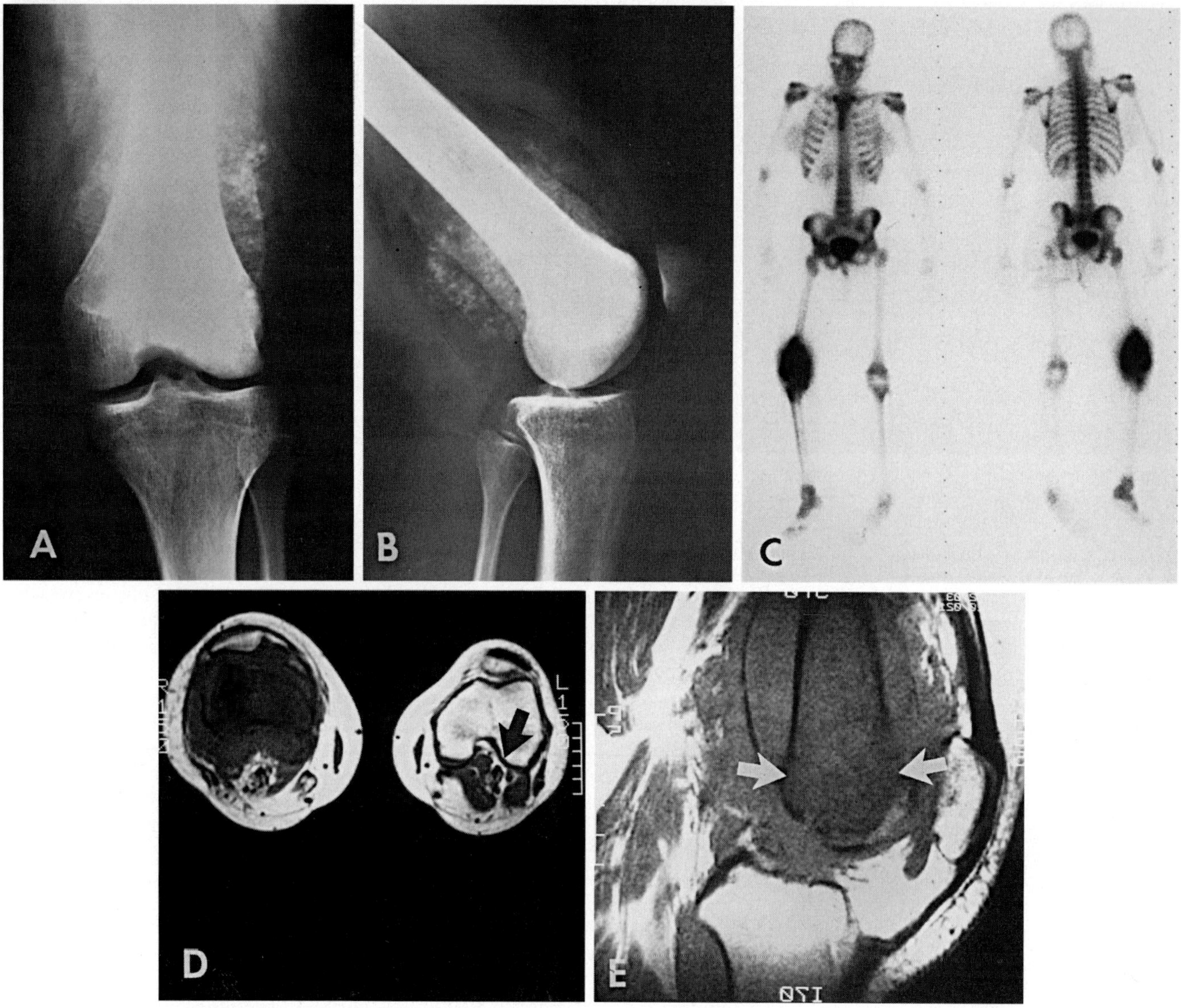

Figure 19–2. *A* and *B,* Dual plain radiographs of 15-year-old girl reveal typical appearance of a malignant aggressive metaphyseal lesion characterized by extensive intraosseous/extraosseous tumor involvement. Surrounding soft tissues are distorted by "sunburst" nature of tumor osteoid and brisk periosteal reaction by host. *C,* Bone scintigraphy reveals unifocal nature of lesion. Additionally, because of the hypervascularity, increased tracer is noted throughout the involved extremity *(left, anterior view; right, posterior view). D* and *E,* T1-weighted images in axial and sagittal planes exhibiting intraarticular *(black arrow)* and epiphyseal extension *(white arrows)* of high-grade osteoblastic osteosarcoma.

thologist to identify the ideal biopsy site on imaging studies before the biopsy is performed.

Since the definitive procedure and open biopsy may not be performed at the same time, the incision site should be placed so as to allow subsequent removal of the biopsy tract en bloc with the underlying tumor. The biopsy incision is in line with the direction of subcutaneous tissue, including muscle and neurovascular structures. For most extremity lesions, longitudinally oriented incisions are preferred. Sharp instruments are used to open the tumor capsule, and extensive dissection and the creation of large flaps are avoided. Generally, the biopsy should be muscle-splitting, with avoidance of interfascial planes. Controlled access to the tumor is obtained with the tourniquet inflated. When a diagnostic sample is obtained, it is deflated to allow coagulation of bleeding vessels.

The obvious advantage of an open biopsy is that sufficient diagnostic material is obtained. This is confirmed by the pathologist with intraoperative frozen section assessment of the specimen. In some cases a definitive diagnosis is possible on frozen section, which allows the surgeon to proceed to reconstructive options for most benign, metastatic, and myeloma lesions. Additionally, frozen section identifies tissue for additional studies using special markers (see Chap. 2). Furthermore, the pathologist can identify acute or granulomatous inflammation; the surgeon can then send additional specimens for cultures. Most open biopsies are incisional; however, in some circumstances, such as

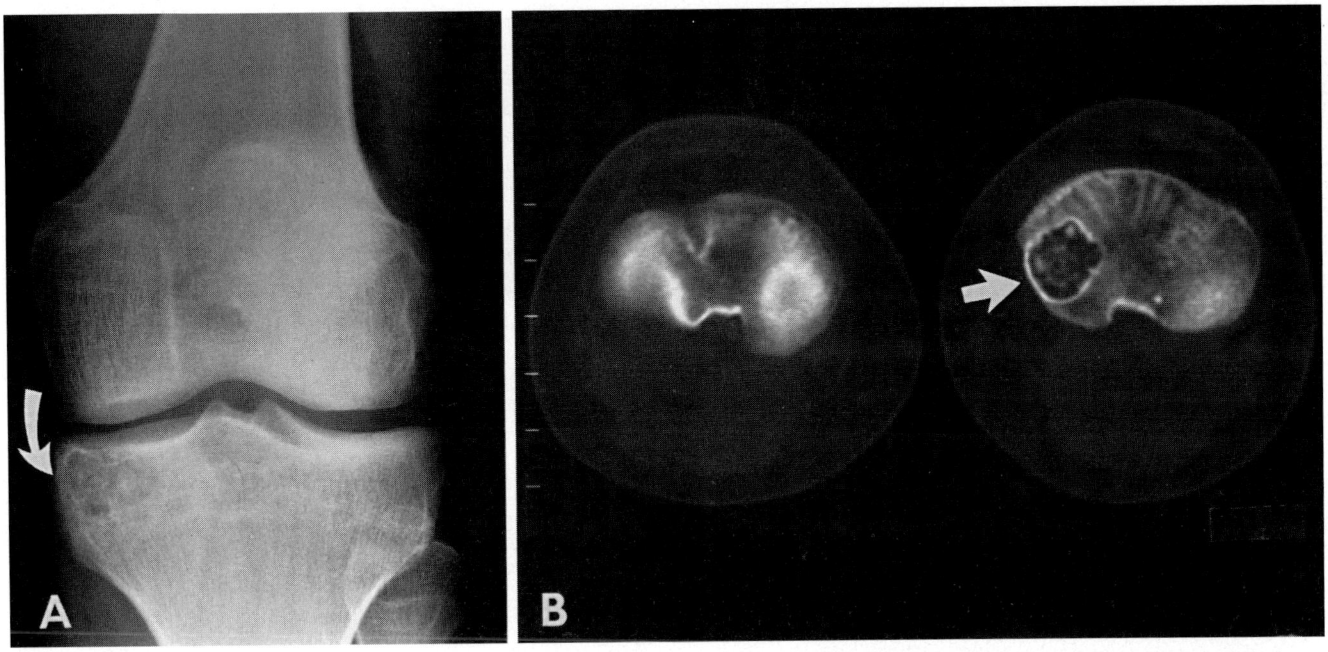

Figure 19–3. *A,* Eccentric epiphyseal lesion *(arrow)* in proximal tibia of a patient at skeletal maturity with progressive closure of epiphyseal plate. *B,* Computed tomography reveals a sclerotic rim separating the lesion *(arrow)* from the host bone and confirms the calcification within the lesion. The anatomic location, age, and radiographic appearance support chondroblastoma, a benign tumor.

an obvious clinical and radiographic low-grade malignant tumor, an excisional biopsy may be performed.

Closed percutaneous needle biopsies have gained popularity.[34–39] The obvious advantages of this technique are cost-effectiveness and no delay in subsequent treatment. It is useful for confirming metastatic disease, local recurrence, myeloma, and Ewing's sarcoma. The major disadvantages include a nondiagnostic aspirate (20%) and the possibility of local recurrence in the needle tract if not excised with the primary tumor (see Chap. 3).[40]

At the time of definitive excision of primary malignant tumors, soft tissue and intramedullary biopsies are performed to assess the adequacy of the margins. It is imperative that the surgeon accurately identify anatomic landmarks on the resected specimen and discuss areas of potential concern with the pathologist. This allows directed biopsy specimens to be evaluated.

Common Conditions of Bone

The following section discusses bone lesions in detail but is confined to the more common conditions of bone. The reader is referred to textbooks on bone tumors for more details on these and other conditions affecting bone.[1]

METASTATIC DISEASE

As previously mentioned, metastatic carcinoma is the commonest neoplasm affecting bone. Most patients with metastatic carcinoma are older adults. A bone lesion in an infant should raise the possibility of metastatic neuroblastoma. The presenting symptom may be bone pain or pathologic fracture. The metastasis may be single, or multiple bones may be involved. Most metastatic tumors involve the central portion of the skeleton, since this is the site of persistent bone marrow. For this reason, metastatic carcinoma is unusual distal to the knee and elbow joints.

Most patients with carcinoma metastatic to bone have a known primary lesion; however, this is not always the case. A small percentage of patients present with metastatic disease. The most common primary malignancies that occur as skeletal lesions are tumors of the lung, breast, prostate, and kidney. Nevertheless, a primary bone lesion is still possible and a biopsy is necessary.

The histologic appearance of the neoplasm may reveal the primary site. Some neoplasms, such as a hypernephroma, have characteristic findings. In most instances, however, a primary site can only be suspected. A high-grade adenocarcinoma of the lung may be identical to a high-grade adenocarcinoma of the gastrointestinal (GI) tract. Immunoperoxidase stains may also be helpful. For example, prostate-specific antigen and prostatic acid phosphatase confirm prostatic origin (see Chap. 2).

The diagnosis of metastatic carcinoma suggests a dismal prognosis; however, there is variation according to primary site. On one end of the spectrum is skeletal metastasis from lung carcinoma, which usually portends death within 6 months. Metastasis from a breast carcinoma may be associated with prolonged survival, especially if the carcinoma is sensitive to hormonal manipulation. If skeletal metastasis is the first sign of a hypernephroma, the prognosis is bleak. However, a skeletal metastasis developing in a patient who has already undergone treatment for hypernephroma may be associated with a long survival time. Whatever the prognosis may be, corrective management of the pathologic fracture or incipient fracture is important. Even if life expectancy is short, pain relief and restoration of function are still worthwhile.

MYELOMA

Myeloma is the commonest primary neoplasm of bone. Most cases are diagnosed by means of a bone marrow aspirate and only about a fifth occur clinically as bone tumors.

Bone pain is the most frequent symptom of myeloma. Patients may present with pathologic fractures. Spine involvement is commonly present, sometimes with cord compression. Patients may also present with systemic disease manifestations, such as weight loss and fatigue. Many patients with myeloma have hypercalcemia, and some hypercalcemic crisis. Laboratory tests usually show anemia, rouleaux formation in the peripheral smear, and increased erythrocyte sedimentation rate. A monoclonal protein can be identified in the serum, urine, or both in almost all patients with myeloma.

Roentgenograms typically show multiple, punched-out, purely lytic lesions in bones (Fig. 19–4). Myeloma is almost never associated with sclerosis. A small percentage of patients with myeloma present with diffuse osteopenia.

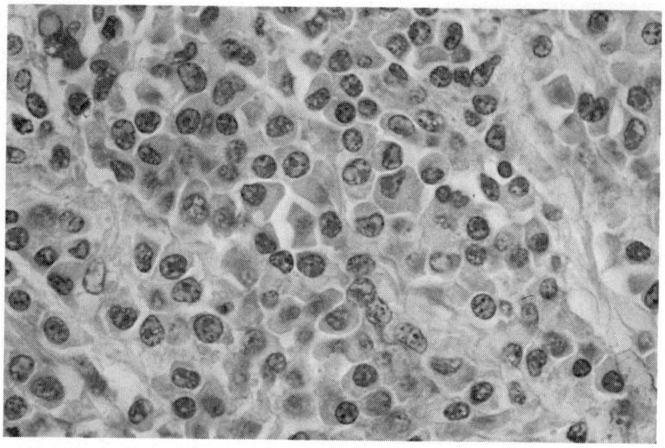

Figure 19–5. "Pure culture" appearance of plasma cells in myeloma. Nuclei are eccentric and there is abundant pink cytoplasm. Hematoxylin and eosin, ×40.

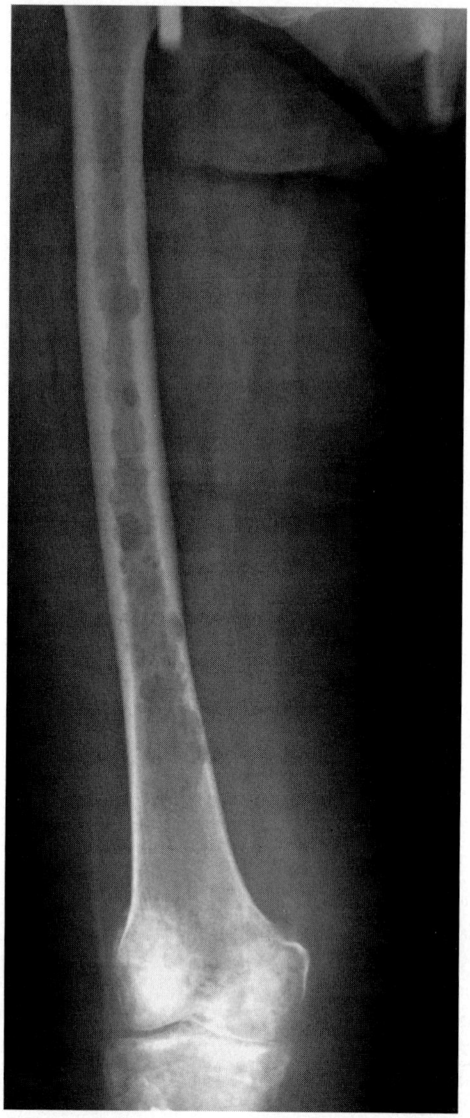

Figure 19–4. Roentgenogram showing multiple lytic areas in a patient with plasma-cell myeloma. There is no associated sclerosis.

Histologically, myeloma consists of sheets of plasma cells. In almost all cases, the plasma-cell nature of the neoplasm is obvious, at least focally (Fig. 19–5). The cells have abundant blue or pink cytoplasm and an eccentrically situated nucleus. The nucleus is round and has clumped chromatin. Double- or triple-nucleated cells are frequently found. Occasionally, the cells are so pleomorphic that the plasma-cell nature of a neoplasm is obscured. Approximately 10 to 15% of myelomas contain deposits of amyloid. The amyloid may be deposited in vessel walls or as masses between tumor cells. Amyloid appears as an amorphous pink material and may incite a giant-cell reaction.

Although most patients present with widespread involvement by multiple myeloma, a few have solitary plasmacytomas. These patients require an exhaustive workup before the diagnosis of solitary myeloma is established. They tend to be younger and may experience a protracted clinical course.[41] Eventually, most patients with solitary myeloma progress to multiple myeloma. The prognosis in multiple myeloma is generally poor. However, this has improved with the advent of chemotherapy. Local radiation is effective for dominant lesions.

MALIGNANT LYMPHOMA

Malignant lymphoma is unusual as a bone tumor; in the Mayo Clinic files, it represents approximately 7% of all malignant bone tumors. There is a slight male predominance, and the disease usually affects both young and old adults. Any portion of the skeleton can be affected, but bones with persisting marrow in them are more often involved. Patients usually present with bone pain or constitutional symptoms such as fever, weight loss, and anorexia. Spinal cord compression may be the clinical presentation of patients with involvement of the spine. Roentgenograms show a permeative, destructive lesion, usually involving the shaft of the bone. An isotopic bone scan is very sensitive for identifying areas involved by lymphoma. Magnetic

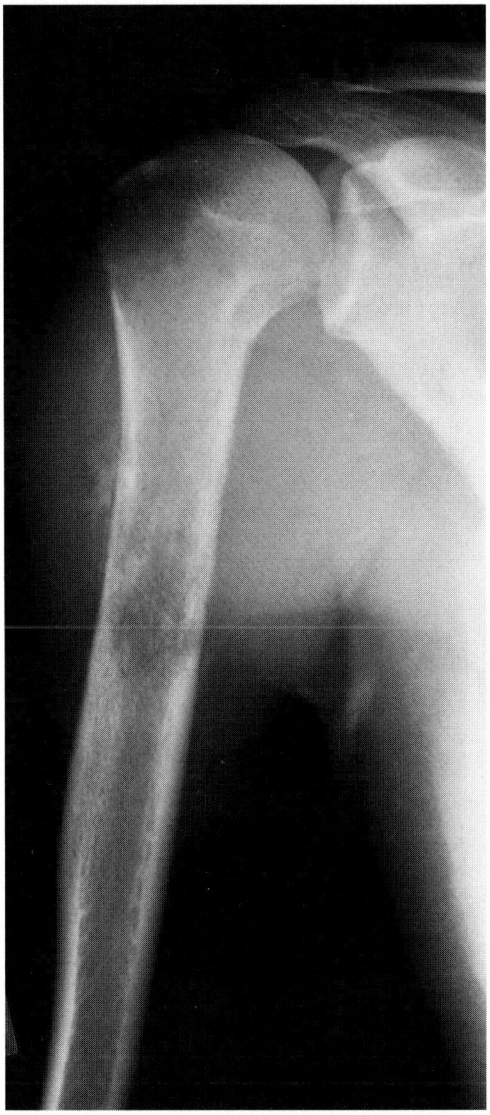

Figure 19–6. Ewing's tumor involving proximal humerus. There is a permeative destructive lesion with periosteal new bone formation.

resonance imaging may also show the lesion when plain roentgenograms do not.

The microscopic appearance of malignant lymphoma of bone varies. The classic appearance is a mixed lymphoid-cell infiltrate. This is accompanied by delicate fibrosis, which may result in a spindled appearance of the tumor cells. At low magnification, malignant lymphoma permeates normal structures such as bony trabeculae and marrow fat. Leukemic infiltrate, especially in a patient with chronic granulocytic leukemia, may occur as a destructive lesion of bone[42] and mimic large-cell lymphoma. Special stains for granulocytic differentiation allow recognition (see Chaps. 2 and 17). The subclassification of malignant lymphoma in bone may be difficult but is often assisted by special methods, such as immunohistochemistry (see Chap. 2). Accurate classification of lymphoma is needed for correct patient management (see Chap. 17). Even when precise classification is not possible, assignment of the process into major prognostic groupings of high, intermediate, or low grade can usually be achieved.

The stage of disease is the single most important prognostic factor for malignant lymphoma.[43] A patient with solitary involvement of a skeletal site, even with high-grade tumor, usually has a good prognosis. About one fifth of patients present with involvement of multiple skeletal sites but without involvement of liver, spleen, or lymph nodes. These patients tend to do well. By contrast, patients with involvement of both skeletal and nonskeletal sites generally do poorly. Therapy consists of radiation and/or chemotherapy. Surgery is indicated only if pathologic fracture is imminent.

EWING'S SARCOMA

Ewing's sarcoma is a rare primary malignant neoplasm of bone. In the Mayo Clinic files, it represents approximately 6% of all malignant bone tumors. The tumor is slightly more prevalent in males. Approximately half of all cases occur in the second decade of life. Ewing's sarcoma is unusual in persons younger than 5 years. Any portion of the skeleton may be involved, but about half of the cases involve the long bones, and the shafts are preferentially involved. Patients present with symptoms such as pain, fever, and malaise, which may lead to a misdiagnosis of osteomyelitis.

Roentgenograms show an extensive permeative lesion, which may involve the entire bone. Periosteal new bone formation is often seen and may have a characteristic "onionskin" pattern (Fig. 19–6). Grossly, Ewing's sarcoma is soft and fleshy, sometimes even liquefied and resembling pus, further supporting the mistaken impression of osteomyelitis. Such a mistake may delay diagnosis if tissue is not obtained for histologic analysis. For this reason, it is important to examine all cases of suspected osteomyelitis to avoid such an error.

The histologic features of classic Ewing's sarcoma are straightforward. The neoplasm is composed of uniform small round cells (Fig. 19–7). Special stains such as periodic acid-Schiff (PAS) with diastase resistance and electron microscopy usually demonstrate glycogen in the cytoplasm.

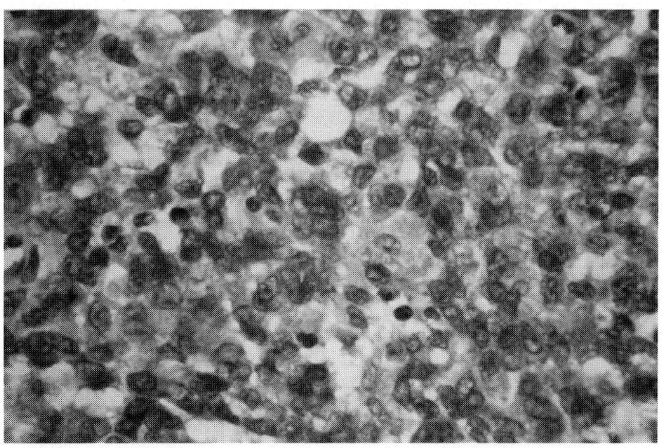

Figure 19–7. Ewing's sarcoma showing proliferation of uniform round cells. Hematoxylin and eosin, ×100.

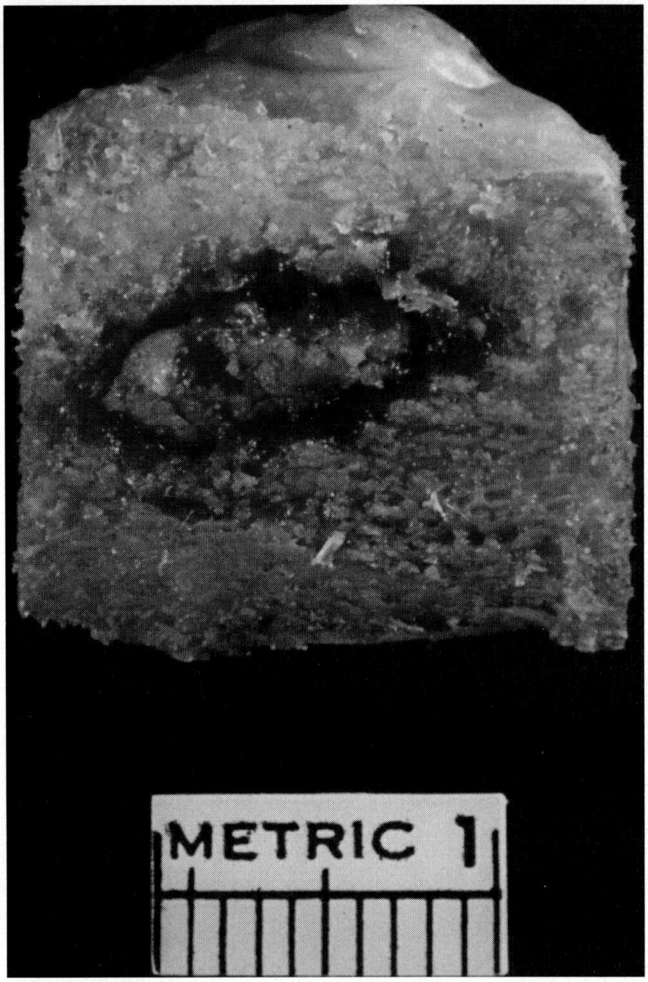

Figure 19–8. Nidus of osteoid osteoma forming an oval nodule situated between the cortex and the medulla.

Approximately 5% of Ewing's sarcomas have larger, more pleomorphic nuclei. However, this characteristic does not seem to affect prognosis.[44]

Before modern radiotherapy and chemotherapy, Ewing's sarcoma carried the worst prognosis of all bone tumors. With modern therapeutic methods, the prognosis has improved considerably. However, radiation and chemotherapy without resection are associated with a significant local recurrence rate. This finding has led to the practice of surgical removal of the involved segment of bone after radiation and chemotherapy. Several studies confirm that this approach improves prognosis.[45]

OSTEOID OSTEOMA

Osteoid osteoma is one of the few bone lesions that can be diagnosed from the clinical presentation alone. Patients present with persistent, localized pain that is characteristically worse at night. The pain is dramatically relieved with the ingestion of aspirin. It is unclear whether osteoid osteoma is a true neoplasm because it certainly has a limited growth potential.

Most patients with osteoid osteomas are in the second decade of life. In addition to the characteristic pain pattern, this tumor may give rise to referred pain. When an osteoid osteoma occurs within the capsule of a joint, synovitis may develop, leading to a mistaken diagnosis of arthritis. Roentgenograms in osteoid osteoma are usually diagnostic. The lesion is associated with extensive sclerosis, which may hinder identification of its characteristic nidus. The nidus is a zone of lucency surrounded by an area of sclerosis (Fig. 19–8). There may be mineral within the zone of lucency. Radionuclide bone scans are especially useful for localizing the lesion. Computed tomography may be necessary to localize the lesion within a given bone.

The gross appearance is typical. When the sclerotic bone overlying the nidus is shaved away, the surgeon unroofs a red, granular area, which is the nidus. The nidus may be very small, never exceeding 2 cm in greatest dimension (Fig. 19–8).

Microscopically, the nidus consists of a network of interlacing osteoid trabeculae lined by osteoblasts (Fig. 19–9). The intertrabecular spaces contain capillaries and a few spindle cells. The bony trabeculae may or may not be mineralized. Under low power, the nidus always has a sharp edge and there is no permeation into surrounding tissues.

In order to identify the nidus during the operation, roentgenograms of both the specimen and the patient will confirm that the lesion has been removed. The patient will confirm that the lesion has been removed because, with an incompletely excised nidus, the pain will persist.

Osteoblastoma is simply a larger osteoid osteoma.[46] By convention, a lesion less than 2 cm is osteoid osteoma; if it is 2 cm or more, it is an osteoblastoma. Osteoblastoma involves the spine more than the appendicular skeleton; it involves the medullary cavity rather than the cortex, and for this reason it is not always associated with a sclerotic reaction. One of the problems with osteoblastoma is that the roetgenographic appearance can mimic that of a malignant tumor. Osteoblastomas can mimic osteosarcomas histologically. Osteoblastomas are always benign, and simple curettage is curative.

OSTEOSARCOMA

Osteosarcoma is the second commonest primary malignant neoplasm of bone, following myeloma. Osteosarcoma

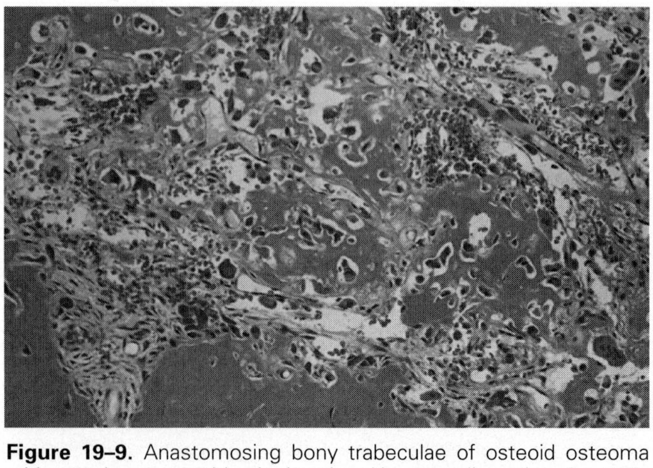

Figure 19–9. Anastomosing bony trabeculae of osteoid osteoma with prominent osteoblastic rimming. Hematoxylin and eosin, ×20.

can be defined simply as a malignant tumor of bone in which the tumor cells produce an osteoid matrix, at least focally. There is great variation in the clinical, roentgenographic, and histologic features of osteosarcomas. Some of these differences have clinical significance, whereas others do not.[47]

Osteosarcoma is a disease of adolescence. Most patients are in the second decade of life. There is a male predominance. Patients usually present with localized pain, usually weeks or months in duration. Occasionally, the patient is asymptomatic until a pathologic fracture occurs. Any portion of the skeleton may be involved, but most tumors are around the knee joint, involving the distal femur or proximal tibia. Most osteosarcomas are metaphyseal. Approximately 10% of osteosarcomas involving long bones are diaphyseal.

The roentgenographic features of osteosarcoma are variable. The tumor usually forms a large area of bony destruction centered on the metaphysis and extending into soft tissue. When the lesion extends into soft tissue, it lifts off the periosteum. Periosteal new bone is formed at this junction, which is termed "Codman's triangle." Rarely, an osteosarcoma is well circumscribed and suggests a benign process. The amount of mineral can be variable. Some osteosarcomas are purely lytic, whereas others are densely sclerotic (Fig. 19–10).

In gross appearance, osteosarcomas are highly variable. They range from a sarcoma resembling fish flesh to a densely ossified mass. Some osteosarcomas have the pearly-white appearance of a cartilage tumor. Others show areas of necrosis and cyst formation. The tumor tends to be well marginated; skip areas of involvement are uncommon (Fig. 19–11).

Great variation exists in the microscopic appearance of osteosarcoma. Most osteosarcomas are highly malignant and can be termed "conventional" osteosarcomas. Approximately 50% of these osteosarcomas produce a large amount of osteoid or bony matrix and can be termed "osteoblastic" osteosarcomas. The osteoid is in the form of a fine network between separate, markedly pleomorphic cells (Fig. 19–12). About 25% of osteosarcomas show predominant chondroid differentiation. The cartilaginous areas show a lobulated growth pattern with marked hypercellularity at the periphery of the lobules. Sheets of spindle cells are formed in these areas, with chondroid matrix production between individual cells. These are called "chondroblastic" osteosarcomas. The remainder show a pure spindle-cell proliferation with only small foci of matrix production. These are termed "fibroblastic" osteosarcomas. These morphologic distinctions lack clinical significance.

Although most osteosarcomas arise in apparently normal bone, a small minority arise in preexisting conditions. Postradiation sarcomas may develop in bones within the field of radiation, usually following a latent period of more than 10 years. Postradiation sarcomas tend to involve the shoulder and pelvic girdles because these areas are frequently radiated for breast or uterine carcinoma. The prognosis for peripherally situated postradiation sarcoma is the same as that for conventional osteosarcoma.[48]

Osteosarcoma occasionally develops in bones affected by Paget's disease. Such osteosarcomas are usually of high grade, with a dismal prognosis.[49]

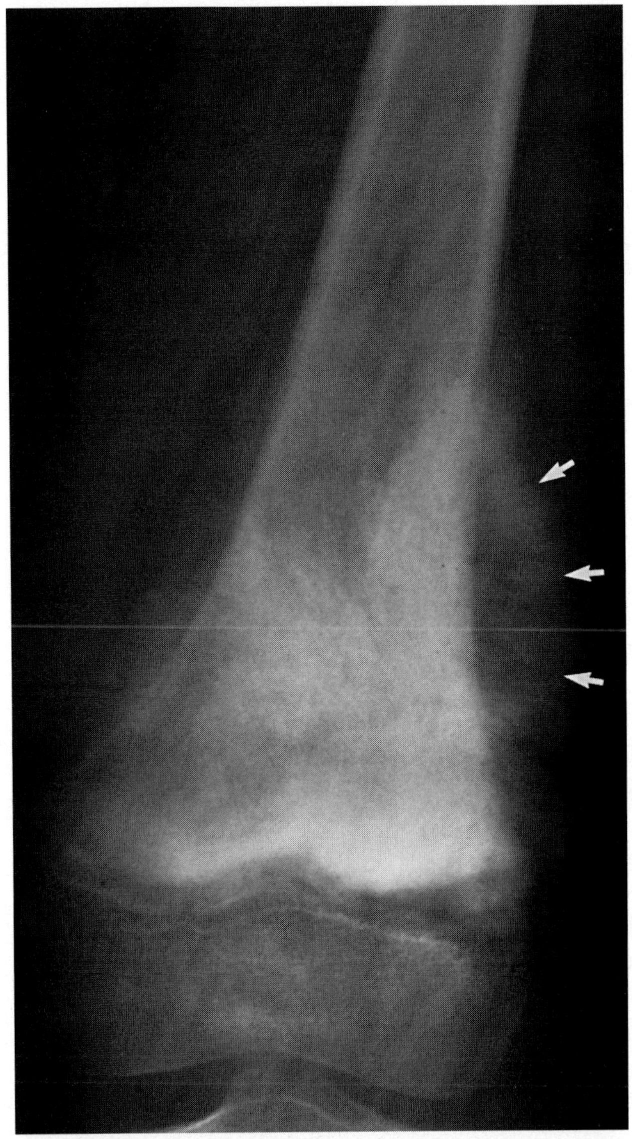

Figure 19–10. Densely sclerotic osteosarcoma of distal femur. Tumor extends into soft tissues where it forms a mineralized mass *(arrows)*.

Before the advent of chemotherapy, the 5-year survival rate for osteosarcoma was only 20%.[50] Some 80% of patients developed pulmonary metastases even if chest radiograph findings were initially negative. Modern chemotherapy has improved the prognosis, so that 5-year survival now ranges from 50 to 60%.

Orthopedic oncologists believe a resectional operation for high-grade osteosarcoma is possible if the patient has received appropriate preoperative chemotherapy. For this reason, most patients with osteosarcoma receive chemotherapy prior to definitive surgery, and the need for amputation for osteosarcoma has declined dramatically. Preoperative chemotherapy also provides a sensitivity test for osteosarcoma. Studies show that the amount of necrosis caused by preoperative chemotherapy correlates well with

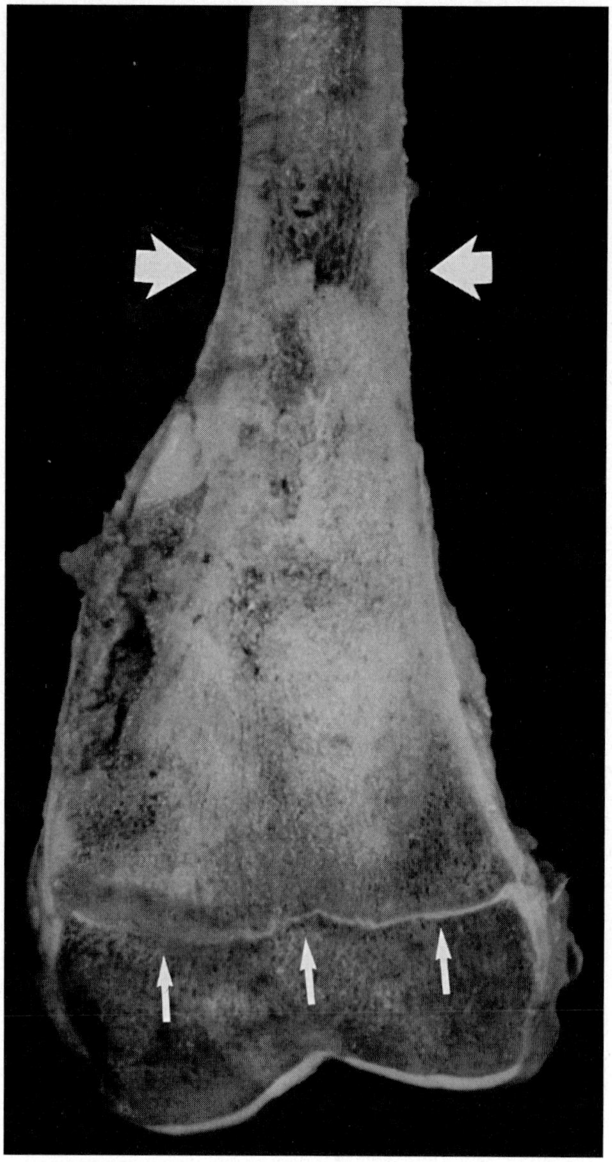

Figure 19–11. Gross specimen of osteosarcoma of distal femur. Epiphyseal plate acts as a relative barrier *(small arrows)*. Proximal margin is also sharply defined *(large arrows)*.

long-term prognosis. Different institutions assess chemotherapy-induced necrosis in varying ways. Although most measure necrosis in a slice of tumor, others use neovascularity on angiography to pinpoint areas of persistent tumor. Patients whose tumors undergo more than 95% necrosis have better prognoses than those whose tumors show less than 95% necrosis.[51]

Most osteosarcomas begin within the medullary cavity but extend into soft tissues by the time they are recognized. However, a small minority of patients have tumors that arise on the surface of bone. The commonest is parosteal osteosarcoma, which was first described as an osteoma, reflecting its indolent nature.[52]

About 80% of parosteal osteosarcomas occur as heavily ossified masses on the posterior aspect of the femoral cortex.[53] The tumors are usually painless and large. Patients usually complain of an inability to flex the knee. Roentgenograms show a heavily calcified mass attached to the underlying cortex without involvement of the bone itself (Fig. 19–13). Microscopically, the tumors are well differentiated and composed of spindle cells with minimal atypia, producing large amounts of trabecular-appearing bone. If the lesion is completely removed, prognosis is excellent. Incomplete removal results in local recurrence.

CHONDROMA

Chondromas are benign proliferations of cartilage. Most occur within the medullary cavity and justify the term ''enchondroma.'' A small percentage occur on the surface of bone; they are ''periosteal'' chondromas. Chondromas that occur in soft tissues are effectively limited to the hands and feet.[54]

Most enchondromas that arouse clinical attention involve the small bones of the hands and feet, where they cause pain from pathologic fracture. Enchondromas of larger bones are asymptomatic. For unknown reasons, enchondromas are hot on bone scans and are frequent incidental findings.

The roentgenographic appearance of an enchondroma is diagnostic. The lesion is small, involves the metaphysis or diaphysis, is extremely well circumscribed, and contains mineral that is uniformly distributed throughout the lesion (Fig. 19–14). If an experienced skeletal radiologist diagnoses an enchondroma, no surgical treatment is required.

Enchondromas of the small bones destroy cortex and cause pathologic fractures. Histologically, enchondromas of the small bones are hypercellular, with moderate atypia of the chondrocytes. Out of context, this appearance may suggest chondrosarcomas; however, chondrosarcomas in the small bones of the hands and feet are extremely unusual.[55] The treatment of benign cartilage lesions is simple curettage or observation.

CHONDROSARCOMA

Chondrosarcoma is the third commonest malignant tumor of bone and is about half as common as osteosarcoma.

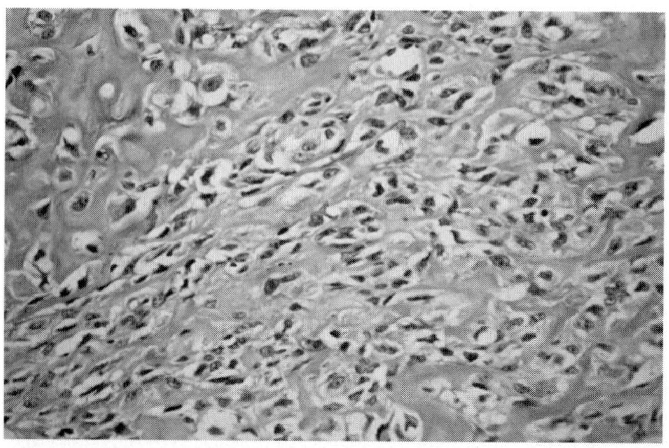

Figure 19–12. Osteoblastic osteosarcoma showing pleomorphic spindle cells with intervening osteoid matrix. Hematoxylin and eosin, ×20.

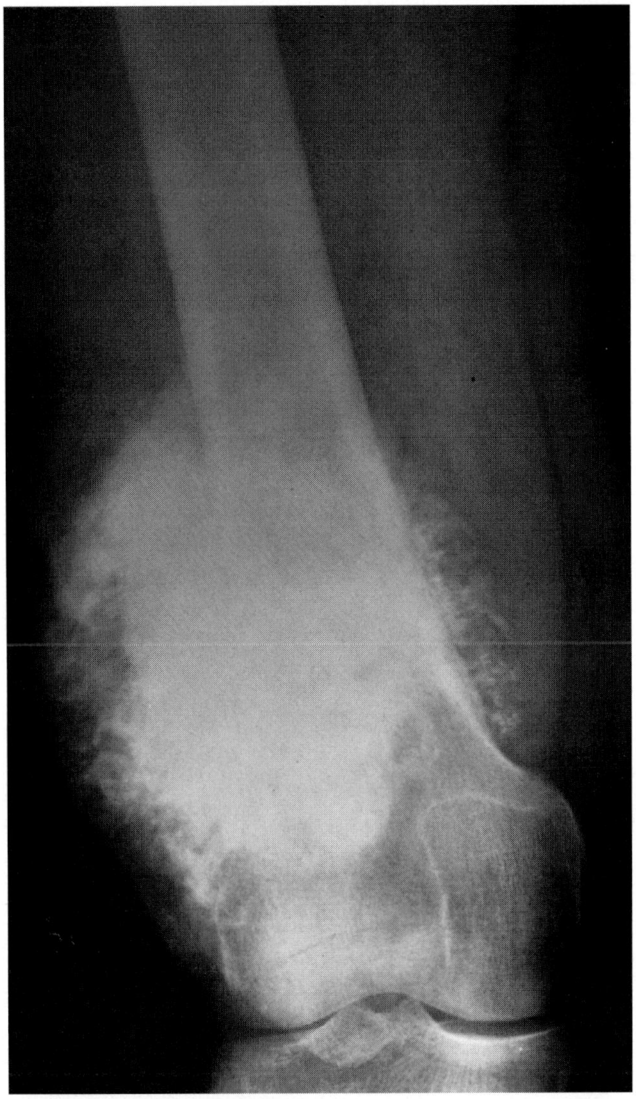

Figure 19–13. Parosteal osteosarcoma presenting as a heavily ossified mass attached to distal femoral cortex.

Like osteosarcoma, chondrosarcoma can be divided into distinct clinicopathologic entities.[56]

Conventional chondrosarcoma affects older adults. Patients report long-standing pain. Bones of the pelvis and shoulder girdles are commonly involved, and for this reason, any cartilaginous tumor involving the pelvis in an adult patient should be considered chondrosarcoma until proved otherwise.

The roentgenographic appearance of chondrosarcoma can be diagnostic. In a long bone, the lesion produces expansion of the bone and thickening of the cortex (Fig. 19–15). The endosteal aspect of the cortex may show erosions. Chondrosarcomas frequently show calcification that tends to be irregularly distributed, unlike calcification in enchondroma, which is more uniform.

The gross appearance of chondrosarcoma is also typical. Cartilage is translucent blue or white, with areas of calcification seen as chalky spots. Areas of myxoid change appear glistening and mucinous (Fig. 19–16) and may liquefy with cystic change. A cystic-appearing cartilage tumor is almost surely chondrosarcoma.

Microscopically, low-grade chondrosarcoma can be difficult to distinguish from benign enchondroma. Chondrosarcomas are more cellular than chondromas and show myxoid change in the matrix. The most important distinguishing feature is the tendency for chondrosarcomas to permeate surrounding bony trabeculae, whereas enchondromas are well circumscribed. Chondrosarcomas are graded from 1 to 3, depending on the cellularity of the lesion and the cytologic atypia of the chondrocytes (Fig. 19–17). Mitotic figures are uncommon in cartilage tumors. Most chondrosarcomas are well differentiated—that is, grade 1 or 2; only rarely are they grade 3.[57] The prognosis in chondrosarcoma is excellent. Complete removal of the lesion with a cuff of surrounding normal tissue is the treatment of choice. Ideally, the surgeon does not encounter tumor at the time of surgery. When the clinical and roentgenographic features are typical, the chondrosarcoma may be resected without prior biopsy. As with most low-grade sarcomas, chemotherapy and radiotherapy have no role in the management of chondrosarcoma.

Rarely, chondrosarcomas arise from a preexisting condition, most commonly osteochondroma.[58] The osteochondroma may be solitary or part of multiple exostoses. When a patient with a known osteochondroma complains of pain and increasing size of the lesion, malignant transformation should be considered. Roentgenographically, the size of the cartilage cap of the osteochondroma and the pattern of

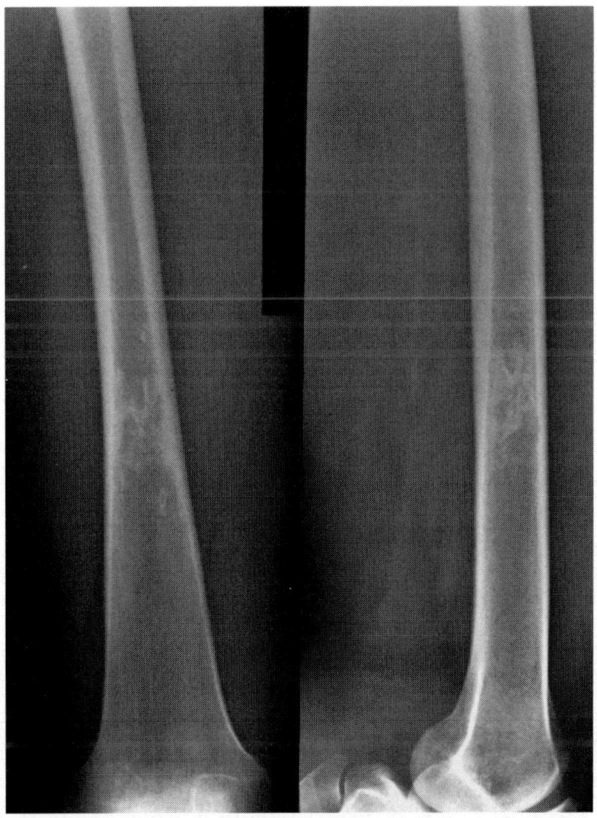

Figure 19–14. Enchondroma involving femoral shaft. The cortex is intact. There is mineralization *(left, anterior view; right, lateral view).*

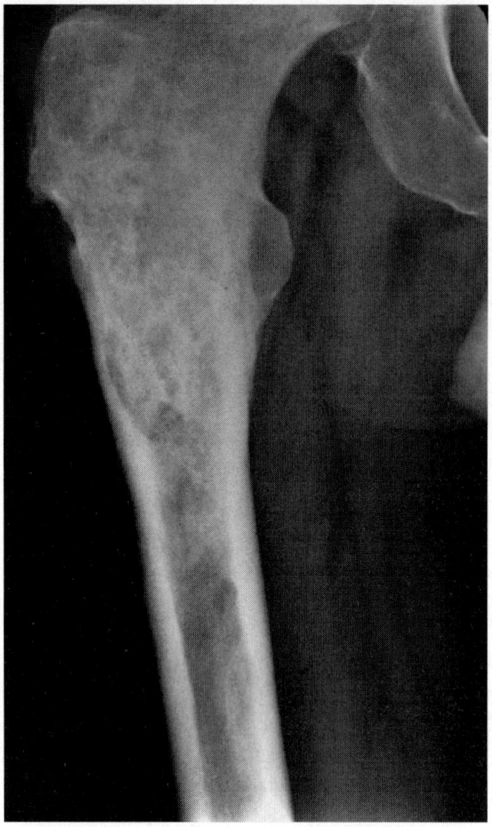

Figure 19–15. Chondrosarcoma of the proximal femur showing widening of the bone and thickening of the cortex.

mineralization are useful distinctions. Most osteochondromas have a thin, regular cartilaginous cap less than 1 cm thick. When a chondrosarcoma develops, the cap becomes irregular, thickened, and lobulated and may show cystic changes (Fig. 19–18). Most secondary chondrosarcomas are low-grade and difficult to recognize as malignancy on histologic grounds. The prognosis in secondary chondrosarcoma is excellent if the lesion can be resected.

About 10% of otherwise ordinary chondrosarcomas dedifferentiate to a high-grade spindle-cell sarcoma.[59] Most patients with dedifferentiated chondrosarcomas are older adults. The lesions tend to involve the same skeletal sites as conventional chondrosarcomas, that is, bones of the pelvis and shoulder girdle. Roentgenograms show a mineralizing mass typical of chondrosarcoma juxtaposed to a nonmineralized, aggressive-appearing neoplasm. The gross appearance also demonstrates this juxtaposition of chondrosarcoma with a high-grade spindle-cell sarcoma that is fleshy and white. Histologically, there is an abrupt change from a well-differentiated chondrosarcoma to a high-grade spindle-cell sarcoma. Dedifferentiated chondrosarcomas have a poor prognosis.

Mesenchymal chondrosarcoma is an uncommon variant of chondrosarcoma.[60] This combines well-differentiated cartilage with a small-cell malignancy suggestive of either malignant lymphoma or Ewing's sarcoma. Typically, the small-cell malignancy has a hemangiopericytomatous pattern. The behavior of mesenchymal chondrosarcoma is unpredictable. Histologic features are not predictive. Some patients present with disseminated disease and die quickly; others may survive for long periods following surgical resection.

MALIGNANT FIBROUS HISTIOCYTOMA

Malignant fibrous histiocytoma is the commonest soft tissue sarcoma. Some workers actually question the independent identity of this neoplasm.[61] The diagnosis of malignant fibrous histiocytoma of bone is made using the same histologic criteria as those for soft tissues (see Chap. 18). The tumor is either a markedly anaplastic spindle-cell neoplasm with a storiform pattern or a pleomorphic sarcoma composed of cells that have abundant pink cytoplasm and an epithelioid appearance. Malignant fibrous histiocytomas

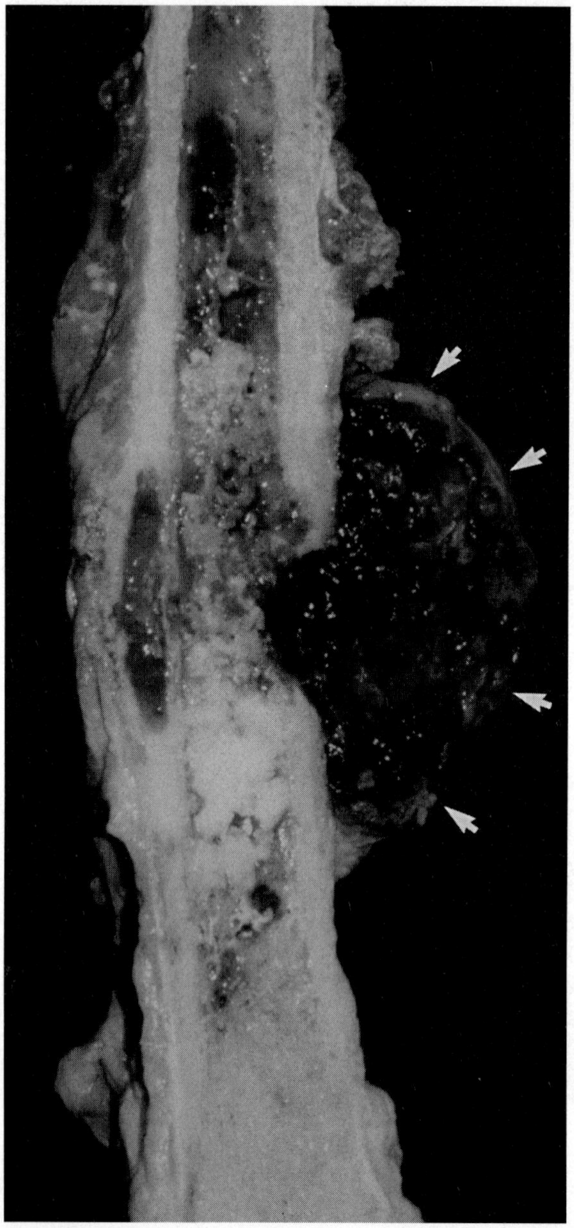

Figure 19–16. Chondrosarcoma of midfemur. Tumor has extended into soft tissues *(arrows)*. Cortex is thickened.

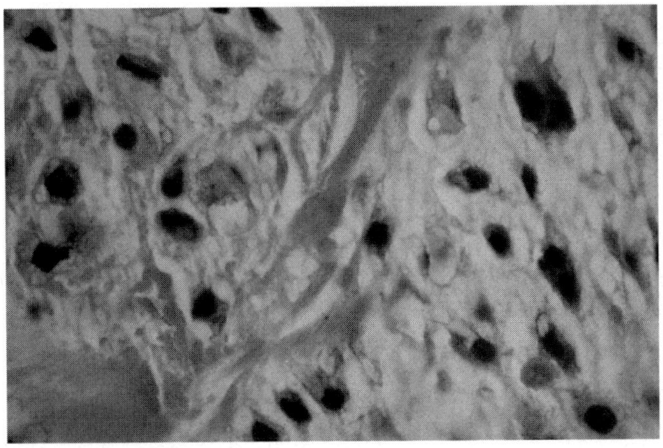

Figure 19–17. Grade 2 chondrosarcoma with several double-nucleated cells, myxoid change in matrix, and moderate cytologic atypia. Hematoxylin and eosin, ×100.

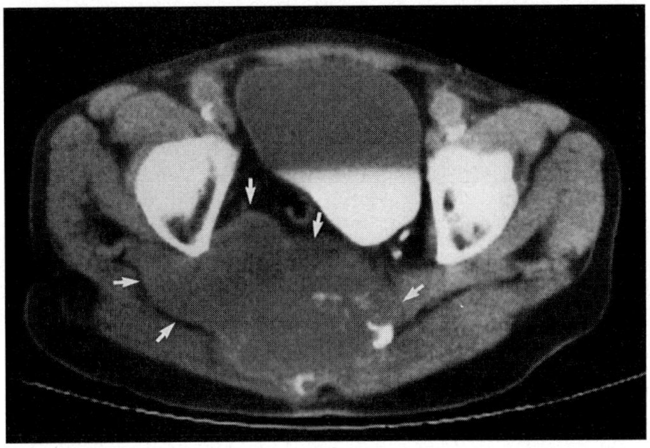

Figure 19–19. Computed tomogram of pelvic chordoma *(arrows)* showing destruction of cortex with formation of soft tissue mass anteriorly.

of bone lack specific roentgenographic or clinical characteristics. They may be difficult to distinguish from osteosarcomas that are producing little bony matrix.

CHORDOMA

Chordoma occurs exclusively along the spinal axis. Just over 50% of chordomas occur in the sacrum and coccyx. Most of the remainder are in the base of the sphenoid, involving the clivus. Primary chordomas of the vertebrae are uncommon. Of these, most occur in the cervical spine.

The clinical presentation of chordoma depends upon the site. Chordoma in childhood is very unusual. Patients with chordomas of the sacrum complain of backaches. Because the sacrum is difficult to visualize on plain roentgenograms, the lesion may be missed initially. In later stages, the patient has symptoms of nerve root compression with loss of bladder and bowel function. Patients with chordomas of the sphenoid present with signs of cranial nerve involvement.

Roentgenographically, chordomas show areas of destruction. Residual osseous trabeculae and calcified material may be seen. Computed tomography and MRI allow better delineation of sacral chordomas, which on plain roentgenograms are often obscured by overlying gas shadows (Fig. 19–19).

Grossly, chordomas are soft and lobulated and may have a gelatinous appearance.

Microscopically, chordomas are always lobulated. Tumor cells lie in a myxoid matrix and form lobules separated by fibrous septa. The tumor cells are small and round and are arranged in cords within a myxoid stroma (Fig. 19–20). Some chordomas show marked cytologic atypia. This finding has no prognostic significance. The cytoplasm of the tumor cells may have a bubbly appearance, thus the term ''physaliferous'' cell.

Chordomas involving the clivus show prominent chondroid differentiation and are termed ''chondroid chordomas.'' The prognosis of chondroid chordoma is better than that of conventional chordoma.[62] If a biopsy specimen from the base of the skull shows a cartilaginous neoplasm and the roentgenogram shows involvement of the clivus, the diagnosis is a chondroid chordoma. Controversy exists in the literature concerning this term. Some workers believe that these lesions are chondrosarcomas, whereas others believe

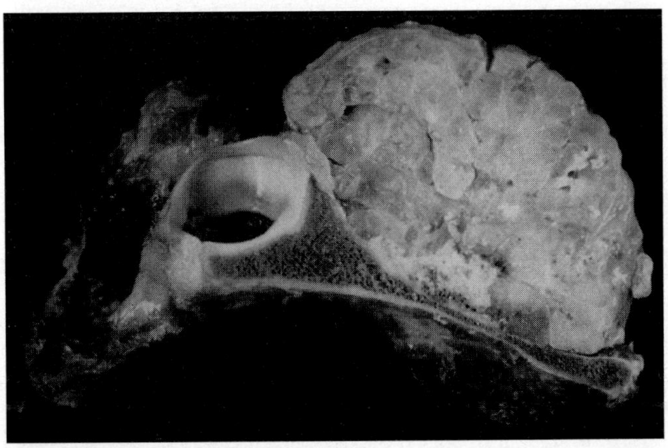

Figure 19–18. Internal hemipelvectomy done for chondrosarcoma arising within osteochondroma. Much of neoplasm is composed of cartilage.

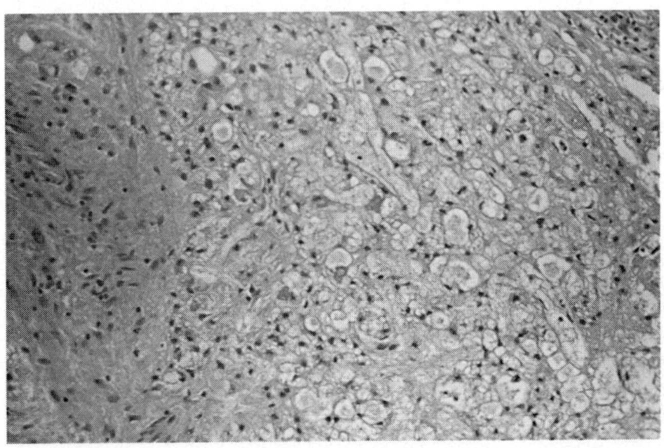

Figure 19–20. A lobule of chordoma showing tumor cells arranged in chords in a myxoid stroma. Hematoxylin and eosin, ×20.

that chondroid chordomas are chordomas. In either case, they should be recognized as a distinct entity because of the favorable prognosis.

Treatment recommendations for chordoma have changed. Technique advances allow radical resections of tumors involving the sacrum and, if the tumor can be removed without spillage, the prognosis is excellent.[63] Of course, chordomas of the base of the skull are not surgically resectable. Nevertheless, many patients, especially those with chondroid chordomas, do well with subtotal removal and postoperative radiation therapy.

BENIGN GIANT-CELL TUMOR

Any lesion of bone may contain giant cells. However, when a tumor is composed of benign giant cells and mononuclear cells, the diagnosis is giant-cell tumor. Giant-cell tumor is one of the few bone tumors with a predilection for women. The lesion occurs in skeletally mature individuals around 20 years of age. Giant-cell tumor is uncommon in persons younger than 15 years, and affected patients between 15 and 20 years are females whose skeletons are mature. Any portion of the skeleton may be involved; however, the commonest sites in order of incidence are the distal femur, proximal tibia, distal radius, and sacrum. Neoplasms in the distal end of the radius are unusual, and although giant-cell tumors are relatively common in the sacrum, they are extremely uncommon in the spine above the level of the sacrum. Roentgenograms usually show a purely lytic destructive lesion that extends to the articular cartilage (Fig. 19–21). The lesion tends to be poorly defined, at least focally, and there is little mineralization.

The gross appearance of a giant-cell tumor can be diagnostic. The tumor is usually solid and soft and has a characteristic dark-brown color (Fig. 19–22). Secondary changes such as yellow discoloration, necrosis, and cyst formation may also be seen. Microscopically, giant-cell tumors show a proliferation of benign giant cells containing between 10 and 40 nuclei. The giant cells tend to be uniformly distributed throughout the lesion—a feature that distinguishes it from giant-cell reparative granuloma, in which the giant cells tend to cluster (Fig. 19–23). Between the giant cells are proliferating mononuclear cells. These are oval-shaped cells with nuclei similar to those of the giant-cell nuclei. Although mitotic figures are common in the mononuclear cells, there is no cytologic atypia. Bone formation is unusual within the lesion; however, when the lesion involves the surrounding soft tissues, reactive bone forms a shell around the lesion. Foam-cell change of the mononuclear cells is common. Secondary aneurysmal bone cysts may occur as either small cysts or the dominant lesion.

The treatment of giant-cell tumors is surgical. When clinical and radiologic findings suggest giant-cell tumor, intraoperative frozen section confirmation justifies immediate, thorough curettage. Both surgeon and pathologist should inspect the appearance of curettage material to as-

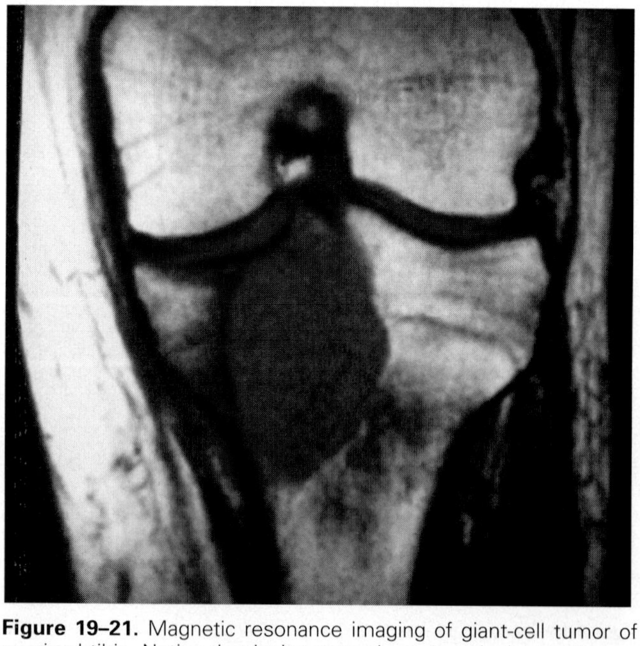

Figure 19–21. Magnetic resonance imaging of giant-cell tumor of proximal tibia. Notice that lesion extends up to articular cartilage.

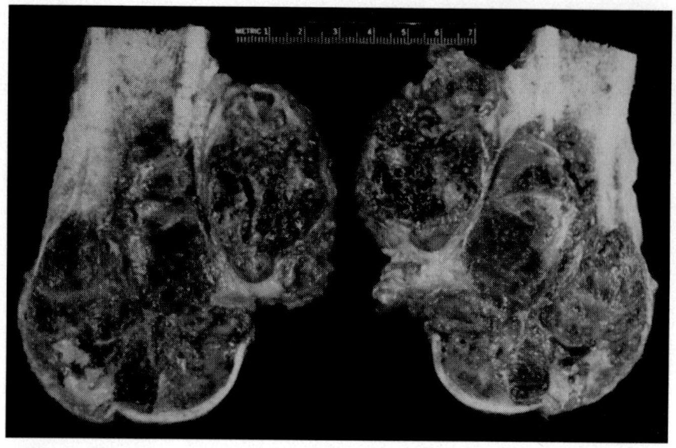

Figure 19–22. Gross appearance of giant-cell tumor of distal femur. The tumor fills the bone, destroys the cortex, and extends into soft tissues.

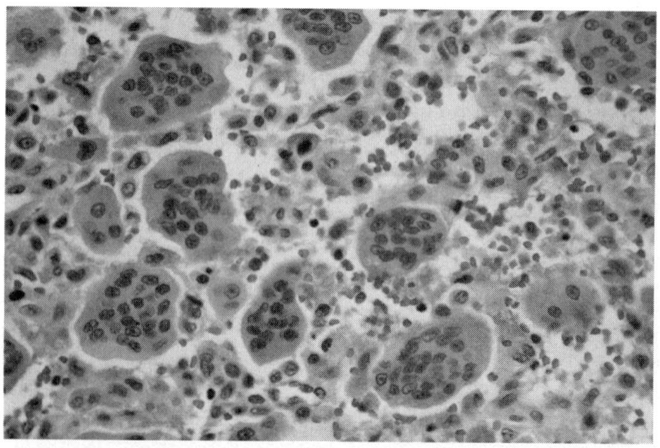

Figure 19–23. Microscopic appearance of giant-cell tumor. Giant cells are distributed more or less uniformly through the lesion. Nuclei of the mononuclear cells are similar to those of the giant cells. Hematoxylin and eosin, ×100.

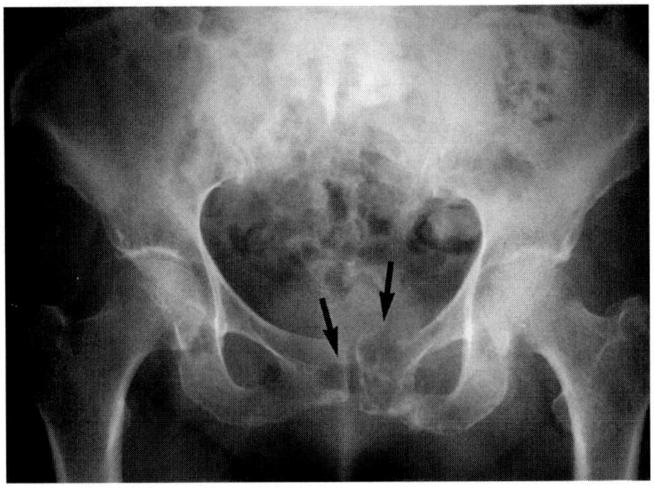

Figure 19–24. Insufficiency fractures of pelvis and sacrum in a postmenopausal woman. Note the destructive-appearing lesion of the pubic symphysis *(arrows)*.

sure that there is no other lesion present that simulates giant-cell tumor by virtue of eliciting an intense giant-cell reaction. The recurrence rate is high because of the tendency for giant-cell tumors to permeate surrounding bone. However, the lesion should be thoroughly curettaged before more extensive procedures such as resections are done. Giant-cell tumors may recur in adjacent soft tissues. In such cases, the roentgenograms show eggshell calcification around the tumor.

Conditions That Simulate Primary Neoplasms of Bone

In addition to the tumors described, nonneoplastic conditions may simulate a neoplasm clinically, roentgenographically, and microscopically.

FRACTURE CALLUS

Fracture callus is usually not a diagnostic problem. When the lesion is traumatic, the diagnosis is obvious. The roentgenographic features also show a clear-cut fracture. However, some fractures are not clinically or roentgenographically straightforward. Stress fractures frequently involve the small bones of the feet and the tibia. Stress fractures are produced by repetitive activity such as long marches or jogging. The patient usually complains of localized pain. The findings on the roentgenograms may be alarming, with extensive periosteal new bone formation simulating the appearance of a small-cell malignancy such as Ewing's sarcoma. The fracture line may not be obvious.

Insufficiency fractures probably represent stress fractures due to osteoporosis. They occur in the pelvic bones of postmenopausal women and are being increasingly recognized.[64] The patients complain of pain in the pelvic area. Patients may have a history of malignancy, such as endometrial carcinoma, and may even have had radiation therapy in this area. A bone scan shows multiple hot spots involving the sacrum, ilium, and pubic bones. Plain roentgenograms may show a destructive-appearing lesion, especially involving the pubic symphysis (Fig. 19–24). Biopsy specimens will show areas of reactive new bone formation but no tumors. Typical roentgenographic and clinical features allow the diagnosis, and a biopsy is thus avoided.

The pathologist examining a fracture callus should make sure that the patient does not have a pathologic fracture. A biopsy may not sample an underlying lesion, and close correlation between the roentgenographic appearance and the histology is necessary to avoid missing a tumor.

A fracture callus usually shows proliferation of cartilage that matures to trabecular-appearing bone. The cartilage may be so cellular that it is mistaken for chondrosarcoma. However, the dwindling of maturation to bone allows the correct diagnosis. As always, communication among the surgeon, radiologist, and pathologist is critical for avoiding such an error.

Myositis ossificans (also called heterotopic ossification) is a variant of fracture callus, occurring in soft tissues (see Chap. 18). Some patients report a history of trauma. Patients complain of a rapidly developing mass lesion. The findings on plain roentgenograms are usually negative in the early stages. After about 3 weeks, mineral appears in the lesion, which tends to be at the periphery, whereas the central areas are lucent. This zonation phenomenon is better shown by CT (Fig. 19–25). By comparison, MRI scans are misleading in heterotopic ossification because margination is not demonstrated, resulting in the appearance of an invasive process.

Grossly, myositis ossificans shows an extremely well-circumscribed mass. The periphery of the lesion may be ossified, giving the lesion the appearance of an eggshell. Microscopically, the zonation phenomenon is seen (Fig. 19–26).[65] The center of the lesion is hypercellular and may show brisk mitotic activity; however, the cells lack atypia and are loosely arranged. At the periphery of the lesion, cells are more polygonal and assume the form of osteoblasts producing osteoid, which matures into bone. When recognized, this lesion will require no treatment, eventually becoming smaller and resolving completely.

ANEURYSMAL BONE CYST

Several cystic conditions of bone mimic neoplasm. Aneurysmal bone cysts may be primary or secondary.[66] Pri-

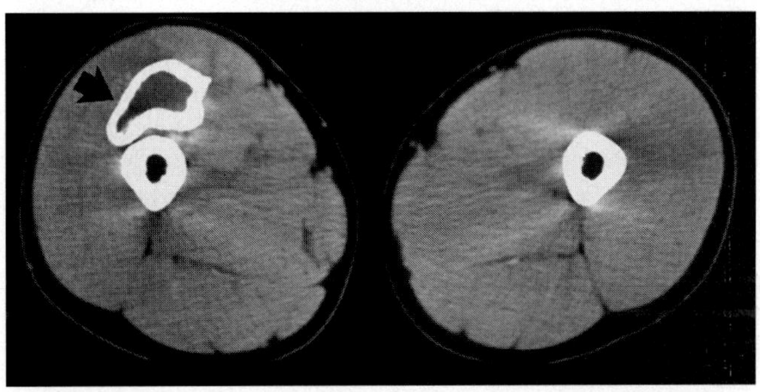

Figure 19–25. Computed tomogram of myositis ossificans of thigh. Note that lesion *(arrow)* is separate from the bone. There is central lucency and peripheral mineralization.

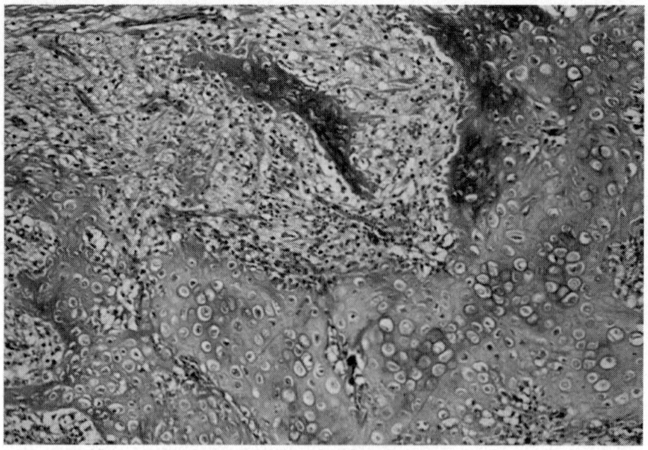

Figure 19–26. Myositis ossificans (heterotopic ossificans) showing loose spindle-cell proliferation and formation of bone and cartilage at periphery. Hematoxylin and eosin, ×16.

mary aneurysmal bone cysts occur in young patients, usually younger than 20 years, and involve the metaphysis of long bones or the posterior elements of the spine. The lesion usually grows rapidly. Involvement of the spine may cause spinal cord compression. Roentgenograms show an eccentrically situated mass that destroys bone and extends into soft tissue (Fig. 19–27). However, at the point where the lesion extends into soft tissue, it produces a shell of ossification. This shell may be highlighted on CT, which also reveals layers of blood products and serum. Magnetic resonance imaging usually shows septa within the lesion.

Grossly, aneurysmal bone cysts show spaces separated by septa. The spaces contain either clear fluid or blood. The lesions bleed profusely, making removal of a vertebral lesion hazardous.

Microscopically, aneurysmal bone cysts are composed of spaces separated by septa. A vascular spindle-cell proliferation with benign giant cells makes up the septa and may show brisk mitotic activity; however, there is no cytologic atypia (Fig. 19–28). Aneurysmal bone cysts are benign. Only rarely, if there is a history of radiation, does malignant transformation occur.

Secondary aneurysmal bone cysts refer to cystic changes occurring in primary neoplastic or tumorlike lesions of bone. The aneurysmal bone cystlike areas may be prominent or may be a minor component of the lesion. Most secondary aneurysmal bone cysts are associated with benign lesions of bone, such as chondroblastoma, giant-cell tumor, or fibrous dysplasia. A secondary aneurysmal bone cyst associated with an underlying malignancy is extremely unusual.

Another cystic condition of bone that may resemble a neoplasm is a simple cyst. This usually occurs in children younger than 10 years and involves the proximal humerus or the proximal femur. Patients typically present with pathologic fracture. Roentgenograms show a cystic lesion that appears trabeculated. The lesion extends to the epiphyseal plate and down the shaft of the bone but is usually no wider than the involved epiphyseal plate (Fig. 19–29). Grossly, the bone shows a cyst lined by thin fibrous tissue and contains clear straw-colored fluid. Most simple cysts are treated with aspiration and injection of methylprednisolone acetate.[67] Hence, simple cysts are rarely seen by the pathologist.

FIBROUS DYSPLASIA

Fibrous dysplasia is not a true neoplasm but rather a defect in ossification. It may be solitary or multifocal. Multifocal fibrous dysplasia is part of Albright's syndrome. Associated features include skin pigmentation, endocrine abnormalities, and precocious puberty, especially in girls.[68] Most patients with solitary fibrous dysplasia are children or young adults. The proximal femur, ribs, and bones of the skull and face are commonly affected. A patient with a

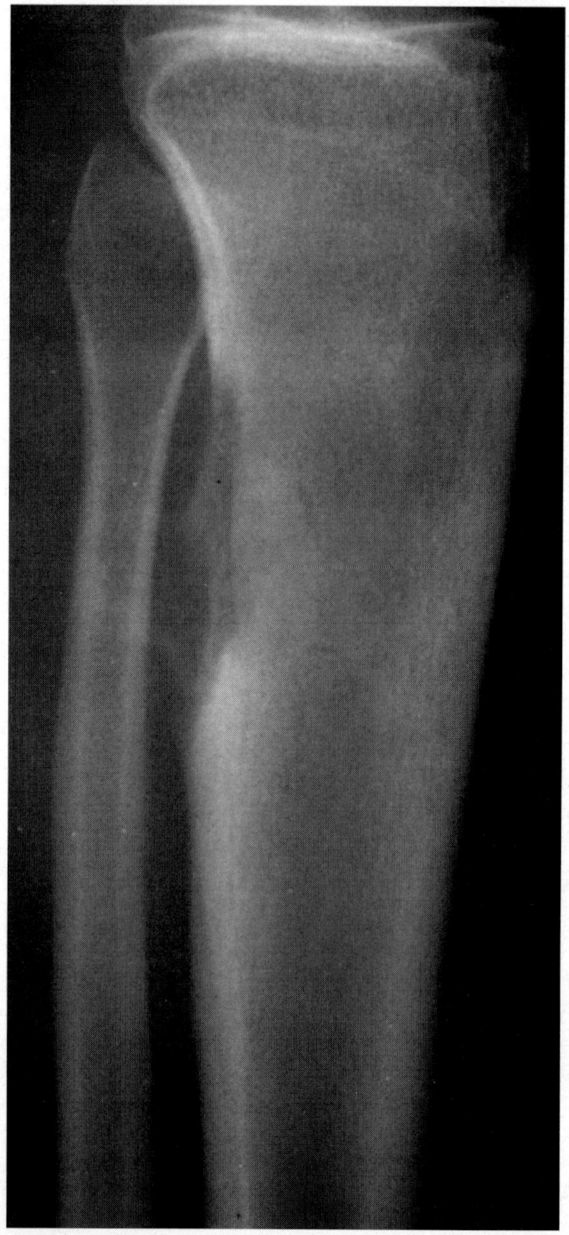

Figure 19–27. Aneurysmal bone cyst of proximal tibia showing a purely lytic eccentric lesion that extends into soft tissues.

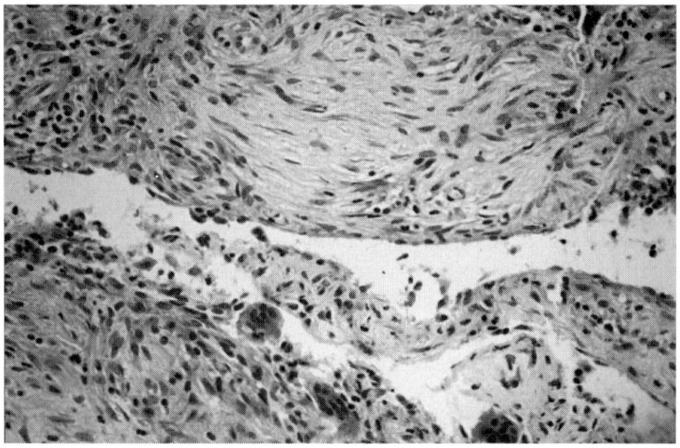

Figure 19–28. Aneurysmal bone cyst showing septa separating spaces. Septa are composed of loosely arranged spindle cells and benign giant cells. Hematoxylin and eosin, ×20.

lesion of the proximal femur may present with a pathologic fracture. Lesions of the ribs are usually encountered as an incidental finding on chest roentgenograms. Fibrous dysplasia of the jaws produces deformities such as facial asymmetry.

Roentgenograms show a well-circumscribed bony lucency which appears somewhat hazy. The term ''ground-glass'' appearance has been given to this. The margins are well defined, with a sclerotic rind (Fig. 19–30).

Microscopically, fibrous dysplasia shows a combination of spindle cells and bone formation. The spindle-cell proliferation is hypocellular, and collagen is produced around the individual cells. The osseous component lacks the orientation seen in normal bone (Fig. 19–31).

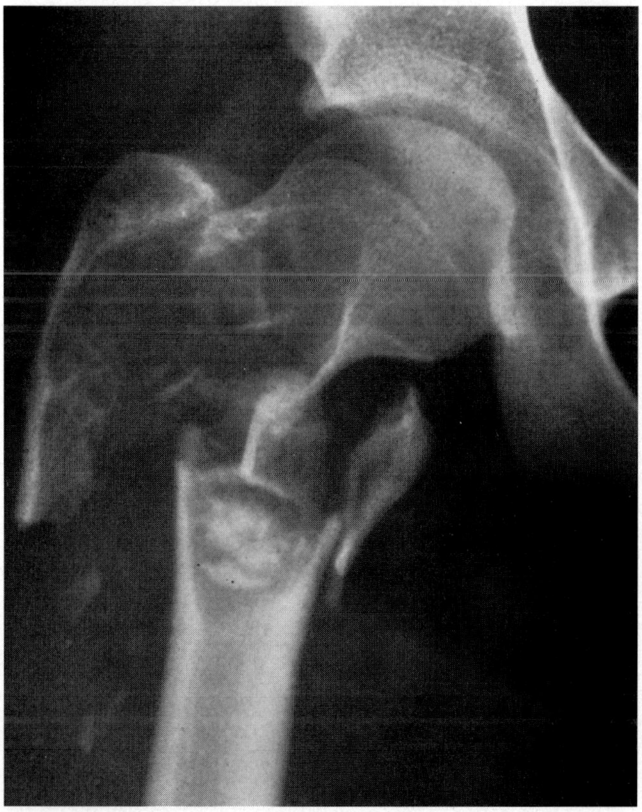

Figure 19–29. Simple cyst of bone involving proximal femur and giving rise to pathologic fracture.

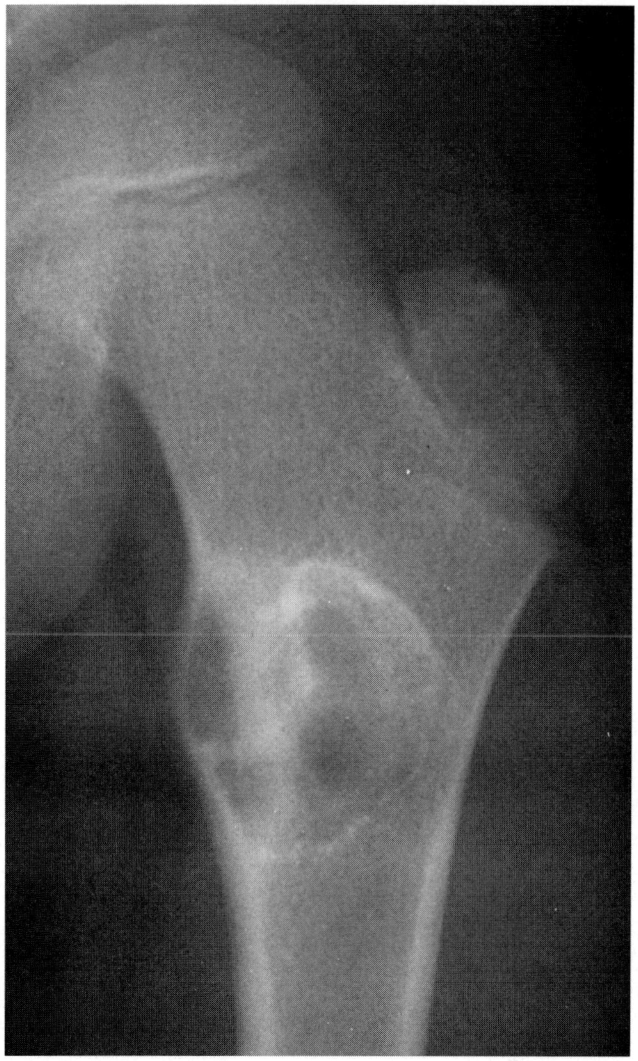

Figure 19–30. Typical appearance of fibrous dysplasia involving proximal femur in a 6-year-old boy. Lesion is well defined and shows a sclerotic rind.

Treatment is necessary only for pathologic fracture or impending pathologic fracture. In fibrous dysplasias of the jawbones, frequent shavings of the bone may be necessary to correct deformities. Malignant transformation in fibrous dysplasia is rare and usually associated with prior radiation. However, examples of sarcomas arising in fibrous dysplasia without prior radiation are well documented.[69]

A rare variant of fibrous dysplasia called osteofibrous dysplasia occurs almost exclusively in the tibia of patients in the first decade of life. The lesion involves the cortex and may be associated with deformities and pathologic fractures. Roentgenograms show a longitudinal lesion involving the tibial cortex with a mixture of lysis and sclerosis. Histologically, osteofibrous dysplasia is similar to fibrous dysplasia except that osteoblastic rimming of bony trabeculae is more prominent. Osteofibrous dysplasia is a

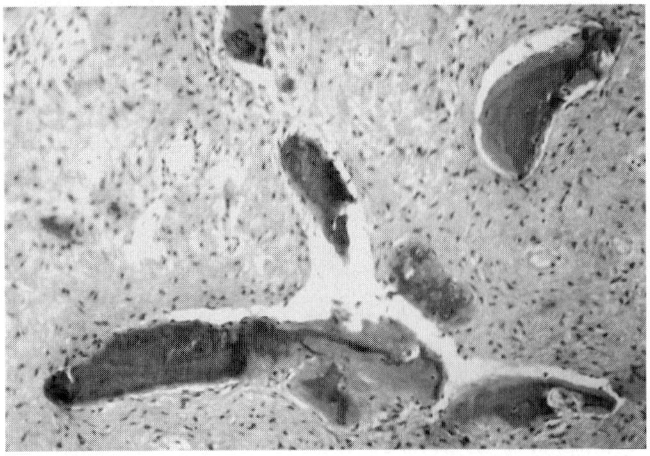

Figure 19–31. Hypocellular spindle-cell proliferation and metaplastic bone formation typical of fibrous dysplasia. There is no osteoblastic rimming of bony trabeculae. Hematoxylin and eosin, ×40.

self-limited disease, and the lesions regress after the patient becomes skeletally mature.[70]

METAPHYSEAL FIBROUS DEFECT

Metaphyseal fibrous defect (also called nonossifying fibroma) is also a defect in ossification. As the name implies, it always occurs in the metaphyses of long bones. Because of some histologic features, it has also been called a fibrous histiocytoma; however, this term should be avoided, because these are not true neoplasms.

Metaphyseal fibrous defects are common. They are asymptomatic when they are small. However, if the lesion becomes large, they may give rise to pathologic fractures. The roentgenographic appearance is typical, and no treatment is necessary. Roentgenograms show a well-defined lucent defect in the metaphysis of a long bone. It may involve the cortex or both the cortex and medullary cavity. The lesion has a characteristic sclerotic margin with a scalloped appearance. If the roentgenograms show these features, a biopsy is unnecessary (Fig. 19–32).

Grossly, metaphyseal fibrous defects are dark brown and granular with focal areas of yellow discoloration. Microscopically, metaphyseal fibrous defects consist of spindle cells arranged in a loose, storiform pattern. Benign giant cells are usually found, but the histologic appearance is rarely mistaken for that of a benign giant-cell tumor.

OSTEOMYELITIS

Osteomyelitis continues to produce clinical problems throughout the world. Patients with osteomyelitis usually present with pain, fever, increased erythrocyte sedimentation rate, and other systemic symptoms. The clinical diagnosis is usually obvious. However, both acute and chronic ostemyelitis can mimic a neoplasm. The systemic symptoms are similar to those of Ewing's sarcoma. Chronic osteomyelitis can mimic an osteoid osteoma.

Most cases of osteomyelitis are hematogenous in pathogenesis, commonly due to *Staphylococcus aureus*. Osteomyelitis can also be caused by fungi and mycobacteria, and immunocompromised patients can be afflicted by a wide range of unusual organisms.

The roentgenographic appearance of osteomyelitis may mimic a round-cell sarcoma. The lesion involves the metaphysis or diaphysis, and a long segment of the bone may be involved. The process shows a permeative, destructive lesion with periosteal new bone formation. With chronic osteomyelitis, an area of lucency surrounded by an area of sclerosis is seen, suggesting the diagnosis of osteoid osteoma. Chronic osteomyelitis can also present as a geographic area of destruction and simulate a neoplasm (Fig. 19–33).

The gross appearance of acute osteomyelitis is typical, and when the lesion is entered, frank pus is encountered. However, it is necessary to confirm the diagnosis with a frozen section. If frozen-section analysis confirms osteomyelitis, material for culture should be obtained. It is best to obtain this material in the surgical suite. Acute osteomyeli-

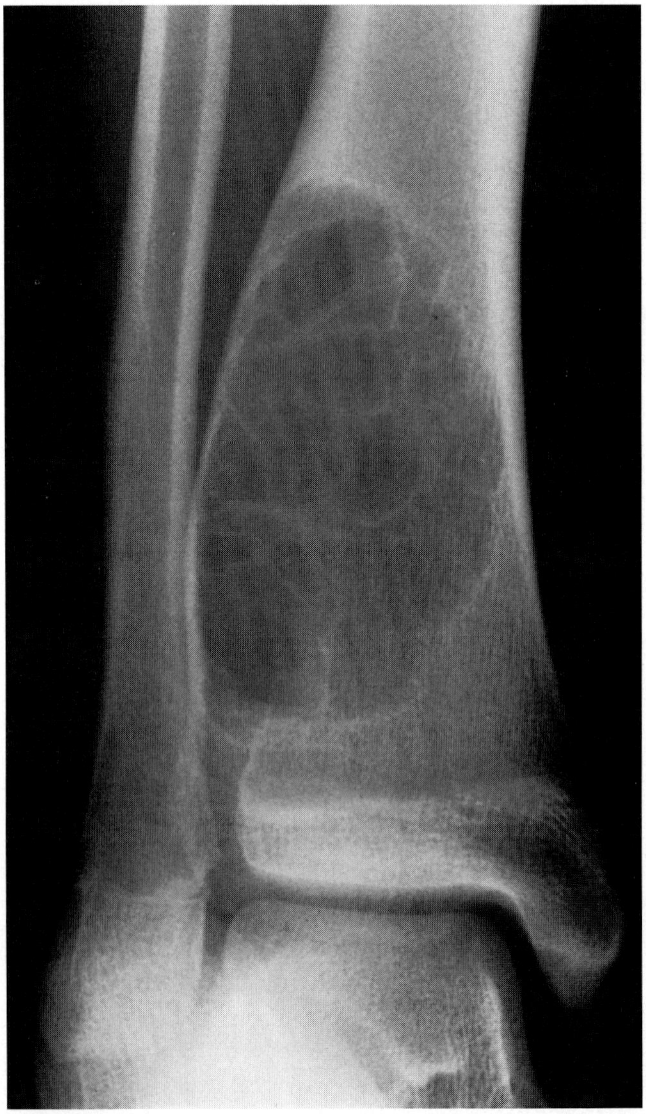

Figure 19–32. Metaphyseal fibrous defect of distal tibia. Lesion has a scalloped, sclerotic rim.

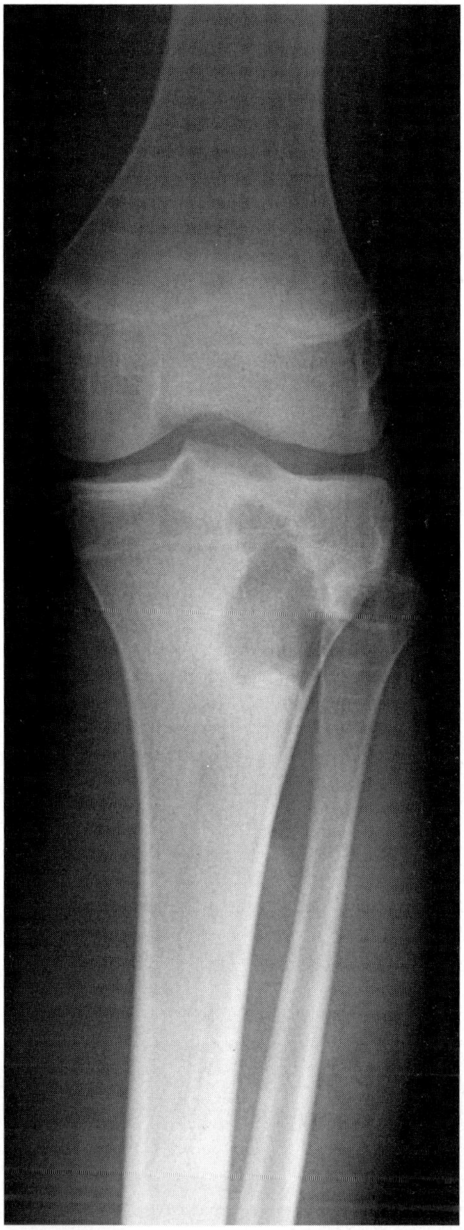

Figure 19–33. Chronic osteomyelitis involving proximal tibia. There is a geographic area of destruction with surrounding sclerosis.

tis shows a mixture of acute and chronic inflammatory cells and capillary proliferation (Fig. 19–34). Granulomatous osteomyelitis may be difficult to discern because the granulomas may not be well formed. The lesion may be mistaken for a neoplasm, especially malignant lymphoma. Although special stains can identify organisms, appropriate microbiologic cultures and sensitivity tests are vital.

The diagnosis of osteomyelitis can be difficult. Unfortunately, some pathologists render this diagnosis nonspecifically when no other pathologic condition is evident. This is a disservice to the patient, because the diagnosis of osteomyelitis results in expensive and time-consuming treatment.

Rarely, a patient with chronic osteomyelitis may have persistent cutaneous sinus tract. A patient who has a long-standing sinus tract on an extremity and complains of increased pain, swelling, and foul discharge may have developed squamous cell carcinoma as a complication.[71] Such carcinomas are usually well differentiated and difficult to recognize histologically. However, when squamous epithelium extends into bone, it is diagnostic of carcinoma. These lesions usually require amputation, after which the patients have an excellent prognosis.

Diseases of Joints

Joints can be involved by conditions that affect other organ systems, such as infections, degenerative diseases, and tumorlike lesions. True neoplasms of the joint are extremely uncommon.

DEGENERATIVE JOINT DISEASE

Degenerative joint disease, or osteoarthritis, is common in our society. This may simply reflect an aging population. Orthopedic procedures to treat osteoarthritis are often performed and are costly.

Symptoms include joint pain and loss of mobility. Roentgenograms show decreased width of the joint space, and subchondral bone appears denser than normal. There are also excrescences from the bone surface called osteophytes.

The gross specimen of a femoral head removed for degenerative joint disease demonstrates the disease process. The articular cartilage is lost, especially over weight-bearing areas. This loss gives rise to sclerosis of the underlying bone, which has the appearance of ivory, termed "eburnation." Osteophytes are bony outgrowths that occur at the junction between the femoral head and neck. The subchondral bone may show myxoid change and cystic degeneration. The sites of cystic degeneration can be so large that they mimic a neoplasm.

The histologic features of degenerative joint disease are not distinctive. In the early stages, there may be fissures in the articular cartilage. However, these are hard to distinguish from artifact. The overlying synovium may be thickened and appear villous. There is usually a nonspecific

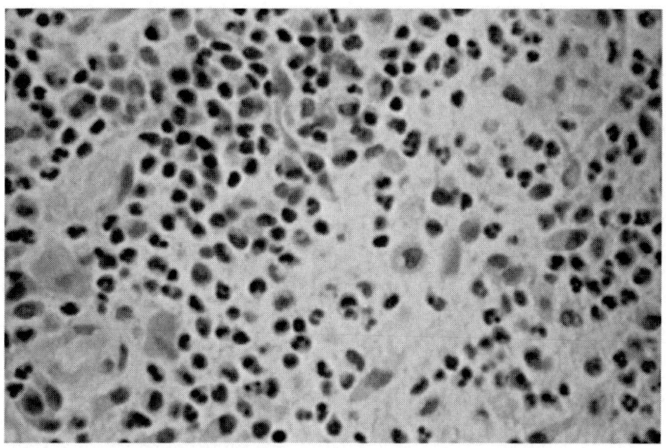

Figure 19–34. Osteomyelitis showing a mixed inflammatory-cell infiltrate and capillary proliferation.

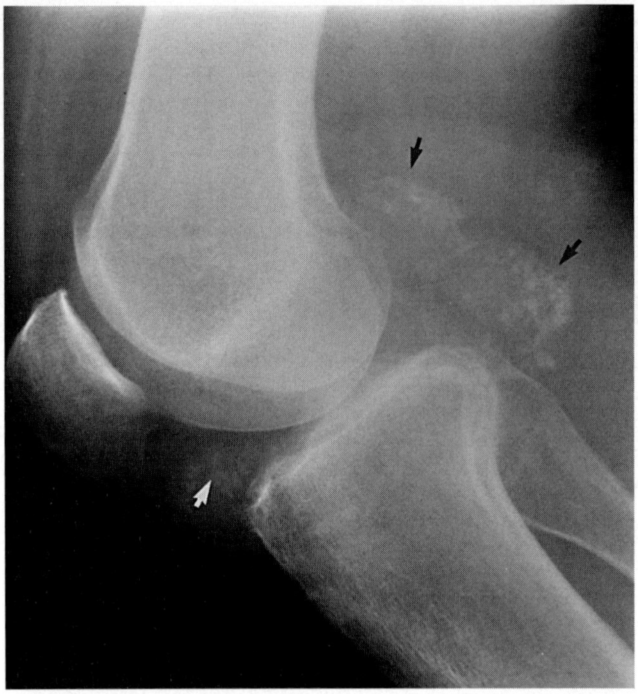

Figure 19–35. Synovial chondromatosis showing calcific densities within joint *(arrows)*.

chronic synovitis. When joint replacements are planned, frozen sections are done to rule out infections. There are no guidelines for correlating numbers of polymorphonuclear leukocytes and likelihood of infections. Other evidence of infection, such as fibrosis, capillary proliferations, and inflammatory cell infiltrates, should be noted. A scattering of polymorphonuclear leukocytes may simply be a reaction to anesthesia.

RHEUMATOID ARTHRITIS

Rheumatoid arthritis is a multisystem disease of unknown cause. It is mediated by autoimmune phenomena. Patients usually complain of joint pain and swelling. Small joints of the hands and feet are frequently involved. It is extremely uncommon for rheumatoid arthritis to involve a single joint. Roentgenograms usually show joint swelling. Histologic features are usually not specific. The synovium appears thickened and boggy and may indeed have a villous architecture. It is unusual to see rheumatoid granulomas within synovium. The usual finding is a dense infiltrate of plasma cells in a perivascular distribution. This inflammatory response is called a pannus, and it spreads along the articular cartilage. If it destroys the articular cartilage, it causes secondary degenerative joint disease.

SYNOVIAL CHONDROMATOSIS

Synovial chondromatosis is a disease of unknown cause characterized by a proliferation of nodules of cartilage within the synovium. The disease is almost always monoarticular, and large joints such as the knee and the hip are commonly affected.[72] Small joints such as the temporomandibular may also be involved. Patients usually complain of pain, swelling, and limited mobility. Roentgenograms show only diffuse swelling of the joint. If the chondroid nodules in the synovium are mineralized, they can be visualized on plain roentgenograms (Fig. 19–35). Grossly, the synovium shows marked thickening. The metaplastic cartilage is embedded in the synovium, producing the thickening (Fig. 19–36). Nodules of cartilage may also be seen floating free in the joint cavity.

Microscopically, synovial chondromatosis consists of nodules of cartilage within synovium. In some sections, flattened out synovial cells overlying the nodule of cartilage are identified. The nodules are composed of chondrocyte clusters separated by a chondroid matrix. The chondrocyte often shows moderate atypia. However, if the process is known to arise from the joint, malignancy is not a consideration.

The prognosis in synovial chondromatosis is excellent. However, the disease is diffuse, and a total synovectomy may be necessary to eradicate it. Hence, local recurrence is not uncommon. Malignant transformation is rare.[73]

PIGMENTED VILLONODULAR SYNOVITIS

Pigmented villonodular synovitis diffusely involves major joints. The disease is almost always monoarticular.[74] Rarely, pigmented villonodular synovitis occurs localized to a single area in a joint, analogous to a giant-cell tumor of tendon sheath. Pigmented villonodular synovitis shows a slight female predominance, and the patients are usually young adults. Patients complain of pain, swelling, or limitation of movement. Generally, the symptoms are of long duration, usually 5 years or more.

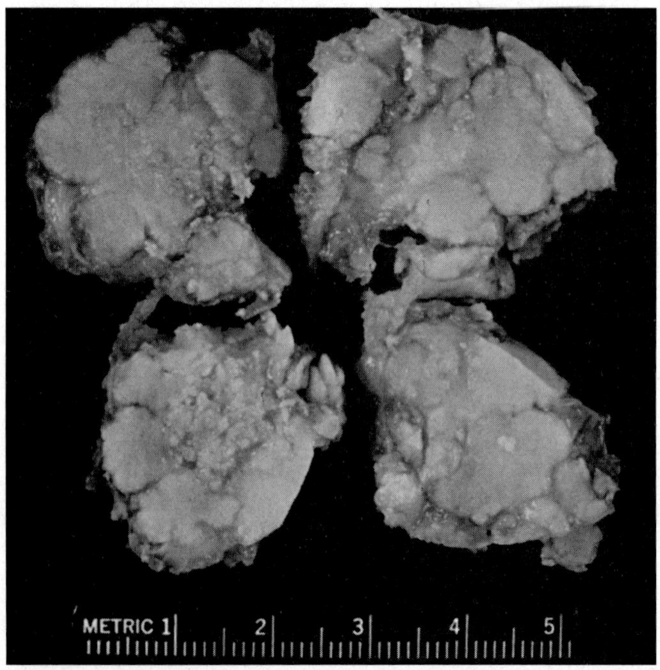

Figure 19–36. Gross appearance of synovial chondromatosis of knee showing thickening of synovium with nodules of cartilage embedded within.

The roentgenographic appearance of pigmented villonodular synovitis may or may not be diagnostic. There is usually diffuse swelling of the joint. In typical cases, there are bony erosions of both sides of the joint. Magnetic resonance imaging may show the characteristic dark color of iron pigment and hence may be diagnostic.

The gross appearance of pigmented villonodular synovitis is typical. The synovium is markedly thickened and shows villous structures on the surface. The synovium is diffusely brown with areas of discoloration.

Microscopically, pigmented villonodular synovitis shows prominent villi on the synovial surface due to proliferation of synovial cells. Giant cells, foam cells, and pigment are seen (Fig. 19–37). The proliferating synovial cells may form nodules in the subsynovial tissues.

The differential diagnosis includes other hyperplastic conditions of the synovium. The presence of villi is not sufficient to diagnose pigmented villonodular synovitis. Villous proliferation may also occur in degenerative joint disease and rheumatoid synovitis; however, in pigmented villonodular synovitis, villous proliferation is due to proliferation of the mononuclear synovial cells.

The prognosis of pigmented villonodular synovitis is excellent. With the localized form, simple excision through an arthroscope may be curative. With the diffuse form, a total synovectomy is necessary. Local recurrences are common. Malignant transformation is extremely rare.

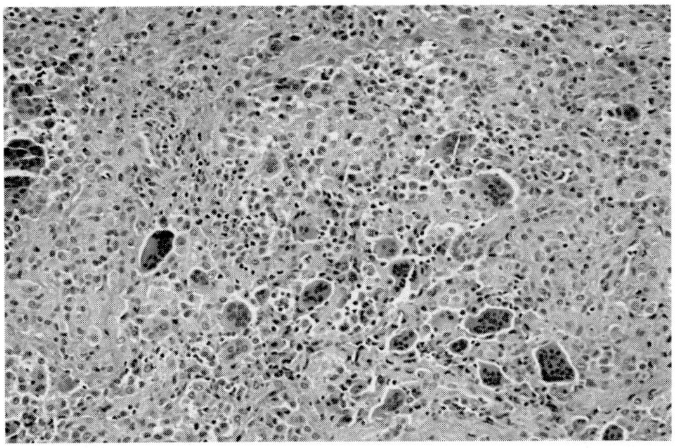

Figure 19–37. Villous proliferation in pigmented villonodular synovitis showing proliferation of synovial cells, foam cells, and giant cells. Hematoxylin and eosin, ×10.

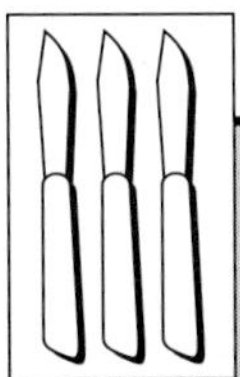

PITFALLS FOR THE SURGEON

1. Attempting to biopsy a lytic bone lesion without evaluating the patient for primary malignancy elsewhere.
2. Performing biopsy of a suspected malignant bone lesion without planning the path. Implanting malignant tumor in critical tissues along the path may preclude limb-sparing surgery.
3. Doing an open biopsy without intraoperative pathologic consultation (or in some cases intraoperative radiologic studies, such as in osteoid osteoma) to ensure adequacy of excision and proper tissue allocation.
4. Failing to consider osteomyelitis in the differential diagnosis and not submitting sampled tissue for microbial culture and sensitivity when indicated.
5. Failing to approach a pathologic fracture correctively in a patient with known past malignancy. The lesion may not be metastatic disease; even if it is, the patient's comfort and short-term survival are affected.
6. Proceeding with a joint prosthesis procedure when hyperemic, edematous synovium is encountered. Infection should be ruled out by frozen section.

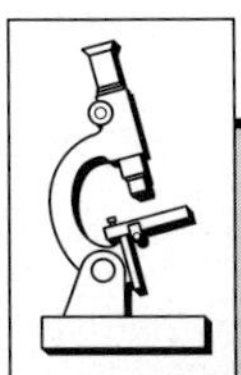

PITFALLS FOR THE PATHOLOGIST

1. Interpreting a bone biopsy without clinical and radiologic information.
2. Misinterpreting the cellular atypia of proliferating bone callus or myositis ossificans and diagnosing a malignancy (osteosarcoma or chondrosarcoma) in lieu of clinical and radiologic evidence.
3. Refusing to attempt intraoperative evaluation because a specimen is bony. In some cases, small bits of soft tissue are available for study or touch preps can be made. If osteomyelitis is suspected, the tissue should be handled accordingly.
4. Placing inadequate emphasis on gross examination of specimen. In many cases, microscopic interpretation depends on correct gross assessment.
5. Missing acute inflammation in synovium because of failure to sample the softest, most cellular component.

FURTHER READING

Berquist TH. Magnetic resonance imaging of musculoskeletal neoplasms. *Clin Orthop.* 1989;244:101.

Enneking WR. The issue of biopsy (editorial). *J Bone Joint Surg [Am].* 1982;64:1119.

Harrington KD. *Orthopaedic Management of Metastatic Bone Disease.* St. Louis: Mosby; 1988.

Mankin HJ, Lange TA, Spanier SS. The hazards of biopsy in patients with malignant primary bone and soft-tissue tumors. *J Bone Joint Surg [Am].* 1982;64:1121.

Sim FH, ed. *Diagnosis and Management of Metastatic Bone Disease: A Multidisciplinary Approach.* New York: Raven Press; 1988.

Simon MA. Biopsy of musculoskeletal tumors. *J Bone Joint Surg [Am].* 1982;64:1253.

Simon MA, Biermann JS. Biopsy of bone and soft-tissue lesions. *J Bone Joint Surg [Am].* 1993;75:616.

Simon MA, Finn HA. Diagnostic strategy for bone and soft-tissue tumors. *J Bone Joint Surg [Am].* 1993;75:622.

REFERENCES

1. Dahlin DC, Unni KK. *Bone Tumors: General Aspects and Data on 8,542 Cases,* 4th ed. Springfield, IL: Charles C Thomas; 1986.
2. Sim FH, ed. *Diagnosis and Management of Metastatic Bone Disease: A Multidisciplinary Approach.* New York: Raven Press; 1988.
3. Harrington KD. *Orthopaedic Management of Metastatic Bone Disease.* St. Louis: Mosby; 1988.
4. Ewing J. *Neoplastic Diseases: A Treatise on Tumors,* 3rd ed. Philadelphia: Saunders; 1928.
5. Silverberg E, Boring CC, Squires TS. Cancer statistics. *CA Cancer J Clin* 1990;40:9.
6. Willis RA. *The Spread of Tumours in the Human Body,* 3rd ed. London: Butterworth; 1973.
7. Abrams HL, Spiro R, Goldstein N. Metastases in carcinoma: Analysis of 1000 autopsied cases. *Cancer.* 1950;3:74.
8. Simon MA, Bartucci EJ. The search for the primary tumor in patients with skeletal metastases of unknown origin. *Cancer.* 1986;58:1088.
9. Simon MA, Finn HA. Diagnostic strategy for bone and soft-tissue tumors. *J Bone Joint Surg Am.* 1993;75:622.
10. Sim FH. Management of primary malignant tumors of bone. In: Galasko CSB, Noble J, eds. *Current Trends in Orthopaedic Surgery.* Manchester, NY: University Press; 1988:48.
11. Coman DR, deLong RP. The role of the vertebral venous system in the metastasis of cancer to the spinal column: Experiments with tumor cell suspensions in rats and rabbits. *Cancer.* 1951;4:610.
12. Lodwick GS. *Tumors of Bone and Soft Tissues.* Chicago: Year Book; 1965:49.
13. Belliveau RE, Spencer RP. Incidence and sites of bone lesions detected by ^{99m}Tc-polyphosphate scans in patients with tumors. *Cancer.* 1975;36:359.
14. Kirchner PT, Simon MA. Radioisotope evaluation of skeletal disease. *J Bone Joint Surg [Am].* 1981;63:673.
15. McNeil BJ. Rationale for the use of bone scans in selected metastatic and primary bone tumors. *Semin Nucl Med.* 1978;8:336.
16. Wahner HW, Brown ML. Role of bone scanning. In: Sim FH, ed. *Diagnosis and Management of Metastatic Bone Disease: A Multidisciplinary Approach.* New York: Raven Press; 1988:51.
17. Simon MA, Kirchner PT. Scintigraphic evaluation of primary bone tumors: Comparison of technetium-99m phosphonate and gallium citrate imaging. *J Bone Joint Surg [Am].* 1980;62:758.
18. Enneking WF, Chew FS, Springfield DS, et al. The role of radionuclide bone-scanning in determining the resectability of soft-tissue sarcomas. *J Bone Joint Surg [Am].* 1981;63:249.
19. Bowers TA, Murray JA, Charnsangavej C, et al. Bone metastases from renal carcinoma: The preoperative use of transcatheter arterial occlusion. *J Bone Joint Surg [Am].* 1982;64:749.
20. Hudson TM, Haas G, Enneking WF, et al. Angiography in the management of musculoskeletal tumors. *Surg Gynecol Obstet.* 1975;141:11.
21. Norman A. The value of tomography in the diagnosis of skeletal disorders. *Radiol Clin North Am.* 1970;8:251.
22. deSantos LA, Goldstein HM, Murray JA, et al. Computed tomography in the evaluation of musculoskeletal neoplasms. *Radiology.* 1978; 128:89.
23. McLeod RA, Stephens DH. Computed tomography of pelvic musculoskeletal neoplasm. *Contemp Orthop.* 1979;1:36.
24. Chang AE, Schaner EG, Conkle DM, et al. Evaluation of computed tomography in the detection of pulmonary metastases: A prospective study. *Cancer.* 1979;43:913.
25. Muhm JR, Brown LR, Crowe JK. Detection of pulmonary nodules by computed tomography. *AJR.* 1977;128:267.
26. Rougraff BT, Kneisl JS, Simon MA. Skeletal metastases of unknown origin: A prospective study of a diagnostic strategy. *J Bone Joint Surg [Am].* 1993;75:1276.
27. Osteen RT, Kopf G, Wilson RE. In pursuit of the unknown primary. *Am J Surg.* 1978;135:494.
28. Berquist T. Magnetic resonance imaging of musculoskeletal neoplasms. *Clin Orthop.* 1989;244:101.
29. Zimmer WD, Berquist TH, McLeod RA, et al. Bone tumors: Magnetic resonance imaging versus computed tomography. *Radiology.* 1985;155:709.
30. Petasnick JP, Turner DA, Charters JR, et al. Soft-tissue masses of the local motor system: Comparison of MR imaging with CT. *Radiology.* 1986;160:125.
31. Kransdorf MJ, Moser RP Jr, Vinh TN, et al. Primary tumors of the patella: A review of 42 cases. *Skeletal Radiol.* 1989;18:365.
32. Simon MA. Biopsy of musculoskeletal tumors. *J Bone Joint Surg [Am].* 1982;64:1253.
33. Mankin HJ, Lange TA, Spanier SS. The hazards of biopsy in patients with malignant primary bone and soft-tissue tumors. *J Bone Joint Surg [Am].* 1982;64:1121.
34. Hajdu SI, Melamed MR. Needle biopsy of primary malignant bone tumors. *Surg Gynecol Obstet.* 1971;133:829.
35. Craig FS. Vertebral-body biopsy. *J Bone Joint Surg [Am].* 1956;38:93.
36. Stoker DJ, Cobb JP, Pringle JAS. Needle biopsy of musculoskeletal lesions: A review of 208 procedures. *J Bone Joint Surg [Br].* 1991;73:498.
37. Moore TM, Meyers MH, Patzakis MJ, et al. Closed biopsy of musculoskeletal lesions. *J Bone Joint Surg [Am].* 1979;61:375.
38. Schajowicz F, Derqui JC. Puncture biopsy in lesions of the locomotor system: Review of results in 4050 cases, including 941 vertebral punctures. *Cancer.* 1968;21:531.
39. White VA, Fanning CV, Ayala AG, et al. Osteosarcoma in the role of fine-needle aspiration: A study of 51 cases. *Cancer.* 1988;62:1238.
40. Davies NM, Livesley PJ, Cannon SR. Recurrence of an osteosarcoma in a needle biopsy track. *J Bone Joint Surg [Br].* 1993;75:977.
41. Frassica DA, Frassica FJ, Schray MF, et al. Solitary plasmacytoma of bone: Mayo Clinic experience. *Int J Radiat Oncol Biol Phys.* 1989;16:43.
42. Meis JM, Butler JJ, Osborne BM, et al. Granulocytic sarcoma in nonleukemic patients. *Cancer.* 1986;58:2697.
43. Ostrowski ML, Unni KK, Banks PM, et al. Malignant lymphoma of bone. *Cancer.* 1986;58:2646.
44. Nascimento AG, Unni KK, Pritchard DJ, et al. A clinicopathologic study of 20 cases of large-cell (atypical) Ewing's sarcoma of bone. *Am J Surg Pathol.* 1980;4:29.
45. Wilkins RM, Pritchard DJ, Burgert EO Jr, et al. Ewing's sarcoma of bone: Experience with 140 patients. *Cancer.* 1986;58:2551.
46. Dahlin DC, Johnson EW Jr. Giant osteoid osteoma. *J Bone Joint Surg [Am].* 1954;36:559.
47. Dahlin DC, Unni KK. Osteosarcoma of bone and its important recognizable varieties. *Am J Surg Pathol.* 1977;1:61.
48. Weatherby RP, Dahlin DC, Ivins JC. Postradiation sarcoma of bone: Review of 78 Mayo Clinic cases. *Mayo Clin Proc.* 1991;56:294.
49. Wick MR, Siegal GP, Unni KK, et al. Sarcomas of bone complicating osteitis deformans (Paget's disease): Fifty years' experience. *Am J Surg Pathol.* 1981;5:47.
50. Dahlin DC, Coventry MB. Osteogenic sarcoma: A study of six hundred cases. *J Bone Joint Surg [Am].* 1967;49:101.
51. Raymond AK, Ayala AG. Specimen management after osteosarcoma chemotherapy. *Contemp Issues Surg Pathol.* 1988;11:157.
52. Geschickter CF, Copeland MM. Parosteal osteoma of bone: A new entity. *Ann Surg.* 1951;133:790.
53. Unni KK, Dahlin DC, Beabout JW, et al. Parosteal osteogenic sarcoma. *Cancer.* 1976;37:2466.

54. Dahlin DC, Salvador AH. Cartilaginous tumors of the soft tissues of the hands and feet. *Mayo Clin Proc.* 1974;49:721.
55. Dahlin DC, Salvador AH. Chondrosarcomas of bones of the hands and feet—A study of 30 cases. *Cancer.* 1974;34:755.
56. Dahlin DC. Chondrosarcoma and its "variants." *Monogr Pathol.* 1976;17:300.
57. Pritchard DJ, Lunke RJ, Taylor WF, et al. Chondrosarcoma: A clinicopathologic and statistical analysis. *Cancer.* 1980;45:149.
58. Garrison RC, Unni KK, McLeod RA, et al. Chondrosarcoma arising in osteochondroma. *Cancer.* 1982;49:1890.
59. Dahlin DC, Beabout JW. Dedifferentiation of low-grade chondrosarcomas. *Cancer.* 1971;28:461.
60. Nakashima Y, Unni KK, Shives TC, et al. Mesenchymal chondrosarcoma of bone and soft tissue: A review of 11 cases. *Cancer.* 1986;57:2444.
61. Fletcher CDM. Pleomorphic malignant fibrous histiocytoma: Fact or fiction? A critical reappraisal based on 159 tumors diagnosed as pleomorphic sarcoma. *Am J Surg Pathol.* 1992;16:213.
62. Heffelfinger MJ, Dahlin DC, MacCarty CS, et al. Chordomas and cartilaginous tumors at the skull base. *Cancer.* 1973;32:410.
63. Kaiser TE, Pritchard DJ, Unni KK. Clinicopathologic study of sacrococcygeal chordoma. *Cancer.* 1984;53:2574.
64. Cooper KL, Beabout JW, Swee RG. Insufficiency fractures of the sacrum. *Radiology.* 1985;156:15.
65. Ackerman LV. Extra-osseous localized non-neoplastic bone and cartilage formation (so-called myositis ossificans): Clinical and pathological confusion with malignant neoplasms. *J Bone Joint Surg [Am].* 1958;40:279.
66. Martinez V, Sissons HA. Aneurysmal bone cyst: A review of 123 cases including primary lesions and those secondary to other bone pathology. *Cancer.* 1988;61:2291.
67. Scaglietti O, Marchetti PG, Bartolozzi P. The effects of methylprednisolone acetate in the treatment of bone cysts: Results of three years follow-up. *J Bone Joint Surg [Br].* 1979;61:200.
68. Dockerty MB, Ghormley RK, Kennedy RLJ, et al. Albright's syndrome (polyostotic fibrous dysplasia with cutaneous pigmentation in both sexes and gonadal dysfunction in females). *Arch Intern Med.* 1945;75:357.
69. Huvos AG, Higinbotham NL, Miller TR. Bone sarcomas arising in fibrous dysplasia. *J Bone Joint Surg Am.* 1972;54:1047.
70. Campanacci M, Laus M. Osteofibrous dysplasia of the tibia and fibula. *J Bone Joint Surg Am.* 1981;63:367.
71. Fitzgerald RH Jr, Brewer NS, Dahlin DC. Squamous-cell carcinoma complicating chronic osteomyelitis. *J Bone Joint Surg [Am].* 1976;58:1146.
72. Murphy FP, Dahlin DC, Sullivan CR. Articular synovial chondromatosis. *J Bone Joint Surg [Am].* 1962;44:77.
73. Bertoni F, Unni KK, Beabout JW, et al. Chondrosarcomas of the synovium. *Cancer.* 1991;67:155.
74. Schwartz HS, Unni KK, Pritchard DJ. Pigmented villonodular synovitis: A retrospective review of affected large joints. *Clin Orthop.* 1989;247:243.

20

Transplantation Pathology

Michael A. Nalesnik and Hector C. Ramos

The well-being of organ transplant candidates and recipients ultimately depends upon the expertise of the surgeon. The dramatic focal point of a patient's course is the transplant operation itself; however, it is the pretransplantation and posttransplantation management that determines long-term patient and allograft survival.

Pathology provides a powerful tool in the care of this patient population. It is most frequently used to evaluate acute or chronic allograft dysfunction but can also benefit the patient in other ways (Table 20–1).

The pathologic interpretation of results from a single biopsy can immediately affect the course of therapy. For this reason it is essential that clear lines of communication exist between surgeon and pathologist. The surgeon and the pathologist must understand both the strengths and limitations of microscopic diagnosis in the transplantation setting.

This chapter addresses pathologic examination of the pretransplantation donor organ and native organ; this is followed by a discussion of changes seen in the allograft itself. The section on allograft pathology provides a brief overview of the various forms of organ rejection. This section is followed by a discussion of organ harvest injury, mechanical injury, infectious complications, drug toxicity, and neoplasia. The subject of graft-versus-host disease in solid organ transplant recipients is discussed. Next, features unique to heart, lung, liver, kidney, pancreas, and small bowel transplantation are considered. Finally, the pitfalls awaiting the unwary surgeon or pathologist caring for the organ transplant patient are listed. Items related specifically to bone marrow transplantation, autotransplantation, and xenotransplantation are not included.

Pathology of the Organ Transplant Donor

The relative scarcity of usable organs stems from the discrepancy between supply and demand for cadaveric donor organs.[1, 2] Because this dilemma shows no tendency toward resolution, continued pressure to use every offered organ is expected. Current clinical practice is extremely efficient in selecting suitable donors. Even so, the actual number of suitable donors is underestimated by 1996 standards. The chronic shortage of donor organs, as well as the standard use of University of Wisconsin organ perfusion solution,[3] has prompted many centers to accept and transplant organs previously deemed inadequate. Several workers have reported that "marginal" donors are often acceptable.[2, 4] Consequently, it is often the transplant pathologist who determines suitability of an individual organ.

Table 20–1. Contributions of Histopathology/Cytopathology to the Care of the Organ Transplant Recipient

Assistance in the clinical evaluation of the donor organ
Detection of occult disease in the resected native organ
Evaluation of acute and chronic allograft dysfunction
Monitoring of the effect of alterations in antirejection therapy
Detection of posttransplantation infectious disease
Detection of posttransplantation malignancy
Evaluation for recurrence of native disease
Determination of cause of allograft failure
Determination of cause of patient death

Table 20–3. Simplified Working Formulation for Cardiac Rejection

Diagnosis	Histopathology
No rejection (grade 0)	Preferred diagnosis when findings are equivocal
Focal mild AR (grade 1A)	Focal lymphoid inflammation in perivascular or interstitial location without injury
Diffuse mild AR (grade 1B)	Diffuse lymphoid inflammation in perivascular or interstitial location without myocyte damage
Focal moderate AR (grade 2)	One focus of lymphoid inflammation ± eosinophils with architectural distortion and myocyte injury
Multifocal moderate AR (grade 3A)	Multifocal lymphoid inflammation ± eosinophils with architectural distortion and myocyte injury
Diffuse moderate AR (grade 3B)	Diffuse lymphoid inflammation with eosinophils ± neutrophils and with myocyte damage
Severe AR (grade 4)	Diffuse mixed inflammation with necrosis, usually hemorrhage and vasculitis

From Billingham ME, Cary NRB, Hammond ME, et al. A working formulation for the standardization of nomenclature in the diagnosis of heart and lung rejection: heart rejection study group. *J Heart Transplantation.* 1990; 9:587–593. With permission.

Table 20–5. Simplified NIDDK Grading for Acute and Chronic Liver Rejection

Diagnosis	Histopathology
No AR	
Mild AR	Rejection infiltrates involving and limited to some portal triads
Moderate AR	Rejection infiltrate in most or all portal triads, with or without spillover beyond limiting plate
Severe AR	Changes of A1 or A2 plus moderate to severe lobular inflammation and lobular necrosis and dropout
Mild CR	Bile duct loss in >50% of triads
Moderate CR	Bile duct loss in >50% of triads and any *one* of the following: centrilobular cholestasis, central vein sclerosis, hepatocyte ballooning, hepatocyte necrosis, and dropout
Severe CR	Bile duct loss in >50% of triads and any *two* of the following: centrilobular cholestasis, central vein sclerosis, hepatocyte ballooning, hepatocyte necrosis, and dropout

From Demetris AJ, Seaberg EC, Batts KP, et al. *Hepatology.* 1995; 21:408–416. With permission.

heart-lung, liver-small bowel, or kidney-pancreas), it is possible to see rejection in only one of the organs. Therefore, it is important to assess each organ individually.

Fine needle aspiration biopsy has been recommended as an alternative to core needle biopsy for both kidney and liver allografts (see Chapter 3).[26, 27] The smaller needle allows more frequent samples to be taken, thus providing earlier diagnosis of rejection as well as closer cytologic monitoring of the course of the rejection episode. The drawback of this technique is its lack of architectural features, needed for recognition of such conditions as chronic rejection. Interpretation requires a skilled and seasoned cytopathologist.

Table 20–4. Simplified Working Formulation for Lung Rejection

Diagnosis	Histopathology
No AR (grade A0)[a]	
Minimal AR (grade A1)	Occasional perivenular inflammatory cuffing, about two or three cells thick
Mild AR (grade A2)	More frequent and obvious perivenular and periarteriolar lymphoid cuffing with eosinophils, "endothelialitis"
Moderate AR (grade A3)	Similar to grade 2, with eosinophils, occasional neutrophils, and extension of inflammation into alveolar septa and air spaces
Severe AR (grade A4)	Similar to grade 3 with alveolar pneumocyte damage/necrosis, hyaline membranes, may have infarcts
Chronic airway rejection	Bronchiolitis obliterans may be active (with inflammatory cells) or inactive (fibrosis only)
Chronic vascular rejection	Fibrointimal thickening of vessels

[a]All grades of rejection are based on vascular/perivascular inflammation. Presence or absence of lymphocytic bronchitis/bronchiolitis is noted separately and receives optional grade B0–B4.

From Yousem SA, Berry GJ, Cagle PT, et al. *J Heart Lung Transplant.* In press.

Chronic rejection occurs months to years following transplantation. It is seen more frequently, but not exclusively, in those patients who have had prior acute rejection episodes. The mechanisms of chronic rejection are poorly understood.[28] In most cases, evidence of subacute vascular damage, e.g., intimal thickening and other variants of atherosclerosis, is seen (Fig. 20–10). This causes insidious and progressive organ dysfunction, which is secondary to relent-

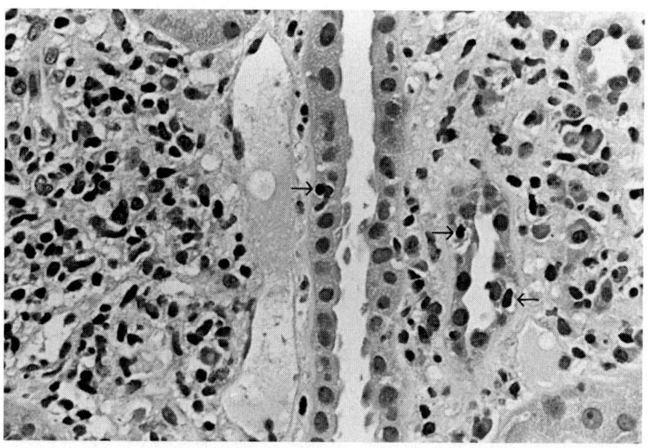

Figure 20–2. Acute cellular rejection, kidney. Several tubules are present and are separated by a widened interstitium that contains numerous inflammatory cells. Small dark nuclei are seen interspersed among the tubular epithelial cells *(arrows)*. These represent infiltrating inflammatory cells, and this process is referred to as tubulitis. Hematoxylin and eosin, ×400.

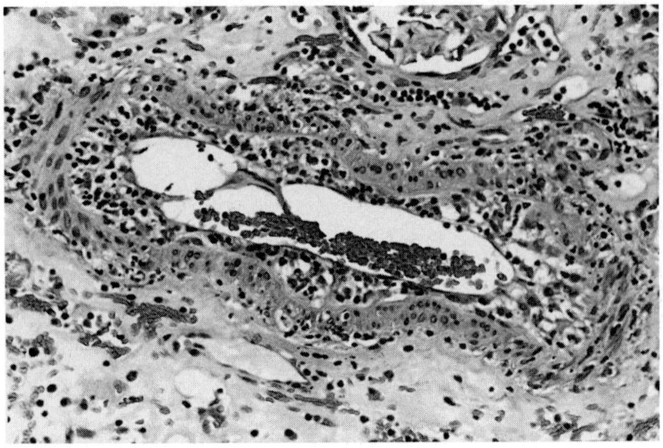

Figure 20–3. Arterial involvement in acute cellular rejection, kidney. A section of a medium-sized artery contains a heavy inflammatory infiltrate in its intimal portion. Arterial components of cellular rejection may lead to organ loss due to ischemia if not rapidly reversed. Hematoxylin and eosin, ×200.

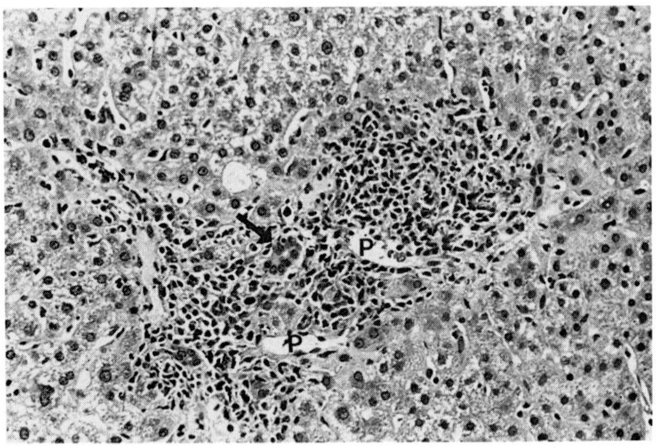

Figure 20–4. Acute cellular rejection, liver. A portal tract contains a heavy infiltrate of inflammatory cells throughout. Despite the intensity of inflammation, the borders of the tract remain fairly well circumscribed (compare with Fig. 20–17). The open space is the lumen of the portal vein *(P)*, the wall of which is infiltrated by the inflammatory cells. The bile duct *(arrow)* is also involved. Hematoxylin and eosin, ×200.

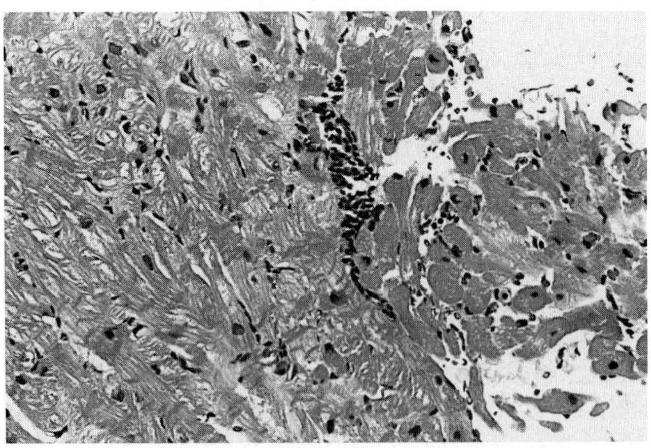

Figure 20–5. Acute cellular rejection grade 1A, heart. A small focus of chronic inflammatory cells aggregates in the interstitium in the vicinity of a small capillary. The presence of occasional infiltrates of this degree of cellularity, or even slightly greater, is consistent with a low-grade type of rejection. Hematoxylin and eosin, ×200.

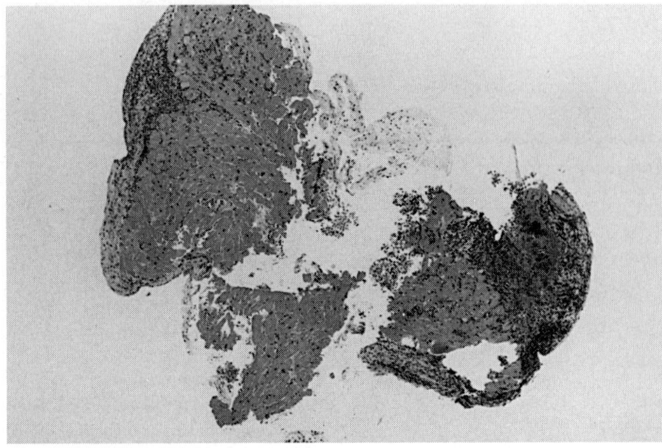

Figure 20–6. Acute cellular rejection grade 3A, heart. In this low-power photomicrograph, two fragments of myocardium are involved with a dense inflammatory infiltrate, which imparts a mottled appearance to the tissue. Hematoxylin and eosin, ×40.

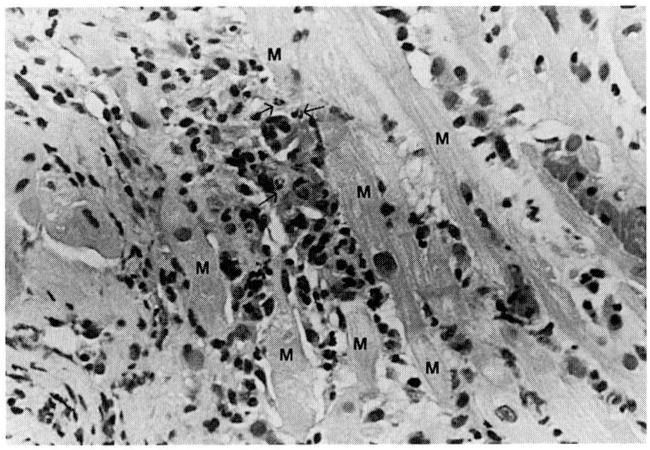

Figure 20–7. Acute cellular rejection grade 3A, heart. At higher magnification, the isolation and separation of myocytes *(M)* by the inflammatory process can be seen. Acute inflammatory cells, i.e., neutrophils, are present as well as lymphocytes and are marked by arrows. Myocytes that were present in the area of inflammation are presumed destroyed. Hematoxylin and eosin, ×400.

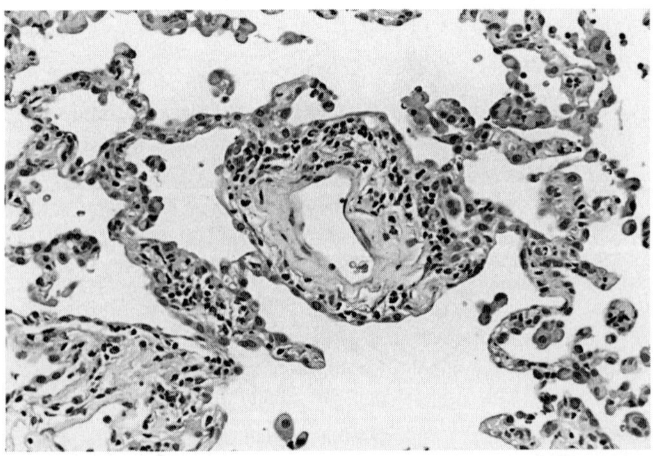

Figure 20–8. Acute cellular rejection, lung. The small vein in the center of the photograph shows a slight cuffing of mononuclear cells with no significant extension of inflammation into the alveolar walls. Inflammation was slightly more prominent elsewhere and the overall grade was A2 (mild acute cellular rejection). Hematoxylin and eosin, ×200. (Specimen supplied by Dr. N.P. Ohori.)

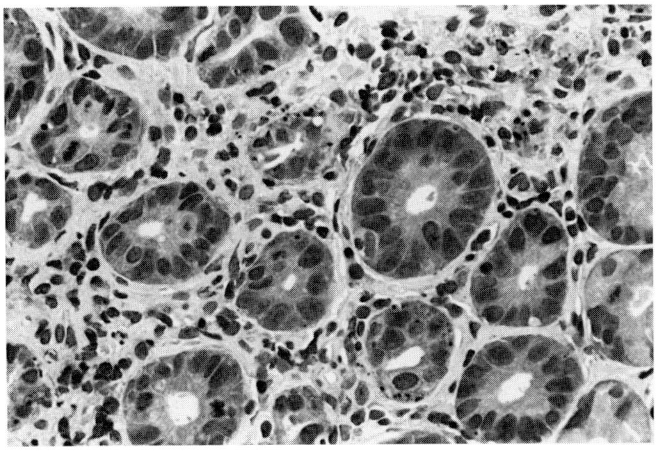

Figure 20–9. Acute cellular rejection, small bowel. The crypts show significant apoptosis, which appears as small dark dots and fragments on the peripheral aspects of the glands. This material represents karyorrhectic nuclear debris. There is also a mild increase of chronic inflammatory cells in the lamina propria. Hematoxylin and eosin, ×400.

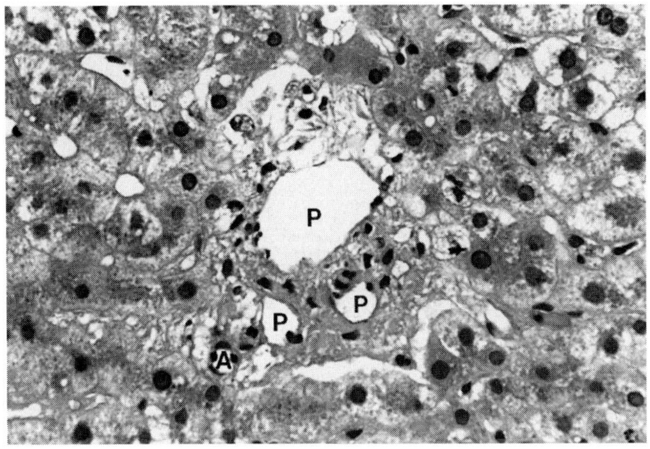

Figure 20–11. Chronic rejection, liver. This small portal tract shows a normal portal vein *(P)* and hepatic artery branch *(A)*. No bile duct is seen. Some nearby hepatocytes show swelling due to interference with bile flow. Note the absence of inflammatory cells. In other cases, a mild, inactive-appearing mononuclear infiltrate may be present in portal tracts. Trichrome, ×400.

less ischemia and fibrosis. There is also a component of parenchymal loss, most likely due to this ischemia as well as to an indolent but a persistent immune reaction unresponsive to current immunosuppressive regimens. In the liver, there is a loss of small bile ducts (Fig. 20–11); in the kidney, a loss of tubules (Fig. 20–12) with possible associated glomerular injury (Fig. 20–13); and in the pancreas, a loss of acini. The lungs show fibrosis and functional loss of small bronchioles, i.e., obliterative bronchiolitis (Fig. 20–14). The clinical consequence of small airway injury outweighs that of vessel damage in this organ. The opposite occurs in the heart, where an accelerated coronary arteriosclerosis is the chief consequence of chronic rejection. In the intestines, the process results in fibrosis of the lamina propria with loss of mucosal and glandular epithelium.

Chronic rejection may be punctuated by episodes of acute rejection or other processes. Indeed, the primary function of the biopsy at this stage is to evaluate the extent of chronic rejection and to rule out other concurrent and more treatable causes of organ dysfunction. Attempts to reverse chronic rejection by maintaining aggressive immunosuppression are futile and only serve to place the patient at increased risk for complications related to such drug therapy.

Because chronic rejection is currently untreatable, prevention is the only tactic. There is no substitute for appro-

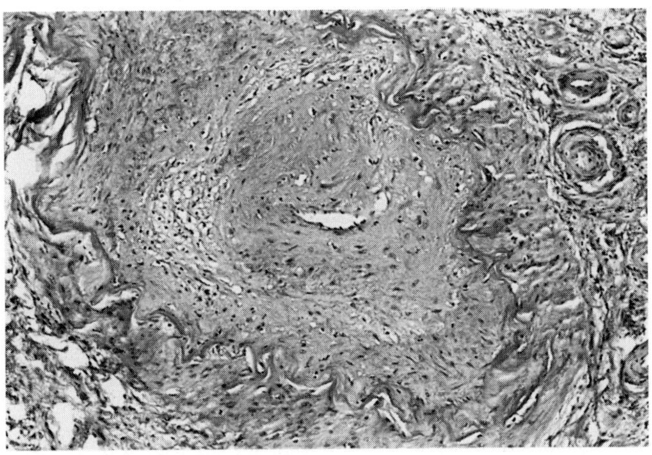

Figure 20–10. Chronic rejection, accelerated arteriosclerosis. Significant intimal thickening with reduction of luminal caliber is seen in this artery and is a common feature of chronic rejection in all organs. The change is often most severe in renal allografts and is of lesser significance in the pulmonary vasculature due to concomitant airway involvement (see Fig. 20–14). Hematoxylin and eosin, ×100.

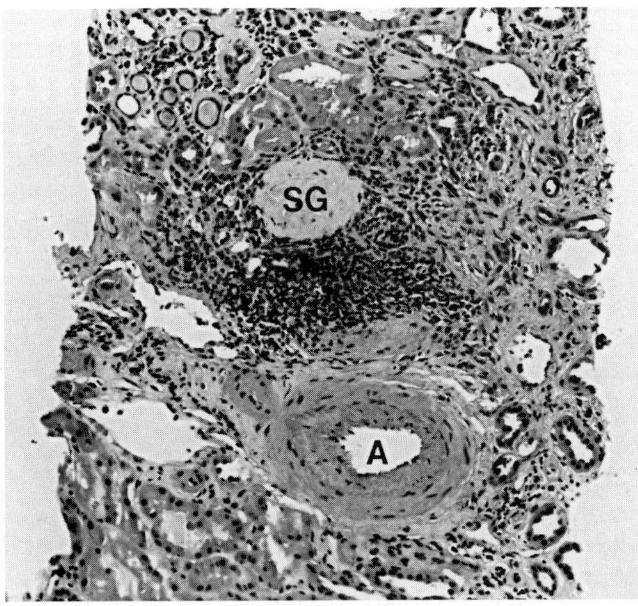

Figure 20–12. Chronic rejection, kidney. This needle biopsy of allograft kidney shows interstitial fibrosis with tubular atrophy. Slight intimal thickening is seen in the artery *(A)* in the lower half of the photograph. A dense chronic inflammatory infiltrate is seen superior to this. This encloses a round body that represents a sclerotic glomerulus *(SG)*. Such periarterial inflammation is common in chronic nephropathy and does not signify a superimposed acute rejection process. Hematoxylin and eosin, ×100.

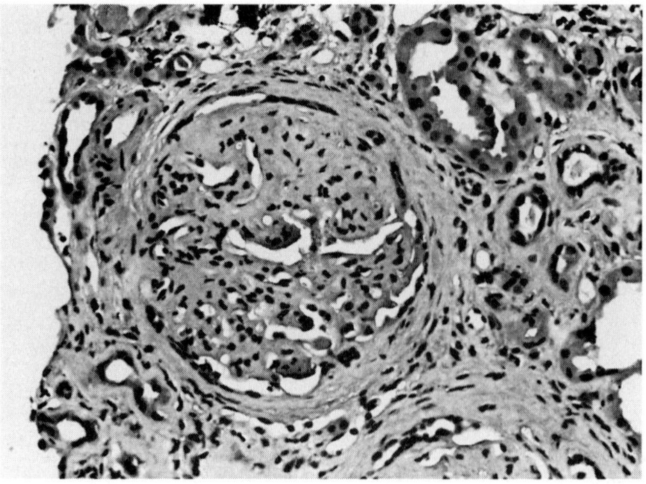

Figure 20–13. Transplant glomerulopathy, kidney. Glomerular disorders may represent recurrent disease, de novo processes, or may be related to ischemia or the rejection process. This is an example of the latter process. The segmental nature of the process in this case is shown by the prominent thickening in the upper as opposed to the lower half of the glomerulus. In some cases, full workup including immunofluorescence and electron microscopy may be necessary to distinguish among the various possibilities. Hematoxylin and eosin, ×200.

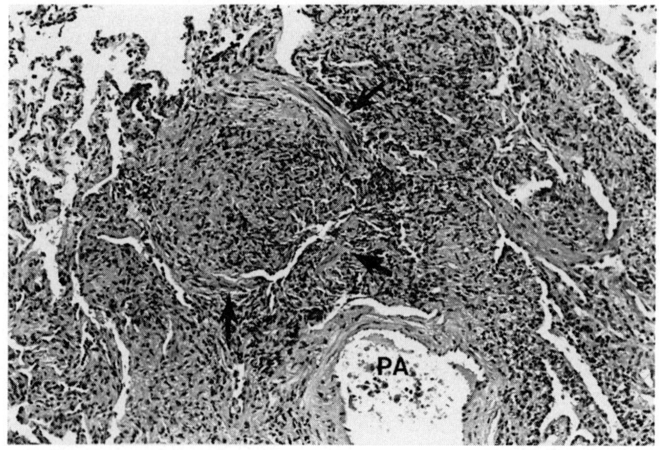

Figure 20–14. Chronic airway rejection (obliterative bronchiolitis), lung. The open area in the lower portion of the photograph represents the lumen of a pulmonary artery branch *(PA)*. Superior and to the left of this is the obliterated lumen of the associated bronchiole. The periphery of this airway segment is recognized by residual smooth muscle bands *(arrows)*. The process is fairly complete at this point but still shows activity in the form of an associated inflammatory infiltrate. Over time these cells will be lost and the former lumen will be marked by a dense fibrous scar. Hematoxylin and eosin, ×100. (Specimen contributed by Dr. N.P. Ohori.)

priate and consistent immunosuppression. In some studies, long-term allograft survival is closely related to the time of onset and severity of the first rejection episode.

Ischemic Injury Related to Organ Procurement ("Harvest" or "Preservation" Injury)

Preservation injury refers to the donor organ damage that occurs between disruption of donor blood supply and allograft anastomosis to the recipient's vascular system. The underlying condition of the donor or the recipient may either enhance or diminish the consequences of these changes. Current preservatives, such as University of Wisconsin solution, minimize hypothermic and oxygen free radical–associated cell injury and provide components to allow rapid resynthesis of ATP, thereby facilitating recovery of organ function.[3] These measures notwithstanding, varying levels of difficulty in organ harvest from individual donors, as well as differences among donors themselves, cause preservation injury as a basis of allograft dysfunction.

This form of injury manifests clinically as primary nonfunction of the engrafted organ. Typically, it occurs to some extent in renal, hepatic, and occasionally pulmonary allografts. Microscopic examination shows ischemic injury of varying degree (Fig. 20–15). Preservation injury may mask a subsequent episode of ACR, and biopsy may be useful in sorting out this problem.

Mechanical Problems

Mechanical problems most commonly manifest as acute episodes of organ dysfunction or nonfunction occurring in the short-term posttransplantation period and following an interval of function. They occur most often in transplants involving small children or patients requiring extensive vascular reconstruction. Immediate surgical intervention may be required for cases of underlying vascular obstruction.

In practice, mechanical complications occur most commonly in liver and kidney allografts. In the case of liver, the biliary tree is particularly susceptible to injury because it is dependent upon hepatic arterial, not portal, circulation (Fig. 20–16). Parenchymal necrosis may also occur, with

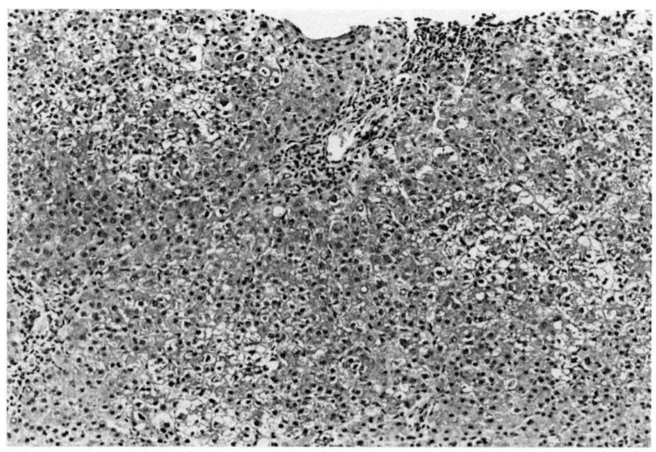

Figure 20–15. Postperfusion ischemia, liver. This low-power photomicrograph of a needle biopsy of liver shows the regularly distributed swollen and pale hepatocytes of mild ischemia. The aggregates of such cells in this photograph mark the centrilobular zones, where the injury is most marked. More significant injury would result in frank centrilobular-based necrosis and a reparative process associated with ductular proliferation at the edges of the portal tracts. Hematoxylin and eosin, ×100.

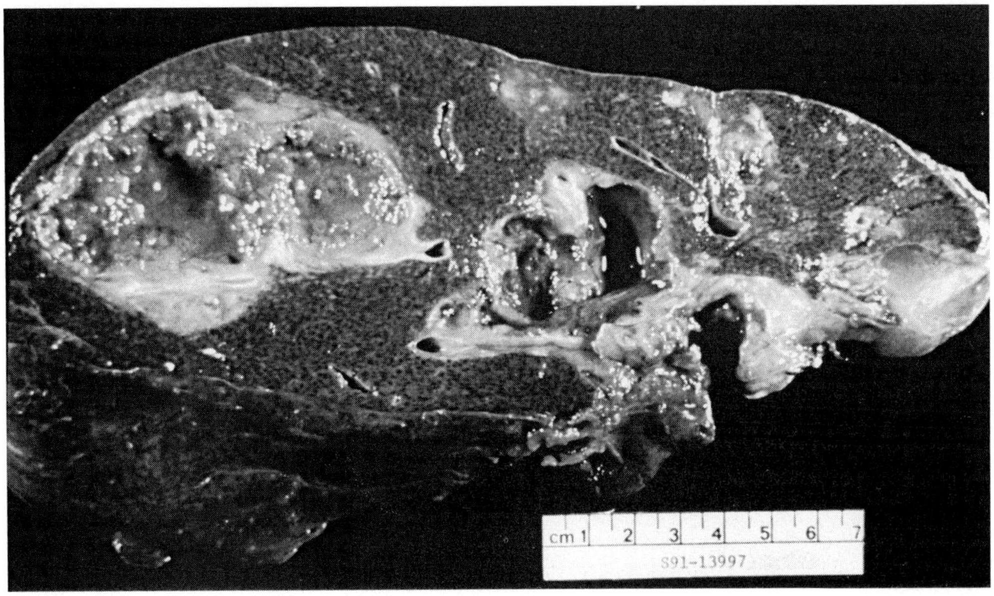

Figure 20–16. Liver allograft failure due to hepatic arterial thrombosis. Preferential damage to the biliary system with necrosis, dilatation, and secondary abscess formation is highlighted in this allograft hepatectomy specimen. The hepatic artery thrombus itself is not well visualized in this view. (Photograph contributed by Mr. F. Fusca.)

subsequent seeding of necrotic foci by intestinal bacteria. Injury related to the portal vein, hepatic vein, or vena cava is rare. In the case of the kidney, ischemic necrosis of renal parenchyma or collecting system may occur. Lymphocele, ureteral obstruction, and reflux may also complicate the operation. In the lung, breakdown of the airway anastomosis was a problem in earlier years but has largely disappeared with improvements in operative techniques.[13]

The sensitivity of biopsy for specifically detecting mechanical injury is low, so that definitive therapy need not await the results of microscopic analysis.

Infections

Infections are a significant cause of morbidity and mortality in organ transplant patients. In this respect, and in many other respects as well, these patients represent an extreme challenge in general principles of postoperative management. Most infections occur in the first three post-transplantation months because of the high levels of immunosuppression used during this period. It has been estimated that 50 to 75% of transplant patients will have one or more episodes of bacterial infection and 30 to 60% will have one or more episodes of viral infection.[29]

Bacterial infections occur early and sometimes represent localized complications of the procedure itself. Such infections typically affect the urinary or respiratory tracts, particularly when organs within those systems are transplanted. Kidneys may develop acute pyelonephritis. Biopsy specimens show acute tubular inflammation, which must be distinguished from rejection infiltrate. The liver may be involved by ascending cholangitis. Alternatively, a secondary infection may involve areas of parenchymal necrosis. The major role of biopsy is to exclude underlying rejection because, if not contraindicated, reduction of immunosuppression is pivotal for controlling infection. However, bacterial and other types of infection in the lungs must be excluded first to make an accurate diagnosis of rejection in this organ because there is overlap in the microscopic appearances of these two different processes.[30]

Of course, these heavily immunosuppressed patients are at risk of developing typical pyogenic bacterial infections at the usual ''barrier'' sites, such as tonsils, perirectal or perianal tissues, or in the region of the ileocecal valve (acute typhlitis). The surgeon must be vigilant for signs or symptoms of such intercurrent problems and be ready to intervene with standard procedures, e.g., incision and drainage for abscess formation.

Virus infections most commonly occur within the first 6 months although they can arise at any time. Cytomegalovirus (CMV) is the most common viral agent in these patients and may manifest as either a localized or disseminated process.

In some cases, the allograft itself serves as the portal of entry. This is particularly true in cases of organs from CMV[31] or EBV-seropositive[32] individuals transplanted into seronegative recipients. In other cases, reactivation infection may occur. This is seen almost universally with liver transplantation for underlying hepatitis B[33] or hepatitis C[34, 35] infection (Fig. 20–17). When the allograft itself is involved, clinical manifestations may be indistinguishable from acute rejection. Biopsy is useful both to establish the diagnosis and to ascertain the presence or absence of concurrent rejection. Sequential biopsies may be extremely helpful in tailoring adjustments of immunosuppressive therapy. Later biopsies are useful in assessing the likely progression of the hepatitic process and in gauging efficacy of antiviral agents such as alpha-interferon. The application of a semiquantitative grading system to the biopsy for chronic viral hepatitis is helpful in this context.[36]

Herpes simplex virus infection usually represents reactivation infection.[29] It tends to be localized but may on occasion occur in a severe disseminated form. Similarly, varicella-zoster virus infection usually represents reactivation and may disseminate in profoundly immunosuppressed patients. Either of these two herpes viruses can produce fulminant hepatitis, either localized or in conjunction with other organ involvement.

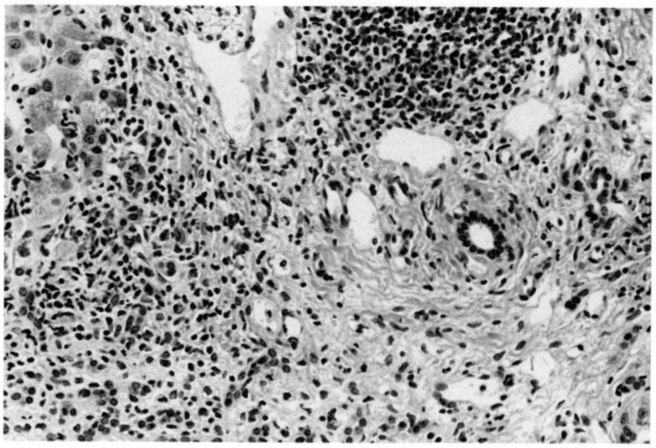

Figure 20–17. Recurrent viral hepatitis, allograft liver. The photograph contains a portal tract with patchy lymphocytic inflammation. The infiltrate spills out beyond the edges of the tract on the left side of the field, giving a ragged appearance typical of the process of piecemeal necrosis. Notice that bile duct and portal vessels are spared involvement (compare with Fig. 20–4). Hematoxylin and eosin, ×200.

Other viruses that may afflict this population include adenovirus and respiratory syncytial virus (RSV). These organisms are most commonly identified in the lungs of the pediatric population. In addition, adenovirus can cause a necrotic form of hepatitis similar to that seen with herpes viruses.[37]

Renal transplant patients may show evidence of papovavirus infection in their allografts, sometimes detectable in urine cytology specimens. This finding has been associated with renal dysfunction in some studies.[38]

Infection with EBV or papillomavirus may lead to neoplasms (lymphomas and epithelial tumors, respectively). These viruses are discussed in the section on neoplasia.

Candida and *Aspergillus* species are the two commonest fungal infections in the transplant patient population. Either occurs in both localized and disseminated forms. Because early detection is crucial for effective therapy, biopsy, including fine needle aspiration sampling, should be obtained whenever there is clinical suspicion (see Chapter 3). *Cryptococcus, Histoplasma, Blastomyces, Coccidioides, Mucor,* and *Rhizopus* species are all detectable by microscopic examination complemented by histochemical stains for fungi. A variety of normal commensal organisms may also act as opportunistic infectious agents in this patient population. It is often not possible to definitively identify the pathogenic species by microscopy alone; microbial cultures are needed for confirmation.

Pneumocystis carinii is the most common protozoan to infect the transplant recipient, restricted to the lungs in the majority of cases. Diagnosis of pulmonary pneumocystosis is facilitated by the use of methenamine silver (Grocott) stain on bronchoalveolar lavage (BAL) fluid specimens. This stain will also detect fungi. In our practice we routinely prepare a hematoxylin and eosin (H&E) stain on BAL specimens in addition to the Grocott stain. In this way we can rapidly screen for *Pneumocystis,* fungi, and CMV infections. A separate portion of the specimen handled by sterile technique is sent to the laboratory for appropriate cultures.

Toxoplasmosis is a rare infectious complication of organ transplantation, and it is seen most commonly in heart or heart-lung recipients. The donor heart is one potential source for infection with this organism.[31] The organism can be identified histologically by endomyocardial biopsy. Management of rejection in a heart transplant patient with cardiac toxoplasmosis is difficult because the inflammation seen in the biopsy sample may be due to either the infection or rejection. Careful clinical correlation and examination of sequential biopsy specimens are requisite for successfully treating these patients.

Drug Toxicity

Cyclosporin A is the main immunosuppressive agent currently in use, and nephrotoxicity remains the primary complication of this drug.[39, 40] Tacrolimus (FK506) shares this same side effect.[39, 41] In the case of renal transplantation, this effect may be compounded in the early posttransplantation phase by concurrent ischemia owing to harvest injury. Biopsy is helpful in evaluating the extent of these changes and in detecting acute rejection, which may be clinically masked by the ischemic/toxic insult.

Acute nephrotoxicity is expressed microscopically as ''isometric'' tubular vacuolization, microthrombi that affect the arterioles or glomeruli, or vascular myocyte injury. Chronic toxicity due to these drugs primarily involves vessels at the arteriolar level. This effect leads to a glassy (hyaline) appearance of these vessels with subsequent glomerulosclerosis and interstitial fibrosis, both due to ischemia (Fig. 20–18). Chronic rejection may lead to similar ischemic injury but tends to involve the larger arterial branches. In some cases, it is not possible to determine the relative effects of drug- or rejection-related injury, and the generic term ''chronic allograft nephropathy'' has been proposed (Fig. 20–12).[24]

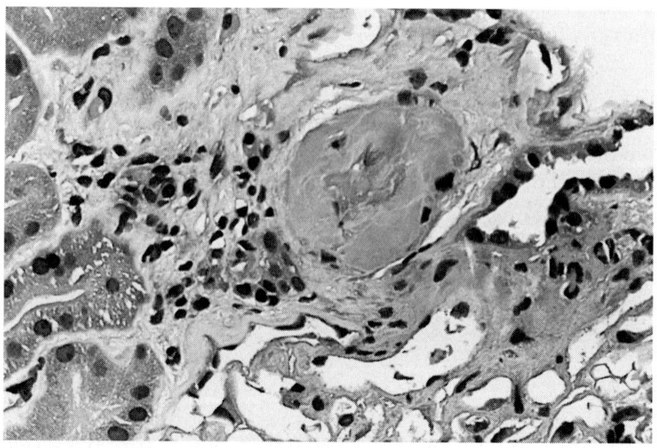

Figure 20–18. Cyclosporine nephrotoxicity, chronic. The arteriole in this photomicrograph is thickened by hyaline material with some nodular features. This form of drug toxicity usually targets vessels of this size whereas cellular and chronic rejection involves larger arteries. Hematoxylin and eosin, ×400.

Neoplasia

As transplanted organs become more commonplace, increasing numbers of patients are subjected to chronic immunosuppression and its attendant complication of neoplasia. The incidence of malignancies in transplanted individuals is estimated to range from 1 to 18% and to average 6%. In the short term this incidence will likely increase in proportion to the increasing longevity of transplant recipients. In the long term, it is hoped that this complication will be avoided when true organ tolerance can be achieved and dependence on relatively nonspecific immunosuppressants diminishes.

Currently used immunosuppressants produce global diminution of the cellular immune response. Reduced antiviral immunosurveillance in particular may result in the emergence of so-called opportunistic virus-related malignancies. The primary offender is EBV, which is associated with closely interrelated lymphoid hyperplasias and malignant lymphomas (Fig. 20–19).[42] Infection with EBV may lead to inapparent infection, a syndrome similar to infectious mononucleosis, single or multiple tumors, or rarely to disseminated and fulminant lymphoproliferation.[43–45] It is important to document the presence of EBV in these growths and to categorize the lesions according to current classification schemes. Both benign and malignant lymphoid proliferations occur, and the pathologist should be familiar with the varying histopathologic patterns that may be encountered.[44–46] It is imperative to discuss any impending biopsy with the pathologist to ensure that the sample is allocated appropriately for the needs of ancillary studies such as DNA analysis of clonality and cytogenetics. These may prove essential to ultimate clinicopathologic correlation. However, clinical management decisions must be initiated on the basis of rapidly available conventional histologic appearance (with or without supportive immunohistochemical studies of cell type and EBV presence), as well as tumor stage and clinical condition of the patient. Such disease can be limited to the allograft organ alone. Clinically, this syndrome may mimic ACR. Because the most effective means for controlling EBV-derived tumors is by reduction of immunosuppression, an erroneous diagnosis of ACR in these circumstances could be of disastrous consequence.

Rare cases of smooth muscle tumors have been observed in transplant patients. Epstein-Barr virus has been found to be present in these proliferations.[47, 48]

Papillomaviruses may be seen in both benign and malignant lesions of the skin such as condyloma acuminatum, premalignant keratosis, Bowen's disease, keratoacanthoma, and squamous cell carcinoma.[49] In female organ transplant recipients, surveillance cervical cytology is important because of the increased risk for dysplasia of the uterine cervix.[50] Skin tumors, which represent the commonest malignancies in the transplant population, are associated as well with sun exposure. Evidence derives from the higher frequency of this form of cancer in transplant patients in geographic areas with strong sunlight than in those patients with less exposure. The relative increase of squamous cell over basal cell carcinomas has been noted.[51] This trend is the opposite of that in nonimmunosuppressed patients.

Hepatitis viruses could in theory lead to posttransplantation hepatomas. However, it appears that most or all of such cases arise from known or occult hepatomas already present at the time of transplantation. Kaposi's sarcoma arises in transplant patients, particularly those of Mediterranean origin. The discovery of herpes virus–like DNA in lesions from AIDS patients suggests that the same viral cofactor may play a role in the genesis of such lesions in transplant recipients.[52]

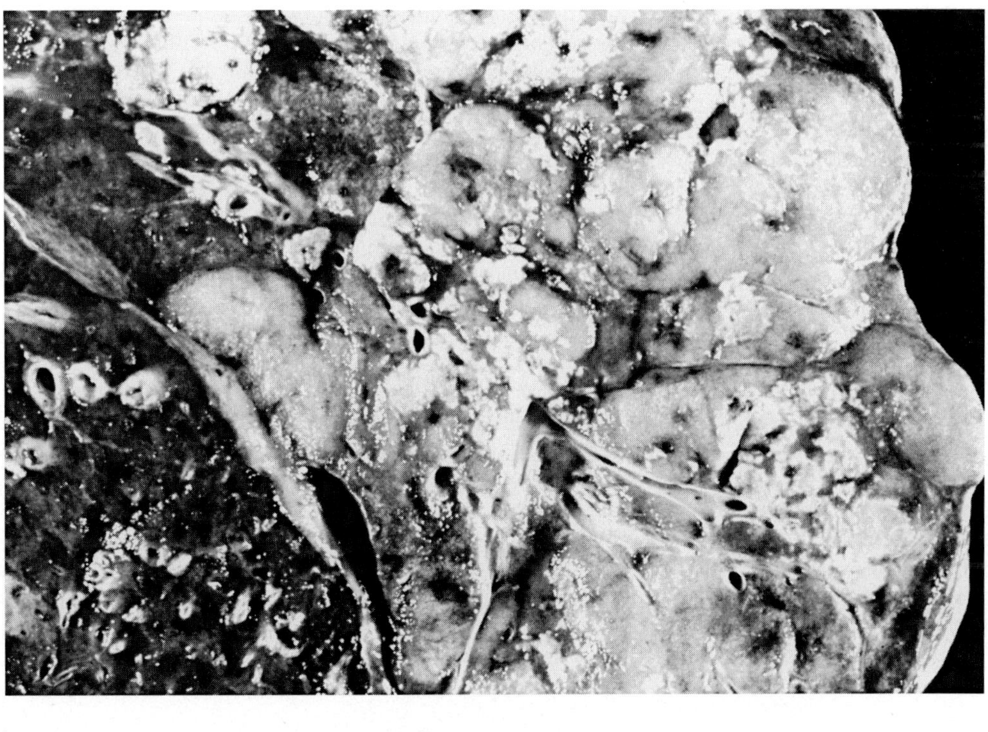

Figure 20–19. Posttransplant Epstein-Barr virus (EBV)-associated lymphoproliferative disorder, lung. This allograft lung was involved with an EBV-associated lymphoproliferation that morphologically resembled large-cell non-Hodgkin's lymphoma ("monomorphic" posttransplant lymphoproliferative disorder). The tumorous nature of the process is apparent. Lighter areas represent regions of necrosis. (Photograph provided by Mr. F. Fusca.)

Graft-Versus-Host Disease

Graft-versus-host disease (GVHD) represents an immune attack against the recipient mediated by donor lymphoid cells.[53] This is a common complication of bone marrow transplantation, in which the recipient's own immune system is intentionally ablated prior to the engraftment.[54] The syndrome has only occasionally been described in solid organ transplantation.[55–57]

The target organs of GVHD (skin, gastrointestinal system, and liver) show changes similar to those described in bone marrow recipients.[58] The presence of a rash should alert the surgeon to the possibility of this condition. Although most rashes are due to drug reactions or other causes, biopsy is often useful for implicating or excluding GVHD.[59] Consultation with the pathologist should precede biopsy because procedures requiring special tissue handling may be needed to specifically uncover the presence of donor inflammation in the target organ.[60, 61] The presence of rare donor cells alone does not constitute prima facie evidence of GVHD. The phenomenon of *microchimerism* is a normal concomitant of organ transplantation and may actually play a beneficial role in the production of mutual immune recognition and hyporeactivity between host and donor.[62, 63]

Points Specific to Individual Allograft Organs

HEART

The heart is relatively resistant to ischemic injury during harvest, although prolonged ischemia as, for example, with donor cardiopulmonary resuscitation, may compromise function.[64] Rejection may be clinically silent in the early stages so that biopsy by protocol is essential for diagnosis (Figs. 20–5 through 20–7). Most surgeons collect four to six biopsy fragments to compensate for the patchy distribution of early rejection.[64] The histologic differential diagnosis of isolated cardiac allograft inflammation is fairly restricted, including toxoplasmosis, lymphoproliferative disease, and myocarditis. In reality, these are extremely rare in comparison with rejection. Endocardial inflammation in the form of so-called Quilty lesions (Fig. 20–20) does not have any immediate therapeutic significance. However, the possibility of endocardial-based rejection must be excluded. The latter tends to have activated lymphocytes, occasional eosinophils, and edema, and lacks the symmetry, small vessels, and uniform small lymphocytes of such Quilty lesions. Prior biopsy sites are associated with inflammation and fibrosis, which must also be distinguished from rejection. A major long-term complication of cardiac transplantation is chronic rejection in the form of symptomatic coronary arteriosclerosis. In patients receiving transplants for amyloidosis, recurrence is common.[65] The only exceptions occur in cases of familial amyloidosis when the amyloid-producing organ, i.e., the liver, is also replaced.

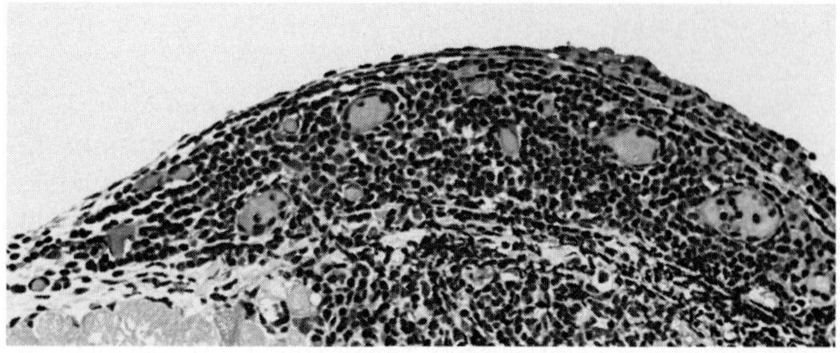

Figure 20–20. So-called Quilty lesion, heart. A symmetric, endocardial-based Quilty lesion is shown. Notice the cellular composition, which consists exclusively of small lymphocytes. The congested capillary-sized vessels are a frequent feature of this lesion. In the lower portion of the field the cells infiltrate a short distance into the underlying myocardium. This is a feature of the less common type B (infiltrating) Quilty lesion. Such lesions are by convention not considered evidence of acute rejection. Hematoxylin and eosin, ×200.

LUNG

Single lung and sequential single lung transplantation, with other technical advances, has markedly reduced the incidence of postoperative complications at the site of tracheal anastomosis.[13] Preservation injury in the immediate posttransplantation period may manifest as diffuse interstitial infiltrates on chest x-ray. The histologic changes range from patchy alveolar injury to diffuse alveolar damage. The possibility of pulmonary infection is a constant confounding variable in the accurate histopathologic diagnosis of rejection. In addition to microbiologic evaluation for bacterial infection, the possibilities of CMV, EBV, and *Pneumocystis* must also be considered. A minimum of five transbronchial biopsy specimens is necessary for reliable pathologic evaluation.[23] Discussion with the pathologist regarding the desirable number and type of specimens is recommended (see Chap. 11). The diagnosis of acute rejection is based on the presence of perivascular inflammation alone (Fig. 20–8); airway inflammation is evaluated separately. The principal long-term complication is obliterative bronchiolitis (Fig. 20–14), which is thought to represent a form of chronic rejection. This is distinct from the often reversible loose intrabronchiolar granulation tissue formation that occurs with resolving infection or other conditions.[13] Accelerated arteriosclerosis also occurs as a component of chronic rejection but is less significant from a clinical standpoint than is obliterative bronchiolitis. Recurrent primary disease is unusual but may occur in such conditions as sarcoidosis, lymphangioleiomyomatosis, or giant cell interstitial pneumonia.[23]

LIVER

Emergent acute rejection must be distinguished from preservation injury in the patient who has just recently received an allograft liver (Figs. 20–4 and 20–15). Later in the recovery period in patients transplanted for end-stage viral hepatitis, the inflammation of recurrent hepatitis must be distinguished from that caused by rejection (Fig. 20–17). Epstein-Barr virus infection can appear either as a hepatitis or as tumorous lymphoid infiltrates (see Fig. 20–19).[66, 67]

In all of these situations, the biopsy, together with liver function studies, can assist in management of immunosuppression in conjunction with therapy for conditions that are not rejection related.

Mechanical problems involving either the hepatic artery or bile duct may lead to biliary dysfunction (Fig. 20–16). In this situation, the biopsy is a relatively insensitive indicator. In the long-term transplantation survivor, partial duct stricture also causes biliary dysfunction.[68] This condition is suggested by low-grade ductular proliferation and neutrophilia in the biopsy. The mixed portal tract inflammation is easily confused with early rejection. Actual loss of bile ducts is most commonly a consequence of chronic rejection.

Recurrent disease is occasionally encountered in relation to primary sclerosing cholangitis, primary biliary cirrhosis, autoimmune hepatitis, and giant cell hepatitis.[68] The recurrence of hepatitis B and C virus infections has already been noted. Recidivism of the alcoholic patient is not unknown.[68] Patients with incidental hepatomas in the native livers should be followed for recurrence. Recurrence is rare for small T1 lesions, but the frequency of recurrence increases in relation to the original tumor stage.

KIDNEY

Primary nonfunction of the allograft kidney is actually a relatively common problem, and biopsy is useful for detecting changes due to ischemia or rejection. It cannot predict when function will commence. Both de novo and recurrent glomerulonephritis may occur,[7] and a thorough pretransplantation review evaluation may assist in this distinction by providing a definitive diagnosis when the diagnosis of the underlying disease was originally uncertain. Transplant glomerulopathy is a form of glomerulonephritis thought to result from the transplant process itself (Fig. 20–13). Chronic rejection is the ultimate fate of many but not all allograft kidneys (Fig. 20–12). Long-term damage may be accelerated by the inherent nephrotoxicity of currently available immunosuppressants. Whether to extend allograft survival or to remove the organ is the surgeon's decision, based upon a synthesis of the clinical picture, renal function tests, all in relation to the histopathologic picture (see Chap. 14).

PANCREAS

Over 5,000 pancreatic transplants had been performed as of 1993.[69] Graft survival appears to be slightly improved when the organ is implanted simultaneously with kidney.[69] This combined approach may stabilize diabetic neuropathy and may forestall the development of diabetic nephropathy in the allograft.[70] A biopsy technique utilizing urinary bladder cystoscopy can be employed when the graft drainage is via a cystoduodenostomy.[71] As it is elsewhere, rejection in this organ is mediated by lymphocytes; however, the case may be complicated by the local release of pancreatic enzymes, with concurrent acute inflammation.[72, 73] Attempts to replace selectively the insulin-producing islet cells via islet cell infusions are also being done at various centers.[70]

SMALL BOWEL

Initial attempts at small bowel transplantation were complicated by lymphoproliferative disease.[74] This lethal complication has been ameliorated by the introduction of Tacrolimus (FK506). However, EBV-associated enteritis and lymphoproliferations are still problems, particularly in the pediatric population. It may be impossible to exclude concurrent rejection in this situation, so that sequential biopsies may be necessary to determine the underlying process. In the adult population, CMV infection can similarly complicate the differential diagnosis of rejection. Again, the biopsy may be the best source of feedback to the surgeon. Pure acute rejection can be diagnosed by endoscopic biopsy (Fig. 20–9). The early stages of this disorder may be extremely subtle, and sequential biopsies may be valuable in following the evolution of a given episode.

Chronic rejection may be seen from months to years after transplantation and is detected histologically as increased fibrous tissue in the lamina propria. This finding probably reflects indolent ischemia secondary to intimal thickening of the donor mesenteric arteries and their branches.

PITFALLS FOR THE SURGEON

1. Failure to coordinate specimen allocation and processing with the pathologist.

   The availability of rapid (same day) specimen processing is the exception rather than the rule because it is dependent upon the availability of mechanical tissue processors, histotechnologists, and other limiting factors. The surgeon and pathologist should work together to ensure that diagnostic turnaround time expectations are realistic and that laboratory resources are both efficiently utilized and responsive to clinical needs.

   Discussing the proper mode of tissue submission (e.g., need for fresh versus fixed tissue, multiple samples) prior to biopsy permits the performance of special procedures such as karyotypic or molecular studies when appropriate.
2. Rigid insistence that all criteria be present or that a single criterion (e.g., myocyte necrosis in the heart) be present to establish a particular histopathologic diagnosis.

   An analogy to physical examination can be made. Lists of signs and symptoms can be

Continued

readily obtained for any disease, yet the art of diagnosis lies in the distillation of these clues and an appreciation of their expression in an individual patient. This concept can be extended to the examination of the case at a microscopic level.

3. Failure to appreciate the diversity of difficulties that complicate microscopic interpretation.

   Similar to the aforementioned, there are "classic" and "atypical" presentations of disease, at both the clinical and histopathologic levels. These present varying challenges to the pathologist's interpretive skill.

4. Insistence on biopsy interpretation in the absence of clinical data.

   This would be akin to performing a physical examination in the absence of any component of the patient history. One could not perform an incisive examination designed to distinguish among various considerations of a logical differential diagnosis. The same holds for the pathologist. Most pathologists first evaluate the specimen without any clinical data, to generate a complete differential diagnosis. However, it is then important to compare this with the relevant clinical and laboratory data. Only in this way can the most specific diagnosis be given. As an example of the importance of clinical data to this process, consider the pathologist who must contemplate the differential diagnosis of inflammation within an organ while not knowing whether it is a native or an allograft.

5. Assumption on clinical/radiologic grounds alone that transplanted organ failure is due to rejection.

   Posttransplantation lymphoproliferative disorders (PTLD), mechanical problems, opportunistic infections, and (in patients with certain original disease processes) recurrences of earlier disease can all affect the organ in ways that clinically simulate rejection closely. Sometimes these are difficult to distinguish *even with* pathologic interpretation of a biopsy. *Without* biopsy diagnostic resolution is very weak. Increased immunosuppression for *presumptive* rejection can worsen PTLD and infectious processes.

PITFALLS FOR THE PATHOLOGIST

1. Failure to commit to a specific diagnosis when possible.

   Descriptive histopathologic diagnoses appear more prevalent in cases of inflammation than in cases of neoplasia. Extensive algorithms exist for the workup of a tumor of unknown primary origin, yet some pathologists may be content to subdivide most nontumorous processes as "mild," "moderate," and "severe" inflammation. In some cases this is unavoidable. In the area of transplant pathology, it is a diagnosis of last resort. The clues to etiology may be subtle, but they are frequently present.

2. Failure to consider causes of inflammation other than rejection.

   In our biopsy experience, rejection is the most common cause of inflammation in allografts. However, the clinical consequences of this diagnosis, i.e., increased immunosuppressive therapy, are immediate. Inflammation due to other causes will generally not respond to this maneuver and may worsen, leading to rapid clinical deterioration. The pathologist must remain cognizant of this and not fall into the trap of making a diagnosis of rejection on the basis of inflammation alone.

3. Failure to obtain relevant clinical information and to compare prior biopsy material with the current specimen.

   As noted, working under this handicap places the pathologist at a distinct disadvantage. Is this a new allograft or has it been in for years? Has there been recent change in immunosuppression? Are any infections suspected? Is this process new or ongoing? Is it getting better or worse? These questions and others should be asked when interpreting the biopsy.

4. Rigid adherence to tabulated criteria for diagnosis.

   The condition of the transplant patient is dynamic, and this is reflected in the biopsy. When viewed sequentially, the biopsy "snapshots" should create a coherent "moving picture" in the mind of the pathologist. It is not to be expected that every possible histologic indicator will be present at every step of evolution of a disease.

5. Failure to closely examine the biopsy specimen for very early evidence of ACR.

   Acute cellular rejection may be seen in association with infection, mechanical problems, and so forth. The successful achievement of a major diagnosis from a biopsy specimen does not excuse the pathologist from searching further for signs of early rejection. Such an approach allows the pathologist to provide guidance to the transplantation team.

6. Misdiagnosis of PTLD as (high-grade) malignant lymphoma.

   By conventional histomorphology alone, PTLD effectively duplicates the features of high-grade lymphoma (see Fig. 20–19). Only with the knowledge that this has arisen in an immunosuppressed transplant recipient can one carefully look for subtle clues to its nonmalignant nature: zones with plasmacytic differentiation, geographic necrosis, apoptosis, and abundant phagocytic histiocytes. Ancillary studies can be useful in demonstrating abundant EBV genome, i.e., in situ hybridization or Southern blot analysis. The distinction is critical because therapeutic indications are in direct conflict for the two considerations. Some cases within the spectrum of the PTLD do attain truly autonomous, malignant behavior; however, these are in the minority and can be recognized or suspected as malignancies on the basis of combined clinical and pathologic findings.

FURTHER READING

Makowka L. *The Handbook of Transplantation Management.* Austin, TX: R.G. Landes; 1991.

Hammond EH. Solid organ transplantation pathology. In: *Major Problems in Pathology.* Vol. 30. Philadelphia: Saunders; 1994.

Sale GE. *The Pathology of Organ Transplantation.* Boston: Butterworth; 1990.

REFERENCES

1. Edwards EB, Guo T, Breen TJ, et al. The UNOS OPTN waiting list for 1988 to 1993. In: Terasaki PI, Cecka JM, ed. *Clinical Transplants 1993.* Los Angeles: UCLA Tissue Typing Laboratory; 1993:71–83.
2. Alexander JW, Vaughn WK. The use of marginal donors for organ transplantation. *Transplantation.* 1991;51:135–141.
3. Belzer FO, Southard JH. Principles of solid-organ preservation by cold storage. *Transplantation.* 1988;45:673–676.
4. Mor E, Klintmalm G, Gonwa TA, et al. The use of marginal donors for liver transplantation. *Transplantation.* 1992;53:383–386.
5. Marsh JW, Esquivel CO, Makowka L, et al. Accidental transplantation of malignant tumor from a donor to multiple recipients. *Transplantation.* 1987;44:449–450.
6. Detry O, Detroz B, D'Silva M, et al. Misdiagnosed malignancy in transplanted organs. *Transplant Int.* 1993;6:50–54.
7. Ramos EL, Tilney NL, Ravenscraft MD. Clinical aspects of renal transplantation. In: Brenner BM, Rector FC, ed. *The Kidney.* 4th ed. Vol. 2. Philadelphia: Saunders; 1991:2361–2407.
8. Starzl TE, Demetris AJ. *Liver Transplantation. A 31-year Perspective.* Chicago: Year Book Medical Publishers; 1990:1–194.
9. Todo S, Demetris A, Makowka L, et al. Primary non-function of hepatic homografts with preexisting fatty infiltration. *Transplantation.* 1989;47:903–905.
10. Dallessandro AW, Kalayoglu M, Sollinger HW, et al. The predictive value of donor liver biopsies for the development or primary nonfunction after orthotopic liver transplantation. *Transplantation.* 1991;51: 157–163.
11. Colvin RB. Cellular and molecular mechanisms of allograft rejection. *Annu Rev Med.* 1990;41:361–375.
12. Mason DW, Morris PJ. Effector mechanisms in allograft rejection. *Ann Rev Immunol.* 1986;4:119–145.
13. Cagle PT. Lung transplant pathology. In: Thurlbeck WM, Churg AM, ed. *Pathology of the Lung,* 2nd ed. New York: Thieme Medical Publishers; 1995:827–849.
14. Starzl TE, Rao AS, Trucco M, et al. Explanation for loss of the HLA matching effect. *Transplant Proc.* 1995;27:57–60.
15. Terasaki PI, Gjertson DW, Cecka JM, Takemoto S. Proposed HLA matching scheme for improved cadaveric kidney allocation. *Transplant Proc.* 1995;27(1):61–63.
16. Demetris AJ, Jaffe R, Tzakis A, et al. Antibody mediated rejection of human orthotopic liver allografts: a study of liver transplantation across ABO blood group barriers. *Am J Pathol.* 1988;132:489–502.
17. Demetris AJ, Nakamura K, Yagihashi A, et al. A clinicopathological study of human liver allograft recipients harboring preformed IgG lymphocytic antibodies. *Hepatology.* 1992;16:671–681.
18. Rose ML, Yacoub MH, ed. *Immunology of Heart and Lung Transplantation.* London: Edward Arnold; 1993.
19. Hall BM, Dorsch SE. Cells mediating allograft rejection. *Transplantation.* 1991;51:1141.
20. Yowell RL, Araneo BA. Mechanisms of allograft rejection. In: Hammond EH, ed. *Solid Organ Transplantation Pathology.* Philadelphia: Saunders; 1994:4–18.
21. Billingham ME, Cary NRB, Hammond ME, et al. A working formulation for the standardization of nomenclature in the diagnosis of heart and lung rejection: heart rejection study group. *J Heart Transplantation.* 1990;9:587–593.
22. Yousem SA, Berry GJ, Brunt EM, et al. A working formulation for the standardization of nomenclature in the diagnosis of heart and lung rejection: lung rejection study group. *J Heart Lung Transplant.* 1990;9:593–601.
23. Yousem SA, Berry GJ, Cagle PT, et al. A revision of the 1990 working formulation for the classification of lung allograft rejection. *J Heart Lung Transplant.* In press.
24. Solez K, Axelsen RA, Benediktsson H, et al. International standardization of criteria for the histologic diagnosis of renal allograft rejection: the Banff working classification of kidney transplant pathology. *Kidney Int.* 1993;44:411–422.
25. Demetris AJ, Seaberg EC, Batts KP, et al. Reliability and predictive value of the National Institute of Diabetes and Digestive and Kidney Diseases liver transplantation database nomenclature and grading system for acute rejection of liver allografts. *Hepatology.* 1995;21:408–416.
26. Hayry P, von Willebrand E. Practical guidelines for fine needle aspiration biopsy of human renal allografts. *Ann Clin Res.* 1981;13:288–306.
27. Lautenschlager I, Hockenstedt K, Hayry P. Fine-needle aspiration biopsy in the monitoring of liver allografts. *Transplant Int.* 1991;4:54–61.
28. Tilney NL, Whitley WD, Diamond JR, et al. Chronic rejection—an undefined conundrum. *Transplantation.* 1991;52:389–398.
29. Ho M, Dummer S, Pasculle AW, et al. Infection in the transplant recipient. In: Makowka L, ed. *The Handbook of Transplantation Management.* Austin, TX: R.G. Landes; 1991:448–516.

30. Tazelaar HD. Perivascular inflammation in pulmonary infections: implications for the diagnosis of lung rejection. *J Heart Lung Transplant.* 1991;10:437–441.
31. Wreghitt TG, Hakin M, Cory-Pearce R, et al. The impact of donor-transmitted CMV and toxoplasma gondii disease in cardiac transplantation. *Transplant Proc.* 1986;18:1375–1376.
32. Cen H, Breinig MC, Atchison RW, et al. Epstein-Barr virus transmission via the donor organs in solid organ transplantation: polymerase chain reaction and restriction fragment length polymorphism analysis of IR2, IR3, and IR4. *J Virol.* 1991;65:976–980.
33. Demetris AJ, Todo S, van Thiel DH, et al. Evolution of hepatitis B virus liver disease after hepatic replacement. Practical and theoretical considerations. *Am J Pathol.* 1990;137:667–676.
34. Loinaz C, Lumbreras C, Gonzalez-Pinto I, et al. High incidence of posttransplant hepatitis and chronic rejection associated with hepatitis C virus infection in liver transplant recipients. *Transplant Proc.* 1995;27:1217–1218.
35. Knoop M, Bechstein WO, Blumhardt G, et al. Recurrent hepatitis C infection after orthotopic liver transplantation. *Transplant Proc.* 1995;27:1208–1210.
36. Knodell RG, Ishak KG, Black WC, et al. Formulation and application of a numerical scoring system for assessing histological activity in asymptomatic chronic active hepatitis. *Hepatology.* 1981;20(5):431–435.
37. Koneru B, Jaffe R, Esquivel CO, et al. Adenoviral infections in pediatric liver transplant recipients. *JAMA.* 1987;258:489–492.
38. Hogan TF, Borden EC, McBain JA, et al. Human polyomavirus infections with JC virus and BK virus in renal transplant patients. *Ann Intern Med.* 1980;92:373–378.
39. Mihatsch MJ, Morozumi K, Strom EH, et al. Renal transplant morphology after long-term therapy with cyclosporine. *Transplant Proc.* 1995;27(1):39–42.
40. Mihatsch MJ, Ryffel B, Gudat F, Thiel G. Cyclosporine nephropathy. In: Tisher CC, Brenner BM, eds. *Renal Pathology with Clinical and Functional Correlations.* Vol. 2. Philadelphia: Lippincott; 1989:1555–1586.
41. Alessiani M, Cillo U, Fung JJ, et al. Adverse effects of FK506 overdosage after liver transplantation. *Transplant Proc.* 1993; 25(1):628–634.
42. Hanto DW, Frizzera G, Purtilo DT, et al. Clinical spectrum of lymphoproliferative disorders in renal transplant recipients and evidence for the role of Epstein-Barr virus. *Cancer Res.* 1981;41:4253–4261.
43. Hanto DW, Frizzera G, Gajl-Peczalska KJ, Simmons RL. Epstein-Barr virus, immunodeficiency, and B cell lymphoproliferation. *Transplantation.* 1985;39:461–472.
44. Nalesnik MA, Jaffe R, Starzl TE, et al. The pathology of post-transplant lymphoproliferative disorders occurring in the setting of Cyclosporine A-prednisone immunosuppression. *Am J Pathol.* 1988;133:173–192.
45. Nalesnik MA, Makowka L, Starzl TE. The diagnosis and treatment of posttransplant lymphoproliferative disorders. *Curr Probl Surg.* 1988;25:365–472.
46. Knowles DM, Cesarman E, Chadburn A, et al. Correlative morphologic and molecular genetic analysis demonstrates three distinct categories of posttransplantation lymphoproliferastive disorders. *Blood.* 1995;85:552–565.
47. Lee E, Dickman PS, Jaffe R, et al. Post-transplant spindle-cell tumor (PTST): an entity associated with Epstein-Barr virus (abstract). *Lab Invest.* 1993;68(1):127A.
48. Lee ES, Locker J, Nalesnik M, et al. The association of Epstein-Barr virus with smooth-muscle tumors occurring after organ transplantation. *N Engl J Med.* 1995;332:19–25.
49. Euvrand S, Chardonnet Y, Pouteil-Noble C, et al. Association of skin malignancies with various and multiple carcinogenic and noncarcinogenic human papillomaviruses in renal transplant recipients. *Cancer.* 1993;72:2198–2206.
50. Busnach G, Civati G, Brando B, et al. Viral and neoplastic changes of the lower genital tract in women with renal allografts. *Transplant Proc.* 1993;25:1389–1390.
51. Penn I. Tumors after renal and cardiac transplantation. In: Antin JH, Shulman LN, ed. *Hematology/Oncology Clinics of North America: Therapy-related Second Malignancies.* Vol. 7. Philadelphia: Saunders; 1993:431–445.
52. Chang Y, Cesarman E, Pessin MS, et al. Identification of herpesvirus-like DNA sequences in AIDS-associated Kaposi's sarcoma. *Science.* 1994;266:1865–1869.
53. Billingham RE. The biology of graft-versus-host reactions. *Harvey Lectures.* 1966;62:21–78.
54. Ferrara JLM, Deeg HJ. Graft-versus-host disease. *N Engl J Med.* 1991;324(10):667–674.
55. Roberts JP, Ascher NL, Lake J, et al. Graft vs. host disease after liver transplantation in humans: a report of four cases. *Hepatology.* 1991;14:274–281.
56. Jamieson NV, Joysey V, Friend PJ, et al. Graft-versus-host disease in solid organ transplantation. *Transplant Int.* 1991;4:67–71.
57. Hunt BJ. Graft versus host disease in heart and/or lung transplantation. In: Rose ML, Yacoub MH, eds. *Immunology of Heart and Lung Transplantation.* London: Edward Arnold; 1993:261–275.
58. Volc-Platzer B, Stingl G. Cutaneous graft-vs.-host disease. In: Burakoff SJ, Deeg HJ, Ferrara J, Atkinson K, eds. *Graft-vs.-Host Disease. Immunology, Pathophysiology, and Treatment.* New York: Marcel Dekker; 1990:245–254.
59. Sale GE, Lerner KG, Barker EA, et al. The skin biopsy in the diagnosis of acute graft-versus-host disease in man. *Am J Pathol.* 1977;89:621–636.
60. Przepiorka D, Gonzales-Chambers R, Winkelstein A, et al. Chimerism studies using in situ hybridization for the Y chromosome after T cell-depleted bone marrow transplantation. *Bone Marrow Transplant.* 1990;5:253–257.
61. Budowle B, Chakraborty R, Giusti AM, et al. Analysis of the VNTR locus D1S80 by the PCR followed by high-resolution PAGE. *Am J Hum Genet.* 1991;48:137–144.
62. Starzl TE, Demetris AJ. Transplantation milestones viewed with one- and two-way paradigms of tolerance. *JAMA.* 1995;273:876–879.
63. Starzl TE, Demetris AJ, Trucco M, et al. Cell migration and chimerism after whole organ transplantation: the basis of graft acceptance. *Hepatology.* 1993;17:1127–1152.
64. Billingham ME. Cardiac transplantation pathology. In: Hammond EH, ed. *Solid Organ Transplantation Pathology.* Philadelphia: Saunders; 1994:69–91.
65. Valantine HA, Billingham ME. Recurrence of amyloid in a cardiac allograft four months after transplantation. *J Heart Transplantation.* 1989;8:337–341.
66. Randhawa PS, Williams PA, Markin RS, et al. Epstein-Barr virus associated syndromes in immunosuppressed liver transplant recipients: clinical profile and recognition on routine allograft biopsy. *Am J Surg Pathol.* 1990;14:538–547.
67. Markin RS. Manifestations of Epstein-Barr virus-associated disorders in liver. *Liver.* 1994;14:1–13.
68. Pappo O, Ramos H, Starzl TE, et al. Structural integrity and identification of causes of liver allograft dysfunction occurring more than 5 years after transplantation. *Am J Surg Pathol.* 1995;19:192–206.
69. Sutherland DE, Moudry-Munns K, Gruessner A. Pancreas transplant results in United Network for Organ Sharing (UNOS) United States of America (USA) registry with a comparison to non-USA data in the International Registry. In: Terasaki PI, Cecka JM, ed. *Clin Transplants 1993.* Los Angeles: UCLA Tissue Typing Laboratory; 1993:47–69.
70. Sutherland DE, Gores PF, Farney AC, et al. Evolution of kidney, pancreas, and islet transplantation for patients with diabetes at the University of Minnesota. *Am J Surg.* 1993;166:456–491.
71. Kuhr CS, Davis CL, Barr D, et al. Use of ultrasound and cystoscopically guided pancreatic allograft biopsies and transabdominal renal allograft biopsies: safety and efficacy in kidney-pancreas transplant recipients. *J Urol.* 1995;153:316–321.
72. Johnson BF, Henry L, Fox M, Raftery AT. Morphology of rejection in experimental pancreas transplantation and its modification by cyclosporin A administration. *Int J Exp Pathol.* 1992;73:751–764.
73. Busing M, Hopt UT, Quacken M, Becker HD, Morgenroth K. Morphological studies of graft pancreatitis following pancreas transplantation. *Br J Surg.* 1993;80:1170–1173.
74. Jaffe R, Trager JDK, Zeevi A, et al. Multivisceral intestinal transplantation: surgical pathology. *Ped Pathol.* 1989;9:633–654.

21

Special Considerations for the Pediatric Patient

Louis P. Dehner

Introduction

Within the last 25 years, pediatric surgery has become established as a surgical subspecialty. Like pediatrics, the emphasis is on the whole patient rather than on a single organ system—the more typical approach in adult patients. It is not uncommon for a pediatric surgeon to be requested to do a biopsy of a neck mass, to repair a tracheoesophageal fistula through the thoracic approach, and to resect a segment of terminal ileum from a neonate with necrotizing enterocolitis. Exceptions are conditions of the brain and spinal cord, which are universally referred to the neurosurgeon, and major disorders of the skeletal system, which are generally referred to the orthopedist.

Unlike the general surgeon who operates on adult patients who suffer from acquired surgical conditions, the pediatric surgeon must be intimately familiar with embryology.[1] Some of the more important surgical disorders of infancy and early childhood result from an abnormal organization of tissue or an entire organ, e.g., multicystic dysplastic kidney; a pattern of anomalies caused by a single event, e.g., oligohydramnios sequence secondary to chronic amniotic fluid leakage, bilateral renal agenesis, or bilateral dysplastic kidneys; or an interruption in organ development, e.g., pulmonary hypoplasia secondary to a congenital diaphragmatic hernia or in utero amputation secondary to a ruptured amniotic sac with the formation of amniotic bands. A detailed discussion of congenital anomalies and malformations is available elsewhere.[2]

Other conditions in the neonatal or early infancy period are congenital or connatal by virtue of age at presentation; however, these disorders are not anomalies or malformations in the same sense as a congenital cardiac defect or a myelomeningocele. For example, stenosis and atresia of the small intestine and meconium peritonitis are regarded by many as a complication of in utero intestinal ischemia rather than a failure in normal intestinal development. Similarly, extrahepatic biliary atresia is a fibroinflammatory condition of unknown etiology resulting in progressive destruction of the biliary tract rather than a primary defect in the development of the common bile duct and hepatic ducts. The question remains unanswered whether Hirschsprung's disease is a migratory defect of precursor cells from the neural crest to the intestine or a secondary loss of ganglion cells in a distal to proximal progression in the colon through some extrinsic mechanism such as ischemia. Some studies indicate that there are intrinsic chromosomal aberrations to explain the pathogenesis of Hirschsprung's disease.[3–5]

Acquired conditions may require either biopsy, for diagnostic purposes, or excision or resection as definitive therapy. Examples include cervical lymphadenopathy and acute appendicitis.

Like other entities of pediatric pathology, many of the neoplasms occur exclusively in this age group and are peculiar in their behavior. In fact, questions remain whether some of these tumors are bona fide neoplasms or whether they represent malformations. Examples of this pathogenetic dilemma are cystic hygroma (lymphangioma) of the neck and cutaneous or soft tissue capillary hemangioma. By convention, these are considered neoplasms, but in most instances they probably represent a defect in normal vascular development. Furthermore, some vascular lesions are a feature of a genetic syndrome, more evidence supporting the pathogenetic argument for their origin as an anomaly in development.[6]

One common characteristic of the more important childhood neoplasms is their microscopic similarity to embryonic and fetal tissue.[7] The resemblance of neuroblastoma to normal fetal neuroblasts and the triphasic Wilms' tumor to the developing kidney are two examples. Exploration of the events that control the development of childhood neoplasms has therefore improved our understanding of normal embryogenesis, and vice versa.[8]

Practice Settings for Pediatric Surgical Pathology

Most large metropolitan areas in the United States have at least one children's hospital. Most pediatric surgeons prefer to operate in these institutions where ancillary services are geared toward the pediatric patient. Such focus applies to anatomic and surgical pathology as well. As a principal consultant to the pediatric surgeon, the pediatric pathologist is a critical participant in patient care.

An active pediatric surgical pathology service in a children's hospital in Canada or the United States may expect an accession of 5,000 to 6,000 cases per year. Of course, a single case ranges from a hernia sac to multiple biopsies from several sites throughout the gastrointestinal tract. A core biopsy of the kidney for primary renal disease requires multifaceted examination including routine light microscopy, electron microscopy, and immunofluorescence. Bone marrow specimens for the diagnosis of acute leukemia and other neoplastic processes are subjected to flow cytometry with many antibodies. Multiple antibody immunohistochemistry is often necessary to differentiate among the various types of primitive small-cell neoplasms of childhood (see Chap. 2).[9]

There are approximately 38,000 accessions per year in our own departmental surgical pathology laboratory. Of these, in excess of 5,000 cases are submitted from patients under 20 years of age. Approximately 45% of such cases are from children under 6 years of age; 20% are from patients 1 year of age and under. Skin biopsies and excisions accounted for almost 35% of our pediatric surgical specimens. These cases included punch biopsies, resections of scars, and staged excisions of congenital melanocytic nevi. Tonsils and adenoids constituted 14% of cases, and hernia sacs represented another 11% of pediatric accessions. A clinically active pediatric gastroenterology service at the St. Louis Children's Hospital has been the source of numerous mucosal biopsies from the upper and lower gastrointestinal tracts. Not surprisingly, the largest number of colorectal biopsies were for suspected Hirschsprung's disease from children under 1 year of age. In later childhood, mucosal biopsies from the rectum and sigmoid colon were performed to establish the diagnosis of idiopathic inflammatory bowel disease or to monitor its activity after primary diagnosis and treatment.

Whether pathologist or surgeon, we all have been affected by the paradigm shift to capitative reimbursement. This has affected our practice regardless of our specialty. One practice that has come into question is the "routine" submission of specimens to the surgical pathology laboratory. A director of laboratories in a major American children's hospital has openly expressed an opinion that is highly provocative.[10] Benjamin suggests that the surgeon should be the one to decide whether a particular specimen should be submitted for formal pathologic examination. Until guidelines have been established on the basis of appropriate retrospective and prospective studies, and issues of medical malpractice tort reform settled, it is probably imprudent to implement his suggestion. Currently, the Joint Commission for Accreditation of Health Organizations requires a formal institutional list of specimens excluded from pathologic examination in by-laws or equivalent documents, rather than allow ad hoc decisions by the surgeon.

Selected Topics for Discussion

Although it is beyond the scope of this chapter to address all facets of pediatric surgical pathology, the more common clinical problems encountered by the surgeon and pathologist are discussed.[11] These include (1) head and neck masses, (2) intrathoracic cysts and tumors, (3) infantile cholestatic liver disease, (4) necrotizing enterocolitis and Hirschsprung's disease, (5) renal neoplasms and neuroblastomas, (6) germ cell neoplasms, and (7) soft tissue neoplasms.

HEAD AND NECK MASSES

The head and neck region is anatomically complex in its structure and organ diversity (see Chap. 6).[12] This site is also the overlapping purview of several surgical specialties. For this reason, the approach to a mass is based upon the presumed site of origin of the tumor. If the swelling is in the oral cavity or oropharynx, either the oral or head and neck surgeon is consulted. If, however, the mass is in the neck, most pediatric surgeons treat the patient themselves. The clinical circumstances influence both the scope and pace of the diagnostic evaluation. For example, an enlarged thyroid is approached differently than a lateral neck mass. In an infant a potentially obstructing lesion of the upper airway is treated emergently, in contrast to a gradually enlarging cyst in the anterolateral neck of a young child.

Persistent cervical lymphadenopathy without other clinical manifestations is an indication for lymph node biopsy.[13] If there is any suspicion of infection, microbiologic cultures should be obtained at the time of the procedure. If lymphoma, including Hodgkin's disease, is in the differential diagnosis, fresh tissue should be reserved for flow cytometry and fresh-frozen tissue for other potential ancillary studies. Fortunately, the commonest finding in a lymph node from a child or an adolescent is benign follicular hyperplasia. Although the etiology is usually unknown, viral infection is suggested if there is an increase in the number of immunoblasts. Extremely intense immunoblastic proliferation is characteristic of acute *Epstein-Barr virus* infection. In contrast, *toxoplasmosis* is associated with a different pattern: parafollicular epithelioid granuloma, follicular hyperplasia, and monocytoid B-cell proliferation. Granulomatous lymphadenitis is relatively common in the pediatric patient. The pattern of inflammation varies with the pathogen: diffuse granulomatous reaction (atypical my-

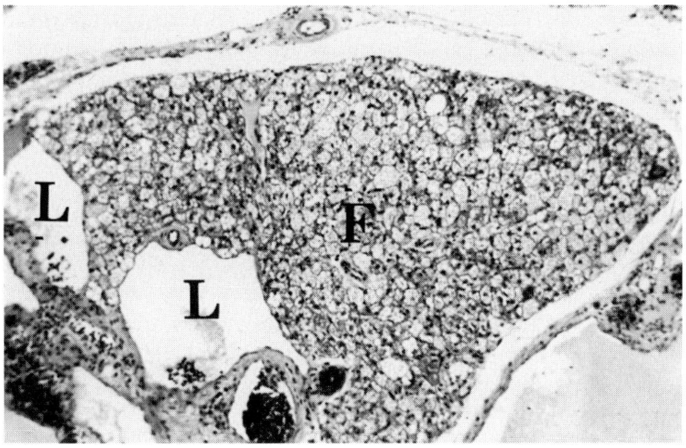

Figure 21–1. Cystic hygroma or lymphangioma with thin-walled vascular spaces surrounding a lobule of immature fat (F) in the soft tissues of the neck in an infant. Note the presence of larger lymphatic spaces (L) pushing the fat aside.

cobacteria), suppurative granulomas with central abscesses (animal-scratch disease, staphylococcal infection with chronic granulomatous disease of childhood), and caseating granulomas (tuberculosis and histoplasmosis).

Cysts and *multicystic lesions* often represent developmental abnormalities, most commonly thyroglossal duct cysts or branchial cleft cysts.[14–16] In one series, congenital cysts accounted for 55% of neck masses in children under 2 years of age.[17] When a cystic lesion is multiloculated, especially in an infant, the presumptive diagnosis is cystic hygroma or lymphangioma. The location determines the nature of a cyst in the neck: thyroglossal duct cyst is midline, branchial cleft cyst is lateral. For the surgeon, when a cyst is the thyroglossal type, more extensive evaluation and, possibly, excision are indicated in relation to the long path of potential midline distribution. Branchial clefts and thyroglossal duct cysts may coexist. Furthermore, branchial cleft cysts are bilateral in 10 to 15% of patients. An uncommon congenital cyst is the *thymic cyst*. These developmental lesions are located in the medial supraclavicular region or lower midline of the neck.[18] Microscopic features useful for differentiating developmental cysts include type of epithelial lining (squamous versus respiratory), presence or absence of subepithelial lymphoid aggregates, and remnants of thyroid follicles. Branchial cleft cysts do not feature Hassall's corpuscles in the midst of the lymphoid aggregates, markings of the thymic cyst. Unfortunately, the type of epithelial lining cannot always determine the nature of the developmental cyst.[19] Only rarely is an aberrant lateral thyroglossal duct cyst seen in a young child without a prior surgical history. Recurrent thyroglossal cysts may be laterally displaced by postoperative fibroinflammatory reaction in the soft tissues of the neck. More uncommon types of developmental and neoplastic cysts include *solid* and *cystic teratomas* of the neck (which occur as large congenital neck masses), *dermoid cysts*, and *enteric duplication cysts*.[15, 20, 21]

Vascular neoplasms, occurring more often in the neck than on the face, constitute as much as 10% of all masses in the head and neck region in children.[6, 17, 20] *Lymphangiomas*, typically cystic hygromas, are more common than hemangiomas. Despite the benign morphologic features of lymphangioma, this lesion can create considerable morbidity owing to widespread soft tissue infiltration of the neck with extension into the floor of the mouth and base of the tongue, mediastinum, and even axilla and chest wall.[20] The extreme form of this process is generalized lymphangiomatosis. In contrast to hemangiomas of the skin and soft tissues, which although nonencapsulated are sharply circumscribed, lymphangiomas can permeate tissues in an aggressive manner—through the adipose tissue, into and through the lymph nodes, and into the septa of the parotid and submandibular glands (Fig. 21–1). No dissection plane can be found around the delicate, readily collapsible cysts with their clear watery contents. There is also minimal soft tissue reaction. Microscopically, cystic hygroma consists of thin-walled cavernous structures lined by flat endothelial cells, with occasional nodules of lymphocytes prolapsing into or adjacent to ectatic vascular spaces (Fig. 21–2). Detecting recurrent lesions, both surgically and microscopically, is often much more difficult due to obscuring reactive fibrosis, inflammation, and alteration in the appearance of the vessels. Vascular spaces may more closely resemble a hemangioma, with a lobular arrangement of blood-filled vessels and large, irregular vessels with thickened fibrous walls. Neutrophilic infiltration of vascular spaces signals lymphangitis, a potentially devastating complication in this lesion.

Hemangiomas, particularly in infants, occur as deforming masses. If located in the larynx, these lesions are potentially life threatening. Sites of predilection for hemangiomas in younger children are the orbital soft tissues, oral cavity, and parotid gland.[22] Although these tumors may infiltrate soft tissues, including the skeletal muscle, similarly to lymphangiomas, these tumors more often appear as multinodular or lobular proliferations superimposed upon a lymph node or the parenchyma of the parotid gland. Grossly, these tumors are solid and multinodular. Depending upon the size of the vascular spaces and their content of erythrocytes, these tumors vary from gray-tan to dark reddish brown (Fig. 21–3). A densely cellular hemangioma with diminutive vascular spaces is recognized

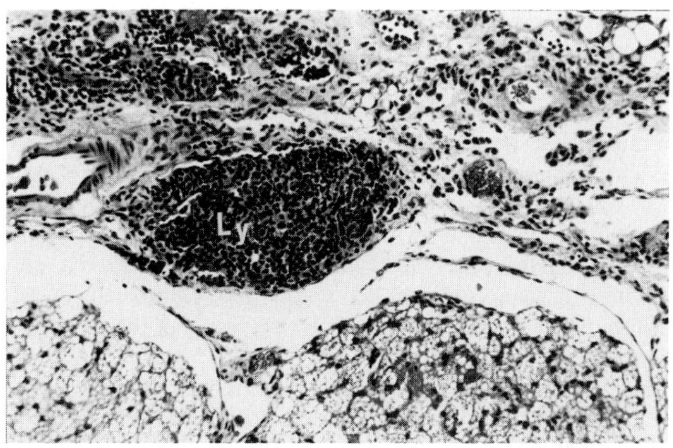

Figure 21–2. Cystic hygroma or lymphangioma with a nodule of small lymphocytes (Ly) adjacent to a vascular space. This relationship of lymphocytes to the vascular spaces of a lymphangioma is a characteristic microscopic feature.

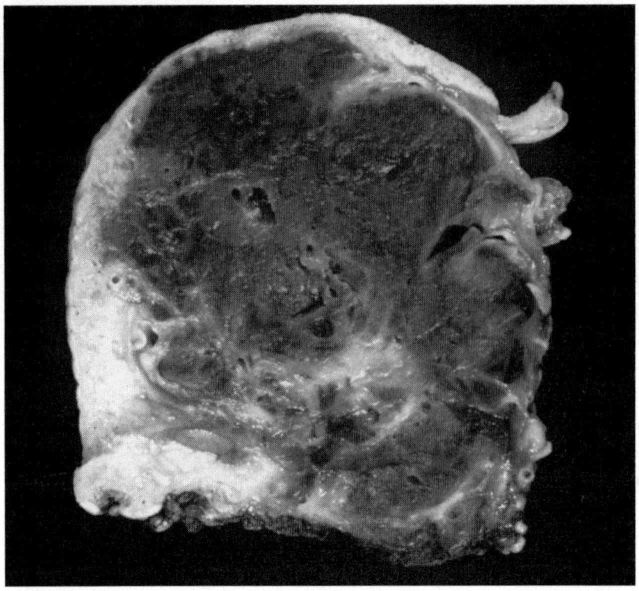

Figure 21–3. Capillary hemangioma in the skin and soft tissues of an infant, showing a multinodular, reddish brown mass with a predominantly solid appearance and focal cystic or cavernous areas.

by its lobular architecture and the presence of larger vascular spaces usually at the periphery of lobules. In exceptional cases microscopy with immunoperoxidase staining may be necessary (Fig. 21–4). It is estimated that 90% of capillary hemangiomas will have undergone involution by the time the child is 10 years old.[6] Spontaneous regression in a hemangioma is characterized by the presence of thrombosis and necrosis. Cognizance of the natural history should temper an overly aggressive approach to these tumors. However, the clinical circumstances of the case may supersede a more sanguine attitude. When the tumor is not obviously vascular in nature, it may be excised for diagnostic as well as therapeutic purposes. Hemangiomas are less likely to recur after resection than lymphangiomas. Hemorrhage is an obvious complication in some hemangiomas; another is the dread, but fortunately rare, occurrence of consumptive coagulopathy and thrombocytopenia of the Kasabach-Merritt syndrome.[23] This disorder depends more upon size and extent of the hemangioma than its site of origin. An exception to this generalization is the retroperitoneal kaposiform infantile hemangioendothelioma, which can induce thrombocytopenia and hemolysis, even when small in size because of its slit-like vessels.[24]

The nomenclature of benign vascular neoplasms in children is confusing. The World Health Organization has recommended the term "capillary hemangioma," but infantile hemangioendothelioma, cellular hemangioma, and juvenile hemangioma or hemangioendothelioma are commonly found in the literature.[25] Hemangioendothelioma has come to be applied to borderline or low-grade malignant vascular neoplasms, which are rare in children.

Other tumors of the head and neck in children include the salivary gland-based neoplasms, nonneoplastic hamartomas (nasal glioma, salivary gland anlage tumor), neuroectodermal neoplasms (classic neuroblastoma, melanotic neuroectodermal tumor of infancy), soft tissue neoplasms (various juvenile fibrous tumors, rhabdomyosarcoma, Ewing's sarcoma, and primitive neuroectodermal tumor), and thyroid-based masses (nodular hyperplasia, adenoma, papillary carcinoma, and medullary carcinoma in the setting of multiple endocrine neoplasia, types IIa and IIb).

CHEST WALL AND INTRATHORACIC CYSTS AND TUMORS

The chest wall and thoracic cavity, with their varied anatomy including soft tissues, bones, and visceral organs, are the sites and sources of a number of developmental and neoplastic disorders in children. Like much of the pathology in children, most of these conditions are distinctive for this age group.

Chest wall masses or lesions in children range from the congenital melanocytic nevus of the so-called bathing trunk or giant type to neoplasms of the soft tissues including lymphangioma, hemangioma, infantile myofibromatosis, congenital infantile fibrosarcoma, lipoblastoma, and Ewing's sarcoma-primitive neuroectodermal tumor (EWS-PNET).[26] Rhabdomyosarcoma infrequently occurs in the soft tissues of the chest wall or thoracic cavity. With the exception of EWS-PNET, most cutaneous and soft tissue neoplasms of the thoracic soft tissues are diagnosed before the patient is 2 years of age.

Osteocentric lesions of the *chest wall* include fibrous dysplasia and chest wall hamartoma, both of which are considered defects in development. The *chest wall hamartoma* is an uncommon lesion in infants that involves one or multiple ribs by an expansile lesion with chondroid, fibroosseous, and aneurysmal bone cyst-like features.[27] *Fibrous dysplasia* is a combination of benign-appearing fibrous tissue and trabecula of woven bone. The critical point in relation to these malformative lesions is that they not be confused with malignancy, in particular osteosarcoma. Most EWSs arise in the rib, whereas most PNETs originate in the soft tissues of the chest wall or within the thoracic space, often in a paravertebral location. A PNET of the chest wall or in the thoracic cavity, in reference to its first observer, has come to be known as the Askin tumor.[28]

The commonest *mediastinal cysts* are a spectrum of

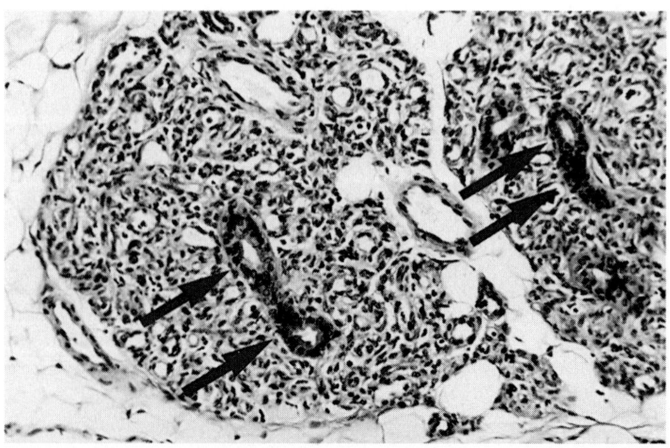

Figure 21–4. Capillary hemangioma in the skin of the back from an infant, showing lobular arrangements of small vessels. The vascular nodules have surrounded sweat ducts *(arrows)*.

lesions collectively referred to as *bronchopulmonary foregut malformation* (BPFM).[29–31] The least complex manifestations of BPFM are the *esophageal duplication cyst* and *bronchogenic cyst*. Some developmental cysts are difficult to categorize based upon histologic features alone. More complex types of BPFM are the foregut cyst with or without fistulous communication with the bronchus, esophagus, or stomach; esophageal atresia; tracheoesophageal fistula; extralobar sequestration; and the so-called esophageal lung. In some cases, there are accompanying vascular malformations.[29] Other cystic lesions of the mediastinum include the lymphangioma; thymic cyst; teratoma; and, by virtue of reactive thymic cyst formation, Hodgkin's disease.

In 60% or more of cases solid tumors of the *mediastinum* are Hodgkin's or non-Hodgkin's lymphoma of the anterior mediastinum or neuroblastic tumor of the posterior mediastinum.[32–35] The principal types of malignant lymphoma occurring as a mediastinal mass in a child are Hodgkin's disease of the nodular sclerosis type, lymphoblastic ("small convoluted–cell") lymphoma, and diffuse large-cell lymphoma with sclerosis. Most children with a mediastinal presentation of malignant lymphoma are over 5 years of age at diagnosis. By contrast, the majority of children with thoracic neuroblastoma are 2 years of age or less. About 10 to 25% of all neuroblastomas occur in the posterior mediastinum.[35] Grossly, the neuroblastoma is well circumscribed and has a connection to or component within the intervertebral foramina. It is generally unnecessary to surgically include this small remnant of tumor. Most neuroblastic tumors in this location have favorable histologic features with evidence of differentiation (abundant neurofibrillary processes, rosette formation, and neuromatous stroma), qualifying them as a differentiating neuroblastoma, an immature ganglioneuroma, or a mature or differentiated ganglioneuroma. Surgical resection alone is sufficient to achieve an excellent prognosis in the majority of patients with thoracic neuroblastomas, and, when total resection is not possible, adjunctive radiotherapy, chemotherapy, or both are also effective.

Congenital cystic lung disorders are important causes of surgically correctable respiratory distress in neonates and infants,[36, 37] the most important being BPFM. Congenital lobar emphysema, adenomatoid malformation, bronchopulmonary sequestration, bronchogenic cyst, and bronchial atresia are the various morphologic expressions of BPFM. Resection of the malformed tissues is necessary to correct compression of normal structures and vascular shunting.

Adenomatoid malformation (congenital cystic adenomatoid malformation, CCAM) is one of the more common types of BPFM. Three classic pathologic types (CCAM types I, II, and III) and two additional types (types 0 and IV) have been described; however, 85 to 90% of cases are either type I or type II.[38] Type I CCAM is the most common form (70 to 75% of cases) and usually occurs within the first 2 months of life as progressive respiratory distress. Radiographic findings of CCAM I are air-filled or air- and fluid-filled cysts, which compress the adjacent lung and/or depress the diaphragm with or without shift of the mediastinum. The cystic character of CCAM II is less impressive radiographically and pathologically than that of CCAM I. However, CCAM II is the more ominous anomaly because it is accompanied by more serious malformations in other organ systems in 25 to 30% of cases. The large cysts (1 to 10 cm) of CCAM I are more readily appreciated in the gross examination in contrast to the smaller cysts (<2 cm) of CCAM II, which merge with the adjacent normal parenchyma. The CCAM type II may thus be overlooked in the microscopic examination (Fig. 21–5 *A* and *B*).

Pulmonary sequestration is defined by its anatomic relationship to the lung, connection (without function) to the tracheobronchial tree, and pulmonary vascular supply.[38] Arguments persist over the existence of a true intralobar sequestration. The more common extralobar sequestration typically occurs as a cystic or solid mass in the posterobasal segment of the lower lobe and has a left-sided predilection. Rarely, an extralobar sequestration is observed in the upper abdomen and retroperitoneum as a suprarenal mass simulating a neuroblastoma.[39] Equally uncommon are extralobar sequestrations with anatomic continuity or connection with the esophagus or stomach as another expression of bronchopulmonary foregut malformation.[10] Communication with the tracheobronchial tree is a rare occurrence, but there is a systemic blood supply from the thoracic or abdominal aorta in 85 to 90% of cases.[41] A defect in the diaphragm is found in as many as 15 to 20% of cases, and another related or unrelated malformation is found in 50 to 60% of cases of extralobar sequestration.[38] Distinguishing pathologic features of extralobar sequestration are (1) one or more arteries without an accompanying major airway and (2) lung parenchyma with the histologic features of CCAM II (Fig. 21–6). Unfortunately, only 25 to 30% of cases have these characteristic findings.[42] Otherwise, the histology of the extralobar sequestration is remarkable for the presence of thick-walled systemic arteries and the absence of a major airway. The distal parenchyma is often normal appearing.

Congenital lobar emphysema (CLE) is the least frequent of the three types of congenital cystic lung disease in infants. The affected lobes, more commonly the left upper lobe (40% of all cases), is overexpanded by a demonstrable or presumed bronchial obstruction that creates a ball-valve effect with distal air trapping.[43] The lung parenchyma is normally developed, unlike its appearance in CCAM. The etiology of the bronchial obstruction is not apparent in all cases even after a thorough gross and microscopic examination. Incomplete development of the bronchial cartilage or bronchial atresia is found in some, but not all, cases. On occasion, there is extrinsic compression of the bronchus by an aberrant vessel. The so-called polyalveolar lobe with the radiographic features of CLE or one of the other cystic disorders has bronchial atresia as an accompanying malformation.[38] Bronchial atresia has also been implicated in the pathogenesis of CCAM. Complete obstruction of the larynx or trachea results in a lethal congenital disorder known as total sequestration or pulmonary hyperplasia. In these cases, there is bilateral expansion of the lungs causing surface impressions of the ribs—so-called accordion lungs.

In comparison to adults, *neoplasms* of the *lung* are uncommon in children. *Inflammatory myofibroblastic tumor* (IMT, inflammatory pseudotumor, plasma-cell granuloma)

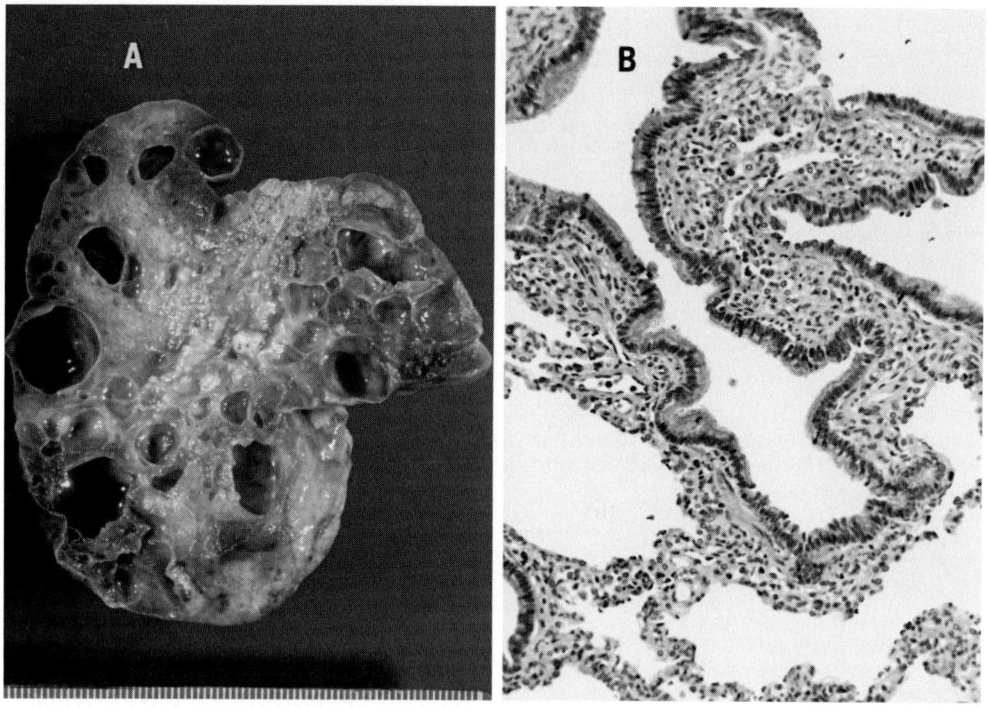

Figure 21–5. *A*, Congenital cystic adenomatoid malformation, showing multiple cysts measuring 1 to 2 cm in diameter. *B*, Ciliated respiratory mucosa lines the abnormally formed distal airways.

accounts for 40 to 50% of pulmonary tumors in the pediatric age population.[44] Most IMTs of the lung occur in children between the ages of 6 and 10 years as a solitary mass in the lower lobe. These tumors are benign processes, but on occasion the tumor locally infiltrates the visceral pleura with involvement of the thoracic cavity and invasion of the parietal pleura. Less often, an IMT appears as a pleural-based mass that must be differentiated from the solitary fibrous tumor of the pleura. Uncommonly IMT appears as an endobronchial mass and is confined to the lobe. Lobectomy is the treatment of choice. An IMT with local growth beyond the involved lobe may represent serious difficulties for complete resection in a manner analogous to desmoid tumor of the soft tissues. A well-circumscribed, firm, gray-yellow to tan mass with or without grossly visible calcifications occupies the greater part of

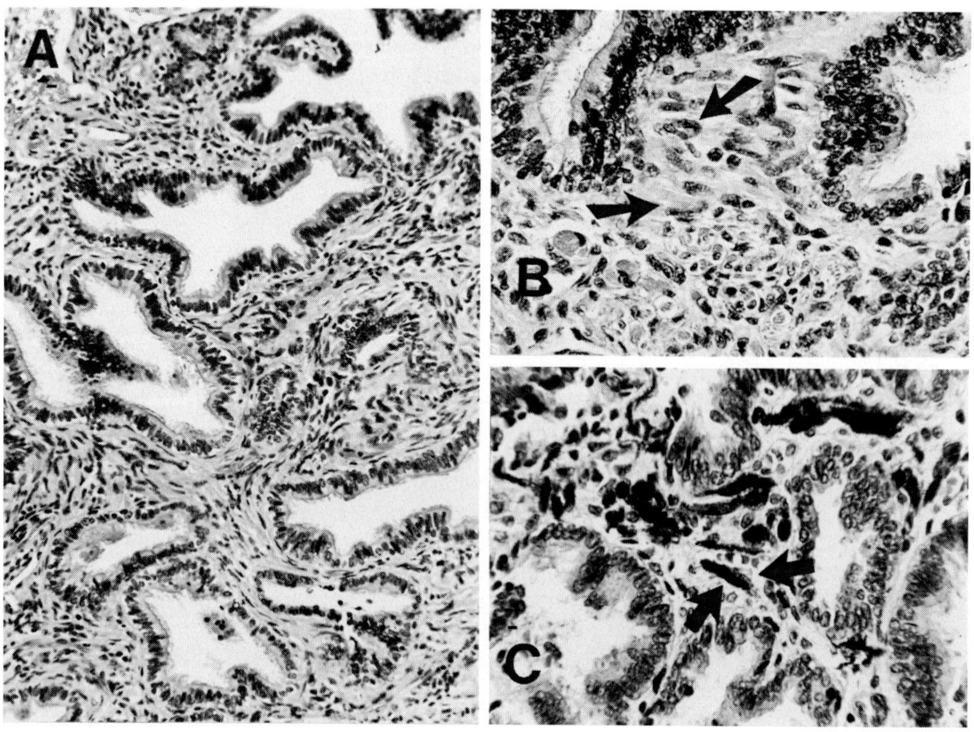

Figure 21–6. *A*. Extralobar pulmonary sequestration with the microscopic features of an adenomatoid malformation, type II. *B*. The stroma is composed of immature skeletal muscle cells *(arrows)*. *C*. An immunoperoxidase stain for muscle-specific actin reacts with the skeletal muscle fibers *(arrows)*.

the resected lobe. Microscopically, there is a spindle cell proliferation representing myofibroblasts, variable numbers of plasma cells and lymphocytes, and dense hypocellular collagen. Numerous histiocytes in an IMT may raise concern about a fibrous histiocytoma.

Bronchial carcinoid is the most common primary malignant neoplasm of the lung in childhood. However, unlike many pediatric tumors, this tumor is not unique to children. In contrast, the so-called pleuropulmonary blastoma (PPB) is seen only in the lung and thoracic cavity of children.[45] Although this neoplasm may appear to be cystic, with imaging features indistinguishable from CCAM or bronchogenic cyst, the more frequent presentation is as a solid mass in the chest of a child between 3 and 4 years of age. Unlike pulmonary blastoma in the adult with its biphasic epithelial and mesenchymal elements, the solid PPB is a complex intermixture of blastema, spindle cells, immature rhabdomyoblasts, chondrosarcomatous nodules, and individual anaplastic cells.[45] The cystic form of PPB has a limited array of neoplastic tissues with a predominant embryonal rhabdomyosarcomatous pattern. There is morphologic evidence that the PPB originates in a developmental lung cyst with the features of CCAM type I. The prognosis for the solid, or predominantly solid, PPB is poor.[45]

CHOLESTATIC LIVER DISEASE IN THE NEONATE

Prolonged conjugated hyperbilirubinemia in a neonate signals serious underlying hepatic and/or biliary tract disease in the overwhelming majority of cases.[46] A serum-conjugated bilirubin level greater than 1.5 mg/dL or 20% of the total bilirubin is the threshold for initiation of evaluation. There is some urgency in the initiation of the diagnostic process, especially in the neonate with suspected extrahepatic biliary atresia.

There are two major categories of neonatal cholestatic liver disease: surgical and nonsurgical disorders. In the former category, most cases are extrahepatic biliary atresia, and less than 5% are choledochal cysts. Numerous nonsurgical conditions of an infectious, metabolic, and toxic nature result in hepatocellular injury. Less easily classified liver disorders include the cholestasis of parenteral hyperalimentation, ischemia, and severe passive congestion secondary to congenital heart disease or sepsis. Overall, extrahepatic biliary atresia accounts for 25 to 30% of cholestatic disease in the neonatal period. The remainder are either idiopathic (35 to 40% of cases) or one of the "medical" causes. The latter include α-1-antitrypsin deficiency and intrahepatic cholestatic syndromes with ductopenia (Alagille and Byler syndromes).

Extrahepatic biliary atresia (EBA) complicates 1 in 10,000 to 15,000 live births.[46] Other congenital malformations may be associated with EBA. Despite intense investigation, the precise etiology of EBA remains essentially unknown, but reovirus serotype 3 is one of the more likely candidates. Numerous procedures to reestablish the drainage of bile from the liver to the small intestine have been developed over the history of pediatric surgery.[47] Prior to the introduction of the hepatoportoenterostomy (Kasai's procedure), only 20% of EBAs were theoretically correctable; however, in reality only half that number could be surgically corrected.[47] The hepatoportoenterostomy is the procedure of choice in infants without visible remnants of the common bile duct or a gallbladder that could be utilized as a conduit for bile drainage. The immediate and short-term results with the Kasai procedure have steadily improved over the past 25 years, now with 3-year survivals of 65 to 70%.[48] However, the liver eventually fails in many of these children, making liver transplantation necessary. In fact, biliary atresia is the most common indication for liver transplantation in children.[49] Approximately 70% of children who have received liver allografts at St. Louis Children's Hospital originally had biliary atresia.

Infants with biliary atresia derive maximum benefit from the hepatoportoenterostomy if they are operated on within the first several weeks rather than several months into their clinical course.[48] The presumed explanation for the difference in outcome is the nature of the pathologic process, progressing to the destruction of the common bile duct in EBA. Chronic inflammation and fibrosis are present in the porta hepatis, which causes the formation of a fibrous mass. In the early stages, duct remnants are accompanied by acute and chronic inflammation within the lumen and in the surrounding tissues.[50] Residual ductal epithelial cells show degenerative as well as regenerative features. Over a relatively brief time, all ductal remnants are destroyed and the active inflammatory process diminishes.[50] The surrounding soft tissues become increasingly fibrotic as the interstitial edema resolves. In the early stages of active bile duct injury, there is sufficient preservation of structural and functional integrity of the remnant structures to allow bile excretion to occur into the small intestine after the hepatoportoenterostomy. The amount of the residual ductal remnants in the porta hepatis correlates with the short-term function of the hepatoportoenterostomy in some but not all studies.[50]

Intraoperative frozen section examination of biopsies from the porta hepatis is used to assist in the decision to perform a hepatoportoenterostomy; however, most surgeons do not wait for the results of frozen section but instead come to a decision on the basis of bile flow in the porta hepatis following transection. Anecdotal experiences describe successful hepatoportoenterostomy even when bile duct remnants were judged "very small" or "absent" on frozen section examination. However, the severity of hepatic fibrosis, which often borders on overt cirrhosis, correlates with the lack of bile drainage. If several weeks have elapsed between the initial liver biopsy and the hepatoportoenterostomy, it is wise to perform needle and wedge biopsies of the liver. Hepatocellular injury is an active process that progresses from seemingly mild to severe bridging fibrosis and the formation of regenerative hepatic nodules over a relatively brief period.

The differentiation of EBA and other forms of surgical jaundice from the nonstructural causes of conjugated hyperbilirubinemia is reliable in most cases on the basis of a needle biopsy.[51] On the basis of proliferation of interlobular bile ducts in the portal tracts and marked cholestasis, EBA is distinguished from the metabolic hepatopathies and idiopathic neonatal hepatitis. Prolonged parenteral nutrition and inborn errors of bile acid synthesis often cause proliferation of small bile ducts in the portal tracts and produce a histologic pattern of liver injury mimicking EBA.

INTESTINAL DISORDERS OF NEONATES AND INFANTS

Many surgical conditions of the gastrointestinal tract become evident early in life. This section focuses on necrotizing enterocolitis, an acquired process, and Hirschsprung's disease or aganglionosis, a congenital disorder. Other important conditions include esophageal atresia and tracheoesophageal fistula with several anatomic configurations, pyloric stenosis, stenosis and atresia of the small intestine, mid-gut malrotation with its worst complication of volvulus and subsequent infarction of the small intestine, intussusception, duplication anomalies, and meconium ileus and peritonitis.

Necrotizing enterocolitis (NEC) is the most common cause of small and/or large intestinal perforation in the neonatal period.[52] The majority of infants who develop NEC are premature by dates (90% of all cases). The remaining cases occur in term infants who have complications in the postnatal period.[53, 54] Between 5 and 15% of premature infants under 1,500 g develop NEC. Typically this occurs within the first 2 weeks of life, but delayed presentations are also well documented.[54, 55] Approximately 25 to 30% of infants with NEC require surgical intervention. Clinical signs that require surgery are pneumoperitoneum, erythema of the abdominal wall, decline of overall clinical status, air in the portal vein, and localized mass.[56] The mortality rate ranges from 10 to 40% in various series. The degree of prematurity and birth weight affect the mortality rate in NEC. The extent of intestinal involvement also determines outcome; infants with extensive NEC have an extremely poor prognosis. Infants at or below 1,000 g have a higher incidence of NEC and are also more likely to require surgery. In the United States, NEC is the cause of death in 13 per 100,000 live births—approximately 4,000 infants are lost each year.[57] Although NEC is listed as the immediate cause of death, these infants often have other major findings at autopsy. These include hyaline membrane disease—bronchopulmonary dysplasia (BPD), severe cholestatic liver disease (in part ascribed to total parenteral nutrition), and one or more sites of infection (either as bronchopneumonia superimposed upon BPD or interloop abscesses between loops of necrotic intestine).

Infants who survive the acute episode of NEC are at risk for subsequent intestinal strictures reported in 15 to 35% of cases.[53] Strictures may also develop in an infant who was premature but did not have clinical NEC in the immediate neonatal period. NEC may also appear late, by definition at 21 days of age or older. Premature infants with delayed-onset NEC are less likely to have had severe neonatal respiratory distress. In fact, with the prevention of surfactant deficiency syndrome and its complications, there has been a corresponding increase of NEC in the somewhat older premature infant.

The pathology of NEC is dominated by ischemic changes.[57] The involved segment of intestine, which is usually the ileum and sometimes a contiguous segment of proximal and distal intestine, has an intense dark red to reddish purple serosa. The serosa has often lost its glistening appearance. This latter feature does not necessarily imply transmural necrosis. The normal pinkish tan mucosal surface now has a dull hemorrhagic appearance that blends with the submucosa and muscularis propria, obscuring the boundaries between the mucosa, submucosa, and muscularis propria. Some specimens are so friable and thin that they disrupt during gross examination. Such fragility is an operative problem for the surgeon. The extent and severity of the necrosis are difficult to gauge by direct visual examination. Furthermore, the cystic lesions of pneumatosis cystoides intestinalis are difficult to recognize. For this reason, the margins of resection should receive particular attention from the pathologist, including microscopic determination of viability.

Intraoperative frozen section consultation to evaluate margins is generally not utilized by the surgeon because one of the primary surgical goals is the preservation of as much intestine as possible, even at the risk of marginal viability. Furthermore, a particular margin that appears viable during surgery may subsequently undergo ischemic change. Oftentimes some revision of the ostomy sites takes place during a second or third procedure. If a primary anastomosis is contemplated, an argument for frozen section is then a relevant one, but is still infrequently necessary. Stricture formation is a relatively common complication at the anastomotic sites or areas of marginal ischemia.

Three pathologic stages of NEC are based upon histologic features that reflect progression in the evolution of NEC.[59, 60] The first is the *acute stage* with coagulative necrosis of one or more layers of the bowel wall, beginning with the mucosa (Fig. 21–7). If present, perforations are found in areas of transmural necrosis. In addition to necrosis, there are congested vessels and interstitial hemorrhage. Clear spaces in the submucosa indicate pneumatosis cystoides intestinalis (Fig. 21–8). At this stage, inflammatory reaction is inconspicuous. The *healing stage* shows mucosal restriction; however, the architecture is simpler than normal small intestinal mucosa. Reepithelialization begins approximately 72 hours after the acute insult. A granulation tissue response with fibroblastic ingrowth occurs over the next several days. The final or *third stage* of NEC is characterized by submucosal fibrosis. This process may extend to involve the muscularis propria. In some cases, there is a disproportionate degree of fibrosis in the muscularis propria when compared with the submucosa. The mucosa continues to show architectural abnormalities. In fact, small foci of mucosal necrosis may persist, reflecting marginal blood supply to the constricted segment.

Although 90 to 95% of cases of NEC in infancy are related to prematurity, a minority of infants instead have a history of exchange transfusions, umbilical artery catheterization, diarrhea, congenital heart disease, Hirschsprung's disease, or maternal cocaine abuse.

Hirschsprung's disease (HRSD, aganglionosis) occurs in 1 per 5,000 live births.[61] The favored hypothesis is failure of the normal cranial-to-caudal population of the intestinal tract by neural crest-derived progenitors of ganglion cells. This failure results in an absence of ganglion cells in the submucosal (Meissner) and myenteric (Auerbach) plexi.[62] The aganglionic segment of rectum, rectum and sigmoid

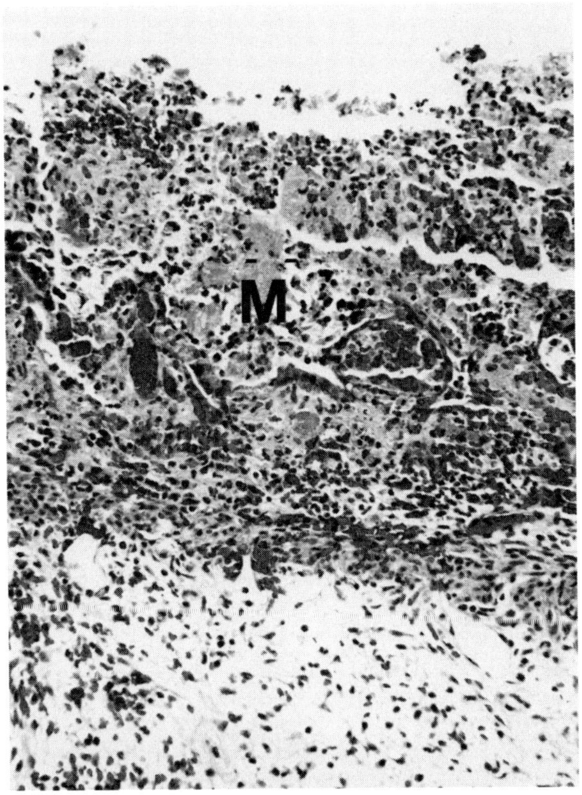

Figure 21–7. Necrotizing enterocolitis in the acute phase with coagulative necrosis confined to the mucosa (M) with intact muscularis mucosae.

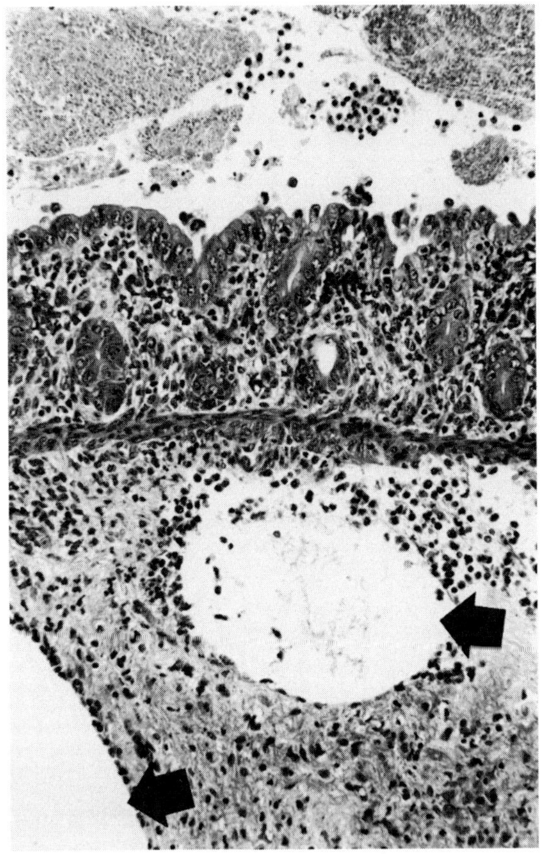

Figure 21–8. Necrotizing enterocolitis, showing pneumatosis cystoides intestinalis *(arrows)* in an area of viable mucosa with the simplified architecture of regenerating mucosa.

colon, and, in severe cases, an even longer segment of bowel lacks normal innervation. Clinical presentation in the neonatal period and early childhood includes (1) failure to pass meconium within 72 hours, (2) intestinal obstruction, and (3) chronic constipation.

In the more common short-segment form, there is a male predilection (M:F, 3:1 to 4:1). However, the sex ratio approaches 1:1 in long-segment HRSD. There is also an increased risk in siblings in the long-segment HRSD, the overall risk being 4 to 19%. HRSD is thought to be a multigenic disorder with mutations in the *RET* oncogene, an affected locus on chromosome 10, and a missense mutation of the endothelin-B receptor gene on chromosome 13.[3–5]

Accurate assessment of a child suspected of having HRSD requires clear communication between the pathologist and the clinician. For the pathologist, the paradigm of "looking for something" is reversed to "looking for nothing"! It must be stressed that rectal tissue with transitional or cloacogenic mucosa is normally aganglionic, and absence of ganglion cells may be the result of a biopsy obtained immediately proximal or distal (1 to 2 cm) to the pectinate line.[61]

Two types of biopsies are generally obtained to establish the diagnosis of HRSD. The less morbid is the rectal suction biopsy. Biopsy adequacy is determined by having as much submucosa as mucosa. The biopsy requires proper orientation in the paraffin block so that the sections are perpendicular to the mucosal surface. Serial sections should also be examined. Ganglion cells in the submucosa are coincidental to those in the deeper myenteric plexus (Fig. 21–9) and are often present as individual cells unaccompanied by the circumferentially arranged smaller Schwann cells. Another question that may arise in some cases during the examination of a rectal suction biopsy is whether the ganglion cells that are present are numerically adequate. One ganglion cell excludes the diagnosis of HRSD.

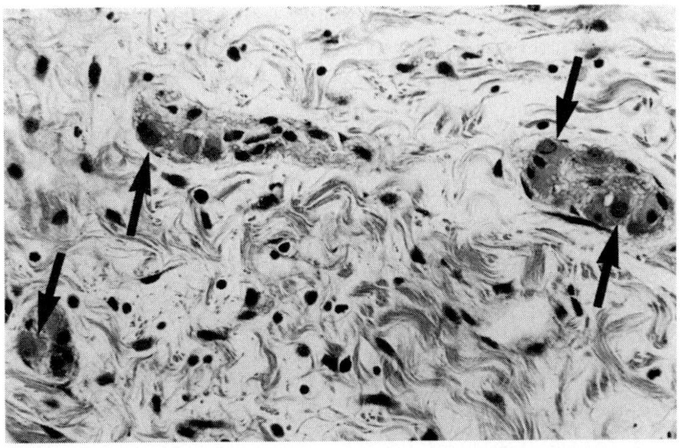

Figure 21–9. Three submucosal plexi with ganglion cells *(arrows)*. These ganglion cells are somewhat immature as noted by their relatively small size and micronucleolus.

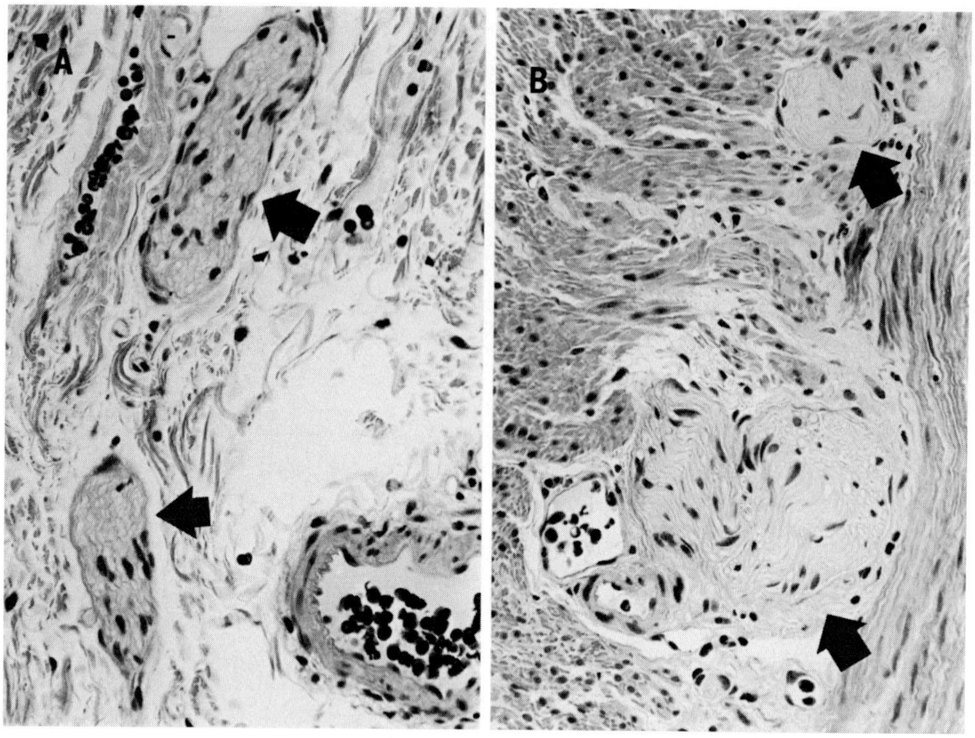

Figure 21–10. *A.* Hirschsprung's disease, showing two hypertrophied nerve bundles *(arrows)* devoid of ganglion cells in the submucosa. *B.* Markedly enlarged nerve bundles of the myenteric plexus *(arrows).*

The second type of biopsy is the full-thickness specimen that includes the muscularis propria. This procedure requires anesthesia and carries greater morbidity than the rectal suction biopsy. The obvious advantage is a more confident diagnosis based upon more tissue and a greater opportunity to identify ganglion cells or to better appreciate the hypertrophied nerve bundles (Fig. 21–10*A* and *B*). This type of specimen also allows easier recognition of ganglion cells, which are generally larger and more mature in the myenteric plexus. The prominent nucleolus of the mature ganglion cell is a micronucleolus in the smaller, less-mature submucosal ganglion cells.[63] While evaluating the biopsy for ganglion cells, crypt dilatation and cryptitis should not be overlooked. Almost 25% of infants with HRSD have enterocolitis as well.[64, 65]

The primary diagnosis of HRSD should not be attempted on frozen section; however, frozen section evaluation is appropriate for determining proximal extent of aganglionosis during colostomy placement. The muscularis propria is sampled through the serosa to allow microscopic examination of the myenteric plexi. If successive biopsy specimens show no ganglion cells and nerve elements are absent between the longitudinal and circular smooth muscle layers, total colonic HRSD must be strongly considered (Fig. 21–11).[61] Subsequent biopsy specimens should be obtained from the ileocecal valve. If ganglion cells are found, the hepatic flexure or transverse colon should then be sampled. We have had the experience of identifying the first ganglion cells at the mid-jejunum or at the ligament of Treitz. In some cases, the appendix is submitted for frozen section evaluation. This has potential pitfalls. The surgeon and pathologist must be cautious, especially in proceeding in the absence of ganglion cells.

It is impractical for the pathologist to serial section rectal biopsy specimens at the time of frozen section. Ganglion cells, not apparent at frozen section, may emerge in deeper levels of the processed, previously frozen colonic biopsy. If the pathologist is uncertain about the presence of ganglia at frozen section, another biopsy may be necessary.

RENAL NEOPLASMS AND NEUROBLASTOMA

Primary renal neoplasms (particularly Wilms' tumor) and neuroblastoma account for approximately 75% or more of intraabdominal malignant neoplasms in children. Less common intraabdominal malignancies include non-Hodgkin's malignant lymphoma of the small noncleaved cell type (Burkitt's and Burkitt's-like B-cell lymphoma),

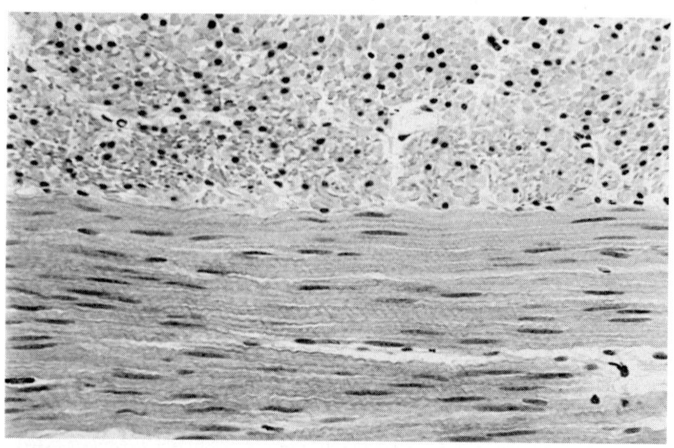

Figure 21–11. Total colonic Hirschsprung's disease, showing absence of nerve bundles between the longitudinal and circular smooth muscle of the muscularis propria.

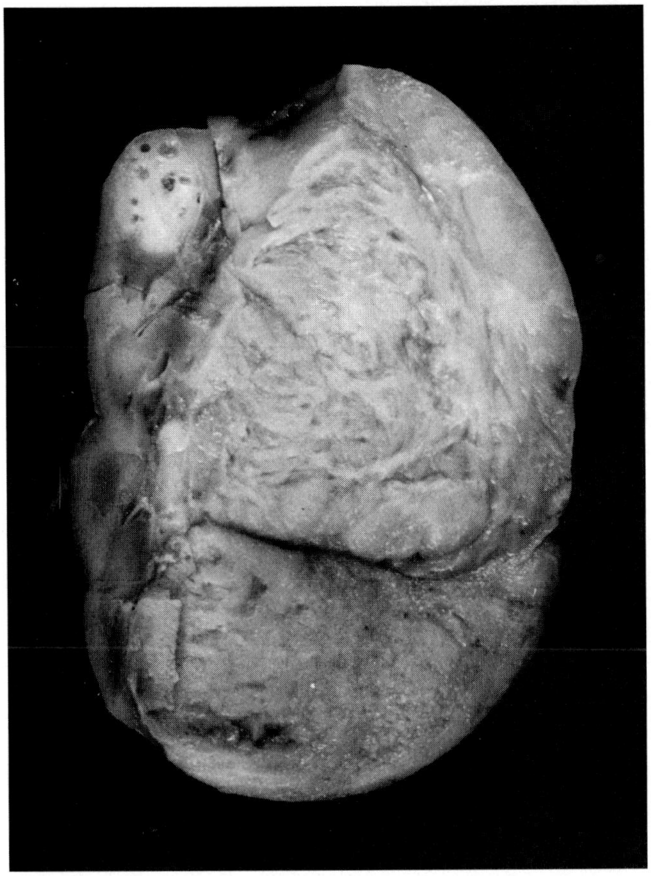

Figure 21–12. Wilms' tumor, showing near complete replacement of the kidney by a soft gray-tan mass.

hepatoblastoma, ovarian malignant germ-cell neoplasm (dysgerminoma, endodermal sinus tumor), rhabdomyosarcoma (bladder, prostate, and retroperitoneum), intraabdominal desmoplastic small-cell tumor, pancreatoblastoma, and Ewing's sarcoma-primitive neuroectodermal tumor (pelvis and retroperitoneum).

In the past, *Wilms' tumor* was the designation for virtually all primary renal neoplasms in children, excluding the rare renal-cell carcinoma and angiomyolipoma. Based upon pathologic studies of renal neoplasms submitted to the National Wilms' Tumor Study (NWTS), it became apparent that Wilms' tumor was not as simple as had been thought previously.[66] Beckwith delineated a spectrum of lesions. While some may regress and are clinically inconsequential, others progress to become a malignant process with the potential to recur or metastasize.[67] Two tumor types with poor prognostic implications emerged that had previously been regarded as sarcomatous variants of Wilms' tumor: clear cell sarcoma of the kidney (CCSK) and malignant rhabdoid tumor (MRT). Together these two neoplasms represented less than 10% of all renal tumors referred to the NWTS.[66] However, CCSK and MRT account for a disproportionate number of treatment failures and tumor-related deaths. Both neoplasms are histogenetically distinct from Wilms' tumor and its congeners. Although the prognosis of CCSK has steadily improved with intensified therapy, MRT remains one of the most treatment-resistant neoplasms of childhood.[68]

Approximately 400 to 500 renal neoplasms are newly diagnosed in children each year in the United States. Overall, 1 child per 10,600 develops a primary tumor of the kidney. This is a Wilms' tumor in 90% of cases.[69] Current therapy includes nephrectomy and chemotherapy with or without adjuvant radiation, depending upon the pathologic stage. The disease-free survival of children with Wilms' tumor is at least 80%.

Classic Wilms' tumor is a unilateral, circumscribed neoplasm that largely replaces the kidney with an eccentric compressed rim of renal tissue at the periphery of the mass (Fig. 21–12). These tumors often weigh in excess of 300 g. Wilms' tumor is quite soft and is sometimes cystic and hemorrhagic. For these reasons, resection risks intraoperative rupture and spillage of tumor into the peritoneal cavity—an event that changes a potential stage I (a completely resected Wilms' tumor with an intact renal capsule and confined to the hilar plane) to stage III (an incompletely resected Wilms' tumor).[70]

The nephrectomy specimen should be submitted to the surgical pathology laboratory intact and unopened.[70] Prior to sectioning, the external surface should be marked with India ink. This allows microscopic evaluation for invasion through the capsule.

Studies of the ontogeny of Wilms' tumor have identified a group of nephroblastic proliferations that are either progenitors of Wilms' tumor or have failed to evolve into a frankly malignant Wilms' tumor. A careful search for these lesions is important because their presence indicates risk for Wilms' tumor in the contralateral kidney (Fig. 21–13).[67] On histologic grounds, it may be difficult to distinguish between a hyperplastic nephrogenic rest and an early Wilms' tumor.

The pathologic examination of a Wilms' tumor establishes the stage of disease (in the absence of distant metastasis) on which treatment decisions and prognosis are based.[70] Prior to the era of effective multimodality therapy, many investigators attempted to correlate the histologic grade of Wilms' tumor with prognosis. Wilms' tumor is often morphologically complex with a classic triphasic pattern (blastema, tubules and glomeruli, and stroma). His-

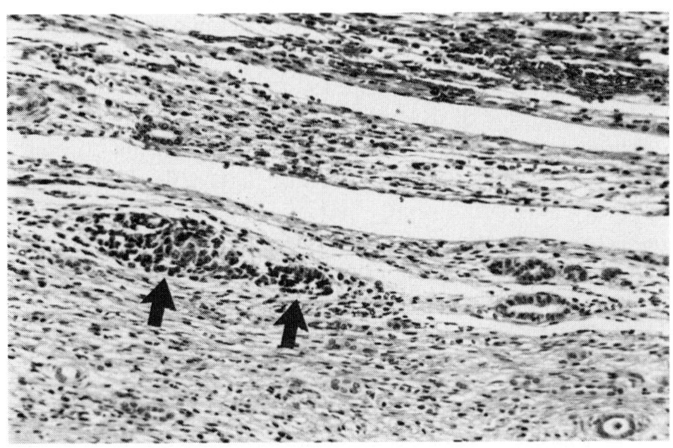

Figure 21–13. Perilobar nephrogenic rests *(arrows)* in the grossly normal appearing kidney adjacent to a Wilms' tumor.

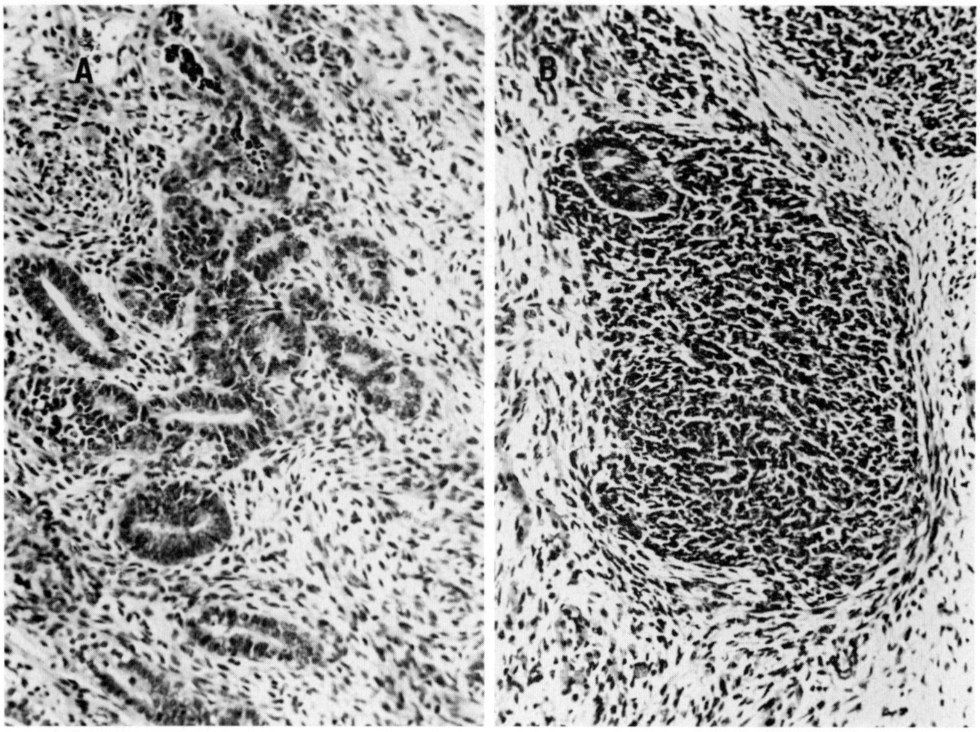

Figure 21–14. *A.* Neoplastic tubules in a spindle-cell stroma with focal areas of rhabdomyomatous differentiation in a classic Wilms' tumor. *B.* A focus of primitive small cells forming a blastemal island that is surrounded by a spindle cell stroma. Both microscopic fields represent favorable histology in a Wilms' tumor.

tologic variations include tumors with a predominant blastemal, stromal, or epithelial tubular pattern. Presumably, for this reason, histologic-survival correlation was not strong (Fig. 21–14*A* and *B*). It was realized that these early grading schemes had borderline significance at best in predicting outcome because the prognosis for Wilms' tumors in general was poor. The most reliable prognostic indicator proved to be the presence of large, bizarre cells with atypical mitotic figures, i.e., anaplasia.[66, 70] The extent of cellular anaplasia is also valuable for prognosis. Although the significance of focal anaplasia has diminished as a prognostically unfavorable finding with increasing therapeutic effectiveness, diffuse anaplasia still carries a poor outcome.[66, 70] Fortunately, diffuse anaplasia is seen in less than 5% of all classic Wilms' tumors.[70]

Mesoblastic nephroma, CCSK, and MRT are the three monophasic neoplasms of the kidney in children.[71] As previously mentioned, the latter two neoplasms have histologic features distinct from those of classic Wilms' tumor.[66] Clear cell sarcoma of the kidney metastasizes to the skeletal system (40% of cases). In contrast, bony metastases are documented in only 3 to 4% of classic Wilms' tumor.[70] With the recognition of CCSK, an aggressive therapeutic approach has substantially reduced the frequency of bony metastasis, resulting in improved prognosis. In contrast, the MRT, a renal tumor typically diagnosed in children under 2 years of age, continues to be a treatment-resistant neoplasm.[68] Grossly, CCSK and MRT resemble classic Wilms' tumor. Microscopic examination allows distinction (Fig. 21–15). Although it is important for the pathologist to note specific features for pathologic staging of CCSK and MRT, these are less critical for making a treatment decision. These tumors are managed aggressively regardless of stage. This approach also applies to the classic Wilms' tumor with diffuse anaplasia.

Congenital mesoblastic nephroma (CMN) was the first of the primary renal neoplasms of childhood to be recognized as an entity separate from classic Wilms' tumor.[71] In the past, CMN was referred to as ''congenital Wilms' tumor'' or ''spindle-cell Wilms' tumor.'' Not all CMNs are congenital; however, most are diagnosed in the first year of life as renal-based abdominal masses. It is estimated that 2.5 to 5% of all pediatric renal tumors are CMNs.[70] Grossly, the CMN replaces most of the affected kidney as a solitary circumscribed mass whose borders blend into the adjacent parenchyma. This is in contrast to the sharply demarcated periphery of a Wilms' tumor. The cut surface

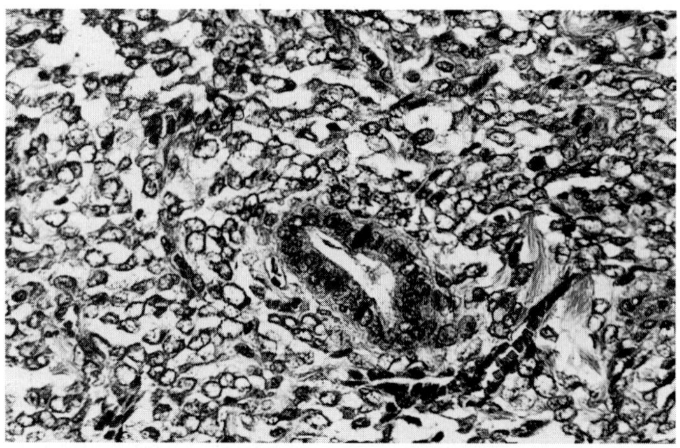

Figure 21–15. Clear-cell sarcoma of the kidney, showing the characteristic monotonous cells with nuclear clearing. An atypical appearing tubule is surrounded by malignant cells.

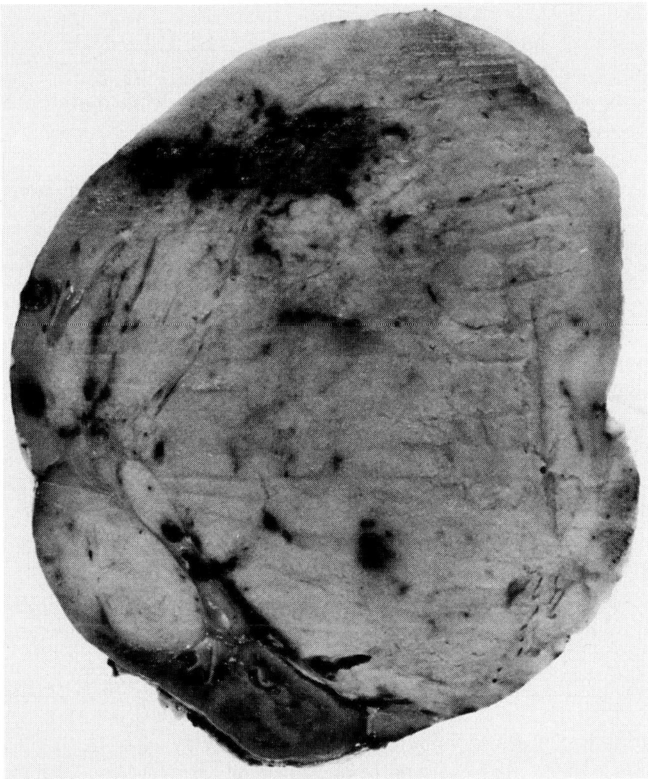

Figure 21–16. Congenital mesoblastic nephroma, presenting as an abdominal mass in a neonate. Note the areas of hemorrhage that are seen more often in the cellular variant.

is gray-white to tan and is trabeculated, resembling a leiomyoma of the uterus. A variant of CMN, the atypical or cellular mesoblastic nephroma, is more homogeneous, white, and glistening, with gross features resembling classic Wilms' tumor (Fig. 21–16). Microscopically, the CMN is composed of fascicles of uniform fusiform to ovoid spindle cells with entrapped tubules and glomeruli at the infiltrating interface (Fig. 21–17). The cellular mesoblastic nephroma does not have a fascicular pattern; instead, the cells are arranged in sheets and possess darker nuclei, less cytoplasm, and more abundant mitotic activity than in typical CMN. Extension of the tumor to involve surrounding perirenal soft tissues is a feature of both CMN and cellular mesoblastic nephroma. Nephrectomy is the treatment of choice. Local recurrences occur only occasionally, and metastasis is rare, sometimes solitary to the lung. The prognosis is excellent, and adjuvant therapy is rarely indicated.

Neuroblastoma is the second commonest solid malignant neoplasm of childhood. It is exceeded in frequency only by brain tumors.[69] In the past 10 years, progress has been made in the understanding of neuroblastomas from the perspective of molecular biology.[72] Most neuroblastomas show deletion of the short arm of chromosome 1 and amplification of N-*myc* oncogene on chromosome 2. Nuclear aneuploidy in a neuroblastoma connotes a favorable outcome. This is in stark contrast to the ominous implications carried by aneuploid tumors in adults. Despite the advances in understanding of these tumors on a molecular biologic level, the prognosis has not improved over the past 25 to 30 years.[73]

A spectrum of neuroblastic tumors exists ranging from poorly differentiated neuroblastoma to mature ganglioneuroma.[74] Approximately 40% of neuroblastic tumors arise in the adrenal gland. The remainder arise in extraadrenal sites: retroperitoneum (25%), posterior mediastinum (15%), pelvis (5%), and neck (5%).[73] A palpable abdominal mass is the commonest clinical presentation. Other presenting signs and symptoms include hepatomegaly, bone pain, Horner's syndrome, and subcutaneous nodules.[75] Among pediatric malignancies, neuroblastoma is one of the most diagnostically confounding upon presentation, and, unfortunately, approximately half of afflicted children have metastatic disease at the time of diagnosis. Neuroblastoma, more so than any other solid malignancy of childhood, occurs with metastasis and an occult primary source. Bone marrow, bone, lymph nodes, and liver are the likeliest metastatic sites. Urinary catecholamine levels are elevated in more than 90% of children with neuroblastoma, facilitating preoperative diagnosis.

In contrast to the surgeon's role in the definitive diagnosis and excision of Wilms' tumor, the surgeon's role in the management of patients with neuroblastoma is less clear-cut. Unlike Wilms' tumors, which are often amenable to complete resection, only a minority of cases of neuroblastoma are completely resectable. In most cases, the surgeon is asked to excise residual tumor following nonoperative therapy. Resection of these tumors is often technically demanding due to marked retroperitoneal fibrosis and matting of lymph nodes. Calcifications may be a prominent feature of the soft tissue surrounding neuroblastomas, even in those tumors that have not been preoperatively treated. Surgical margins are virtually impossible to assess because these tumors are excised piecemeal.

Although several histologic grading systems have been proposed over the last 40 years, none have been reliable for predicting outcome, and, like Wilms' tumors, neuroblastic tumors may show microscopic heterogeneity. For instance, ganglion cells may be present focally, whereas the remainder of the tumor has primitive or poorly differentiated features or a predominantly ganglioneuromatous appear-

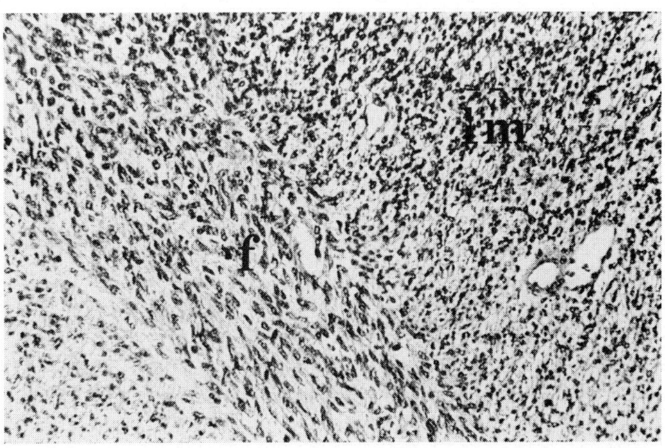

Figure 21–17. Congenital mesoblastic nephroma, showing the classic fascicular pattern (f) adjacent to the less mature cellular pattern (lm).

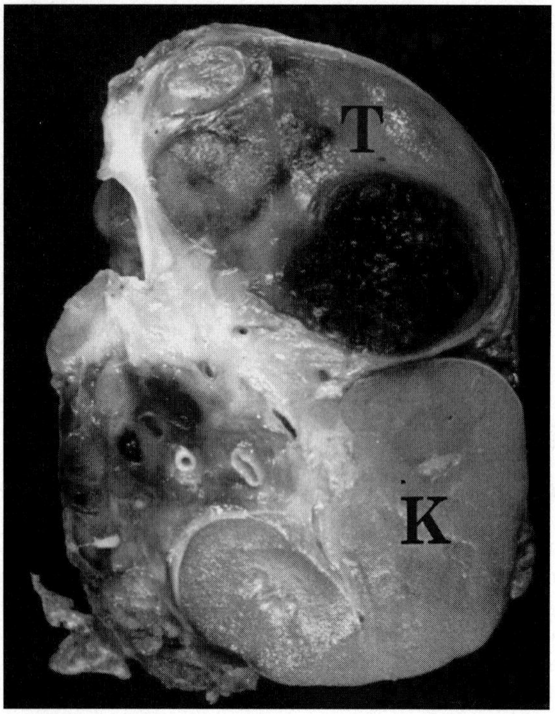

Figure 21–18. Adrenal neuroblastoma, showing the main tumor mass (T) above the kidney (K) and extensive infiltration of the perirenal and hilar soft tissues. The dark nodule in the suprarenal mass is a focus of poorly differentiated neuroblastoma.

ance with aggregates of neuroblasts (Fig. 21–18). No uniform histopathologic criteria exist for separating "differentiating neuroblastoma" from ganglioneuroblastoma. Three indicators of poor prognosis are (1) lack of differentiation, (2) high mitotic activity, and (3) macroscopically visible nodules of neuroblasts surrounded by ganglioneuroma (nodular, stroma-rich neuroblastoma, composite ganglioneuroblastoma) (Fig. 21–19).[73] However, the most reliable prognostic indicators are age at diagnosis (less than or greater than 1 year old) and pathologic stage.[76] A child under 1 year of age with localized resectable tumor has the most favorable outcome.

GERM-CELL NEOPLASMS—TERATOMA AND RELATED NEOPLASMS

Growths presumably derived from the primordial germ cells (ovum and spermatogonium) are the quintessential tumors of childhood, with overlapping features of maldevelopment and of neoplasia and with attention to detail critical for proper management.[77] Among congenital neoplasms that are detectable in utero by ultrasonographic examination, the sacrococcygeal teratoma is the commonest.[78, 79] Isaacs reviewed the literature on congenital tumors and determined that neuroblastoma and teratomas account for 50% of all cases.[80] Soft tissue neoplasms, congenital leukemias, and brain tumors make up another 30 to 35% of congenital tumors.

Whether in children or adults, germ-cell neoplasms are divided into distinct tumor types based upon microscopic features. These include pure teratoma, germinoma, embryonal carcinoma, endodermal sinus tumor (yolk sac carcinoma), and choriocarcinoma or a mixed pattern with two or more type components.[77] By definition, any germ-cell neoplasm with more than one pattern or type is malignant and is therefore designated as a malignant mixed germ-cell neoplasm.

Although similar in microscopic appearances, the anatomic sites of germ-cell neoplasms vary between the child and adult. In adults, 65 to 70% of neoplasms arise in either the ovary or testis. In children, the same percentage of germ-cell tumors originate in extragonadal locations in the following order of frequency: sacrococcygeum, mediastinum, central nervous system, head and neck, and retroperitoneum.[77, 80] Tumors of the sacrococcygeal and head and neck regions typically occur in children under the age of 2 years, whereas germ-cell neoplasms in other extragonadal sites typically occur at a later age. Teratomas of the stomach and pericardium are almost exclusively seen in infants.

Sacrococcygeal teratoma accounts for 40% or more of germ-cell neoplasms in children.[77] In the reported experience of Children's Hospital of Los Angeles, 69% of all teratomas were sacrococcygeal.[80] This is one condition associated with nonimmune hydrops fetalis without a clear pathophysiologic explanation. Females are affected more commonly than males in a ratio of 3:1 to 4:1. A mass is apparent in 65 to 75% of cases at or shortly after birth.[81–83] Less than 50% of sacrococcygeal teratomas are purely postsacral; most of the rest have a presacral component. Lesions that are entirely presacral are potentially undetectable in the neonatal period. When children present at 1 to 2 years of age, almost always with either obstructive symptoms or neurologic signs, malignant transformation or overgrowth has already occurred. Only 2 to 3% of sacrococcygeal teratomas diagnosed in the neonatal and early infancy period have evidence of malignancy, usually in the form of endodermal sinus tumor (Fig. 21–20). In contrast, 50% of sacrococcygeal teratomas prove malignant when the tumor is recognized after 1 year of age, and virtually all tumors are malignant if they escape detection until the patient is 4 to 5 years old.[77–82] It is extremely uncommon for a previously resected neonatal sacrococcygeal teratoma to recur as an endodermal sinus tumor. More commonly, what is thought to represent a recurrent sacrococcygeal teratoma instead proves to be a subcutaneous nodule of mature gliomatous tissue in the postsacral soft tissues.

Grossly, sacrococcygeal teratomas vary from a 6- to 12-cm mass composed of multiple collapsible cystic structures with mucoid contents to a much smaller cystic and solid or exclusively solid tumor (Fig. 21–21). The neuroepithelial component of the tumor corresponds grossly to soft gray-tan to white tissue with cerebroid features. Firm, infiltrative areas of hemorrhage and necrosis should raise concern about malignancy. However, in most cases of neonatal malignant sacrococcygeal teratomas, features indicating malignancy are difficult to appreciate by gross inspection.

As is true for all large tumors, thorough sampling of a sacrococcygeal teratoma is necessary. In general, one microscopic section is taken for each centimeter of maximum dimension of the tumor. One potential pitfall in the microscopic assessment of these large tumors is missing focal immature teratomatous elements, especially primitive

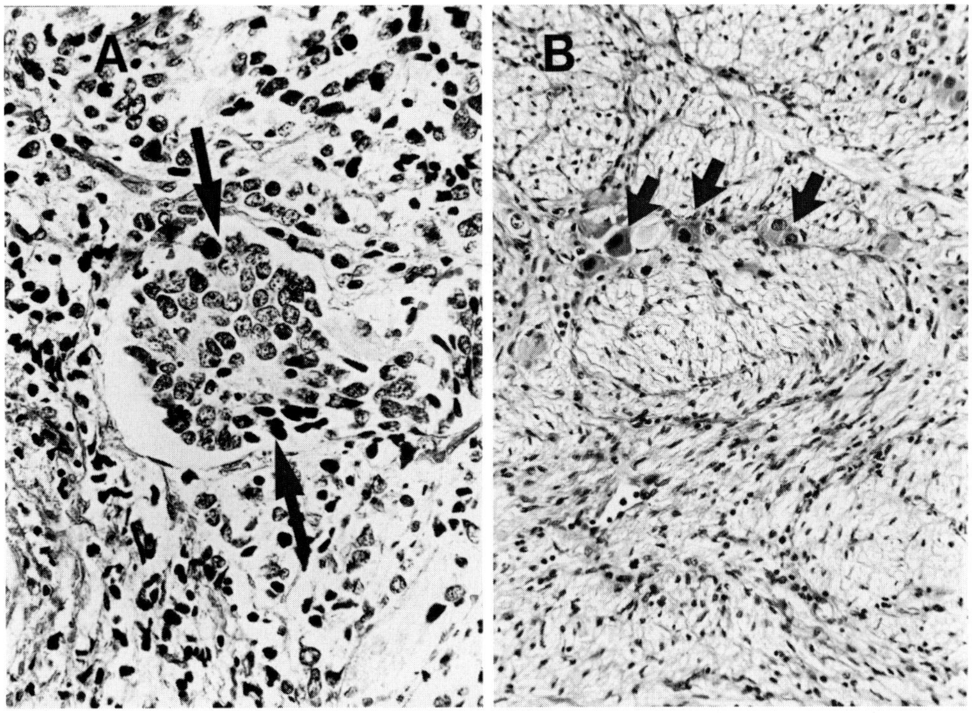

Figure 21–19. *A.* Classic neuroblastoma, showing a central nest of neuroblasts *(arrows)*. *B.* Other areas of the tumor, showing neuromatous stroma and ganglion cells *(arrows)* in various stages of maturation.

neuroectoderm with foci of embryonic appearing neural tubes and sheets of neuroblastic cells. These areas may be virtually indistinguishable from neuroblastoma (Fig. 21–22). Some sacrococcygeal teratomas are dominated by immature neuroepithelium. More commonly, there is a mixture of immature and mature somatic tissues (Fig. 21–23). Approximately 50% of tumors are composed entirely of mature tissues. These are often the purely cystic tumors; the cysts are lined by squamous, respiratory, and enteric mucosa (Fig. 21–24). Bone, cartilage, smooth muscle, and fat are the various differentiated mesenchymal tissues. Immature mesenchyme, kidney, and liver are other fetal-type tissues.

Microscopic grading of sacrococcygeal teratomas based upon a semiquantitative estimation of immature somatic tissues has been evaluated as a prognostic determinant. However, unlike the solid teratoma of the ovary, testis, and anterior mediastinum in which the presence of immature teratomatous tissues has negative prognostic implications, both immature and mature teratomas of the sacrococcygeal region have excellent prognoses.[84] The maturational stage of a sacrococcygeal teratoma mirrors the developmental stage of the host. Although the pathologist may be asked to grade a sacrococcygeal teratoma, this exercise lacks prognostic significance. By contrast, the pathologist must carefully look for microscopic foci of endodermal sinus tumor in a teratoma in a neonate. Most sacrococcygeal teratomas in later infancy or early childhood are predominantly endodermal sinus tumor complete with Schiller-Duval bodies. This finding contrasts with neonatal tumors in which any malignant foci are relatively inconspicuous and are interspersed with immature teratomatous tissues.

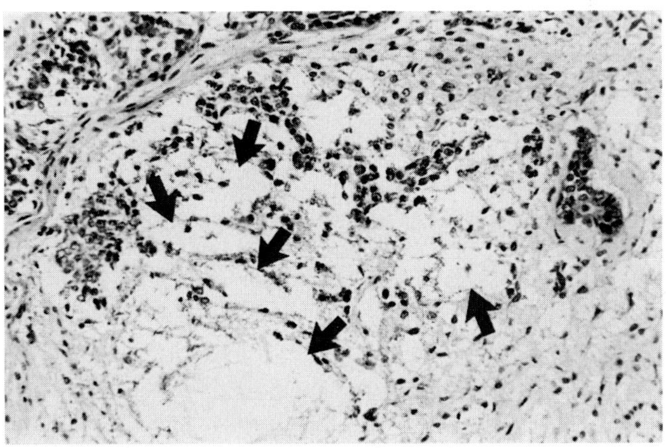

Figure 21–20. Microscopic focus of endodermal sinus tumor in a sacrococcygeal teratoma presenting in a neonate. Note long delicate spaces resembling endodermal sinus structures *(arrows)*.

SOFT TISSUE NEOPLASMS

Soft tissue malignancies comprise a relatively insignificant portion of a pediatrician's practice—approximately 8.5 soft tissue sarcomas per million children between the ages of 0 and 14 years were seen in the Surveillance, Epidemiology, and End Results Program. This compares with 35 to 40 cases of acute leukemia, 20 to 25 cases of brain and spinal cord tumors, 11 or 12 cases of neuroblastoma, and 10 or 11 cases of Wilms' tumor.[69]

In a review from the Minnesota Pediatric Soft Tissue Data Base of 944 soft tissue neoplasms that occurred in the first 2 decades of life, approximately 30% of all tumors were of vascular origin, consisting principally of capillary hemangiomas and cystic lymphangiomas.[85] Nerve sheath, fibrous, myofibroblastic, and rhabdomyogenic neoplasms

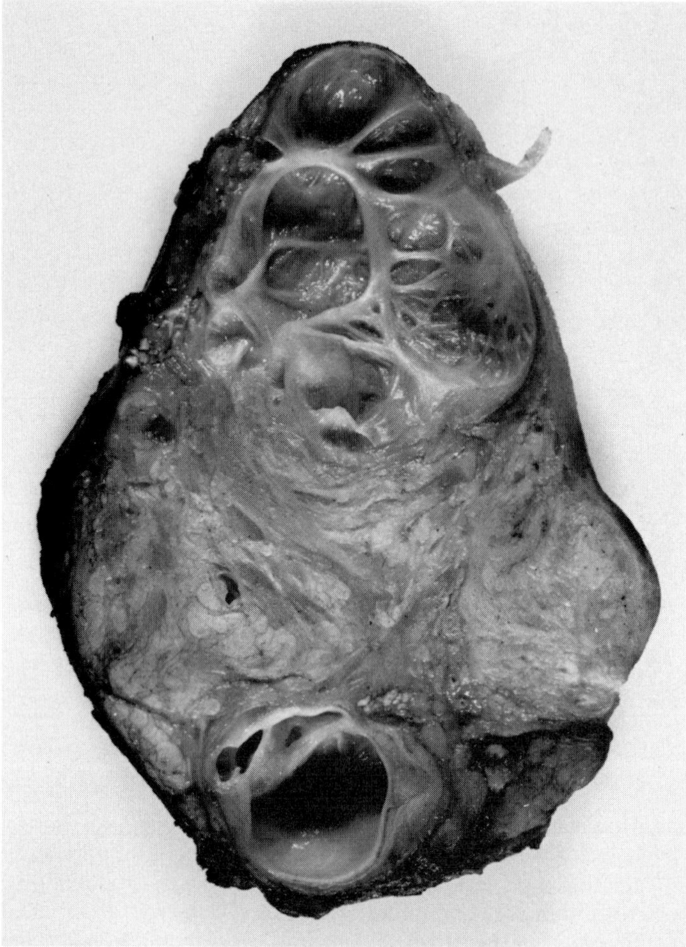

Figure 21–21. Sacrococcygeal teratoma, presenting in a newborn female showing solid and cystic features. Many of the solid areas were composed of mature neuroglial tissue.

together accounted for 14% of the total. When the age at diagnosis was restricted to the first year of life, vascular tumors were still the largest category (34% of cases), with the fibrous and myofibroblastic tumors representing 27% of all tumors.[86]

Juvenile fibrous tumors actually encompass several distinct neoplasms that have a predilection for children, especially those who are less than 7 years old. Of the 108 fibrous and myofibroblastic tumors in our series, half were diagnosed at or before 1 year of age.[85] The commonest type of juvenile fibrous tumor is *infantile myofibromatosis* (22% of cases). This lesion occurs in infants as a solitary, firm cutaneous and/or subcutaneous mass measuring 1 to 3 cm in diameter (Fig. 21–25). Less commonly, the disease is multifocal. The patient presents with multiple soft tissue masses and/or lytic lesions in the bone. The generalized

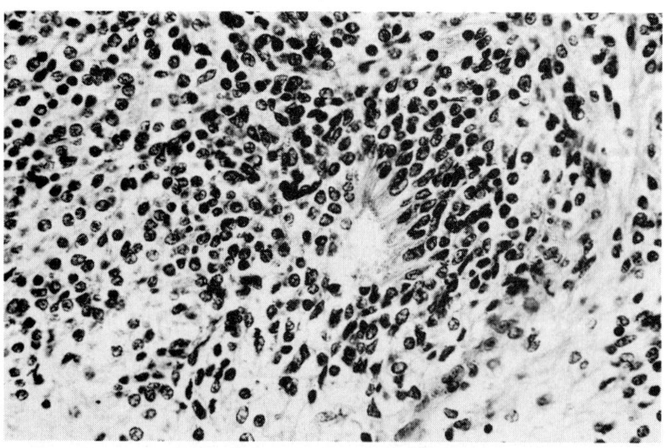

Figure 21–22. Sacrococcygeal teratoma, showing immature neural tissue that has no prognostic significance.

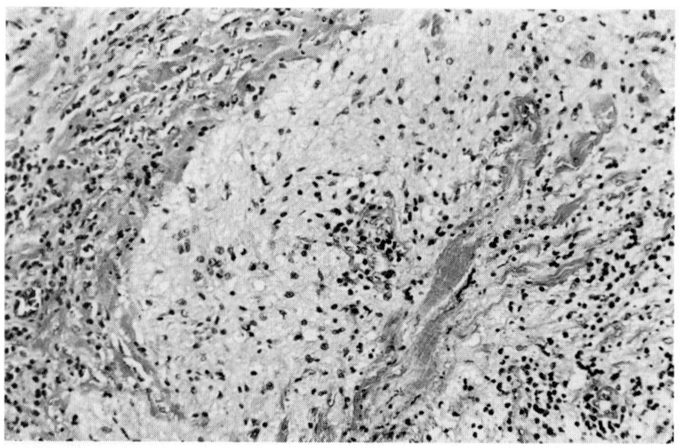

Figure 21–23. Sacrococcygeal teratomas, showing mature neuroglial tissue.

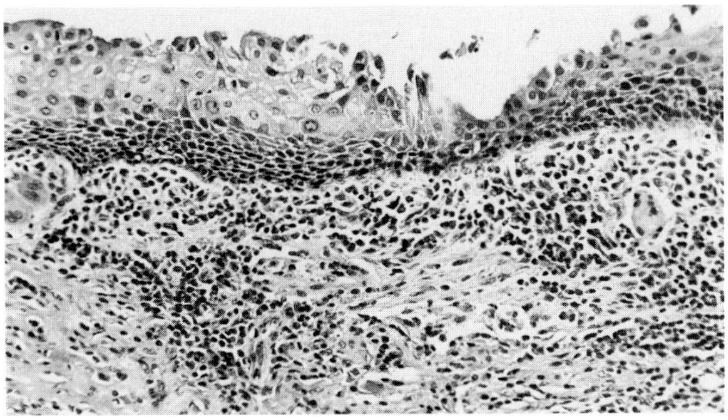

Figure 21–24. Sacrococcygeal teratoma, showing a portion of a cyst lined by squamous epithelium.

form of infantile myofibromatosis has lesions in multiple organs, in addition to the soft tissues and bone. Obstruction of the pulmonary veins by myofibromatous nodules may prove lethal. Microscopically, the tumor is composed of compact bundles or fascicles of spindle cells, less cellular areas with a hyalinized stroma, and, in some tumors, hemangiopericytoma-like foci (Fig. 21–26). Necrosis and calcification reflect the tendency of these tumors to undergo spontaneous regression.

Other types of juvenile fibromatosis have distinctive clinical and pathologic manifestations. These include fibromatosis colli, infantile digital fibromatosis, fibrous hamartoma of infancy, juvenile aponeurotic fibroma, and congenital-infantile fibrosarcoma. The latter neoplasm is a disturbing one in terms of its size, location, and microscopic features. Despite these disquieting aspects, the prognosis is excellent, with 90 to 95% cure rate.[85]

Rhabdomyosarcoma of the embryonal and alveolar subtypes is the commonest soft tissue sarcoma in the first 2 decades of life.[87] Multiinstitutional study groups and registries report that 45 to 55% of childhood sarcomas are rhabdomyosarcomas.[88] In the past, the category of ''undifferentiated sarcoma'' or ''malignant small-cell tumor of indeterminate histogenesis'' was the second most frequent type of soft tissue sarcoma in children. Later studies have permitted the correct identification of most of these tumors as either soft tissue Ewing's sarcoma or primitive neuroectodermal tumor (EWS-PNET). It is interesting that tumors previously called undifferentiated sarcoma comprised 15 to 20% of all soft tissue sarcomas. This is almost identical to the percentage of EWS-PNET identified in current prospective series.

An important clinical difference between soft tissue sarcomas in children and adults is the anatomic distribution of the tumors. The majority of soft tissue sarcomas in adults occur as a mass in an extremity or the retroperitoneum. Juvenile rhabdomyosarcomas, in particular the embryonal type (50 to 60% of cases), have a predilection for the head and neck region (45% of cases) and genitourinary tract (25% of cases).[87] Embryonal rhabdomyosarcoma may appear as a polypoid mass (so-called sarcoma botryoides) in the middle ear, nasopharynx, urinary bladder, and vagina or as a solid mass (Fig. 21–27). A minority of embryonal rhabdomyosarcomas (5% of cases) have the gross features of a sarcoma botryoides. Another distinction is that liposarcoma and malignant fibrous histiocytoma, which constitute 35 to 45% of all adult soft tissue sarcomas, are uncommon in children.

Alveolar rhabdomyosarcoma is the particularly aggressive, potentially lethal type of juvenile rhabdomyosarcoma. Long-term survival is only 40 to 50%. This contrasts with the more favorable embryonal rhabdomyosarcoma that has an overall survival of 70%. Approximately 20% of juvenile rhabdomyosarcomas are the alveolar type. Patients with this type of tumor are generally older (late childhood, adolescence, and young adulthood) than children with embryonal rhabdomyosarcoma, who are usually diagnosed before 10 years of age.[89] Although this tumor tends to occur in the extremities, particularly the distal aspects, it may also occur in the head and neck region, sometimes with regional lymphadenopathy. A small subset of patients presents with disseminated alveolar rhabdomyosarcomas. Such clinical presentation can mimic hematopoietic neoplasms, with generalized lymphadenopathy, bone lesions, and pleural effusions. Likewise, a biopsy or needle aspiration sample may be misinterpreted microscopically, since the cells are delicate and uniform and may lack an obvious alveolar pattern. Differential immunohistochemistry and cytogenetics allow recognition as alveolar rhabdomyosarcoma with its expression of myogenous filament proteins and characteristic reciprocal translocation, t(2;13) (q35;q14), respectively (see Chap. 2).

Ewing's sarcoma-primitive neuroectodermal tumor (EWS-PNET) is now considered a single family of closely related small round-cell neoplasms.[28, 90] These tumors have a common reciprocal translocation, t(11;22) (q24;q12) in 80 to 90% of cases. Typically, the tumor is greater than 6 to 8 cm and is often cystic and hemorrhagic. Microscopically, there is either a geographic arrangement of cohesive small cells with or without rosette formation or formless sheets or nests of infiltrating cells. When strict microscopic criteria are applied to distinguish between EWS and PNET, the latter is the more aggressive of the two neoplasms.[91] Electron microscopy, immunohistochemistry, and cytogenetics accurately differentiate EWS-PNET from the other small-cell neoplasms of childhood (see Chap. 2). Because

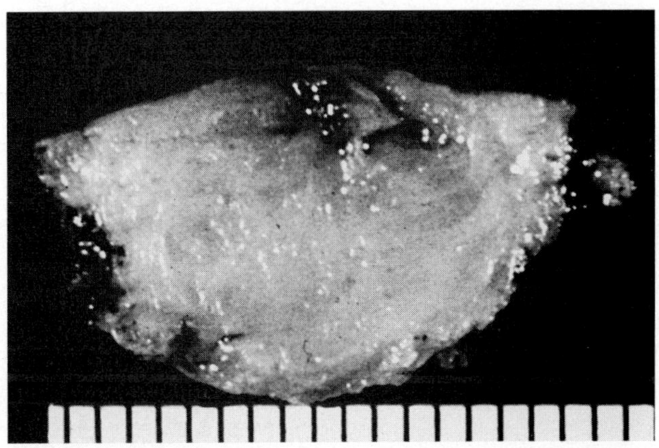

Figure 21–25. Infantile myofibromatosis of the neck in an infant. The cut surface has a glistening trabeculated appearance and a nodular periphery.

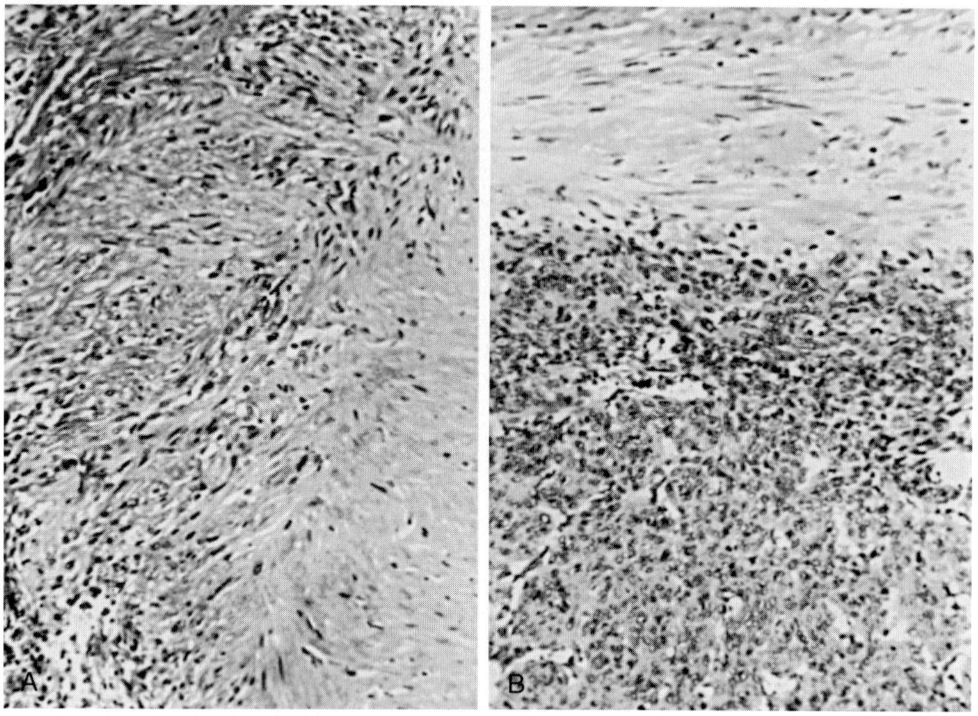

Figure 21–26. *A.* Infantile myofibromatosis, showing contiguous spindle-cell and hyalinized areas. *B.* Another area of the same tumor showing a hemangiopericytoma-like pattern.

EWS-PNETs typically spread hematogenously early in their course, and because of their sensitivity to both radiation and chemotherapy, resection alone is no longer accepted for clinical management.

Conclusions

This chapter discusses some of the most critical and demanding, if not necessarily the most common, conditions that bring the surgeon and pathologist together in the care of a child. With a few exceptions, these developmental and acquired conditions come to clinical attention in childhood, often in infants and very young children. The sense of anxiety and urgency associated with a sick child is profoundly different from that with an adult, even one with a serious illness. It is not difficult to identify with the anguish of the parents. The purpose of this chapter is to enhance the surgeon's understanding of pathology with the ultimate goal of improving communication between the surgeon and pathologist in achieving optimal treatment of these children.

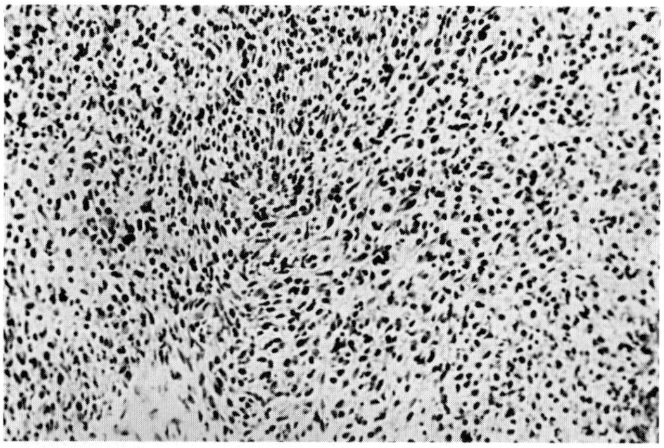

Figure 21–27. Embryonal rhabdomyosarcoma of the nasopharynx, showing the uniform primitive cellular composition of this neoplasm.

PITFALLS FOR THE SURGEON

1. Diagnosing and treating childhood disease, especially neoplasms, according to principles of adult surgical management.
2. Being unaware of the lack of pediatric experience of a pathologist who is involved in a critical pediatric case.
3. Failure to submit a portion of a biopsied lymph node for microbial culture, particularly in a child with associated inflammatory manifestations.
4. Intervening aggressively in the case of vascular tumors of the head and neck region in an infant whose tumor is likely to undergo spontaneous regression.
5. Aggressively resecting a thoracic lymphoma, when nonsurgical therapeutic modalities are more effective.
6. Delay in surgically intervening in a suspected case of extrahepatic biliary atresia.
7. Resecting excessive or insufficient lengths of bowel for necrotizing enterocolitis. If margins are in doubt, intraoperative frozen section consultation should be obtained.
8. Submitting rectal biopsies too close to the pectinate line (the region that is normally aganglionic) for diagnosis of suspected Hirschsprung's disease.
9. Rupturing a cystic or hemorrhagic Wilms' tumor during resection, with consequent upstaging of the neoplasm from stage I to stage III.
10. Delay in resecting a sacrococcygeal teratoma in an infant, in the hopes that it will mature. With increasing age, the *likelihood of malignancy increases.*
11. Attempting to determine whether a teratoma contains malignant elements by biopsy alone: a positive finding *is* conclusive, but a *negative* finding does not exclude the possibility of unsampled malignant elements.

PITFALLS FOR THE PATHOLOGIST

1. Interpreting microscopic findings in pediatric cases only on the basis of one's understanding of adult pathology.
2. Failing to properly allocate a lymph node biopsy sample for microbial culture and for either flow immunophenotyping or frozen tissue bank (for the option of future frozen section immunostains or molecular probe analysis).
3. Failing to report acute inflammation in a recurrent lymphangioma ("cystic hygroma"); lymphangitis is a potentially devastating complication in this setting.
4. Misinterpreting inflammatory myofibroblastic tumor of the lung as a true malignancy.
5. Misinterpreting a liver biopsy as extrahepatic biliary atresia when the underlying problem is an inborn error of bile acid synthesis or prolonged parenteral nutrition.
6. Failing to appreciate that a case of necrotizing enterocolitis is on the basis of Hirschsprung's disease rather than prematurity.
7. Rendering a diagnosis of aganglionic megacolon without completely sampling the tissue block with serial sections.
8. Failing to recognize the presence of nephrogenic rests in the otherwise normal renal parenchyma around a Wilms' tumor; this finding indicates an increased risk for the development of a contralateral Wilms' tumor.
9. Mistaking immature somatic elements in a sacrococcygeal teratoma from a neonate as evidence of malignancy.

Continued

10. Failing to thoroughly sample a sacrococcygeal teratoma for microscopic foci of malignancy, commonly endodermal sinus tumor.
11. Misinterpreting a distinctive variant of juvenile fibromatosis as malignancy, e.g., (calcifying) juvenile aponeurotic fibroma. The microscopic appearance alone can be misleading, especially in a case of congenital infantile fibrosarcoma.
12. Misinterpreting alveolar rhabdomyosarcoma (with dissemination upon presentation) as malignant lymphoma or another type of hematolymphoid malignancy.

FURTHER READING

Dehner LP. *Pediatric Surgical Pathology*, 2nd ed. Baltimore: Williams & Wilkins; 1987.

Skandalakis JE, Gray SW, eds. *Embryology for Surgeons*, 2nd ed. Baltimore: Williams & Wilkins; 1994.

Stocker JT, Dehner LP, eds. *Pediatric Pathology*. Philadelphia: Lippincott Co.; 1992.

REFERENCES

1. Skandalakis JE, Gray SW, eds. *Embryology for Surgeons*, 2nd ed. Baltimore: Williams & Wilkins; 1994.
2. Gilbert-Barness E, Opitz JM. Congenital anomalies and malformation syndromes. In: Stocker JT, Dehner LP, eds. *Pediatric Pathology*. Philadelphia: Lippincott Co.; 1992:73.
3. Romeo G, Ronchetto P, Luo Y, et al. Point mutations affecting tyrosine kinase domain of the RET proto-oncogene in Hirschsprung's disease. *Nature*. 1994;367:377.
4. Edery P, Lyonnet S, Mulligan LM, et al. Mutations of the RET proto-oncogene in Hirschsprung's disease. *Nature*. 1994;367:387.
5. Puffenberg EG, Hosoda K, Washington SS, et al. A missense mutation of the endothelin-B receptor gene in multigenic Hirschsprung's disease. *Cell*. 1994;79:1257.
6. Silverman RA. Hemangiomas and vascular malformations. *Pediatr Clin North Am*. 1991;38:811.
7. Bolande RP. Neoplasia of early life and its relationships to teratogenesis. *Perspect Pediatr Pathol*. 1976;3:145.
8. Coppes MJ, Haber DA, Grundy PE. Genetic events in the development of Wilms' tumor. *N Engl J Med*. 1994;331:586.
9. Schmidt D, Harms D, Pilon VA. Small-cell pediatric tumors: histology, immunohistochemistry and electron microscopy. *Clin Lab Med*. 1987;7:63.
10. Benjamin D. How much is necessary? *Pediatr Pathol*. 1994;14:755.
11. Dehner LP. *Pediatric Surgical Pathology*, 2nd ed. Baltimore: Williams & Wilkins; 1987.
12. Skandalakis JE, Gray SW, Todd NW. The pharynx and its derivatives. In: Skandalakis JE, Gray SW, eds. *Embryology for Surgeons*, 2nd ed. Baltimore: Williams & Wilkins; 1994:17.
13. Bodenstein L, Altman RP. Cervical lymphadenitis in infants and children. *Semin Pediatr Surg*. 1994;3:134.
14. Guariso JL. Congenital head and neck masses in infants and children: part 1. *Ear Nose Throat J*. 1991;70:40.
15. Guariso JL. Congenital head and neck masses in infants and children: part 2. *Ear Nose Throat J*. 1991;70:75.
16. Roback SA, Telander RL. Thyroglossal duct cysts and branchial cleft anomalies. *Semin Pediatr Surg*. 1994;3:142.
17. Torsiglieri AJ, Tom LWC, Ross AJ III, et al. Pediatric neck masses: guidelines for evaluation. *Int J Pediatr Otorhinolaryngol*. 1988; 16:199.
18. Spigland N, Bensoussan AL, Blanchard H, et al. Aberrant cervical thymus in children: three case reports and review of the literature. *J Pediatr Surg*. 1990;25:1196.
19. Sonnino RE, Spigland N, Laberge J-M, et al. Unusual patterns of congenital neck masses in children. *J Pediatr Surg*. 1989;24:966.
20. Filston HC. Hemangiomas, cystic hygromas, and teratomas of the head and neck. *Semin Pediatr Surg*. 1994;3:147.
21. Ward RF, April M. Teratomas of the head and neck. *Otolaryngol Clin North Am*. 1989;22:621.
22. Coffin CM, Dehner LP. Vascular tumors in children and adolescents: a clinicopathologic study of 228 tumors in 222 patients. *Pathol Annu*. 1993;28(pt 1):97.
23. El-Dessouky M, Azmy AF, Raine PAM, et al. Kasabach-Merritt syndrome. *J Pediatr Surg*. 1988;23:109.
24. Zukerberg LR, Nickoloff BJ, Weiss SW. Kaposiform hemangioendothelioma of infancy and childhood. An aggressive neoplasm associated with Kasabach-Merritt syndrome and lymphangiomatosis. *Am J Surg Pathol*. 1993;17:321.
25. Weiss SW. *Histological Typing of Soft Tissue Tumours*, 2nd ed. Berlin: Springer-Verlag; 1994:31.
26. Shamberger RC, Grier HE. Chest wall tumors in infants and children. *Semin Pediatr Surg*. 1994;3:267.
27. Baretton G, Stehr M, Nerlich A, et al. Chest wall hamartoma in infancy: a case report with immunohistochemical analysis of various interstitial collagen types. *Pediatr Pathol*. 1994;14:3.
28. Dehner LP. Primitive neuroectodermal tumor and Ewing's sarcoma. *Am J Surg Pathol*. 1993;17:1.
29. Clements BS, Warner JO. Pulmonary sequestration and related congenital bronchopulmonary-vascular malformations: nomenclature and classification based on anatomical and embryological considerations. *Thorax*. 1987;42:401.
30. Haddon MJ, Bowen AD. Bronchopulmonary and neurenteric forms of foregut anomalies. *Radiol Clin North Am*. 1991;29:241.
31. Fowler CL, Pokorny WJ, Wagner ML, et al. Review of bronchopulmonary foregut malformations. *J Pediatr Surg*. 1988;23:793.
32. Azarow KS, Pearl RH, Zurcher R, et al. Primary mediastinal masses. A comparison of adult and pediatric populations. *J Thorac Cardiovasc Surg*. 1993;106:67.
33. Mullen B, Richardson JD. Primary anterior mediastinal tumors in children and adults. *Ann Thorac Surg*. 1986;42:338.
34. Saenz NC, Schnitzer JJ, Eraklis AE, et al. Posterior mediastinal masses. *J Pediatr Surg*. 1993;28:172.
35. Adams GA, Shochat SJ, Smith EI, et al. Thoracic neuroblastoma: a Pediatric Oncology Group study. *J Pediatr Surg*. 1993;28:372.
36. Schneider JR, St Cyr JA, Thompson TR, et al. The changing spectrum of cystic pulmonary lesions requiring surgical resection in infants. *J Thorac Cardiovasc Surg*. 1985;89:332.
37. Nuchtern JG, Harberg FJ. Congenital lung cysts. *Semin Pediatr Surg*. 1994;3:233.
38. Stocker JT. Congenital and developmental diseases. In: Dail DH, Hammar SP, eds. *Pulmonary Pathology*, 2nd ed. New York: Springer-Verlag; 1993:155.
39. Brink DA, Balsara ZN. Prenatal ultrasound detection of intra-abdominal pulmonary sequestration with postnatal MRI correlation. *Pediatr Radiol*. 1991;21:227.
40. Lewis JE, Murray RE. Pulmonary sequestration with bronchoesophageal fistula. *J Pediatr Surg*. 1968;2:575.
41. John PR, Beasley SW, Mayne V. Pulmonary sequestration and related congenital disorders: a clinico-radiological review of 41 cases. *Pediatr Radiol*. 1989;20:4.
42. Zangwill BC, Stocker JT. Congenital cystic adenomatoid malformation within an extralobar pulmonary sequestration. *Pediatr Pathol*. 1993;13:309.
43. Stigers KB, Woodring JH, Kanga JF. The clinical and imaging spectrum of findings in patients with congenital lobar emphysema. *Pediatr Pulmonol*. 1992;14:160.
44. Stocker JT, Dehner LP. Acquired neonatal and pediatric diseases. In: Dail DH, Hammar SP, eds. *Pulmonary Pathology*, 2nd ed. New York: Springer-Verlag; 1993:191.
45. Dehner LP, Watterson J, Priest J. Pleuropulmonary blastoma: a unique intrathoracic-pulmonary neoplasm of childhood. *Perspect Pediatr Pathol*. 1995;18:214.

46. Trivedi P, Mieli-Vergani G, Mowat AP. Cholestasis in infancy and childhood: an overview. In: Lentze M, Reichen J, eds. *Paediatric Cholestasis. Novel Approaches to Treatment.* Dordrecht The Netherlands: Kluwer Academic Publishers; 1992:129.
47. Hoffman MA. Perspectives on biliary atresia. In: Hoffman MA, ed. *Current Controversies in Biliary Atresia.* Austin, TX: Landes Co.; 1992:1.
48. Karrer FM. Results of portoenterostomy. In: Hoffman MA, ed. *Current Controversies in Biliary Atresia.* Austin, TX: R. G. Landes Co.; 1992:73.
49. Rosenthal P, Podesta L, Sher L, et al. Liver transplantation in children. *Am J Gastroenterol.* 1994;89:480.
50. Witzleben CL. Pathology of biliary atresia. In: Hoffman MA, ed. *Current Controversies in Biliary Atresia.* Austin, TX: R. G. Landes Co.; 1992:28.
51. Lai M-W, Chang M-H, Hsu S-C, et al. Differential diagnosis of extrahepatic biliary atresia from neonatal hepatitis: a prospective study. *J Pediatr Gastroenterol Nutr.* 1994;18:121.
52. Tan CEL, Kiely EM, Agrawal M, et al. Neonatal gastrointestinal perforation. *J Pediatr Surg.* 1989;24:888.
53. Kosloske AM, Musemeche CA. Necrotizing enterocolitis of the neonate. *Clin Perinatol.* 1989;16:97.
54. Uauy RD, Fanaroff AA, Korones SB, et al. Necrotizing enterocolitis in very low birth weight infants: biodemographic and clinical correlates. *J Pediatr.* 1991;119:630.
55. Covert RF, Neu J, Elliott MJ, et al. Factors associated with age of onset of necrotizing enterocolitis. *Am J Perinatol.* 1989;6:455.
56. Ross MN, Wayne ER, Janik JS, et al. A standard of comparison for acute surgical necrotizing enterocolitis. *J Pediatr Surg.* 1989;24:998.
57. Holman RC, Stehr-Green JK, Zelasky MT. Necrotizing enterocolitis mortality in the United States, 1979–85. *Am J Public Health.* 1989;79:987.
58. Caplan ME, MacKendrick W. Necrotizing enterocolitis: a review of pathogenetic mechanisms and implications for prevention. *Pediatr Pathol.* 1993;13:357.
59. Ballance WA, Dahms BB, Shenker N, et al. Pathology of neonatal necrotizing enterocolitis: a ten-year experience. *J Pediatr.* 1990; 117(Suppl):6S.
60. Joshi VV. *Common Problems in Pediatric Pathology.* New York: Igaku-Shoin; 1994:114.
61. Joshi VV. *Common Problems in Pediatric Pathology.* New York: Igaku-Shoin; 1994:202.
62. Kapur RP. Contemporary approaches toward understanding the pathogenesis of Hirschsprung disease. *Pediatr Pathol.* 1994;13:83.
63. Qualman SJ, Murray R. Aganglionosis and related disorders. *Hum Pathol.* 1994;25:1141.
64. Teitelbaum DH, Qualman SJ, Caniano DA. Hirschsprung's disease. Identification of risk factors for enterocolitis. *Ann Surg.* 1988; 207:240.
65. Teitelbaum DH, Caniano DA, Qualman SJ. The pathophysiology of Hirschsprung's-associated enterocolitis: importance of histologic correlates. *J Pediatr Surg.* 1989;24:1271.
66. Beckwith JB, Palmer NF. Histopathology and prognosis of Wilms tumor. Results from the First Wilms' Tumor Study. *Cancer.* 1978;41:1937.
67. Beckwith JB, Kiviat NB, Bonadio JF. Nephrogenic rests, nephroblastomatosis and the pathogenesis of Wilms' tumor. *Pediatr Pathol.* 1990;10:1.
68. Weeks DA, Beckwith JB, Mierau GW, et al. Rhabdoid tumor of kidney. A report of 111 cases from the National Wilms' Tumor Study Pathology Center. *Am J Surg Pathol.* 1989;13:439.
69. Robison LL. General principles of the epidemiology of childhood cancer. In: Pizzo PA, Poplack DG, eds. *Principles and Practice of Pediatric Oncology*, 2nd ed. Philadelphia: Lippincott Co.; 1993:3.
70. Beckwith JB. Renal neoplasms of childhood. In: Sternberg SS, ed. *Diagnostic Surgical Pathology*, 2nd ed. New York: Raven Press; 1994:1741.
71. Kissane JM, Dehner LP. Renal tumor and tumor-like lesions in pediatric patients. *Pediatr Nephrol.* 1992;6:365.
72. Brodeur GM. Molecular biology and genetics of human neuroblastoma. In: Pochedly C, ed. *Neuroblastoma: Tumor Biology and Therapy.* Boca Raton, FL: CRC Press; 1989:31.
73. Brodeur GM, Castleberry RP. Neuroblastoma. In: Pizzo PA, Poplack DG, eds. *Principles and Practice of Pediatric Oncology*, 2nd ed. Philadelphia: Lippincott Co.; 1993:739.
74. Dehner LP. Pathologic anatomy of classic neuroblastoma: including prognostic features and differential diagnosis. In: Pochedly C, ed. *Neuroblastoma: Tumor Biology and Therapy.* Boca Raton, FL: CRC Press; 1989:112.
75. Harms D, Schmidt D, Leuschner I. Abdominal, retroperitoneal and sacrococcygeal tumours of the newborn and the very young infant. *Eur J Pediatr.* 1989;148:720.
76. Brodeur GM, Pritchard J, Berthold F, et al. Revisions of the International Criteria for Neuroblastoma diagnosis, staging and response to treatment. *J Clin Oncol.* 1993;11:1466.
77. Dehner LP. Gonadal and extragonadal germ cell neoplasms— teratomas in childhood. In: Finegold M, ed. *Pathology of Neoplasia in Children and Adolescents.* Philadelphia: Saunders Co.; 1986:282.
78. Stevens MCG. Neonatal tumours. *Arch Dis Child.* 1988;63:1122.
79. Werb P, Scurry J, Ostor A, et al. Survey of congenital tumors in perinatal necropsies. *Pathology.* 1992;24:247.
80. Isaacs H Jr. *Tumors of the Newborn and Infant.* St. Louis: Mosby Year Book; 1991:13, 43.
81. Schropp KP, Lobe TE, Rao B, et al. Sacrococcygeal teratoma: the experience of four decades. *J Pediatr Surg.* 1992;27:1075.
82. Bilik R, Shandling B, Pope M, et al. Malignant benign neonatal sacrococcygeal teratoma. *J Pediatr Surg.* 1992;28:1158.
83. Keslar PJ, Buck JL, Suarez ES. Germ cell tumors of the sacrococcygeal region: radiologic-pathologic correlation. *Radiographics.* 1994; 14: 607.
84. Joshi VV. *Common Problems in Pediatric Pathology.* New York: Igaku-Shoin; 1994:333.
85. Coffin CM, Dehner LP. Fibroblastic-myofibroblastic tumors in children and adolescents: a clinicopathologic study of 108 examples in 103 patients. *Pediatr Pathol.* 1991;11:569.
86. Coffin CM, Dehner LP. Soft tissue tumors in first year of life: a report of 190 cases. *Pediatr Pathol.* 1990;10:509.
87. Raney RB, Tefft M, Hays DM et al. Rhabdomyosarcoma and the undifferentiated sarcomas. In: Pizzo PA, Poplack DG, eds. *Principles and Practice of Pediatric Oncology*, 2nd ed. Philadelphia: Lippincott Co.; 1993:769.
88. Harms D. Soft tissue sarcomas in the Kiel Pediatric Tumor Registry. *Curr Top Pathol.* 1995;89:31.
89. Harms D. Alveolar rhabdomyosarcoma: a prognostically unfavorable rhabdomyosarcoma type and its necessary distinction from embryonal rhabdomyosarcoma. *Curr Top Pathol.* 1995;89:273.
90. Delattre O, Zucman J, Melot T, et al. The Ewing family of tumors—a subgroup of small-round-cell tumors defined by specific chimeric transcripts. *N Engl J Med.* 1994;331:294.
91. Schmidt D, Herrmann C, Jurgens H, et al. Malignant peripheral neuroectodermal tumor and its necessary distinction from Ewing's sarcoma. A report from the Kiel Pediatric Tumor Registry. *Cancer.* 1991;68:2251.

Index

Note: Page numbers in *italics* refer to illustrations; page numbers followed by (t) refer to tables.